PET/CT in Lymphomas

John A. Andreou • Paris A. Kosmidis
Athanasios D. Gouliamos
Editors

PET/CT in Lymphomas

A Case-Based Atlas

In collaboration with
Effimia P. Vrakidou
Vassilios K. Prassopoulos
Theodoros P. Vassilakopoulos

Springer

Editors
John A. Andreou
Imaging Department
Hygeia and Mitera Hospitals
4 Erythrou Stavrou Street
and Kifisias Avenue
15123 Athens
Greece

Paris A. Kosmidis
Medical Oncology Department
Hygeia Hospital
4 Erythrou Stavrou Street
and Kifisias Avenue
15123 Athens
Greece

Athanasios D. Gouliamos
Professor of Radiology (emeritus)
National and Kapodistrian
University of Athens
76, Vas. Sophias Avenue
11527 Athens
Greece

In collaboration with
Effimia P. Vrakidou
Department of Hematology
Hygeia Hospital
4 Erythrou Stavrou Street
and Kifisias Avenue
15123 Athens
Greece

Vassilios K. Prassopoulos
Department of Nuclear Medicine
Hygeia Hospital
4 Erythrou Stavrou Street
and Kifisias Avenue
15123 Athens
Greece

Theodoros P. Vassilakopoulos
Department of Haematology
and Bone Marrow Transplantation
National and Kapodistrian University
of Athens
Laikon General Hospital
Agiou Thoma 17
11527 Athens
Greece

ISBN 978-3-319-27378-5 ISBN 978-3-319-27380-8 (eBook)
DOI 10.1007/978-3-319-27380-8

Library of Congress Control Number: 2016934602

Printed on acid-free paper

This Springer imprint is published by Springer Nature
The registered company is Springer International Publishing AG Switzerland

Ἐς δὲ τὰ ἔσχατα νουσήματα αἱ ἔσχαται θεραπεῖαι ἐς ἀκριβείην, κράτισται

For extreme diseases extreme strictness of treatment is most efficacious

Hippocrates Med. et Corp, Aphorismi 1.6.1[1]

[1] Hippocrates, with an English translation by W. H. S. Jones, Litt. D., ST. Catharine's College, Cambridge, Vol IV, London, William Heinemann LTD, Cambridge, Massachusetts, Harvard University Press, MCMLIX.

Preface

Two years after publishing the book *Imaging in Clinical Oncology*, we have decided to rewrite Part VI on Lymphomas and present it in the form of an atlas.

This entirely new editorial work has been accomplished with the collaboration of Theodore Vassilakopoulos and Effimia Vrakidou, Department of Hematology, and Vassilis Prassopoulos, Department of Nuclear Medicine, all of whom contributed valuable criticisms and suggestions during the preparation of the book.

Several staging systems of lymphoma have been proposed and revised. Dedicated criteria have been developed for evaluating response to treatment. The most recent one is the Lugano classification system proposed for staging and response assessment. The new Lugano classification represents a consensus of experts in lymphoma diagnosis and management. These changes resulted in revision of our concepts and are reflected in the present volume.

In the past 10 years, the use of FDG PET/CT in the initial evaluation, monitoring, and follow-up of lymphoma patients has integrated new knowledge in our clinical practice. The aim of this atlas is to understand the role and limitations of FDG/PET and PET/CT in the evaluation of patients with lymphoma, in order to effectively use this imaging tool in management decisions.

Characteristic examples of FDG PET/CT imaging in patients with lymphoma are presented. The authors of this book have selected cases from the various types of Hodgkin and non-Hodgkin lymphoma in adults, children, and adolescents illustrated with FDG PET/CT imaging. After a short clinical introduction, each case is presented in a uniform fashion.

Review of the numerous cases which are presented will help the radiologists and clinicians as members of the multidisciplinary teams to understand the different aspects of lymphoma patients and become true partners in patient care.

Athens, Greece

John A. Andreou
Paris A. Kosmidis
Athanasios D. Gouliamos

Acknowledgments

The editors gratefully acknowledge all the authors who contributed in the completion of this atlas providing a series of cases, representative of Hodgkin and non-Hodgkin lymphoma.

We also like to express our gratitude to the staff of Springer Verlag Italia, Milan, for their continuous support and especially to Antonella Cerri who guided our first steps into the subject of this book and Alessandra Born for her assistance during the preprint process.

Saanthi Shankhararaman and Venkatramani Kalpana provided outstanding production services.

Finally, we would like to thank Ioanna Konti for her secretarial assistance.

Contents

Part I

Introduction to Lymphomas

The 2008 WHO Classification of B-Cell Lymphomas by the Pathologist's Clinical Point of View

1

Dimitra S. Anagnostou

Classifications of diseases have been reasonably characterized as the language of medicine given that categorization of entities facilitates understanding among pathologists, clinicians and basic scientists while also providing at the same time a framework for the clinical practice and genesis of new data and concepts. *The World Health Organization (WHO) Classification of Tumours of Haematopoietic and Lymphoid Tissues* (4th edition) was a collaborative project of the European Association for Haematopathology and the Society for Hematopathology [1]. The WHO classification of tumours of haematopoietic and lymphoid tissues, published as monograph in 2001 (3rd edition) [2] and updated in 2008 (4th edition) [1], represents a worldwide consensus in regard to the diagnosis of these tumours. Historically, both classifications are recognized as functional in the sense that lymphoma cells are related to the cells of the normal immune system; this constitutes a tumultuous revolution and a significant breakthrough in the field of haematopathology given that previous traditional classification schemes were based merely or entirely on morphology. Their worldwide approval relies on their clinical relevance, reproducibility and practicality, but more importantly, it depends on their solid biological background. Moreover, they have been used in clinical trials and in pathologic and epidemiological studies. Likewise, new genetic and molecular investigations rely upon these classifications.

Changes and modifications concerning the 2001 WHO classification, as well as new information, concepts and proposals, were to emerge after the publication of the 3rd, 2001, WHO classification and are presented in the updated 2008 WHO classification. This updated WHO classification incorporates new defining criteria for some diseases, biological or clinical categories or groups and provisional entities. These accomplishments resulted from new insights into clinical and laboratory research, the tremendous progression made in technology and the successful partnership of laboratory workers and clinicians. The participation in the lymphoma advisory committees of haematopathologists, clinical specialists and haematologists/oncologists led to a multiparameter approach to lymphoma diagnosis and management. Thus although histopathology remains the cornerstone in the diagnosis of lymphomas, equally critical are clinical data, immunophenotypical studies and flow cytometry in almost all circumstances, while molecular, genomic and cytogenetic techniques and, more recently, next-generation sequencing, have an increasingly important diagnostic impact.

This chapter will refer to the process and rationale for the 2008 WHO classification

D.S. Anagnostou, MD, PhD
Department of Haematopathology, Referral Center, Evaggelismos Hospital, Athens, Greece
e-mail: dimit.anagnostou@gmail.com

J.A. Andreou et al. (eds.), *PET/CT in Lymphomas: A Case-Based Atlas*,
DOI 10.1007/978-3-319-27380-8_1

focusing selectively on those B-cell-origin diseases on which changes that have been made have had an effect in terms of the diagnostic approach and management of the patient. Moreover, in light of the fact that since 2008, new information from published studies has been presented, and new concepts have emerged, an effort will be made to selectively highlight those with clinical implications.

1.1 Principles of the Updated 2008 WHO Classification

The major principle of the 2008 WHO classification is the stratification of neoplasms primarily according to (a) their cell lineage, namely, myeloid, lymphoid B-, T-/NK- and histiocytic/dendritic cell origin, and (b) their derivation from precursor lymphoid cells, such as lymphoblastic leukaemias/lymphomas, or mature (peripheral) lymphoid cells including mature B-cell, mature T-cell and NK-cell neoplasms [3]. A normal counterpart is postulated for each neoplasm. The different types of neoplasms are listed according to (a) their clinical features; age, dissemination of disease, leukaemic picture, nodal versus extranodal localization, specific anatomic site of involvement, clinical behaviour (indolent or aggressive), history of cytotoxic or other therapies and (b) the stage of differentiation of the neoplastic cellular population, when this could be postulated. Though the 2008 WHO classification deliberately does not distinguish lymphomas by grade of malignancy, traditionally mature B-cell lymphomas composed mainly of small lymphocytes have been called low-grade lymphomas. It has been reported that, since the period of 2001–2008, the number of categories of mature B- and T-cell-origin neoplasms has almost doubled, while at the same time about 25 % more pages have been added in the updated WHO monograph (WHO) [3].

In general the updated WHO classification refined definitions of already existing diseases, identified new entities and variants, introduced new concepts and questioned the validity of some established beliefs [4, 5]. Moreover, some of the interventions that have been made are related to several discrete issues: (1) greater attention and appreciation of early or in situ lesions in the context of revealing and defining early steps in the process of evolution or transformation of a lesion, (2) introduction of new entities, (3) acceptance of age as a determining factor in the pathobiology of some diseases, (4) significant role of site-specific consequences on disease definitions, (5) initiation of provisional categories and diseases with uncertainties in definitional clinical and/or biological criteria and (6) incorporation of minor changes in terminology [6].

1.2 Aggressive B-Cell Lymphomas

Aggressive B-cell lymphomas are a diverse group of neoplasms that arise at different stages of B-cell development and by various mechanisms of transformation [7]. They include both precursor lymphoid neoplasms (B lymphoblastic leukaemia/lymphoma) and an increased number of mature B-cell neoplasms such as diffuse large B-cell lymphoma (DLBCL) with its subtypes and variants, Burkitt lymphoma (BL), mantle cell lymphoma and its blastoid variant, effusion lymphoma and B-cell lymphoma unclassifiable with features intermediate between DLBCL and BL [7].

1.3 Diffuse Large B-Cell Lymphoma (DLBCL)

According to the updated WHO classification, diffuse large B-cell lymphoma (DLBCL) is defined as a neoplasm of large B-lymphoid cells with a nuclear size equal to or exceeding normal macrophage nuclei or more than twice the size of a normal lymphocyte. In some subtypes, such as T-cell-/histiocyte-rich large B-cell lymphoma, small non-neoplastic lymphocyte and histiocytes may outnumber the large B-cell component [1]. DLBCL is the most common type of non-Hodgkin's lymphomas (NHLs) accounting for 30 % of all adults NHLs in Western countries with 40 % encountered in extranodal sites at stage I or II. It represents about 20 % of NHLs in children under 14 years and up to 37 % in adolescents aged 15–19 years [8]. DLBCL is one of the most heterogeneous groups of tumours and includes several types, subtypes and variants classified together on the basis of their clinical features, morphology, immunophenotype, genetic alterations and clinical behaviour. This unique clinical and biological heterogeneity of DLBCL, which is observed not only between but even within lymphoma subtypes, may explain its substantial variability to antitumour activity by novel therapeutic agents [9]. Approximately 40 % of the patients have refractory disease to chemotherapy or relapse after an initial response, while the majority of patients who relapse will succumb to the disease. It is understood that appropriate therapy presupposes stratification of the different subtypes in a clinically valid scheme.

Some DLBCLs exhibit a predilection for specific anatomic sites of presentation such as primary DLBCL of the central nervous system (CNS), primary cutaneous DLBCL leg type and primary mediastinal large B-cell lymphoma (PMBCL). However, the majority of DLBCLs without specific clinical or pathologic features are included in the group of '*not otherwise specified (NOS) lymphoma*', a histological group to which special attention will be paid in this chapter [10]. DLBCL NOS is subclassified according to the morphology (centroblastic or immunoblastic), site of primary involvement (nodal, extranodal) and clinical background (normal or compromised immunity). DLBCL can arise as de novo or in the context of progression or transformation in patients with low-grade lymphomas including chronic lymphocytic leukaemia/small-cell lymphocytic lymphoma (CLL/SCL), follicular lymphoma (FL) and marginal zone lymphoma (MZL).

1.3.1 Cell of Origin (COO) in DLBCL

The idea of distinguishing lymphomas into clinical grades (high, intermediate, low) dates back to the mid-1970s. Since then separating lymphomas has become progressively more complex; gene expression profile (GEP) has opened up a new window characterizing DLBCLs by cell of origin (COO) into biologically distinct molecular groups: (a) those with gene expression reminiscent of germinal centre B-cells (GCB-like group) (b) those with gene expression similar to activated B-cells (ACB-like group) accounting for 50 % of the cases, and (c) small number of unclassifiable cases, named 'type 3' [11]. Genes that are associated with the GCB subtype include markers of germinal centre differentiation, such as CD10 and the BCL6 gene. In the ABC type the nuclear factor kappa B (NF-kB) pathway is constitutively active, with the expression of NF-kB genes. The clinical interest of the above two subsets lies in their specific genetic alterations, different molecular signalling pathways, different clinical outcomes and potential therapeutic implications. According to gene expression signatures, most DLBCLs can be identified as prognostically favourable (GCB) or prognostically unfavourable (ABC) subtypes, both of which respond differently to therapeutic agents [12, 13]. Some authors are optimistic that eventually treatment of DLBCL will be guided by the genetic profile of tumour cells. However the wide complexity, concerning the applicability of different methods and techniques for routine use and lack of reproducibility that has been revealed by genomic studies, does not seem very encouraging at least at this point in time [1, 14]. In this context rather than applying gene expression profiling as a routine diagnostic test, several algorithms have been proposed based on immunohistochemical staining or tissue microarray analysis as purportedly useful surrogates for the classification of DLBCL subsets. In their published report from the International DLBCL Rituximab-CHOP Consortium Program Study, Visco C and colleagues introduced a new immunophenotypical algorithm called 'Visco-Young' [15]. The authors supported that using an algorithm based on the combined expression of three markers (CD10, FOXP1, BCL6) could classify DLBCL into GCB and non-GCB subgroups with high specificity and that their method can predict an outcome similar to that of GEP analysis in R-CHOP-treated patients. A short time later 17 centres from Europe, the USA and Canada successfully tested a new method for COO assignment of DLBCL that differentiated ABC from GCB applying NanoString technology to formalin-fixed paraffin-embedded tissues in the routine diagnostic workflow [16]. However, in a study published in 2015, some investigators indicate that none of the immunohistochemical algorithms alone is sufficient to predict the outcome of patients with DLBCL especially those receiving R-CHOP therapy [17].

1.3.2 CD30-Positive DLBCL

A novel subgroup of CD3O-positive DLBCL with favourable prognosis and distinct gene expression signature was recently reported by the International DLBCL Rituximab-CHOP Consortium Program Study [18]. This study demonstrated that patients with CD30+ DLBCL had superior, 5-year, overall survival *(CD30+ 79 % versus CD30− 59 %, P = .001)* and progression-free survival *(P = .003)* in a cohort of 903 de novo DLBCL patients. CD30 was expressed in approximately 14 % of DLBCL cases. Notably, this favourable outcome was observed regardless of COO (GCB, ABC) stratification of cases [18]. Moreover, CD30 expression was predictive of superior 5-year progression-free survival within R-CHOP-treated de novo DLBCLs in a population-based study from British Columbia where the lymphoma cells were germinal centre B-cell-like (GCB) [19]. Thus CD30 immunohistochemistry was proposed as a useful prognostic marker.

1.3.3 Epstein-Barr Virus (EBV)-Positive DLBCL of the Elderly

The 2008 updated WHO classification recognized a new provisional entity defined as EBV + DLBCL of the elderly in the sense of an EBV+ monoclonal lymphoproliferative disorder arising in immunocompetent patients of advanced age encountered commonly in Asia and less frequently in North America and Europe [1]. An arbitrary cut-off of 50 years has been recommended in the updated WHO classification. EBV-positive DLBCL of the elderly is also known as age-related EBV B-cell lymphoproliferative disorder or senile EBV-associated B-cell lymphoproliferative disorders. Seventy percent of the patients presented with extranodal involvement. Morphologically the neoplastic cells may mimic Hodgkin/Reed-Sternberg cells and present marked pleomorphism [6]. Most cases demonstrate an activated ABC immunophenotype [20]. As a risk factor, EBV positivity is reported in about 10 % of DLBCL. EBV-positive DLBCL of the elderly is considered as an EBV-driven lymphoma with an aggressive clinical course in which clonality of the immunoglobulin genes and EBV can usually be detected by molecular techniques. It has been assumed that EBV+ DLBCL of the elderly might be caused by the senescence of the immune system, a phenomenon which could possibly be interpreted in the context of the normal ageing process and where the adaptive immune system is preferentially affected in contrast to the innate immunity [21]. EBV+ DLBCL may also be associated with long-standing pyothorax and may well be seen in other instances of prolonged inflammation. As EBV+ DLBCL in the elderly is still considered a provisional entity, special attention is required in distinguishing it from other EBV-related disorders including reactive lesions, EBV+ classic Hodgkin's lymphoma and the more recently described mucocutaneous ulcer.

1.3.4 The Impact of Microenvironment in DLCBCL

There is increasing evidence that in the DLBCL not only the malignant cells of the tumour but the cellular composition of the tumour microenvironment may affect survival. Similarly, stromal signatures of the tissue background and host factors may give information regarding the pathogenesis and clinical behaviour of DLBCL [7]. It is postulated that cells in the microenvironment may promote cell growth and survival or may represent part of the host response against the tumour. Lenz and colleagues [22] demonstrated an increased survival for patients with DLBCL in these cases that the microenvironment expressed a group of genes, namely, stromal-1 genes; they identified two patterns of stromal signature: the prognostically favourable stromal-1 signature related to extracellular matrix deposition and histiocytic infiltration and the unfavourable stromal-2 signature expressing tumour blood vessel density. Additionally, genes expressed by the immune microenvironment such as TNFRSF9 and immunostains for stromal markers such as SPARC (acidic and rich in cysteine) can be used for prognostic purposes [23, 24].

1.4 Borderline Malignancies

Most lymphomas can be accurately classified as one of the currently recognized distinct disease entities. Nonetheless a group of lymphomas present with overlapping or borderline, histological, immunophenotypical, biological and clinical features between various types of lymphomas. The major overlaps occur between nodular sclerosis Hodgkin's lymphoma (cHL-NS) and primary mediastinal large B-cell lymphoma (PMBCL), lymphocyte-rich Hodgkin's lymphoma (LRcHL) and nodular lymphocyte-predominant Hodgkin's lymphoma (NLPHL) and NLPHL and T-cell-/histiocyte-rich LBCL (THRLBCL). These lymphomas have been reported with different terms such as borderline lymphomas, B-cell lymphomas unclassifiable and grey zone lymphomas (GZLs). The term 'grey zone lymphoma' was firstly introduced in 1998 at the 'Workshop report on Hodgkin's disease and related diseases'. This term was further extended to lymphomas with transitional features between Burkitt lymphoma (BL) and DLBCL [25]. In the updated 2008 WHO classification, this group of lymphomas was assigned to two provisional categories called *'B-cell lymphoma unclassifiable with features intermediate between DLBCL and classical Hodgkin's lymphoma (cHL) and B-cell lymphoma unclassifiable with features intermediate between DLBCL and Burkitt lymphoma (BL)'* [26, 27]. It is apparent that the intention of proposing such a category was to maintain the 'integrity' of the well-defined categories in the updated WHO classification and more importantly to proceed with further studies concerning their identity. This group of lymphomas comprises a heterogeneous array group of lymphoma types with variable clinical courses and a spectrum of genetic lesions. Although most grey zone lymphomas are associated with mediastinal disease, it should be noted that similar cases have also been reported in peripheral lymph nodes without mediastinal involvement [28]. The use of gene expression profiling studies further confirmed the biological relationship of the above group of diseases [28]. A representative example of this category of grey zone lymphoma is PMBCL and cHL-NS (mediastinal grey zone lymphoma (MGZL)). The use of gene expression profiling studies demonstrated that the profile of PMBCL differs from that of non-mediastinal DLBCL but is more closely related to cHL; thus this phenomenon may indicate true biological relationship between these two diseases [29]. Both, DLBCL and cHL, also show clinical, histopathological and molecular similarities and have been reported sequentially in the same patient, while in the scheme of composite lymphoma, they have been observed in the same anatomic site [30]. They both present as an anterior mediastinal mass with involvement of the thymus and/or supraclavicular lymph nodes; they affect young adults, preferentially men, and appear to have a more aggressive clinical course and poorer outcome than either PMBCL or cHL separately. Immunophenotypical findings that may play a misleading role in their diagnostic approach and in parallel justify their inclusion in the borderline category of lymphoma are [31, 32] as follows: CD30, an essential diagnostic marker for cHL, is also expressed in more than 80 % of cases of PMBCL but usually is weak and heterogeneous compared to cHL; CD15 presents in the majority of cHL (75–85 %) but may be detected in PMBCL; Reed-Sternberg-like cells and sclerosis, as part of the histological profile in PMBCL, intensify the difficulties in regard to its differential diagnosis from cHL-NS; MAL protein is expressed in 70 % of PMBCL and 10 % of cHL, a marker which indicates their histogenetical link with the thymic asteroid medullary B-cells [25]. As a rule the neoplastic cells in PMBCL express B-cell markers; they are typically CD23 positive (70 %) and lack expression of HLA class I antigens and surface immunoglobulin (Ig). Moreover, in contrast to cHL, expression of Ig-associated transcription factors (BOB1, OCT2, PU1), is preserved. One of the major dilemmas is the interpretation of CD20 expression in cHL. As immunohistochemical standards have improved, CD20 positivity in Reed-Sternberg cells is no longer a rare finding, although its expression is usually weak and heterogeneous. Strong and uniform CD20 expression in cHL should alert the pathologist to proceed to complete immunophenotypical investigation of a particular case [33].

1.4.1 Biological Insights in Mediastinal Grey Zone Lymphoma (MGZL)

Recent studies have noticed a number of common immunophenotypical features and genetic alterations that link cHL-NS and PMBCL. There are rather relatively ample data supporting this close relationship as well as noteworthy data concerning dilemmas in the therapeutic approach of this category of lymphomas [34]. Both entities were found to be similarly positive for cyclin E (75 % and 93 %, respectively) and p63 (50 % and 53 %, respectively) performed on tissue microarray sections [28]. Classical HLs show frequent gains of regions 2p, 9p, 16p and 8q, and similar aberrations were also recognized in PMBCL [28, 35, 36]. Two of the PMBCL distinction genes, CD30 and TARC, are both expressed in the malignant Hodgkin-Reed-Sternberg (R-S) cells [37, 38]. It is intriguing that PMBCL gene signature appears to relate more to cHL gene signature than to most other DLBCLs, a finding that may support a true biological overlapping between these two diseases [29]. Similarly, analysis of methylation profiling of MGZL by Eberle and colleagues [39] showed a close epigenetic relationship between MGZL, cHL and PMBCL but in parallel demonstrated a unique epigenetic signature for MGZL, which seems to justify its classification in WHO 2008 as a separate disease entity. Moreover, in a very recent study by Steidl and colleagues [40], whole genome sequencing showed a gene fusion involving the MHC class transactivator CIITA in both cHL and PMBCL, a finding which further underscores their biological relationship.

1.5 Double-Hit (DH) B-Cell Lymphomas

Double-hit or triple-hit lymphomas are rare subtypes of lymphomas which were initially defined as mature B-cell neoplasms bearing concurrent rearrangements of the BCL2/18q21 and MYC/8q24 loci. The emergence of cumulative clinical and biological data led to the definition of double-hit lymphomas being expanded to encompass any aggressive mature B-cell neoplasm with a chromosomal breakpoint affecting MYC locus and one or more additional rearrangements recurrently associated with lymphoma, most commonly BCL2, BCL6 or CCND1 [41]. Additionally, B-cell lymphomas with more than two lymphoma-specific chromosomal abnormalities are described as triple- or quadruple-hit lymphomas [33]. MYC translocation, characteristic biological marker of BL, can also be detected, though in relatively lower frequencies, in other B-cell lymphomas such as follicular lymphoma, DLBCL and B-cell lymphoma unclassifiable with features intermediate between DLBCL and BL. It should be mentioned that there are some essential differences between the MYC translocation in BL and in other mature B-cell lymphomas. More precisely, in BL the MYC translocation always involves one of the immunoglobulin loci and is considered a disease-initiating event which occurs in the context of a rather simple karyotype [42]. In contrast MYC translocation in other mature B-cell lymphomas, most often involving non-IG partners, are mostly found in complex karyotypes, and they possibly occur during disease progression, rather than disease initiation [42]. Gene profiling studies have shown that some double-hit cases have a profile with features intermediate between DLBCL and *BL* [27]. In principle, this group of lymphomas is genetically defined and their incidence increases with age. All other lymphomas with a MYC breakpoint, irrespective of the presence of other aberrations, are termed 'single-hit' lymphomas. Though relatively rare, the double-hit category of lymphomas has drawn the attention of clinicians and pathologists due to their aggressive course, early relapse and resistance to treatment even when treated with R-CHOP or high-intensity chemotherapy [43]. No unifying pathologic features of double-hit lymphomas have been described in the sense that in the majority of the cases the morphological and immunophenotypical findings do not correspond with established diagnostic entities; they usually present a spectrum of pathologic features overlapping with BL, DLBCL and B lymphoblastic leukaemia/lymphoma [4]. Double-hit lymphomas have the double disadvantage of MYC (proliferation) and BCL2 (antiapoptosis). This could explain the poor prognosis and the minimal or absent response to therapy. Most patients (80–85 %) present de novo disease, while in 15–20 % of patients double-hit lymphoma develops secondarily as a result of transformation of an indolent lymphoma, most often grade 1–2 follicular lymphoma [44]. Double-hit lymphomas represent a necessary but temporary category, until more refined criteria become available.

1.6 Follicular Lymphoma (FL)

Follicular lymphoma (FL) is the second most common type of B-cell NHL comprising approximately 25 % of NHLs worldwide [45]. The vast majority of cases manifest as systemic disease involving lymph nodes. FL is characterized by the t(14;18)(q21;q32) chromosome translocation, presented in up to 80–90 % of cases. It arises from germinal centre (GC) B-cells and is composed of follicle centre (germinal centre) B-cells with morphological profile of centrocytes and large transformed cells/centroblasts. By definition, the tumour shows at least a partial follicular growth pattern. Histological grading of FL has been a matter of discussion given that this issue has been related to the outcome and the overall clinical management of the patient. The 2008 WHO classification subdivides FL into three (1,2,3) histological grades according to the relative proportion of small centrocytes and large centroblasts within the neoplastic follicles [45]. Moreover, the updated WHO classification groups grades 1 and 2 together (FL1-2), according to the presence of few centroblasts, while grade 3 (>15 % centroblasts/hpf) has been further subdivided into types A (FL3A) and B (FL3B) based on the proportion of centrocytes. More specifically centrocytes are still present in grade 3A, while in grade 3B follicles are composed entirely of large blast cells (centroblasts or immunoblasts). Additionally, the updated 2008 classification recommends that any diffuse area in an FL consisting entirely or predominantly of large blastic/transformed cells should be reported as DLBCL, as primary diagnosis, with a parallel estimate of the proportion of DLBCL and FL cell components [45].

The prognostic value of the WHO classification grading system for FL remains controversial. FL grades 1–2 and 3A have been considered as indolent, 'low-grade' lymphomas, while FL grade 3 has been connected with a more aggressive clinical behaviour [46]. However, others failed to support these findings [47]. In a recent study including the largest number of purely follicular lymphomas grade 3B (FL3B), the cytogenetic and immunohistochemical findings defined FL grade 3B as a distinct category with infrequent BCL2 and BCL6 translocations (9 % and 17 %, respectively), CD10(−) IRF4/MUM1(+) compared with FL grades 1, 2 and 3A which have shown frequent BCL2 translocations and CD10(+) IRF4/MUM1 (−) [48]. Interestingly, in a currently published study, and notably one of the few conducting studies in patients undergoing rituximab-containing therapy, overall survival and progression-free survival did not significantly differ between patients with FL grade 3 and those with FL grades 1–2 [49].

The conflicting results among various reports of FL grade 3 could be attributed to several factors: small patient cohorts, lack of reproducibility among pathologists, differences in the diagnostic approach of the biopsy material extending from strictly morphological criteria to molecular or genetic studies and the fact that most studies were retrospective in nature. More importantly, variability in the treatment approach and the era of rituximab versus pre-rituximab and anthracycline-containing chemotherapy may have prognostic implications.

1.6.1 Follicular Lymphoma Transformation

Follicular lymphoma, initially an indolent and responsive to therapy disease, remains largely incurable [50]. A crucial event in the natural history of FL is the histological transformation to more aggressive malignancies, typically represented by a DLBCL, though transformation to lymphoblastic leukaemia/lymphoma and B-cell lymphoma unclassifiable with features between DLBCL and BL has also been documented [50] Transformation of FL to DLBCL has been reported to occur in 16–70 % of patients over time with a consensus rate of 3 % per year and is associated with a mean survival post-transformation of less than 2 years [14]. Histological transformation is usually associated with a rapidly progressive clinical course, treatment resistance and poor survival. An unequivocal definition of transformation presupposes histological confirmation of a FL diagnosis and demonstration of a clonal relationship between the original FL and the subsequently developed neoplasm. The median time from diagnosis to transformation ranges from 40 to 66 months with the earliest transformation reported at 2 months and the latest at 5 years.

The biological mechanisms which are responsible for this phenomenon of transformation are not completely understood. According to recent data on the biology of transformation of FL, it is assumed that chromosomal abnormalities associated with transformation of the disease may impair immune surveillance, activate the nuclear factor-kB pathway and deregulate P53 and B-cell transcriptor factors [51]. Moreover, whole exome sequencing and copy number analysis revealed that the dominant clone of FL and transformed FL arises by divergent evolution from a common mutated precursor cell through acquisition of distinct genetic effects [52]. Currently, Kiaii and colleagues [53] showed altered gene expression in tumour-infiltrating T-cells in FL and demonstrated that altering the immune microenvironment in FL affects overall survival and time to transformation process.

1.6.2 Variants of Follicular Lymphoma

1.6.2.1 Paediatric Follicular Lymphoma

The updated WHO classification recognizes certain distinctive clinical and genetic subtypes such as paediatric FL and primary intestinal FL.

Paediatric FL in children, even in the early stage of the disease, presents with grade 3 histology [45]. It shares many histological features with those of adult FL but lacks BCL2/IGH translocation and does not express BCL2 protein. Though paediatric FLs are of high histological grade [3], they usually present with localized disease. According to the European Intergroup for Childhood Non-Hodgkin Lymphoma and the International Berlin-Frankfurt-Münster Study Group, treatment outcome in pFL seems to be excellent with risk-adapted chemotherapy or after complete resection and ‘a watch and wait’ strategy [54].

1.6.2.2 Primary Intestinal Follicular Lymphoma

The majority of cases of primary gastrointestinal (duodenum) follicular lymphoma occur in the small intestine and most often in the duodenum, the second portion being a frequent location. Most cases are diagnosed at endoscopy. It presents as solitary or multiple small polyps and in most patients as localized disease (stage IE-IIE). Histologically the atypical follicles are found in the mucosa and submucosa, and the cellular population of the follicles consists almost entirely of centrocytes which carry the t(14;18) translocation. Duodenum FL has an indolent clinical course, and the risk of progression and dissemination is less than 5 years [6].

1.7 Early Lymphoid Lesions

The widespread use of immunohistochemistry, multicolour flow cytometry and molecular techniques on tissue biopsy samples together with the expansion in knowledge of the genetic and phenotypic alterations of specific disease entities led to the recognition of 'early' lymphoid lesions which carry some, but not all, necessary characteristics of their malignant counterparts, and their biological behaviour is uncertain [55].

Lymphoproliferative disorders associated with an indolent behaviour can be broadly separated into two groups [56]: (a) clonal proliferations that share genetic and molecular features with well-defined lymphoid neoplasms such as a monoclonal gammopathy of undefined significance (MGUS) and multiple myeloma, monoclonal B-cell lymphocytosis (MBL) and chronic lymphocytic leukaemia/small-cell lymphocytic lymphoma(CLL/SLL), follicular lymphoma in situ and follicular lymphoma(FL) and mantle cell lymphoma in situ and mantle cell lymphoma (MCL) and (b) clonal lymphoid proliferations resembling lymphomas and diagnosed as a lymphoma which do not have a counterpart among established lymphoma subtypes and are associated with an indolent clinical behaviour in the context that may represent an exaggerated antigenic response, clonal, but self-limiting [56]. This particular group includes the paediatric variants of nodal FL and nodal MZL and also the breast implant-associated anaplastic large-cell lymphoma (ALCL).

These 'early' lymphoid lesions represent an incidental finding that may be observed in asymptomatic individuals, and their biological behaviour is uncertain. Though these lesions have been reported as 'indolent', it is not clear whether they will ever progress to clinically overt lymphoma or represent self-balanced benign clonal proliferations [57, 58]. More precisely clonal lymphoid proliferations pertain to minimal infiltrates of clonal B-cells, observed and confined within apparently reactive lymphoid tissues, with some of the phenotypic and genetic features of specific B-cell lymphoma subtypes and the distinctive topographical localization of the particular lymphoma type.

Early and possibly neoplastic or pre-neoplastic lymphoid proliferations with the immunophenotypical and molecular profile of FL have been defined as 'in situ FL'. The term 'in situ neoplasia', initially applied to epithelial tumours, was later extended to the lymphoma setting. In situ FLs are characterized by the scattered presence, among their normal counterparts, of atypical lymphoid cells expressing strong BCL2+ and CD10+, positivity for CD20 and BCL6, but not IgD, and carrying t(14;18)(q32;q21) translocation. Detection of monoclonality by microdissecting BCL2+ follicles followed by polymerase chain reaction may confirm the diagnosis. The atypical lymphoid cells are strictly confined to their normal anatomic sites, usually isolated germinal centres, without any sign of invasion to the surrounding structures [59]. Cases of in situ FL have also been referred to in the 2008 WHO classification as intrafollicular neoplasia. In a similar way, in situ mantle cell lymphoma (MCL) is detected exclusively in the mantle zone of the follicles where the clonal B-cell proliferations carry some of the molecular hallmarks of its malignant counterpart such as t(11;14)(q13;q32) translocations. The concept of 'early' lymphoma is used only for cases where minimal disease extends beyond the boundaries of the follicular structures [59]. The progression of these lesions to overt lymphoma occurs rarely and may require the accumulation of additional genetic interventions. The genetic events underlying the progression from in situ FL to FL are currently unknown. Very recently Green and colleagues [60] provided evidence that IgH-BCL2 translocations and CREBBP mutations are early events during disease evolution, while MLL2 and TNFRSF14 mutations may represent late events. Moreover in addition to genetic events, microenvironmental factors may also be implicated in the process of evolution. A genomic instability has been suggested even in the very early stages of an apparently benign lymphoid lesion.

1.8 Mantle Cell Lymphoma (MCL)

Mantle cell lymphoma is a B-cell neoplasm accounting for approximately 6 % of all NHLs. It is characterized by t(11;14)(q13;32) chromosome translocation leading to overexpression of cyclin D1 and cell cycle dysregulation in almost all cases. Cell cycle dysregulation combined with chromosomal instability and activation of cell survival mechanisms are implicated in the pathogenesis of the disease [61]. MCL presents with extensive disease and is generally composed of monomorphic small to medium-sized lymphoid cells with irregular nuclear contours. A spectrum of morphological variants of MCL with blastoid and pleomorphic histologies are also of important clinical significance [62]. To a large extent, MCL cells are CD20+, usually CD5+, FMC7+ and CD43+, but negative for CD10 and BCL6. All cases are BCL2 protein positive and in the majority of cases cyclin D1 positive. CD23 is negative or weakly positive. The cells express relatively intense surface IGM/IGD with CIgλ>CIgκ. Recently [63], the transcription factor SOX11 has been described as being expressed in most MCLs, including cyclin D1-negative cases. Aberrant phenotypes have also been described. Even though SOX11 has been characterized as a powerful tool in MCL diagnosis, its interpretation requires caution, and strict criteria should be applied given that positive SOX11 cases of DLBCL and splenic lymphoma have been reported. MCL is an aggressive disease [64]; it is considered as an incurable subtype of NHLs which, despite remissions, presents a relapse rate of approximately 50 %. Currently published studies propose that the MCL-initiated cells (MCL-ICs) are the main reason for relapse and chemoresistance of MCL. Tumour-initiated cells also referred to as cancer stem cells (CSCs) are a small fraction of cells within tumours that have been implicated in the growth, progression and relapse of several tumour subtypes [65]. It has been shown that MCL-ICs are resistant to genotoxic agents vincristine, doxorubicin and the newly approved Bruton's tyrosine kinase inhibitor (ibrutinib). A brief reference is made to a recent study with cyclin D1-positive DLBCL with IGH-CCND1 translocation and BCL6 rearrangement [66] that aimed to alert diagnosticians to its differential diagnosis from blastoid and pleomorphic variants of mantle cell lymphoma.

1.8.1 Indolent Mantle Cell Lymphoma/Leukaemia

Early studies found that leukaemic involvement in MCL was associated with aggressive disease and poor prognosis. However, a growing body of investigation studies have identified a subset of MCL, designated indolent mantle cell leukaemia, with a more indolent disease course and significantly prolonged survival, often 7–10 years, even without therapy and slow or absent clinical progression [67]. More specifically, most cases present with a leukaemic picture, absence of lymphadenopathy and hepatosplenomegaly and less frequent minimal nodal infiltration. All these cases were identified in asymptomatic patients with lymphocyte counts ranging between 4.5 and 14.2×10^9/L, and all were characterized by t(11;14) translocation. The circulating atypical cells are of small to medium size with a high nuclear to cytoplasmic ratio and slight nuclear irregularities expressing in flow cytometric analysis CD5, CD19 and CD20. However, in contrast to MCL, the indolent subtype of MCL discloses on immunohistochemistry on flow cytometry a meaningful proportion of CD23+ cells. Similarly, as opposed to typical MCL, there is a striking kappa immunoglobulin light chain restriction in most cases [68], while expression of SOX11 was absent, significantly lower than in typical MCL or only weakly expressed. Bone marrow biopsies demonstrate limited, interstitial, neoplastic infiltration. Indolent MCL presenting solely with lymphocytosis has been estimated to be just 3 % among all MCLs diagnosed during the same period.

1.9 Bone Marrow Biopsy versus FDG-PET/CT

1.9.1 General Aspects

Examination of bone marrow (BMB) has been considered as a standard procedure for the diagnosis, staging and monitoring of lymphomas. This presupposes the following [69]: Bone marrow specimens or samples, ordinarily from the posterior iliac crest, should fulfil optional quantitative and qualitative standards; the pathology lab should respond to the current technological advances; pathologists are specialized to the field of haematopathology and collaboration with the clinician is a must. In most cases morphological and immunophenotypical findings allow a definitive diagnosis. However, selected cases are supplemented with cytogenetics and interphase fluorescence in situ hybridization (FISH). Concerning treatment response measurements, which target the detection of a limited number of tumour cells, namely, minimal residual disease (MRD), molecular tests are designed to detect specific translocations or specific DNA sequence of the antigen receptor of a particular lymphoma [69] A monolateral long (3–4 cm) cylinder, ordinarily taken from the posterior iliac crest, is considered sufficient for an accurate diagnosis and sufficiently reliable to detect focal BM involvement in patients particularly in those with Hodgkin's disease.

1.9.2 Relevance of BMB versus FDG-PET/CT in Lymphomas

Bone marrow biopsy has been a reference standard procedure in lymphoma staging, and marrow histology has been incorporated into the new National Comprehensive Cancer Network International Prognostic Index. However, through the years positron emission tomography (PET) using fluorodeoxyglucose (FDG) with computed tomography (CT) has become an established modality for staging newly diagnosed lymphomas particularly FDG-avid lymphomas, nodal and extranodal, including bone marrow assessment [70]. The major advantages imputed to FDG-PET/CT over BMB by its supporters include: noninvasiveness of the procedure, absence of sampling errors given that BMB assesses only a very small portion of the entire bone marrow and thus focal BM involvement can be missed by BMB, its capacity to distinguish viable tumour from scars and fibrosis and less time consuming considering the preparation procedures needed for fixation and decalcification stages [71]. An impressive number of articles presenting new data on the role of FDG-PET/CT in the evaluation of BM in HL and DLBCL, including lately follicular and paediatric lymphomas, have seen the light in recent publications [72]. Hence, the high sensitivity of PET/CT for BM involvement has recently prompted many authors to question the continued use of BMB in some histologies. The response was given recently at the 12th International Conference on Malignant Lymphoma in Lugano, Switzerland, in June 2013 where the initially developed criteria for staging and response for HLs and NHLs were revised [73]. As a result, establishment of modernized recommendations for initial evaluation, staging and response assessment in patients with HLs and NHLs was recorded. Additionally, FDG-PET/CT was formally incorporated into standard staging for FDG-avid lymphomas, whereas CT scan was indicated for non-avid histologies. In summary the conclusions drawn at this conference concerning BMB are the following [73]: (1) If a PET/CT is performed, a BMB is no longer indicated for routine staging of HL, (2) a BMB is only needed for DLBCL in the event that PET is negative and identifying a discordant histology in DLBCL lymphomas is important for patient management. Moreover, a 2.5 cm unilateral BMB was recommended along with immunohistochemistry and flow cytometry, whereas a preference to excisional biopsy was proposed. It is intriguing that in April 2015, a letter to the editor by Adams JA and Kwee TC, headed 'Do Not Abandon the Bone Marrow Biopsy Yet in DLBCL', expressed the opinion that whether FDG-PET/CT can replace BMB has yet to be proven both from a diagnostic and prognostic perspective [74]. Interestingly, in a large international cohort study to better define the use of PET in DLBCL, Cerci and colleagues [75] concluded that neither BM histology nor PET alone is a reliable indicator of poor-risk marrow disease and that the most consistent indicator is marrow involvement identified by both PET scan and histology. It should be clarified that in regard to other lymphoma histologies, the existing data is considered insufficient to permit similar changes in practice as in HL and DLBCL HL. Thus BMB continues to be recommended for staging all other lymphoma histologies providing that it would affect treatment.

1.9.3 Prognostic Impact of BM Histological Subtypes in DLBCL

Approximately 10–25 % of patients with DLBCL exhibit BM involvement at diagnosis. BM histology in DLBCL has been incorporated in the National Comprehensive Cancer Network. In many patients with DLBCL, BMB presents histology similar (concordant) to that of the primary site of involvement, i.e. infiltration with large B-cells. In 40–72 % of patients the histology at the time of staging is discordant in the sense that BM in contrast to lymph node histology is infiltrated by small B-lymphocytes [76]. In this context it is presumed that the DLBCL may have developed as a transformation of an occult small B-cell lymphoma or alternatively two unrelated lymphomas are present [77]. A recently published large retrospective population-based study represents the first comprehensive analysis [76] on the prognostic impact of BM involvement in 795 unselected patients with DLBCL treated with R-CHOP, based on the histological type of the infiltration, concordant or discordant. It was demonstrated in this study that the outcomes of patients with concordant BM involvement were inferior to the outcomes of those with no marrow involvement or those with discordant lymphoma. More precisely, the negative prognostic impact of discordant BM involvement affects progression-free survival (PFS), but not overall survival (OS), and it is adequately represented by the International Prognostic Index (IPI) score. In contrast, concordant BM involvement is characterized by a negative impact both on the PFI and OS independently of the IPI. Concordant BM involvement was associated with poor performance status with elevated lactate dehydrogenase, advanced stage, an increased number of extranodal sites and older age patients. Nonetheless the effects of discordant lymphomas, in regard to patient's outcome, are controversial; some studies claim that discordant BM involvement does not affect patient's outcome, while others support a higher rate of delayed relapses.

1.10 Hodgkin's Lymphoma (HL)

Hodgkin's lymphoma is a lymphoid tumour that represents about 1 % of all de novo neoplasms occurring every year worldwide. In the 1990s it was recognized that the neoplastic cells of Hodgkin's lymphoma (originally designated as disease) were of B-cell lineage. The diagnostic criteria for Hodgkin's lymphoma (HL) have been refined in the 3rd and 4th editions of the WHO Classification of Tumours of Haematopoietic and Lymphoid Tissues [78]. Based on clinical, biological and histological findings and the microenvironmental surroundings, it has been shown that HL consists of two distinct disease entities [79, 80], namely, nodular lymphocyte-predominant Hodgkin's lymphoma (NLPHL) and classical Hodgkin's lymphoma (cHL) with the latter comprising the following histological subtypes: lymphocyte rich (LRHL), nodular sclerosis (NSHL), mixed cellularity (MCHL) and lymphocyte depleted (LDHL). There are basic distinctions between NLPHL and cHL in clinical presentation, behaviour, morphology, phenotype, molecular profile and composition of the cellular background. In this context NLPHL deserves special attention, and thus, in the interest of space, it will be given a more generous reference comparatively to cHL and its subtypes. NLPHL represents 4–5 % of all HL cases and histologically may present several distinct immunoarchitectural patterns. However, according to the current WHO classification, at least a partial nodular pattern is required for its diagnosis. NLPHL, in contrast to cHL, has no relationship with EBV infection, patients are predominantly middle-aged males and the disease is localized (stages I–II in 70–80 %), usually affecting single cervical, axillary or inguinal nodes. Many patients may present with very large solitary masses with no other signs or symptoms of lymphoma. Bone marrow and mediastinum are rarely involved. The disease shows a very indolent course with prolonged disease-free period and high rates of relapses. The characteristic cell for the disease is the lymphocyte-predominant (LP) cell [79] which is a large mononuclear cell with a polylobular appearance, finely dispersed chromatin and multiple, small, basophilic nucleoli, while it only occasionally may show features of Hodgkin's-Reed-Sternberg cell. LP cell presents a germinal centre (GC) phenotypic profile with expression of GC markers together with expression of transcriptor factors such as OCT-2 and BOB-1. Lymphocyte-predominant cells are positive for the epithelial membrane antigen (EMA), and in contrast to cHL, they are CD15 negative and generally lack CD30, although a small subset may be CD30 positive since CD30 is an activation marker. Heavy and light chains of immunoglobulins are frequently expressed, and in particular IgD positivity identifies a subgroup of cases with peculiar epidemiological, phenotypic and clinical features [81]. Occasionally, NLPHL may be confused with an atypical form of follicular hyperplasia, namely, follicular hyperplasia with progressive transformation of germinal centres (PTGC) [79, 82]. This lesion is observed particularly in children and young adults and may precede, concur or follow NLPHL. Its pre-neoplastic nature has not been confirmed, though it seems to be associated with a slightly higher risk of evolving to NLPHL. Notably, BM involvement in NLPHL may not be strictly related to the disease stage, as BM involvement has also been recorded even in stage IA patients, a situation that is associated with aggressive clinical behaviour.

Progression of NLPHL, commonly to a clone-related DLBCL, occurs between 6 months and 24 years after NLPHL diagnosis. In the past 20 years, simultaneous or secondary transformation of NLPHL into DLBCL has been reported in up to 30 % of cases [83]. With the exception of one study [84], several authors have suggested that patients with NLPHL and DLBCL, simultaneously presented in the same lymph node, will have a favourable clinical outcome [83, 85]. Additionally, patients with sequential transformation have shown a nonsignificant tendency towards worse overall and progression-free survival compared to patients with simultaneous presentation of NLPHL and DLBCL. The morphological and phenotypic features of the DLBCL deriving from NLPHL are heterogeneous, a phenomenon that could possibly explain the different mechanisms involved in the transformation process [83]. Recently, germline mutations of the *NPAT* gene have been recognized as a risk factor for NLPHL in the Finnish population [86], and there are also reports about a high familial risk in first-degree relatives of NLPHL patients [87].

Classical Hodgkin's lymphoma [79] shows a bimodal age distribution. It is characterized by dissemination and presents variable correlation with EBV in 30–40 % of cases, depending on the histotype of the disease. All histological subtypes of cHL are characterized by the presence of Hodgkin's and Reed-Sternberg cells and variants. They all express the same phenotypic profile: CD45−, CD30+, CD15+/− (positivity in 75–80 % of cases), CD79−, CD20− (variably + in 20 %), IRF4+, EMA−, BCL6−, PAX5/BSAP+ (with a few exceptions) and Ig-transcription factor. The diagnosis of cHL is based on the identification of the characteristic for the disease neoplastic cellular component (lacunar cells, mononuclear Hodgkin's and multinucleated Hodgkin's-Reed-Sternberg cell) and the tissue background (inflammatory milieu, collagen bands, the proportion of small reactive lymphocytes). HRS cells even diagnostic are not exclusive for HL. Though the neoplastic components in cHL, as in NLPHL, are related to germinal centre B-cells, the former display high load of somatic mutations becoming subsequently stable, while in the latter ongoing mutations are detected in about half of the cases [88].

References

1. Swerdlow SH, Campo E, Harris NL, Jaffe E, Pileri SA, Stein H, Thiele J, Vardiman JW (eds) (2008) WHO classification of tumours of haematopoietic and lymphoid tissues. IARC Press, Lyon
2. Jaffe ES, Harris NL, Stein H, Vardiman JW (eds) (2001) Tumours of haematopoietic and lymphoid tissue, 3rd edn. IARC Press, Lyon
3. Harris NL, Campo E, Jaffe ES et al (2008) Introduction to the WHO classification of tumours of haematopoietic and lymphoid tissues. In: Swerdlow SH, Campo E, Harris NL (eds) WHO classification of tumours of haematopoietic and lymphoid tissue, 4th edn. IARC Press, Lyon, pp 14–15
4. Campo E, Swerdlow SH, Harris N et al (2011) The 2008 WHO classification of lymphoid neoplasms and beyond: evolving concepts and practical applications. Blood 117(19):5019–5032
5. Swerdlow SH (2013) Lymphoma classification and the tools of our trade: an introduction to the 2012 USCAP long Course. Mod Pathol 26:S1–S14
6. Jaffe ES (2009) The 2008 WHO classification of lymphomas: implications for clinical practice and translational research. Hematology Am Soc Hematol Educ Program 2009:523–531
7. Said JW (2013) Aggressive B-cell lymphomas: how many categories do we need? Mod Pathol 26:S42–S56
8. Oschlies I, Klapper W, Zimmrmann M et al (2006) Diffuse large B-cell lymphoma in pediatric patients belongs predominantly to the germinal center type B-cell lymphomas: a clinicopathologic analysis of cases included in German BFM (Burlin-Franfurt-Munster) multicenter trial. Blood 107:4047–4052
9. Nowakowski GS, Czuczman MS (2015) ABC, GCB, and double hit diffuse large B-cell lymphoma: does subtype make a difference in therapy selection? Am Soc Clin Oncol Educ Book 35:e449–e457
10. Menon MP, Pittaluga S, Jaffe ES (2012) The histological and biological spectrum of diffuse large B-cell lymphoma. Cancer J 18(5):411–420
11. Scott DW (2015) Cell-of- origin in diffuse large cell lymphoma: are assays ready for the clinic? Am Soc Clin Oncol Educ Book 35:e458–e466
12. Dunleavy K, Wyndham H (2014) Appropriate management of molecular subtypes of diffuse large B-cell lymphoma. Oncology 28(4):326–334
13. Carbone A, Gloghini A, Kwong Y-L, Younes A (2014) Diffuse large B-cell lymphoma: using pathologic and molecular biomarkers to define subgroups for novel therapy. Ann Hematol 93(8):1263–1277
14. Montono S, Fitzgibbon J (2011) Transformation of indolent B-cell lymphoma. J Clin Oncol 29(14):1827–1834
15. Visco C, Li Y, Xu-Monette ZY et al (2012) Comprehensive gene expression profiling and immunohistochemical studies support application of immunophenotypic algorithm for molecular subtype classification in diffuse large B-cell lymphoma: a report from the International DLBCL Rituximab-CHOP Consortium Program Study. Leukemia 26(9):2103–2113
16. Scott DW, Wright GW, Williams PM et al (2014) Determining cell-of-origin subtypes of diffuse large B-cell lymphoma using gene expression in formalin – fixed paraffin-embedded tissue. Blood 123(8):1214–1217
17. Lu T-X, Gong Q-X, Wang L et al (2015) Immunohistochemical algorithm alone is not enough for predicting the outcome of patients with diffuse large B-cell lymphoma treated with R-CHOP. Int J Clin Exp Pathol 8(1):275–286
18. Hu S, Xu-Monette ZY, Balasubramanyam A et al (2013) CD30 expression defines a novel subgroup of diffuse large B-cell lymphoma with favourable prognosis and distinct gene expression signature: a report from the International DLBCL Rituximab –CHOP Consortium Program Study. Blood 121(14):2715–2724
19. Slack GW, Steidi C, Sehn LH, Gascoyne RD (2014) CD30 expression in de novo diffuse large B-cell lymphoma: a population based study from British Columbia. Br J Haematol 167(5):608–617
20. Castillo JJ, Beltran BE, Miranda RN et al (2011) Epstein –Barr-Virus –positive diffuse large B-cell lymphoma of the elderly: what we know so far. Oncologist 16(1):87–96
21. Ok CY, Papathomas TG, Medeiros LJ, Young KH (2013) EBV-positive diffuse large cell lymphoma. Blood 122(3):328–340
22. Lenz G, Wright G, Dave SS et al (2008) Stromal gene signatures in large B-cell lymphoma. N Engl J Med 359(22):2313–2323
23. Alizadeh AA, Gentles AJ, Alencar AJ (2011) Prediction on survival in diffuse large B-cell lymphoma based on the expression of 2 genes reflecting tumor and microenvironment. Blood 118(5):1350–1358
24. Meyer PN, Fu K, Greiner T et al (2011) The stromal cell markers SPARC predicts survival in patents with diffuse large B-cell lymphoma treated with rituximab. Am J Clin Pathol 135(1):54–61
25. Quintanilla-Martinez L, de Jong D, de Mascarel A et al (2009) Gray zones around diffuse large B-cell lymphoma. Conclusions based on the workshop of the XIV meeting of the European Association for Hematopathology and the Society of Hematopathology in Bordeau, France. J Hematopath 2(4):211–236
26. Jaffe ES, Stein H, Swerdlow SH et al (2008) B-cell lymphoma unclassifiable, with features intermediate between diffuse large B-cell lymphoma and classical Hodgkin lymphoma. In: Swerdlow SH, Campo E, Harris NL et al (eds) WHO classification of tumours of haematopoietic and lymphoid tissues, 4th edn. IARC Press, Lyon, pp 267–268
27. Kluin P, Harris NL, Stein H et al (2008) B-cell lymphoma unclassifiable, with features intermediate between diffuse large B-cell lymphoma and Burkitt lymphoma. In: Swerdlow SH, Campo E, Harris NL

(eds) WHO classification of tumours of haematopoietic and lymphoid tissues, 4th edn. IARC Press, Lyon, pp 265–266
28. Eberle FC, Salaverria I, Steidl C et al (2011) Gray zone lymphoma: chromosomal aberrations with immunophenotypic and clinical correlations. Mod Pathol 24(12):1586–1597
29. Savage KJ, Monti S, Kutoc JL (2003) The molecular signature of mediastinal large B-cell lymphoma differs from that of other diffuse large B-cell lymphomas and shares features with classical Hodgkin lymphoma. Blood 102(12):3871
30. Küppers R, Dührsen U, Hansman ML (2014) Pathogenesis, diagnosis, and treatment of composite lymphomas. Lancet Oncol 15:e435–e446
31. Hoeller S, Copie-Bergman C (2012) Grey zone lymphomas with intermediate features. Adv Hematol. Article ID 460801, 7 pages. http://dx.doi.org/10.1155/2012/460801
32. Harris NL (2013) Shades of gray between large B-cell lymphomas and Hodgkin lymphomas: differential diagnosis and biological implications. Mod Pathol 26(Suppl 1):S57–S70
33. Quintanilla-Martinez L, Fend F (2011) Mediastinal gray zone lymphoma. Haematologica 96(4):496–499
34. Dunleavy K, Steidl C (2015) Emerging biological insights and novel treatment strategies in primary mediastinal large B-cell lymphoma. Semin Hematol 52(2):119–125
35. Wessendorf S, Bath TFE, Viardot A et al (2007) Further delineation of chromosomal consensus regions in primary mediastinal B-cell lymphomas: an analysis of 37 tumor samples using high-resolution genomic profiling (array-CGH). Leukemia 21(12):2463–2469
36. Steidl C, Telenius A, Shah SP et al (2010) Genome-wide copy number analysis of Hodgkin Reed-Sternberg cells identifies recurrent imbalance with correlations to treatment outcome. Blood 116(3):418–427
37. Rosenwald A, Wright G, Leroy K et al (2003) Molecular diagnosis of primary mediastinal B-cell lymphoma identifies a clinically favourable subgroup of diffuse large B-cell lymphoma related to Hodgkin lymphoma. J Exp Med 198(6):851–862
38. Peh SC, Kim LH, Poppema S (2001) TARC, a CC chemokine, is frequently expressed in classic Hodgkin's lymphoma but not in NLP Hodgkin's lymphoma, T-cell rich B-cell lymphoma and most cases of anaplastic large cell lymphoma. Am J Surg Pathol 225(7):925–929
39. Eberle FC, Rodriguez-Canales J, Wei L et al (2011) Methylation profiling of mediastinal gray zone lymphoma reveals a distinctive signature with elements shared by classical Hodgkin's lymphoma and primary mediastinal large B-cell lymphoma. Haematologica 96(4):558–566
40. Steidl C, Shah SP, Woolcock BW et al (2011) MHC class transactivator CIITA is a recurrent gene fusion partner in lymphoid cancers. Nature 471(7338):377–381
41. Coleman Lindsley R, LaCasce AS (2012) Biology of double hit lymphomas. Curr Opin Hematol 19(4):299–304
42. Aukema SM, Kreuz M, Kohler CW et al (2014) Biological characterization of adult MYC-translocation-positive mature B-cell lymphomas other than molecular Burkitt lymphoma. Hematologica 99(4):726–735
43. Aukema SM, Siebert R, Schuuring ED et al (2011) Double hit lymphomas. Blood 117(8):2319–2331
44. Xu X, Zhang L, Wang Y et al (2013) Double- hit lymphomas arising from follicular lymphoma following acquisition of MYC: report of two cases and literature review. Int J Clin Exp Pathol 6(4):788–794
45. Harris NL, Swerdlow SH, Jaffe ES et al (2008) Follicular lymphoma. In: Swerdlow SH, Campo E, Harris NL et al (eds) WHO classification of tumours of haematopoietic and lymphoid tissues, 4th edn. IARC Press, Lyon, pp 220–226
46. Wahlin BE, Oe Y, Kimby E et al (2012) Clinical significance of follicular lymphoma in a population-based cohort of 505 patients with long follow- up times. Br J Haematol 156(2):225–233
47. Shustik J, Quinn M, Connors JM et al (2011) Follicular non-Hodgkin lymphoma grades 3A and 3B have similar outcome and appear incurable with anthracycline-based therapy. Ann Oncol 22(5):1164–1169
48. Horn H, Schmelter C, Leich E et al (2011) Follicular lymphoma grade 3B is a distinct neoplasm according to cytogenetic and immunohistochemical profiles. Haematologica 96(9):1327–1334
49. Maeshima AM, Taniguchi H, Nomoto J et al (2013) Prognostic implications of histologic grade and intensity of Bcl-2 expression in follicular lymphoma undergoing rituximab-containing therapy. Hum Pathol 44(11):2529–2535
50. Lossos IS, Gascoyne IS (2011) Transformation of follicular lymphoma. Best Pract Res Haematol 24(2):147–163
51. Bouska A, Mckeithan TW, Deffenbacher KE et al (2014) Genome-wide copy-number analyses reveal genomic abnormalities involved in transformation of follicular lymphoma. Blood 123(11):1681–1690
52. Pasqualucci L, Khiabanian H, Fangzio M et al (2014) Genetics of follicular lymphoma transformation. Cell Rep 6(1):130–140
53. Kiaii S, Clear AJ, Ramsey AG et al (2013) Follicular lymphoma cells induce change in T-cell gene expression and function: potential impact on survival risk and risk transformation. J Clin Oncol 31(21):2654–2661
54. Attarbaschi A, Beishuizen A, Mann G et al (2013) Children and adolescents with follicular lymphoma have an excellent prognosis with either limited chemotherapy or with a 'watch and wait' strategy after complete resection. Ann Hematol 92(11):1537–1540
55. Hsi ED, Martin P (2014) Indolent mantle cell lymphoma. Leuk Lymphoma 55(4):761–767
56. Ganapathi KA, Pittaluga S, Odejide OO et al (2014) Early lymphoid lesions: conceptual, diagnostic and clinical challenges. Haematologica 99(9):1421–1432

57. Carvajal-Cuenca A, Campo E (2013) Early neoplastic lymphoid lesions. Semin Diagn Pathol 30(2):146–155
58. Fend F, Cabecadas J, Gaulard P et al (2012) Early lesions in lymphoid neoplasia. J Hematop 5(3). doi:10.1007/s12308-012-0148-6
59. Carbone A, Gloghini A (2014) Emerging issues after the recognition of in situ follicular lymphoma. Leuk Lymphoma 55(3):482–490
60. Green MR, Gentles AL, Nair RV et al (2013) Hierarchy in somatic mutations arising during genomic evolution and progression of follicular lymphoma. Blood 121(9):1604–1611
61. Skarbnik AP, Goy AH (2015) Mantle cell lymphoma: state of the art. Clin Adv Hematol Oncol 13(1): 44–55
62. Swerdlow SH, Campo E, Seto M, Hermelink-Müller HK (2008) Mantle cell lymphoma. In: Swerdlow SH, Campo E, Harris NL et al (eds) WHO classification of tumours of haematopoietic and lymphoid tissue, 4th edn. IARC Press, Lyon, pp 229–232
63. Nakashima MO, Durkin L, Bodo J et al (2014) Utility and diagnostic pitfalls of SOX11 monoclonal antibodies in mantle cell lymphoma and other lymphoproliferative disorders. Appl Immunohistochem Mol Morphol 22(10):720–727
64. Vose JM (2015) Mantle cell lymphoma: 2015 update on diagnosis, risk-stratification and clinical management. Am J Hematol 90(8):739–745
65. Mathur R, Seghal L, Braun FK et al (2015) Targeting Wnt pathway in mantle cell lymphoma – initiating cells. J Hematol Oncol 8:63
66. Al-Kawaaz M, Mathew S, Liu Y et al (2015) Cyclin D1-positive diffuse large B-cell lymphoma with IGH-CCND1 translocation and BCL6 rearrangement: a report of two cases. Am J Clin Pathol 143(2):288–289
67. Ondreika SL, Lai R, Smith SD, Hsi ED (2011) Indolent mantle cell leukaemia: a clinicopathological variant characterized by isolated lymphocytosis, interstitial bone marrow involvement, kappa light chain restriction, and good prognosis. Haematologica 96(8):1121–1127
68. Furtado M, Rule S (2011) Indolent Mantle cell lymphoma. Haematologica 96(8):1086–1088
69. Anagnostou D (2012) Janus-faced lymphoid infiltrates. In: Anagnostou D, Matutes E (eds) Bone marrow lymphoid infiltrates: diagnosis and clinical impact. Springer/Printforce, The Netherlands, pp 113–144
70. Kostakoglu L, Cheson BD (2014) Current role of FDG-PET/CT in lymphomas. Eur J Nucl Med Mol Imaging 41(5):1004–1027
71. Adams HJA, Kwee T, De Keizer B et al (2014) Systemic review and meta-analysis on the diagnostic performance of FDG-PET/CT in detecting bone marrow involvement in newly diagnosed Hodgkin lymphoma: is bone marrow still necessary? Ann Oncol 25(5):921–927
72. Vassilakopoulos TP, Prassopoulos V, Rondogianni P et al (2015) Role of FDG-PET/CT in staging and first-line treatment of Hodgkin and aggressive B-cell lymphomas. Memo 8:105–114
73. Cheson BD, Fisher RI, Barrington SF et al (2014) Recommendations for initial evaluation, staging, and response assessment of Hodgkin and non-Hodgkin lymphoma: the Lugano Classification. J Clin Oncol 32(27):3059–3065
74. Adams HJ, Kwee TC (2015) Do not abandon the bone marrow Biopsy yet in diffuse large B-cell lymphoma. J Clin Oncol 33(10):217
75. Cerci JJ, Györke T, Fanti S et al (2014) Combined PET and biopsy evidence of marrow involvement improves prediction in diffuse large B-cell lymphoma. J Nucl Med 55(10):1591–1597
76. Sehn LH, Scott DW, Chhanabhai M et al (2011) Impact of concordant and discordant bone marrow involvement on outcome in diffuse large B-cell lymphoma treated with R-CHOP. J Clin Oncol 29(11):1452–1457
77. Kremer M, Spitzer M, Mandl-Weber S et al (2003) Discordant bone marrow involvement in diffuse large B-cell lymphoma: comparative molecular analysis reveals a heterogeneous group of disorders. Lab Invest 83(1):107–114
78. Stein H (2008) Hodgkin lymphoma- introduction. In: Swerdlow SH, Campo E, Harris NL et al (eds) WHO classification of tumours haematopoietic and lymphoid tissue, 4th edn. IARCPress, Lyon, p 322
79. Agostinelli C, Pileri S (2014) Pathobiology of hodgkin lymphoma. Mediterr J Hematol Infect Dis 6(1):e2014040. doi:10.4084/MJHID.2014.040
80. Poppema S, Delsol G, Pileri SA et al (2008) Nodular lymphocyte predominant Hodgkin lymphoma. In: Swerdlow SH, Campo E, Harris NL et al (eds) WHO classification of tumours of haematopoietic and lymphoid tissue, 4th edn. IARC Press, Lyon, pp 323–325
81. Prakash S, Fountain T, Raffeld M et al (2006) IgD positive L&H cells identify a unique subset of nodular lymphocyte predominance Hodgkin lymphoma. Am J Surg Pathol 30(5):585–592
82. Smith BL (2010) Nodular lymphocyte predominant Hodgkin lymphoma: diagnostic pearls and pitfalls. Arch Pathol Lab Med 134(10):1434–1439
83. Hartman S, Eray M, Döring C et al (2014) Diffuse large B-cell lymphoma derived from nodular lymphocyte predominant Hodgkin lymphoma presents with variable histopathology. BMC Cancer 14:332. doi:10.1186/1471-2407-14-332
84. Huang JZ, Weisenburger DD, Vose JM et al (2004) Diffuse large B-cell lymphoma arising in nodular lymphocyte predominant Hodgkin lymphoma: a report of 21 cases from the Nebraska Lymphoma Study Group. Leuk Lymphoma 45(8):1551–1557
85. Biasoli I, Stamatoullas A, Meignin V et al (2010) Nodular, lymphocyte- predominant Hodgkin lymphoma; a long term study and analysis of transfor-

mation to diffuse large B-cell lymphoma in a cohort of 164 patients from Adult Lymphoma Study Group. Cancer 116(3):631–639

86. Saarinen S, Aavikko M, Aittomaki K et al (2011) Exome sequencing reveals germline NPAT mutation as a candidate risk factor for Hodgkin lymphoma. Blood 118(3):493–498
87. Saarinen S, Pukkala E, Willenbrock K et al (2013) High familial risk in nodular lymphocyte predominant Hodgkin lymphoma. J Clin Oncol 31(7):938–943
88. Banerjee D (2011) Recent advances in the pathobiology of Hodgkin's lymphoma: potential impact on diagnostic, predictive, and therapeutic strategies. Adv Hematol 2011:439456. doi:10.1155/2011/439456

General Principles of PET/CT Imaging

2

Vassilios K. Prassopoulos
and Roxani D. Efthymiadou

Positron emission tomography (PET) constitutes a relatively novel imaging procedure useful mainly in oncology, but also in cardiology and neurology. PET imaging is based on the detection of annihilation photons produced after positron emission from a radiolabeled tracer, which follows and corresponds to a specific molecular biological or biochemical pathway. Combination with computed tomography (CT) provides both functional and morphological information in one single device.

PET imaging includes positron-emitting isotopes such as F-18, C-11, N-13, Ga-68, etc. After b+decay (isobaric decay) the positron travels (positron range) among material and electron clouds until it loses almost all its energy. At that point the positrons interact with an electron and annihilate each other producing two gamma ray photons (annihilation photons) each 511 keV; energy corresponds to electron and positron mass, which are emitted to opposite directions of ~180o. The annihilation photons are detected and then registered as one event if they reach the detectors within a limited time frame (coincidence detection). It is assumed that the event occurred at the straight line between the two detectors (line of response, LOR). Time of flight (TOF) is a novel technique in newer PET scanners, which incorporates time during coincidence detection. Coincidence detection is the principle basis of PET imaging and in which ideally only the coincidence photons are finally registered while the rest are being rejected. However coincidence events may be provoked from random or scattered events. Photons strike onto detectors (scintillator crystals); their energy is converted into light, which is multiplied through photomultipliers and then converted to electric signal. In each step the energy produced (light, electric signal) is analogous to the one initially deposited by the photons onto scintillators. Data are acquired in a list mode or frame mode, LORs are saved, and a raw data histogram (sinogram) is formatted. Attenuation correction is likely the most important source of errors in PET imaging. In PET/CT scanners correction is accomplished through the application of CT. Finally, through the application of mathematic algorithms, tomographic images are reconstructed and the biodistribution of the tracer is visualized. Several reconstruction methods have been used, with iterative to be preferred and widely applied. Combination of PEt alone and CT alone provides hybrid PET/CT systems that allow the simultaneous anatomic information, as well as

V.K. Prassopoulos (✉)
Department of Nuclear Medicine and PET/CT, "HYGEIA" Hospital, Kifissias Av. and Erythrou Stavrou 4, Maroussi 15123, Greece
e-mail: vprasso@otenet.gr

R.D. Efthymiadou
Director of PET/CT Department, "HYGEIA" Hospital, Erythrou Stavrou 4 and Kifissias, Maroussi 15123, Greece
e-mail: r.efthimiadi@hygeia.gr

J.A. Andreou et al. (eds.), *PET/CT in Lymphomas: A Case-Based Atlas*,
DOI 10.1007/978-3-319-27380-8_2

the correction of attenuated photons, leading to better image quality and resolution. Adding also the development of advanced software and hardware technologies, high spatial resolution has been achieved, resulting to more accurate and confident imaging interpretation. Semiquantitative and volume calculations constitute in everyday practice assistant tools during interpretation (for review see Ref. [1, 2]).

In parallel with the advances in technology and PET scanners, radiochemistry was also developed. The first report of artificial radiation production (N-13) was in 1934, and PET-dedicated cyclotrons were commercially available in the mid-1980s. FDG was developed in the 1970s and was administered to the first humans in 1976, gaining since then a variety of applications, mainly in oncology, but also in neurology and cardiology. FDG is a glucose analogue, resulting from the substitution of an OH- by F-18. FDG is taken intracellularly through facilitated transport by GLUT transporters. Inside the cell it is phosphorylated by hexokinase producing FDG-6-phosphate, which cannot be further metabolized; therefore it is trapped intracellularly. Small to negligible amount is dephosphorylated by glucose-6-phosphatase and facilitated diffused outside the cell. Tumor cells express the glycolytic phenotype (Warburg effect), and FDG is mainly transported into these cells through GLUT1, GLUT3, and GLUT4 transporters, depending on histologic type, subtype, and specific characteristics, as well as tumor grade, proliferation, and aggressiveness. Distribution of FDG reflects the distribution of glucose inside the body [2].

Most cancerous diseases are FDG avid, and therefore FDG-PET/CT is currently widely applied, mainly for evaluation of treatment response and recurrence. Its prognostic information is in several occasions incremental and is reported to alter treatment management in about 1/3 of the cases. For NSCLC, and esophageal cancer before surgical intervention, PET/CT is considered definitive in initial staging as well for treatment decision followed. FDG-PET/CT information is crucial in Hodgkin disease and most cases of non-Hodgkin lymphomas both in adults and children. Solitary pulmonary nodule evaluation is one of the first FDG-PET indications, fever of unknown origin investigation is one of the most common non-tumor FDG-PET/CT applications, while PEt also serves as a unique tool in radiation planning delineation, providing the metabolic information otherwise missed.

Apart from FDG, several other radiopharmaceuticals have been developed, both generator produced, i.e., Ga-68 for labeling peptides in neuroendocrine tumors assessment, and cyclotron produced, i.e., F-18-fluorothymidine for imaging proliferation, F-18- and C-11-choline with main applications in prostate cancer, radiolabeled amino acids for brain tumor imaging, radiolabeled tracers for hypoxia imaging, as well as N-13-NH_3 and O-15-H_2O, and more recently F-18-Flurpiridaz for cardiologic applications, as well as amyloid imaging for neurologic information [3, 4].

References

1. Townsend DW (2004) Physical principles and technology of clinical PET imaging. Ann Acad Med Singapore 33(2):133–145
2. Basu S, Hess S, Nielsen Braad PE, Olsen BB, Inglev S, Høilund-Carlsen PF (2014) The basic principles of FDG-PET/CT imaging. PET Clin 9(4):355–370
3. Jiang L, Tu Y, Shi H, Cheng Z (2014) PET probes beyond (18)F-FDG. J Biomed Res 28(6):435–446
4. Maddahi J, Packard RR (2014) Cardiac PET perfusion tracers: current status and future directions. Semin Nucl Med 44(5):333–343

Anatomic Classification of Lymph Nodes

3

Vassilis C. Koutoulidis, Athanasios D. Gouliamos, and Evaggelia C. Panourgias

3.1 Lymph Nodes of the Neck

One of the most widely used, imaging-based classifications of cervical lymph nodes (LNs) is the one introduced by Som et al., which is based on the clinical classifications of the American Joint Committee on Cancer and the American Academy of Otolaryngology-Head and Neck Surgery [1–3]. This classification system has been shown to be simple and consistent, with nodal levels easily distinguished by radiologists on axial slices of neck CT and MRI exams. Although this system was originally conceived as a nodal mapping guide for selecting the most appropriate neck dissection procedure, its simplicity and reproducibility make it appropriate for other clinical uses, including assessment of lymphoma patients. Indeed, in the case of lymphoma, standardization of lymph node terminology facilitates communication between imagers (radiologists and nuclear physicians) and clinicians (oncologists, hematologists, and radiotherapists) and aids correct evaluation of initial disease extent, treatment planning, and treatment response assessment.

According to the Som classification, the anatomically based terminology that was introduced by Rouviere in 1938 is replaced by a system based on levels, a concept first introduced by Shah et al. in 1981 [4, 5]. Cervical lymph nodes are divided in seven levels, numbered from I to VII. Some node categories of the head and neck region are not included in the numbered system and retain their anatomical names. The anatomic boundaries between nodal levels, as defined on axial slices of neck CT and MRI exams, are the following (Fig. 3.1):

Level I nodes are those located above the hyoid bone, below the mylohyoid muscle, and anterior to a transverse line drawn on each axial CT/MRI image through the posterior edge of the submandibular gland. They are further subdivided into *IA* nodes (formerly classified as submental), and *IB* nodes (previously classified as submandibular). Level *IA* nodes are located between the medial edges of the anterior bellies of the two digastric muscles. Level *IB* nodes lie posterior and lateral to the medial edge of the anterior belly of the digastric muscle and anterior to a transverse line drawn on each axial slice through the posterior surface of the submandibular gland.

V.C. Koutoulidis • A.D. Gouliamos (✉)
E.C. Panourgias
1st Department of Radiology,
National and Kapodistrian University of Athens
School of Medicine, Aretaieion Hospital,
76, Vas. Sophias Ave., 11528 Athens, Greece
e-mail: vkoutoulidis@med.uoa.gr;
agouliam@med.uoa.gr; epanourgias@yahoo.com

J.A. Andreou et al. (eds.), *PET/CT in Lymphomas: A Case-Based Atlas*,
DOI 10.1007/978-3-319-27380-8_3

The next three levels (*II–IV*) comprise the internal jugular nodes. Level *II* nodes extend from the skull base to the lower margin of the hyoid bone. They lie posterior to a transverse line drawn on each axial image through the posterior edge of the submandibular gland (level IB nodes lie anterior to this line). They are also located anterior to a transverse line drawn through the posterior edge of the sternocleidomastoid muscle (level V nodes lie posterior to this line). Nodes situated within 2 cm of the skull base that lie anterior, lateral, or posterior to the carotid sheath are classified as level II. If they lie medial to the internal carotid artery, they are classified as retropharyngeal. Caudal to 2 cm below the skull base, level II nodes are subdivided into *IIA* nodes (those lying anterior, lateral, or medial to the internal jugular vein; formerly classified as upper internal jugular vein nodes) and *IIB* nodes (nodes lying posterior to the vein; formerly classified as upper spinal accessory nodes).

Level III nodes are those formerly classified as mid jugular nodes, and they lie between the level of the lower body of the hyoid bone and the level of the lower margin of the cricoid cartilage arch. They lie anterior to a transverse line drawn on each axial image through the posterior margin of the sternocleidomastoid muscle (this line separates them from level V nodes). They also lie lateral to the medial margin of the common carotid artery or the internal carotid artery (this margin separates them from level VI nodes).

Level IV nodes (previously known as low jugular nodes) lie between the level of the lower margin of the cricoid cartilage arch and the level of the clavicle. A line drawn on axial images through the posterior edge of the sternocleidomastoid muscle and the posterolateral edge of the anterior scalene muscle separates level IV nodes (lying anterior to this line) from level V nodes (posterior to the line). They also lie lateral to the medial margin of the common carotid artery (this margin separates them from level VI nodes).

Level V nodes extend from the skull base, at the posterior border of the attachment of the sternocleidomastoid muscle, to the level of the clavicle. They are subdivided in level *VA* nodes, which extend between the skull base and the level of the lower margin of the cricoid cartilage arch, and *VB* nodes, which lie between the level of the lower margin of the cricoid cartilage arch and the level of the clavicle. *VA* nodes are located posterior to a transverse line drawn on each axial scan through the posterior edge of the sternocleidomastoid muscle (which separates them from level II and III nodes). *VB* nodes lie behind an oblique line through the posterior edge of the sternocleidomastoid muscle and the posterolateral edge of the anterior scalene muscle (which separates them from level IV nodes). An important distinction is between supraclavicular nodes and level V and IV nodes. The Som classification considers the visualized portion of the clavicle, as seen on each of the axial CT/MRI images through the region, as the most reliable imaging marker of the supraclavicular fossa. Thus, when a node is observed in an axial slice where portion of the clavicle is also seen, the node is classified as supraclavicular.

Level VI nodes lie inferior to the lower margin of the hyoid bone, superior to the top of the manubrium, and between the medial margins of the common carotid arteries or the internal carotid arteries.

Level VII nodes are essentially superior mediastinal nodes that lie caudal to the manubrium, between the medial margins of the left and right common carotid arteries, and extend to the level of the innominate veins.

Apart from the above numbered nodes, the following nodal groups of the head and neck are still referred to by their anatomical names: retropharyngeal, parotid (intraglandular and periglandular, both contained within the parotid space fascia), facial, occipital, postauricular, and supraclavicular.

As elsewhere in the body, lymphomatous nodes of the neck tend to be enlarged and homogeneous, although their size may vary from a few millimeters to many centimeters. Multiple nodal levels may be involved. Necrosis and/or signs of extracapsular spread are rare. Calcifications are also very uncommon in untreated patients [6, 7].

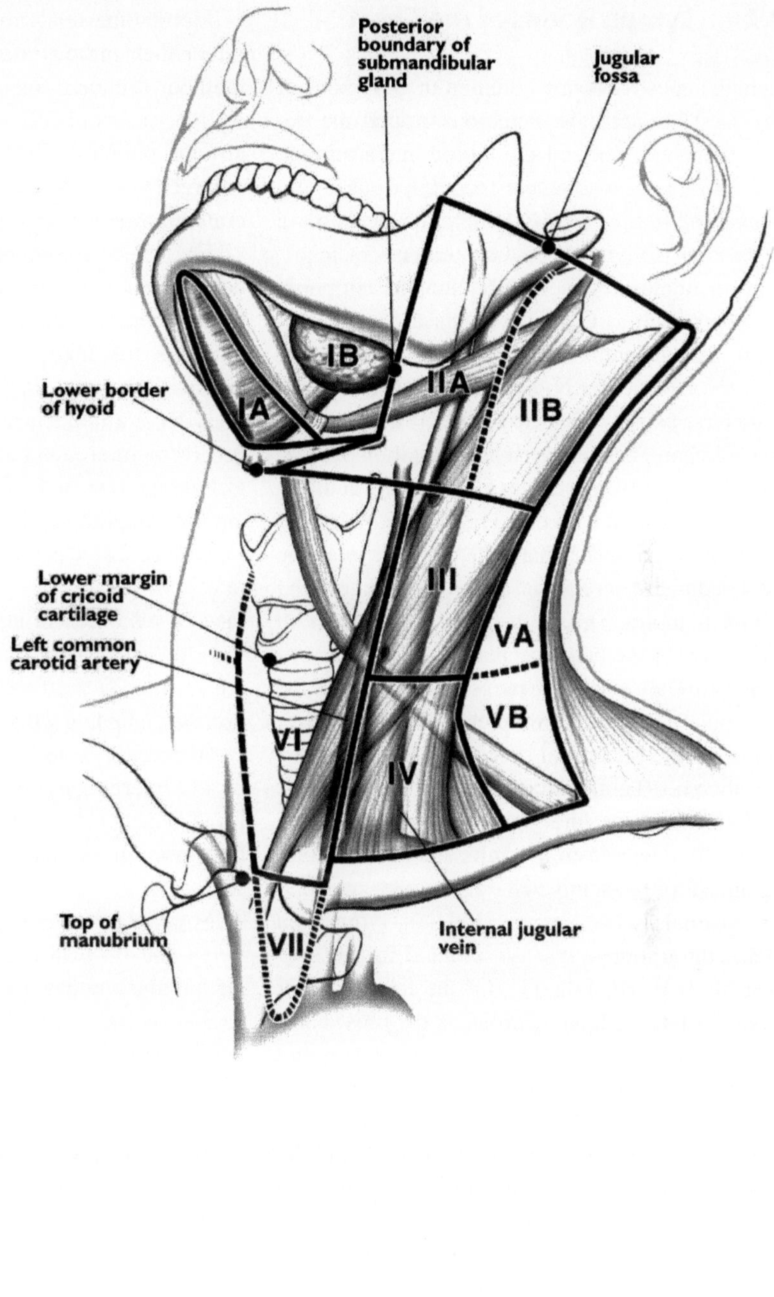

Fig. 3.1 Drawing of neck as seen from left anterior view shows lines of separation between cervical nodal levels (Used with permission from Ref. [1])

3.2 Lymph Nodes of the Chest

Lymph nodes (LNs) are common in all regions of the chest but are most numerous around the tracheobronchial tree and the middle mediastinum. Causes of LN enlargement include primary neoplasms of lymph nodes (lymphoma, leukemia), metastases from intrathoracic or extrathoracic primary malignancies, nonlymphomatous lymphoid disorders such as Castleman's disease and infections. The generally accepted upper limit of normal for short-axis LN diameter is 1.0 cm in the transverse plane, as detected on CT [8]. According to the Lugano classification, the definition of measurable adenopathy includes a longest nodal diameter of greater than 1.5 cm. This is a definition for CT studies. Smaller than 1.0 cm LNs may be involved with lymphoma if found positive on FDG PET/CT studies [9]. LNs in the paraspinal areas, in the region of the brachiocephalic veins and retrocrural area, are smaller, 6 mm or less. Nodes in the aortopulmonary window, pretracheal and lower paratrachial spaces, and subcarinal compartments are often 6–10 mm on transverse CT scan images.

Lymphoma is the most common primary mediastinal neoplasm in adults and can be either localized or disseminated. The most common mediastinal lymphoma is Hodgkin lymphoma (HL). Intrathoracic disease is noted in 60 % of patients with HL [10, 11]. Of the four types of classical HL, nodular sclerosis is the most common and most often is found in the anterior and superior mediastinum. Other types of classical HL (lymphocyte rich, mixed cellularity, and lymphocyte depletion) can involve anterior, middle, and posterior lymph nodal groups. Intrathoracic disease is noted at presentation in 40–50 % of patients with NHL [10, 11]. NHL with mediastinal involvement usually manifests with diffuse lymphadenopathy involving middle mediastinal and hilar nodes. However, aggressive B-cell (the so-called primary mediastinal or thymic large B-cell lymphoma) or lymphoblastic lymphoma can present as an isolated anterior mediastinal mass, which may obstruct the superior vena cava, compress the airway, or invade the chest wall, pericardium, lung parenchyma, and pleura. Juxtaphrenic and posterior mediastinal nodal involvement is considered characteristic in NHL.

Lymphoma tends to expand along or around rather than invade existing structures. CT is the method of choice for identifying and staging as well as means of following the response to therapy of patients with HL and NHL. Discrete enlarged solid LNs or large, lobulated conglomerate masses of nodes are seen.

HL most commonly spreads contiguously between nodes of the anterior mediastinum, paratrachial region, and hilum. Paracardiac, subcarinal, superior diaphragmatic, internal mammary, and axillary nodes are less frequently involved.

NHL is a multifocal disorder, and patterns of involvement are unpredictable and atypical such as lymph nodes of the posterior mediastinum and anterior diaphragm [10, 11].

Diffuse LN calcification is a consequence of radiation therapy or systemic chemotherapy but may be also seen in granulomatous disease. LNs with low attenuation centers and rim enhancement are seen in 20 % of patients and are indicative of necrosis, a finding without prognostic significance.

According to the lymph node map proposed by the International Association for the study of Lung Cancer (IASLC), the following LN stations have been described [12, 13] and are shown in a schematic illustration (Fig. 3.2):

Supraclavicular LNs (Station 1)

1R and 1L. Low cervical, supraclavicular, and sternal notch nodes.

Above the level of the left brachiocephalic vein, the clavicles and the manubrium extending to the lower margin of the cricoid.

Superior Mediastinal LNs (Stations 2–4)

2R. Upper paratracheal

Above the level of the intersection of the caudal margin of the innominate vein with the trachea extending to the apex of the right lung and pleural space

2L. Upper paratracheal

Above the level of the superior border of the aortic arch extending to the apex of the left lung and pleural space

3A. Prevascular

Anterior to the vessels

On the right: anterior the superior vena cava

On the left: anterior to the left carotid artery

Not accessible with mediastinoscopy

3P. Prevertebral

Below the plane tangential to the upper margin of the aortic arch, behind the esophagus, extending to the chest apex. Accessible with endoscopic ultrasound (EUS).

4R. Lower paratracheal

Drain the right paratracheal and pretracheal area from the level of the azygos vein up to the level of the intersection of the caudal margin of the innominate vein with the trachea

4L. Lower paratracheal

Located in the space between the left lateral border of the trachea, medial to the ligamentum arteriosum from the upper rim of the left main pulmonary artery up to the upper margin of the aortic arch

Aortic Nodes (Stations 5–6)

5. Subaortic (aortopulmonary window)

Lateral to the ligamentum arteriosum from the upper rim of the left main pulmonary artery to the lower border of the aortic arch

6. Para-aortic

Anterior and lateral to the ascending aorta, the aortic arch, or the proximal brachiocephalic artery from the lower to the upper border of the aortic arch

Inferior Mediastinal Nodes (Stations 7–9)

7. Subcarinal (beneath the main bronchi within the mediastinal pleura)

Lower border on the right: lower border of the bronchus intermedius

Lower border on the left: upper border of the lower lobe bronchus

8. Paraesophageal

Below the subcarinal nodes extending caudally to the diaphragm

Upper border on the right: the lower border of the bronchus intermedius

Upper border on the left: the upper border of the lower lobe bronchus

9. Pulmonary ligament

Below the inferior pulmonary vein extending caudally to the diaphragm

Nodes outside the mediastinal pleura are:

Hilar, Lobar, Segmental, and Subsegmental LNs (Stations 10–14)

10. Hilar

On the right: from the lower rim of the azygos to the interlobar region

On the left: upper rim of the pulmonary artery to the interlobar region

11. Interlobar

Between the origin of the lobar bronchi

11s: between the upper lobe bronchus and bronchus intermedius on the right

11i: between the middle and lower lobe bronchus on the right

12. Lobar

Adjacent to lobar bronchi

13. Segmental

Adjacent to segmental bronchi

14. Subsegmental

Adjacent to subsegmental bronchi

Hilar nodes are considered N1 nodes and are removed at pneumonectomy

Axillary LNs

Divided in five groups:

Lateral or brachial group
: Located in the inferomedial side of the axillary vein

Anterior or pectoral group
: Located on the lower parts of the pectoralis minor muscle

Posterior or subscapular group
: Located in the groove that separates the teres minor and subscapularis muscles following the course of the subscapular vessels

Central group
: Located inside the central part of the adipose tissue of the axilla

Apical (medial or subclavicular) group
: Located on the upper parts of the pectoralis minor muscle

Chest wall LNs

Internal mammary nodes
: Located at the anterior ends of the intercostal spaces, along the internal mammary vessels

Posterior intercostal LNs
: Located near the head and neck of the posterior ribs

Juxtavertebral (prevertebral or paravertebral) LNs
: Lie along the anterior and lateral aspects the vertebral bodies, from T8 to T12 levels

Diaphragmatic LNs
: Located on or just above the thoracic surface of the diaphragm and divided in three groups:

Anterior (pre-pericardial or cardiophrenic) group

Middle (juxtaphrenic or lateral) group

Posterior (retrocrural) group

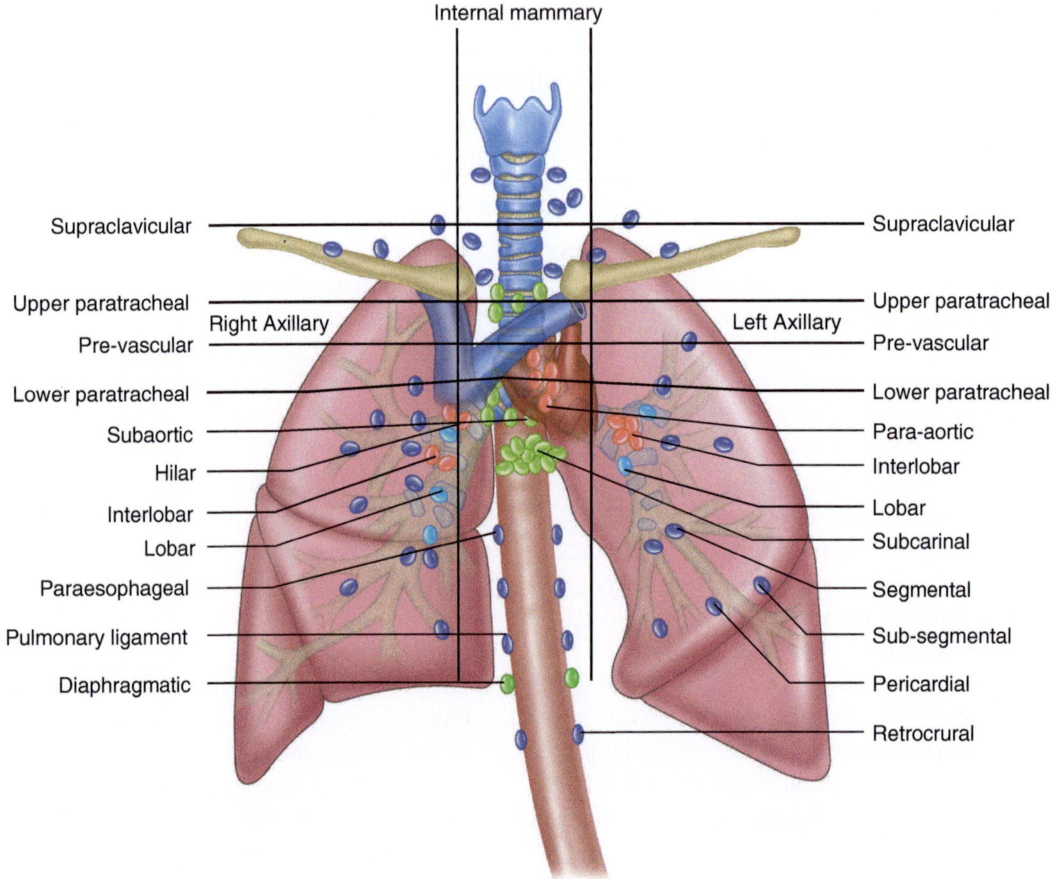

Fig. 3.2 Schematic illustration indicating the anatomical location of the various LN stations in the chest. Used with permission from Ref. [12]

3.3 Abdominal Lymph Node Anatomy

Detection of abdominal lymphadenopathy is facilitated by the widespread use of axial imaging. Knowledge of the network of nodal chains and their complex interconnections is important to correctly diagnose the spread of tumors within the peritoneal cavity.

Criteria based solely on size for the characterization of malignant lymph nodes is a source of false-negative results from CT examinations, as has been described in various published reports.

Lymph nodes within normal limits, with regard to size, may have abnormal internal architecture and enlarged lymph nodes can be nonmalignant. Newer imaging modalities such as PET/CT and MRI with nanoparticles are superior techniques for accurate nodal characterization [14].

3.3.1 Lymphatics of the Abdomen

3.3.1.1 Liver

The hepatic lymphatics can be divided into two sets, superficial and deep. The *superficial lymphatic network* is located subperitoneally, within Glisson's capsule, over the entire hepatic surface. The drainage of superficial lymphatics can be classified into three major groups:

1. Lymph nodes in the hepatoduodenal and gastrohepatic ligaments are the commonest routes (Fig. 3.3a).
2. The diaphragmatic lymphatic plexus either directly at the bare area or indirectly through the coronary and triangular ligaments.
3. From the segments adjacent to the falciform ligament, lymphatics drain into the deep superior epigastric node in the anterior abdominal wall.

Also, some lymph vessels may run through the diaphragm to enter the precardiac, superior phrenic, and juxtaesophageal lymph nodes or accompany the right or left inferior phrenic artery to the celiac nodes. Others run across the anterior margin of the liver to lymph nodes at the porta hepatis. Lymph vessels from the caudate lobe drain into the precaval nodes.

The *deep lymphatics* follow the portal veins and leave the liver through the lymph nodes at the porta hepatis, the hepatic lymph nodes, and to the nodes in the hepatoduodenal ligament. It is possible to distinguish the nodes in the hepatoduodenal ligament: the hepatic artery chain and the posterior periportal chain. The hepatic artery chain accompanies the proper hepatic artery to reach the celiac nodes and then into the cisterna chyli. The posterior periportal chain is located posterior to the portal vein. It drains into the retropancreatic nodes and the aortocaval node and then into the cisterna chyli and the thoracic duct [15].

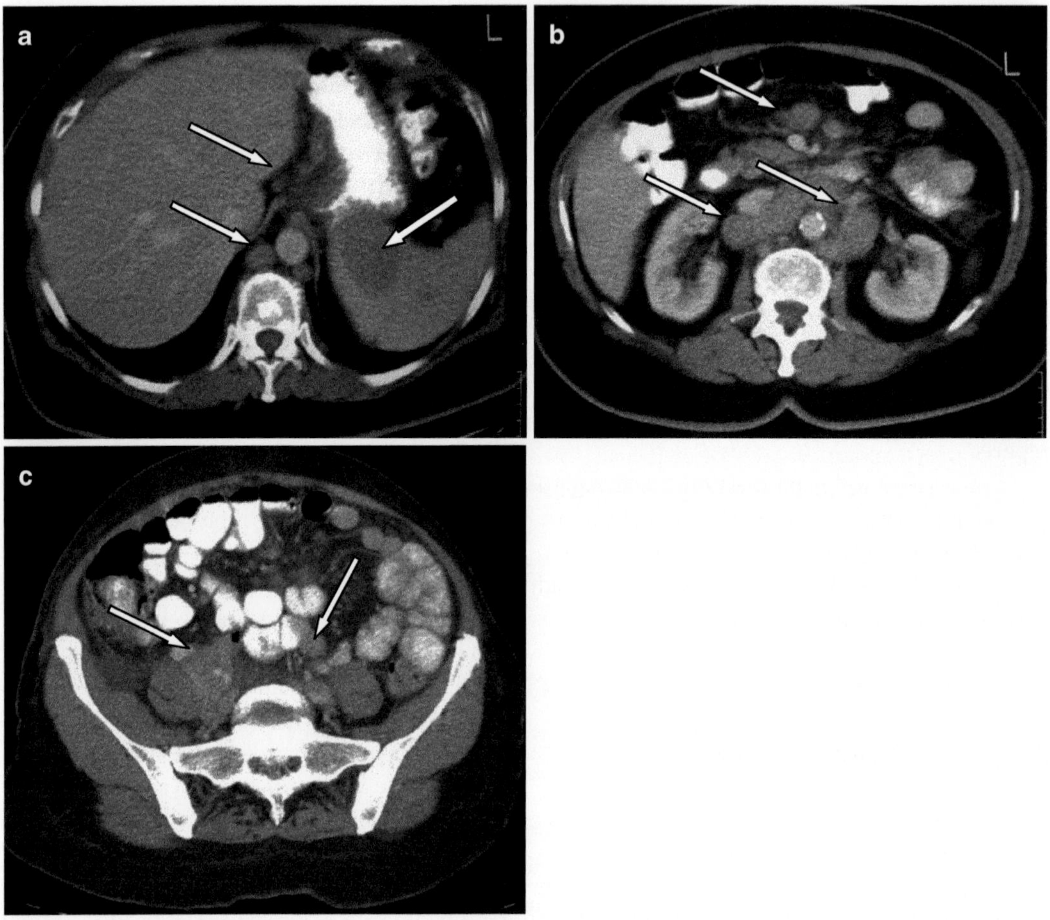

Fig. 3.3 (**a**) Axial CT image in a patient with lymphoma with enlarged hepatogastric and retrocrural lymph nodes and metastatic splenic lesions (*arrows*). (**b**) Axial CT image at the level of the renal hila shows multiple enlarged para-aortic, aortocaval, and mesenteric lymph nodes (*arrows*). (**c**) Axial CT image in a patient with lymphoma demonstrates multiple enlarged common iliac lymph nodes (*arrows*).

3.3.1.2 Stomach

The gastric lymphatic drainage forms a network that follows the course of vessels in various peritoneal ligaments of the stomach and forms four groups of lymph nodes:

1. Left gastric nodal group, which follows the left gastric artery and drains into the celiac nodes. They drain the left side of the lesser curvature of the stomach and the esophagogastric junction area.
2. Short gastric and left gastroepiploic lymphatic vessels drain the proximal part of the greater curvature of the stomach. They follow the left gastroepiploic vessels and drain into the perisplenic nodes. From the splenic hilum, they enter the celiac nodes, coursing along the splenic artery. These nodes are known as pancreaticosplenic nodes.
3. The right half of the greater curvature and the antral portion of the stomach drain into (a) the right gastroepiploic nodes, which in turn drain into the nodes at the gastrocolic trunk and to (b) the subpyloric nodes.
4. Pyloric nodes which drain the pyloric part of stomach to the hepatic, pyloric, and left gastric nodes.

All the vessels enter into the celiac nodes [16]. From these nodes they pass into the intestinal lymph trunks, which then enter the cisterna chyli and into the thoracic duct.

3.3.1.3 Pancreatic Lymph Nodes

Three lymphatic drainage pathways exist for the head of the pancreas and a single corporeo-caudal segment for the rest of the pancreas. The lymphatics arising around the head of the pancreas and the duodenum are sent to the superior and inferior pancreaticoduodenal nodes.

The anterosuperior surface of the head of the pancreas drains by the gastroduodenal route from the anterior pancreaticoduodenal nodes. The lymphatics arising from the posterior surface of the head drain in the posterior pancreaticoduodenal nodes and terminate in the posterior periportal node. The dorsal pancreatic route less commonly collects lymphatic from the medial side of the cephalic portion of the pancreas to the celiac or superior mesenteric artery node [17].

The lymphatics for the body and caudal part of the pancreas follow the dorsal pancreatic artery and reach the nodes situated to the left of the celiac trunk origin and the superior mesenteric artery.

3.3.1.4 Duodenum

Lymphatic vessels of the duodenum drain into the pancreaticoduodenal nodes which are situated between the head of the pancreas and the duodenum. The efferents of these glands drain into the hepatic and the periaortic nodes, around the root of the superior mesenteric artery.

3.3.1.5 Small Intestine and Appendix

The lymphatic vessels of the jejunum and the ileum run within the mesentery and enter the superior mesenteric nodes which drain into the para-aortic nodes (Fig. 3.3b). Likewise, lymphatic drainage of the appendix ends in the superior mesenteric and para-aortic group.

3.3.1.6 Large Intestine

The lymphatic drainage for the cecum, ascending, and transverse colon is via the *epicolic* and *paracolic* nodes, accompanying the marginal vessels. The paracolic nodes drain into the superior mesenteric nodes, at the root of the superior mesenteric artery. The inferior mesenteric lymph nodes drain the epicolic and paracolic group of the left side of the colon and the upper part of the rectum. The lymphatics from the lower rectum transverse the pararectal nodes and pass either toward the mesorectum and mesocolon or, laterally, toward the hypogastric and obturator nodes. These lymph nodes eventually drain into the para-aortic nodes. The lymphatics for the anus drain into the superficial inguinal nodes and then into the deep inguinal nodes. These nodes drain into the external iliac and para-aortic glands [18].

3.3.1.7 Retroperitoneal Lymph Nodes

Three renal lymphatic plexuses drain into the upper para-aortic lymph nodes, cisterna chyli, and mainly the left supraclavicular nodes via the thoracic duct. The lymphatic vessels from the upper portion of the ureter end in the para-aortic nodes. The middle uretral lymphatic drainage is to the common iliac glands, while the intrapelvic portion of the urethra drains into the common and internal iliac nodes. The iliac nodes end in the para-aortic lymph nodes, cisterna chyli, and via the thoracic duct into the left supraclavicular nodes. The lymphatic drainage of the adrenals usually accompanies the suprarenal veins and end in the para-aortic nodes.

3.3.1.8 Bladder

The lymphatic drainage is derived from two plexus, one draining the anterior and another from the posterior surface of the bladder. The former passes into the external iliac nodes and the lymphatic vessels from the posterior surface drain into the common iliac nodes (Fig. 3.3c).

3.3.1.9 Prostate

The lymphatic drainage is from the internal iliac and sacral glands. There is also lymphatic drainage to the external iliac and the para-aortic lymph nodes.

3.3.1.10 Uterus and Ovary

The lymph of the cervix drains to the external iliac, the internal iliac nodes, and the common iliac glands. The lymphatic drainage of the body and fundus of the uterus is via the lateral and para-aortic nodes.

Lymphatics draining the ovary run upward to the lateral and para-aortic nodes.

References

1. Som PM, Curtin HD, Mancuso AA (2000) Imaging-based nodal classification for evaluation of neck metastatic adenopathy. AJR Am J Roentgenol 174:837–844
2. Som PM, Curtin HD, Mancuso AA (1999) An imaging-based classification for the cervical nodes designed as an adjunct to recent clinically based nodal classifications. Arch Otolaryngol Head Neck Surg 125:388–396
3. Robbins KT, Shaha AR, Medina JE et al (2008) Consensus statement on the classification and terminology of neck dissection. Arch Otolaryngol Head Neck Surg 134:536–538
4. Rouvière H (1938) Lymphatic system of the head and neck. Edwards Brothers, Ann Arbor
5. Shah JP, Strong E, Spiro RH et al (1981) Surgical grand rounds. Neck dissection: current status and future possibilities. Clin Bull 11:25–33
6. Lee YY, Van Tassel P, Nauert C et al (1987) Lymphomas of the head and neck: CT findings at initial presentation. AJR Am J Roentgenol 149:575–581
7. Weber AL, Rahemtullah A, Ferry JA (2003) Hodgkin and non-Hodgkin lymphoma of the head and neck: clinical, pathologic, and imaging evaluation. Neuroimaging Clin N Am 13:371–392
8. Glaser GM, Gross BH, Quint LE et al (1985) Normal mediastinal lymph nodes: Number and size according to American Thoracic Society mapping. AJR: Leesburg, USA. Am J Roentgenol 144:261–265
9. Johnson SA, Kumar A, Matasar MJ et al (2015) Imaging for staging and response assessment in lymphoma. Radiology 2:323–338
10. Castellino RA, Blank N, Hoppe RT et al (1986) Hodgkin disease: contribution of chest CT in the initial staging evaluation. Radiology 160:603–605
11. Castellino RA (1991) The non-Hodgkin lymphomas: practical concepts for the radiologist. Radiology 178:315–321
12. Harisinghani MG (2013) Atlas of lymph node anatomy. Springer, New York, pp 31–57
13. Suwatanapongched T, Gierada DS (2006) CT of thoracic lymph nodes. Part I: anatomy and drainage. Br J Radiol 79:922–928
14. Kambadakone AR, Sahani DV (2011) Lymph node imaging techniques. In: Sahani DV, Samir AE (eds) Abdominal imaging, vol 1, set; Expert radiology, chapter 92, Saunders, Elsevier, pp 1001–1016
15. Wolf GL, Gazelle GS, McIntire GL et al (1994) Percutaneous computed tomography lymphography in the rabbit by subcutaneously injected nanoparticulates. Acad Radiol 1:352–357
16. Trutmann M, Sasse D (1994) The lymphatics of the liver. Anat Embryol (Berl) 190:201–209
17. O'Morchoe C (1997) Lymphatic system of the pancreas. Microsc Res Tech 37:456–477
18. Topor B, Acland R, Kolodko V, Galandiuk S (2003) Mesorectal lymph nodes: their location and distribution within the mesorectum. Dis Colon Rectum 46:779–785

4 An Overview of the Clinical Evaluation of Lymphomas According to the WHO 2008 Classification

Theodoros P. Vassilakopoulos
and Effimia P. Vrakidou

4.1 Introduction

Malignant lymphomas are neoplasms of the lymphoid tissue, which are divided into Hodgkin (HL) and non-Hodgkin lymphomas (NHL). They are classified according to the 2008 World Health Organization (WHO) scheme [1], using clinical, morphologic, immunophenotypic, and genetic features to define distinct entities (Table 4.1).

Among all lymphomas, 85–90 % are of B-cell and 10–15 % are of T- or NK-cell origin [1]. Diffuse large B-cell lymphoma (DLBCL) and related disorders including primary mediastinal large B-cell lymphoma (PMLBCL) constitute the most common subtype of B-NHL (40–45 % of total), followed by follicular lymphomas (~30 %), extranodal marginal zone (MALT) lymphomas (9 %), mantle cell lymphoma (7 %), and small lymphocytic lymphoma (12 %, including also cases of chronic lymphocytic leukemia) [1, 2]. Each one of the other subtypes account for 2 % or less of the total cases [1, 2]. The most common subtypes of T-cell lymphomas are peripheral T-cell lymphomas not otherwise specified (NOS), angioimmunoblastic and anaplastic large cell lymphoma [1, 2]. Finally, HL accounts for approximately 10 % of all malignant lymphomas [3] and can be divided into two major types: Classical HL (95 % of all cases) and the nodular lymphocyte predominant subtype, which is much less common and more indolent disease than the classical form.

Extranodal involvement is more common in NHL than in HL; it can be either part of disseminated disease or a primary localization. However, in sharp contrast to the exceedingly rare primary extranodal HL, 20–30 % of NHLs are primarily localized to extranodal sites. Any anatomic site can be involved, but the most common ones included the gastrointestinal tract, skin, and central nervous system [4].

4.2 Clinical Evaluation

The clinical evaluation of patients with malignant lymphomas should establish the precise histologic subtype, the sites, and the extent of the disease and patient's performance status (PS). After the initial histologic diagnosis, a complete medical history should be taken to assess the presence or absence of systemic "B" symptoms (fever, night sweats, weight loss), pruritus, other disease-related symptoms, and the presence of previous or concomitant illnesses.

Aggressive and highly aggressive lymphomas, such as DLBCL, Burkitt lymphoma, most

T.P. Vassilakopoulos (✉)
University of Athens Hematology Clinic, G.N.A. "POP", St. Thomas 17, Athens 11527, Greece
e-mail: theopvass@hotmail.com

E.P. Vrakidou
Hygeia Hospital,
4 Erythrou Stavrou Street and Kifisias Avenue, Athens 15123, Greece
email: e.vrakidou@gmail.com

J.A. Andreou et al. (eds.), *PET/CT in Lymphomas: A Case-Based Atlas*,
DOI 10.1007/978-3-319-27380-8_4

Table 4.1 The 2008 World Health Organization (WHO) classification of lymphoid neoplasms

Hodgkin lymphoma
Nodular lymphocyte predominant Hodgkin lymphoma
Classical Hodgkin lymphoma
Subtypes: nodular sclerosis, lymphocyte rich, mixed cellularity, lymphocyte depleted
Mature B-cell neoplasms
Chronic lymphocytic leukemia/small lymphocytic lymphoma
B-cell prolymphocytic leukemia
Lymphoplasmacytic lymphoma/Waldenstrom's macroglobulinemia
Heavy chain diseases
Hairy cell leukemia
Splenic B-cell lymphoma/leukemia, unclassifiable
Including: splenic diffuse red pulp small B-cell lymphoma, hairy cell leukemia variant
Splenic marginal zone lymphoma
Extranodal marginal zone lymphoma (MALT)
Nodal marginal zone lymphoma
Follicular lymphoma
Follicle center cell lymphoma, primary cutaneous
Mantle cell lymphoma
Diffuse large B-cell lymphoma, NOS (not otherwise specified)
T-cell/histiocyte-rich large B-cell lymphoma
Primary DLBCL of the CNS
Primary cutaneous DLBCL, leg type
EBV-positive DLBCL of the elderly
Primary mediastinal (thymic) large B-cell lymphoma
Intravascular large B-cell lymphoma
DLBCL associated with chronic inflammation
Lymphomatoid granulomatosis
Large B-cell lymphoma arising in HHV8-associated multicentric Castleman disease
ALK-positive large B-cell lymphoma
Plasmablastic lymphoma
Primary effusion lymphoma
Burkitt lymphoma
B-cell lymphoma, unclassifiable, with features intermediate between diffuse large B-cell lymphoma and Burkitt lymphoma
B-cell lymphoma, unclassifiable, with features intermediate between diffuse large B-cell lymphoma and classical Hodgkin lymphoma
Monoclonal gammopathy of unknown significance (MGUS)
Plasma cell myeloma
Solitary plasmacytoma of bone
Extraosseous plasmacytoma
Monoclonal immunoglobulin deposition diseases
Primary amyloidosis, monoclonal light and heavy chain deposition disease, osteosclerotic myeloma (POEMS syndrome)
Mature T- and NK-cell neoplasms
T-cell prolymphocytic leukemia
T-cell large granular lymphocytic leukemia
Chronic lymphoproliferative disorders of NK cells
Aggressive NK-cell lymphoma
Adult T-cell leukemia/lymphoma
Extranodal NK-/T-cell lymphoma, nasal type
Enteropathy-associated T-cell lymphoma
Hepatosplenic T-cell lymphoma
Subcutaneous panniculitis-like T-cell lymphoma
Mycosis fungoides
Sezary syndrome
Primary cutaneous CD30-positive T-cell lymphoproliferative disorders
Primary cutaneous anaplastic large cell lymphoma
Lymphomatoid papulosis
Primary cutaneous γδ T-cell lymphoma
Primary cutaneous CD8-positive, aggressive, epidermotropic, cytotoxic T-cell lymphoma
Primary cutaneous CD4-positive, small/medium T-cell lymphoma
Peripheral T-cell lymphoma, NOS (not otherwise specified)
Angioimmunoblastic T-cell lymphoma
Anaplastic large cell lymphoma, ALK positive
Anaplastic large lymphoma, ALK negative
Systemic EBV-positive T-cell lymphoproliferative disease of childhood
Hydroa vacciniforme-like lymphoma
Precursor lymphoid neoplasms
B-cell lymphoblastic leukemia/lymphoma (either NOS or 7 subtypes with recurrent cytogenetic abnormalities)
T-cell lymphoblastic leukemia/lymphoma

mature T-cell lymphomas, and precursor B- and T-cell lymphoblastic lymphoma typically present with rapidly growing masses and/or systemic B symptoms. Indolent lymphomas, mostly including follicular lymphomas, small lymphocytic lymphoma/chronic lymphocytic leukemia (SLL/CLL), and marginal zone lymphomas, most frequently present with lymphadenopathy, organomegaly, or, less frequently, cytopenias, while B symptoms are rare. However, the clinical presentation may be highly diverse among patients even within the same histologic subtype, depending on disease aggressiveness and the individual, specific anatomic sites of involvement.

Emergency conditions are rather rare at the time of diagnosis of malignant lymphomas. However, events such as the superior vena cava syndrome, pericardial tamponade, acute airway obstruction, intestinal obstruction or perforation, lymphomatous meningitis, hyperviscosity syndrome, severe autoimmune hemolytic anemia, and/or thrombocytopenia, etc., should be promptly recognized and appropriately treated.

4.3 Laboratory Evaluation

Initial laboratory evaluation should include complete blood count and leukocyte differential and complete serum biochemical profile including the assessment of renal and liver function and lactate dehydrogenase (LDH) levels. Peripheral blood smear examination is essential in order to recognize the presence of atypical lymphomatous cells, a finding that is much more frequent in indolent than in aggressive lymphomas and absent in HL. Peripheral blood involvement may not be frankly leukemic, being limited only to a small percentage of circulating lymphocytes. Blood immunophenotype by flow cytometry may uncover low-level leukemic involvement by flow cytometry and can be a very helpful method for the accurate classification of the disease.

Other important laboratory tests to be performed at baseline include serology for HIV, Hepatitis B and C [5, 6], and serum immunoglobulin determination and immunofixation. Paraproteins are frequent in lymphoplasmacytic lymphoma/Waldenstrom's macroglobulinemia as well as in marginal zone lymphomas and hypogammaglobulinemia is of concern in SLL/CLL, but immunoglobulin disorders may be present in any lymphoma subtype.

4.4 Staging

4.4.1 Conventional Staging

In contrast to solid tumors, which are generally staged based on TNM classification schemes, lymphoma staging is based on the Lugano classification [7], which represents a modification of the Ann Arbor staging system that was initially developed mainly for HL [8].

Except for history and physical examination, lymphoma staging generally requires chest X-rays; cervical, chest, abdominal, and pelvic CT imaging; and bone marrow aspiration and biopsy (see below for specific entities). Other conventional imaging studies (MRI, ultrasound, bone scanning) are only used in specific clinical circumstances in order to clarify medical questions. Gastrointestinal endoscopy and lumbar puncture are also used in specific clinical settings (see below).

Integrated position emission tomography with computed tomography (PET/CT) is now increasingly used for baseline staging of malignant lymphomas. Current guidelines recommend its use for staging and posttreatment response assessment of all FDG-avid lymphomas [7, 9]. Further details are provided in a subsequent paragraph and throughout this atlas.

Bone marrow aspiration and biopsy used to be part of the initial staging for all patients with malignant lymphomas [8, 10, 11]. However, recent data suggest that it can be spared in all patients with HL if baseline staging is based on PET/CT [7, 9], because few patients have bone marrow involvement by biopsy, which is not detectable by PET/CT; even in these few cases, treatment is not influenced by bone marrow biopsy. A detailed discussion on the issue of the omission of bone marrow biopsy in HL and aggressive B-cell lymphomas is provided in Chaps. 6 and 7.

Lumbar puncture should undergo in all patients with aggressive lymphomas like Burkitt, lymphoblastic, double HIT lymphomas, in patients with testicular paranasal sinus, epidural or bone marrow involvement [10–12]. These patients are at risk of central nervous system (CNS) involvement. The cerebrospinal fluid (CSF) by lumbar puncture should be exam with cytology and flow cytometry [13].

Except for staging procedures, cardiac assessment and ultrasonography should be performed prior to treatment. Lung function tests are also necessary in specific treatment settings, where pulmonary toxicity is likely to arise. Finally, fertility issues should be discussed and appropriate actions be taken prior to treatment initiation [14].

4.4.2 PET/CT Staging

As already mentioned, PET/CT is recommended for staging and posttreatment response assessment of HL (which is routinely FDG-avid) and all FDG-avid NHL [7, 9, 15]. All histologic subtypes of nodal NHL (including primary extranodal DLBCLs) are considered FDG-avid except for some indolent ones, namely, chronic lymphocytic leukemia/lymphoma, lymphoplasmacytic lymphoma/Waldenstrom's macroglovbulinemia, marginal zone lymphomas, and mycosis fungoides (unless transformation is suspected) [7]. CT remains the preferred imaging method for all these non-FDG-avid lymphoma subtypes. Set of criteria, which are applicable in baseline staging and response assessment in malignant lymphomas, are provided as an Appendix at the end of this atlas. The Deauville 5-point scale (D5-PS) is now the method of choice for the interpretation and reporting of posttreatment PET/CT. D5-PS is briefly described in Chap. 6, Table 6.1, and further details are provided in the Appendix.

During the last decade, increasing data suggest that early interim evaluation, usually after two cycles of chemotherapy, is a strong predictor of the final outcome [16–23]. This is mainly applicable in HL and aggressive B-cell lymphomas, as analyzed in Chaps. 6 and 7. However, interim PET evaluation is not still recommended for use in clinical practice in order to guide early treatment modifications outside clinical trials, because there is no proven benefit of this strategy derived from randomized trials for the time being. However, despite recent recommendations, interim response assessment is already used in everyday practice by many physicians and may become standard practice soon. The D5-PS is now the method of choice for the interpretation and reporting of interim PET as well (mainly in HL), although a semiquantitative assessment based on SUVmax alterations is used in DLBCL. Thus, the optimal criteria are still under evaluation.

FDG-PET/CT before auto-SCT has prognostic value for patients with relapsed/refractory Hodgkin's disease (HD) and diffuse large B-cell lymphoma (DLBCL). There are data indicate that pre-transplant positive (+) PET/CT is significantly associated with inferior OS and may predict shortened PFS in patients undergoing SCT. [24–27]. In contrast, the use of PET/CT for disease surveillance after a PET-confirmed complete remission is discouraged because of the high rate of false-positive results.

Concluding FDG-PET/CT using FDG has been successfully used for staging, treatment planning, response evaluation and follow up examination, in patients with aggressive non-Hodgkin's lymphoma (NHL) and Hodgkin's lymphoma (HD). An early interim FDG-PET/CT scan after one or two cycles of chemotherapy is a very strong predictor of outcome in these patients for further treatment planning of combined chemotherapy or radiotherapy. The use of PET/CT in other lymphoma subtypes, the FDG-avid ones, is rapidly increasing but deserves further evaluation with the accumulation of more clinical experience.

References

1. Swerdlow SH, Campo E (2008) WHO classification: pathology and genetics of tumors of haematopoietic and lymphoid tissues. IARC Press, Lyon
2. Hartge P, Wang SS, Bracci PM, Devesa SS, Holly EA (2006) Non-Hodgkin lymphoma. In: Schottenfeld D, Fraumeni JFJ (eds) Cancer epidemiology and prevention, 3rd edn. Oxford University Press, New York, pp 898–918
3. Jemal A, Siegel R, Ward E et al (2009) Cancer statistics, 2009. CA Cancer J Clin 59:225
4. Chiu BC, Weisenburger DD (2003) An update of the epidemiology of non-Hodgkin's lymphoma. Clin Lymphoma 4(3):161–168

5. D'Addario G, Dieterle A, Torhorst J et al (2003) HIV-testing and newly-diagnosed malignant lymphomas. The SAKK 96/90 registration study. Leuk Lymphoma 44:133
6. National Comprehensive Cancer Network (NCCN) (2014) NCCN Clinical practice guidelines in oncology. http://www.nccn.org/professionals/physician_gls/f_guidelines.asp. Accessed 01 April 2014
7. Cheson BD, Fisher RI, Barrington SF et al (2014) Recommendations for initial evaluation, staging, and response assessment of Hodgkin and non-Hodgkin lymphoma: the Lugano classification. J Clin Oncol 32:3059–3067
8. Carbone PP, Kaplan HS, Musshoff K, Smithers DW, Tubiana M (1971) Report of the Committee on Hodgkin's disease staging classification. Cancer Res 31:1860–1861
9. Barrington SF, Mikhaeel NG, Kostakoglu L et al (2014) Role of imaging in the staging and response assessment of lymphoma: consensus of the International Conference on Malignant Lymphomas Imaging Working Group. J Clin Oncol 32:3048
10. Conlan MG, Bast M, Armitage JO, Weisenburger DD (1990) Bone marrow involvement by non-Hodgkin's lymphoma: the clinical significance of morphologic discordance between the lymph node and bone marrow. Nebraska Lymphoma Study Group. J Clin Oncol 8:1163
11. Foucar K, McKenna RW, Frizzera G, Brunning RD (1982) Bone marrow and blood involvement by lymphoma in relationship to the Lueks-Collins classification. Cancer 49:888
12. Savage KJ, Zeynalova S, Kansara RR et al (2014) Validation of a prognostic model to assess the risk of CNS disease in patients with aggressive B-cell lymphoma. Blood (ASH Annual Meeting Abstracts) 124:394
13. Hedge U, Filie A, Little RF et al (2005) High incidence of occult leptomeningeal disease detected by flow cytometry in newly diagnosed aggressive B-cell lymphomas at risk for central nervous system involvement: the role of flow cytometry versus cytology. Blood 105:496
14. Aw L, Mangu PB, Beck LN et al (2013) Fertility preservation for patients with cancer. American Society of Clinical Oncology clinical practice guideline update. J Clin Oncol 31:2500
15. Juweid ME, Stroobants S, Hoekstra OS et al (2007) Use of positron emission tomography for response assessment of lymphoma: consensus of the Imaging Subcommittee of International Harmonization Project in Lymphoma. J Clin Oncol 25:571
16. Gallamini A, Hutchings M, Rigacci L et al (2007) Early interim 2-[18F]fluoro-2-deoxy-D-glucose positron emission tomography is prognostically superior to international prognostic score in advanced-stage Hodgkin's lymphoma: a report from a joint Italian-Danish study. J Clin Oncol 25:3746–3752
17. Gallamini A, Barrington SF, Biggi A, Chauvie S, Kostakoglou L, Gregianin M et al (2014) The predictive role of interim positron emission tomography for Hodgkin lymphoma treatment outcome is confirmed using the interpretation criteria of the Deauville five-point scale. Haematologica 99:1107–1113
18. Oki Y, Chuang H, Chasen B, Jessop A, Pan T, Fanale M et al (2014) The prognostic value of interim positron emission tomography scan in patients with classical Hodgkin lymphoma. Br J Haematol 165:112–116
19. Kostakoglu L, Coleman M, Leonard JP, Kuji I, Zoe H, Goldsmith SJ (2002) PET predicts prognosis after 1 cycle of chemotherapy in aggressive lymphoma and Hodgkin's disease. J Nucl Med 43:1018–1027
20. Spaepen K, Stroobants S, Dupont P, Vandenberghe P, Thomas J, de Groot T et al (2002) Early restaging positron emission tomography with (18) F-fluorodeoxyglucose predicts outcome in patients with aggressive non-Hodgkin's lymphoma. Ann Oncol 13(9):1356–1363
21. Horning SJ, Juweid ME, Schoeder H et al (2010) Interim positron emission tomography scans in diffuse large B-cell lymphoma: an independent expert nuclear medicine evaluation of the Eastern Cooperative Oncology Group E3404 study. Blood 115:775–777
22. Casasnovas RO, Meignan M, Berriolo-Riedinger A et al (2011) SUVmax reduction improves early prognosis value of interim positron emission tomography scans in diffuse large B-cell lymphoma. Blood 118:37–43
23. Itti E, Meignan M, Berriolo-Riedinger A, Biggi A, Cashen AF, Verra P et al (2013) An international confirmatory study of the prognostic value of early PET/CT in diffuse large B-cell lymphoma: comparison between Deauville criteria and ΔSUVmax. Eur J Nucl Med Mol Imaging 40:1312–1320
24. Moskowitz C, Matasar MJ, Zelenetz AD et al (2012) Normalization of pre-ASCT, FDG-PET imaging with second-line, non-cross-resistant, chemotherapy programs improves event-free survival in patients with Hodgkin lymphoma. Blood 119(7):1665–1670
25. Schot B, van Imhoff G, Pruim J et al (2003) Predictive value of early 18F-fluoro-deoxyglucose positron emission tomography in chemosensitive relapsed lymphoma. Br J Haematol 123:282
26. Sauter CS, Matasar MJ, Meikle J et al (2015) Prognostic value of FDG-PET prior to autologous stem cell transplantation for relapsed and refractory diffuse large B-cell lymphoma. Blood 125(16): 2579–2581
27. Derenzini E, Musuraca G, Fanti S et al (2008) Pretransplantation positron emission tomography scan is the main predictor of autologous stem cell transplantation outcome in aggressive B-cell non-Hodgkin lymphoma. Cancer 113:2496

The Role of PET/CT in Radiotherapy Planning of Lymphoma

5

Kostantinos E. Dardoufas, Ioannis E. Datseris, Chryssa J. Paraskevopoulou, and Christos V. Skarleas

5.1 Introduction

The aim of radiation therapy (RT) is to deliver the maximum dose to the tumor while sparing the surrounding healthy tissues.

RT has a dominant role in cancer treatment and has always been a major part of the effort to cure patients with any pathology lymphoma disease.

The role of RT in lymphomas has changed through time from single modality treatment to adjuvant treatment following chemotherapy. Recent studies have shown that RT improves the overall survival rate for patients of all stages, in adults, or pediatric cases significantly [1–3].

K.E. Dardoufas, MD (✉)
Center of Radiation Oncology,
Hygeia Hospital, 4 Erythrou Stavrou St &
Kifissias Ave, Athens 15123, Greece
e-mail: kdardoufas@hygeia.gr

C.J. Paraskevopoulou, MSc
Department of Medical Physics, Hygeia Hospital,
4 Erythrou Stavrou St & Kifissias Ave,
Athens 15123, Greece
e-mail: c.paraskevopoulou@hygeia.gr

I.E. Datseris, MD
Department of Nuclear Medicine,
Evangelismos Hospital, Athens, Greece
e-mail: datseris@otenet.gr

C.V. Skarleas, MD
Center of Radiation Therapy, Hygeia Hospital,
Athens, Greece
e-mail: cskarleas@hygeia.gr

In this chapter, a case of Hodgkin lymphoma treated with RT as an adjuvant treatment will be presented. Hodgkin lymphoma (HL) is a malignancy that involves both lymph nodes and the lymphatic system. Most patients are diagnosed between the age of 15 and 30 and at the age of 55 or older [4].

PET/CT imaging using the tracer fluoride-6-deoxy-glucose labeled with ^{18}F (^{18}FDG) has become an important tool for staging, prognosis, and treatment evaluation outcome in patients with lymphomas. It provides metabolic mapping of affected nodes and tissue lesions in combination with anatomical information. It is significantly more accurate than conventional imaging modalities. PET/CT can reveal the disease in sites where there is inadequate contrast between lymphoma and healthy tissue or scar on CT only, such as mediastinum, spleen, etc. [5].

Involved site radiation therapy (ISRT) is recommended for targeting the originally involved lymph nodes as well as tissues suspicious for microscopic disease prior to chemotherapy or surgery. Advanced RT techniques should be used in order to deliver the desirable dose to the tumor while minimizing the dose to normal tissue. Dose sparing for organs at risk such as heart, lung, esophagus, and spinal cord reflects best clinical practice [4].

J.A. Andreou et al. (eds.), *PET/CT in Lymphomas: A Case-Based Atlas*,
DOI 10.1007/978-3-319-27380-8_5

5.2 Treatment Planning

The first and most important step of treatment planning procedure is to determine the target to be treated accurately. In order to define the extent of affected tissue, the best imaging modality is chosen according to tumor type.

The target volume includes the gross tumor volume (GTV) and the possible region of microscopic disease called clinical target volume (CTV). The planning target volume (PTV) is defined according to ICRU 62 report and includes GTV, CTV and takes into account internal organ motion and set up errors [6].

CT is the modality of choice suitable to be used for radiation therapy treatment planning because it provides information about tissue density that is used for accurate dose calculation.

PET/CT combines biological and anatomical information and is the basic tool for accurate target determination and definition of the metabolic target volume (MTV). MTV is not defined by anatomical boundaries but from actual metabolic information, reflecting the increased uptake and trapping of ^{18}FDG within the affected lymphatic cells. Thus, PET/CT became an integral part of radiation therapy treatment planning procedure [7]. Target delineation based on hypermetabolic tumor can be substantially different from target delineation if CT only is used. In 35–60 % of cases, target volume is reduced using PET/CT [8, 9].

The standard treatment RT technique is three-dimensional conformal planning (3DCRT) uses static fields of uniform intensity conformed to the planning target volume, delivering a dose, as low as possible, to the surrounding healthy tissues. Recent advances in technology have resulted in more sophisticated planning techniques. Intensity-modulated radiation therapy (IMRT) optimizes the radiation intensity distribution within each beam in order to achieve optimum conformity to irregularly shaped tumors. Volumetric modulated arc therapy (VMAT) is a novel form of IMRT delivery in single or multiple arcs. This type of treatment is dynamic and time efficient.

As the plan dose distribution conforms highly to the target delineated on the planning reference CT, the precision of dose delivery becomes limited by assuming that the planning CT represents each patient's anatomy on the treatment table throughout an extended course of treatment [10, 11]. Organs may change position, size, and shape during treatment due to normal anatomical changes as well as tumor response to RT. In order to accurately deliver IMRT/VMAT treatments, the patient must be positioned in the same way every day. Image-guided radiotherapy (IGRT) is the use of patient imaging on the treatment table to ensure accurate dose delivery to the target, and it helps monitoring all treatment-relevant time-dependent factors throughout the complete treatment course. IGRT is used for fast correction of patient positioning in everyday fraction but also for monitoring tumor response during radiotherapy course. This information is used to improve patient's therapy [11].

Cone beam CT (CBCT), a CT scan of the patient, is obtained on the treatment couch immediately before radiation delivery. The CT scan is co-registered automatically with the planning reference CT to facilitate precise positioning of the patient. Furthermore, CBCT allows monitoring of tumor changes during treatment caused by tumor shrinkage, changes in tumor biology (hypoxia), or patient weight loss. As a result, the initial target delineation and treatment plan could not match the delivered treatment. These are the major factors for target missing and/or over-treating normal tissues. Adaptive radiotherapy is defined as changing the treatment plan delivered to the patient during a course of radiotherapy to account for the above anatomical changes and ensures minimum normal tissue irradiation [12].

In order to account for breathing-induced organ motion during treatment, 4D radiation therapy technique is used. Several systems of motion control have been developed like gating or tracking, i.e., the radiation beam is turned on only during a specified phase of the respiratory cycle [13].

Recent state-of-the-art radiation treatment machines support flattening filter-free (FFF) technology, delivering very high-dose rate treatments in a very short time further minimizing breathing-induced organ motion.

PET/CT can be used to define the residual post chemo disease. Involved site radiation area can be reduced compared to CT target delineation [5]. IMRT/VMAT delivery in combination with IGRT can assure accurate dose delivery to the target while protecting the surrounding healthy tissues. As a result, toxicity and treatment complications are minimized and the possibility of radiation-induced cancer to young patients is decreased.

Table 5.1 Comparison of dose delivered to PTV and organs at risk from 3D and VMAT treatment technique

Structure	Plan	Hot ref (Gy)	%Vol > Hot ref	Difference
PTV Phase I	3D	28.5	98.7	Same coverage
	VMAT	28.5	98.6	
PTV Phase II	3D	34.2	96.6	Same coverage
	VMAT	34.2	99.4	
Both lungs	3D	20	15.13	68 % less volume receiving 20 Gy
	VMAT	20	4.78	
Heart	3D	4.8	50	23 % less mean dose
	VMAT	3.7	50	
Esophagus	3D	28.2	1	14 % less max dose
	VMAT	24.2	1	
Spinal cord	3D	28.2	1	50 % less max dose
	VMAT	14.1	1	

5.3 Future Trends

PET/CT imaging promises to reveal tumor biology. Based on biological principles, tumors are not homogeneous. Tumor subregions may selectively contain an enriched population of cancer stem cells that may be responsible for recurrence and distant metastasis. These regions have different tumor metabolic activity estimated by standard uptake value (SUV) in PET/CT, an important prognostic factor. Studies have shown that high-SUV ($SUV > 13.8$) regions and hypoxic areas are more likely to have local recurrence after a standard dose of radiotherapy [14].

These developments, in combination with new treatment planning techniques that can deliver inhomogeneous dose distributions and thus selectively "paint" dose to subregions within the target, can further enhance radiotherapy success. Dose "painting" or delivery of higher doses to regions with high risk of tumor recurrence may further improve local control and potentially survival [4].

The implementation of new treatment planning techniques (IMRT/VMAT) had improved physical conformality in radiotherapy. The combination of these techniques with functional imaging can further improve the success of radiotherapy by launching a new era of biological conformality [3].

5.4 Case Presentation: Hodgkin Lymphoma Radiation Therapy

A 19-year-old male was referred for adjuvant RT following chemotherapy. Patient was initially diagnosed with nodular sclerosis Hodgkin lymphoma after biopsy. CT scan showed soft tissue mass on mediastinum with multiple infiltrated mediastinum and axillary nodes. In order to evaluate the disease response, PET/CT was performed post chemotherapy treatment showing hypermetabolic nodes of mediastinum – Deauville 4 (Fig. 5.1).

According to NCCN Guidelines, patient was prescribed 36 Gy with 1.8 Gy per fraction. RT scheme consisted of two phases. Phase I that included pre chemo initial disease irradiated to 30 Gy and Phase II that included the post chemo disease irradiated the rest 6 up to 36 Gy.

In order to delineate the involved site radiation area accurately, pre chemo CT was co-registered in the treatment planning system with post chemo CT and PET/CT. Use of PET/CT was critical to evaluate the residual disease (GTV – shown in red in Fig. 5.2) as well as to exclude the adjacent healthy organs. PTV Phase I included initial disease combined with post chemo findings thus sparing adjacent uninvolved organs. Large areas of normal lung and heart were excluded which if PET/CT had not been used, they would have been included in the radiation field. The combination of two examinations led to 37 % target reduction for Phase I and 30 % for Phase II. Figures 5.2 and 5.3 show the difference of the delineated targets with and without the use of PET/CT. In Fig. 5.2 PTV in blue represents the one defined from the combination of two modalities while PTV in purple represents the PTV if CT only was used for delineation. Large volume of lungs and heart are spared. In Fig. 5.3 Phase II PTV was defined from residual hypermetabolic area (green), while if CT only was used PTV would have been much bigger (magenta).

VMAT planning technique was used for both Phase I and Phase II of RT scheme. For each phase a conventional 3D plan was also created. Elekta's Monaco 5.1 treatment planning system was used for both plan types.

In Figs. 5.4 and 5.5, dose distribution for each phase and for each treatment planning technique is shown. Dose-volume histograms of both techniques are presented in Fig. 5.6. As shown in Table 5.1, 95 % of the prescribed dose covers more than 95 % of the PTV for both treatment techniques. The dose reduction to the organs at risk is substantial if VMAT irradiation is used. Volume of both lungs receiving 20 Gy (V_{20Gy}) is 68 % smaller than with the conventional 3D technique. Mean dose to heart is reduced by 23 %, while the maximum dose to spinal cord and esophagus is 50 and 14 % less, accordingly.

Prior to everyday treatment delivery, verification of patient positioning was performed with CBCT in order to carefully monitor the treated area and to avoid risk of tumor "geographic" miss.

Patient tolerated treatment without any acute toxicity or side effects.

PET/CT revolutionized RT treatment planning because it provides accurate and precise target delineation in order to spare surrounding healthy tissues. Advanced radiation therapy techniques such as VMAT have the advantages of tightly conformal doses and steep gradients next to normal tissues. IGRT provides daily monitoring of the irradiated area and ensures accurate treatment delivery. Modern radiation therapy reflects best clinical practice because it combines dose reduction to organs at risk without compromising target coverage, thus decreasing late side effects.

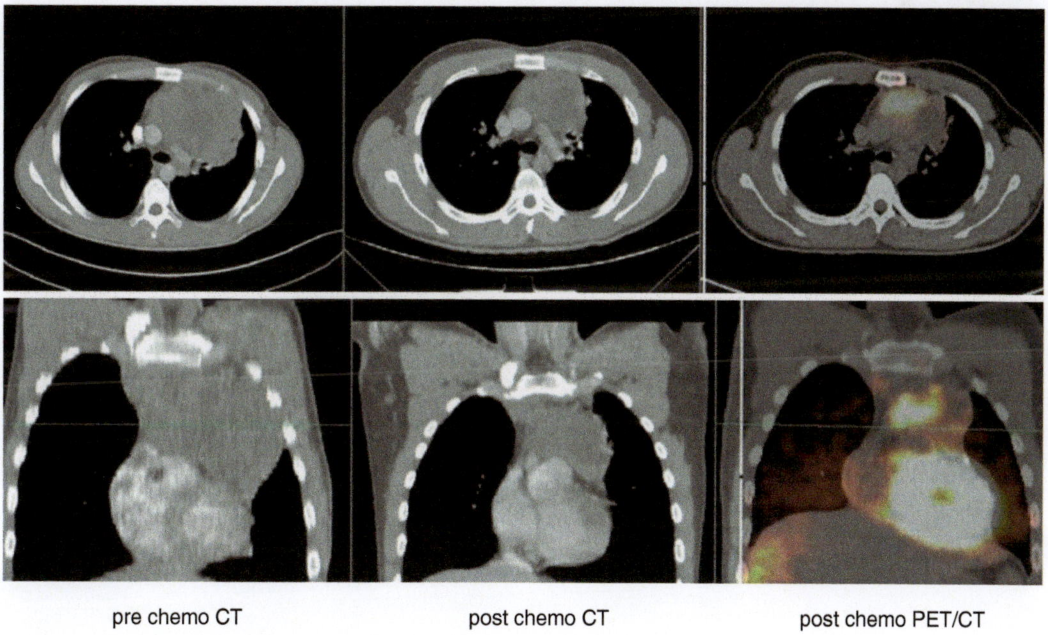

Fig. 5.1 Pre chemo CT, post chemo CT, and post chemo PET/CT results

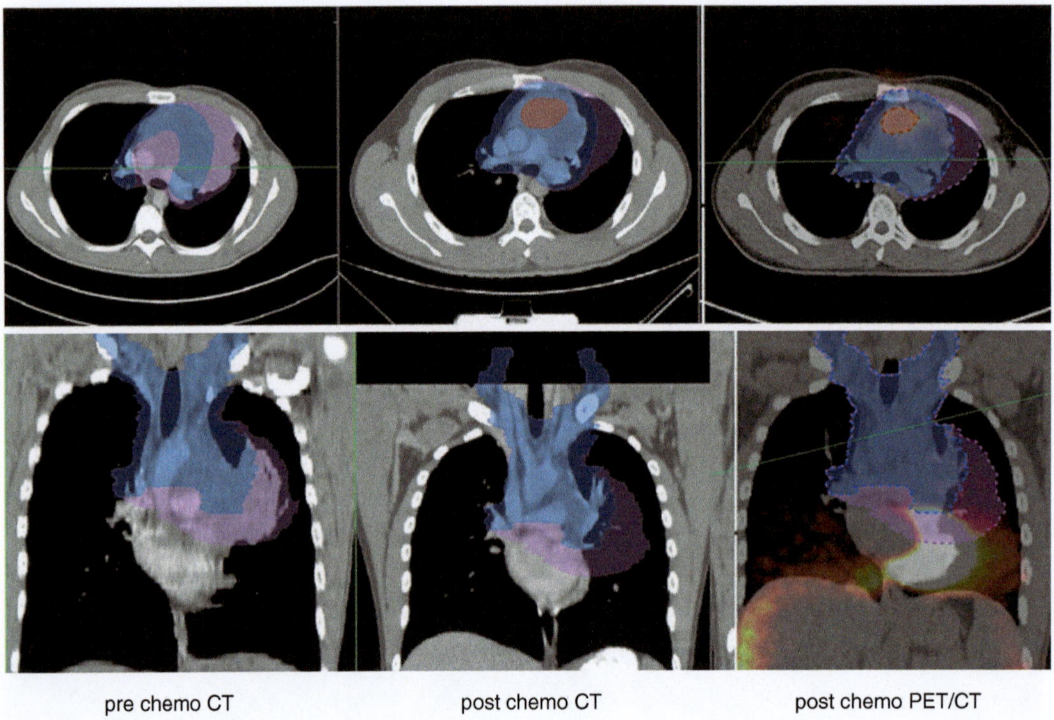

Fig. 5.2 PTV Phase I delineation using PET/CT findings

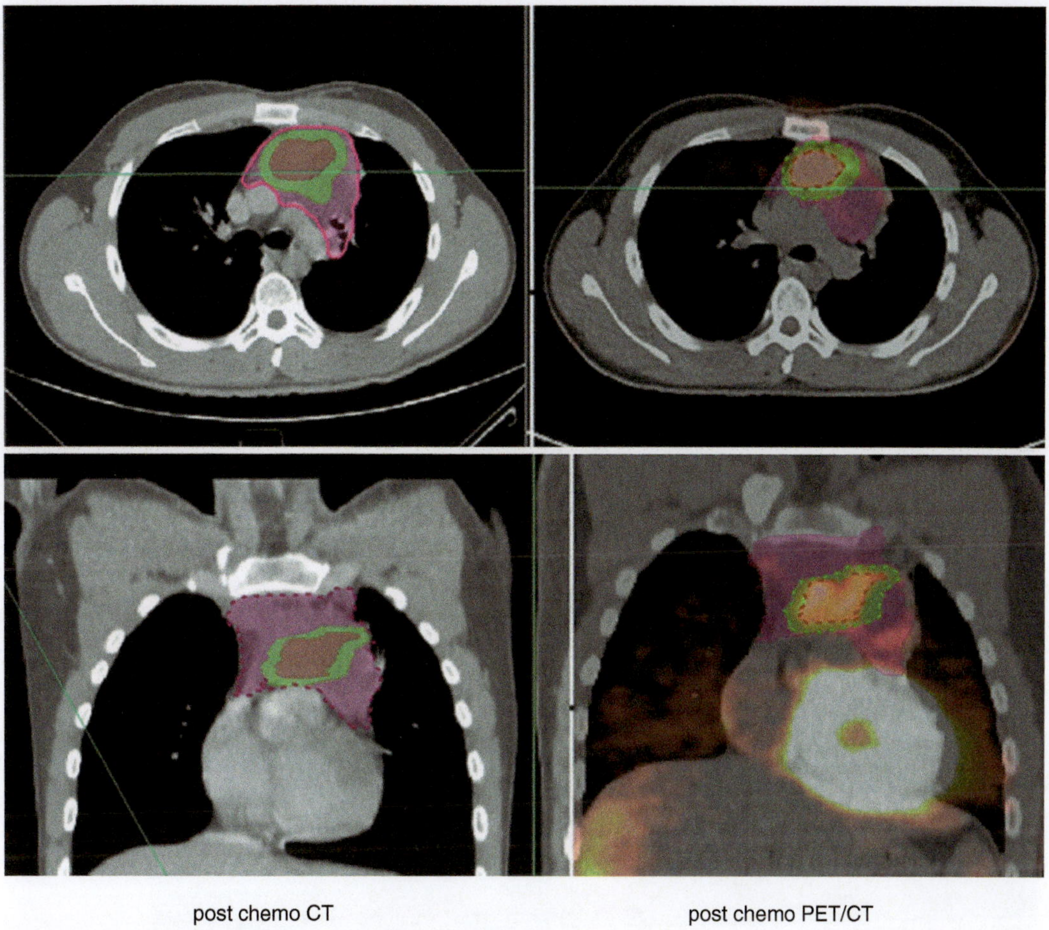

Fig. 5.3 PTV Phase II delineation using PET/CT findings

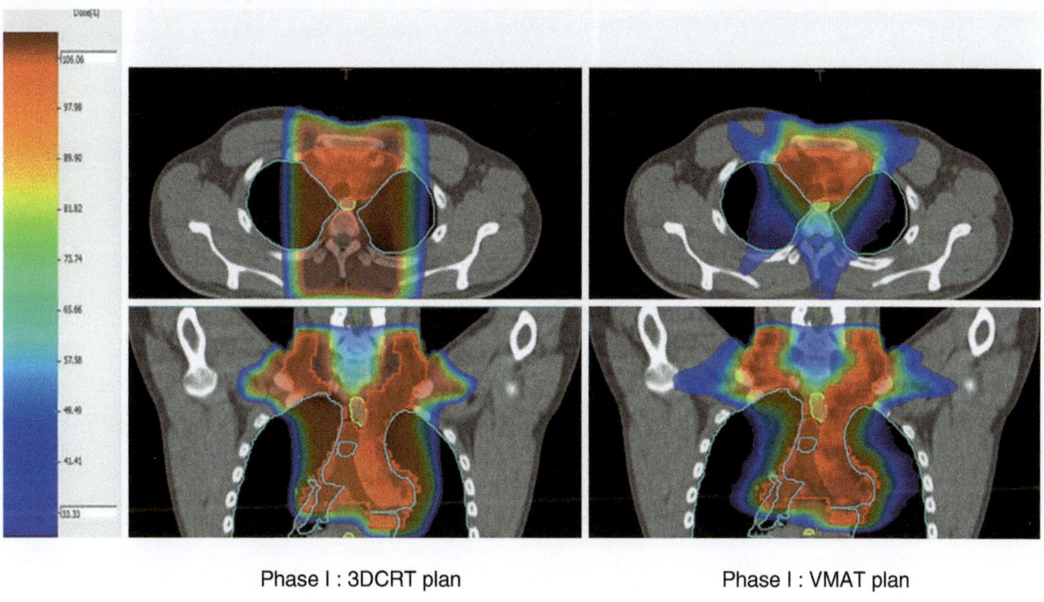

Fig. 5.4 Dose distribution with 3D and VMAT planning technique for Phase I

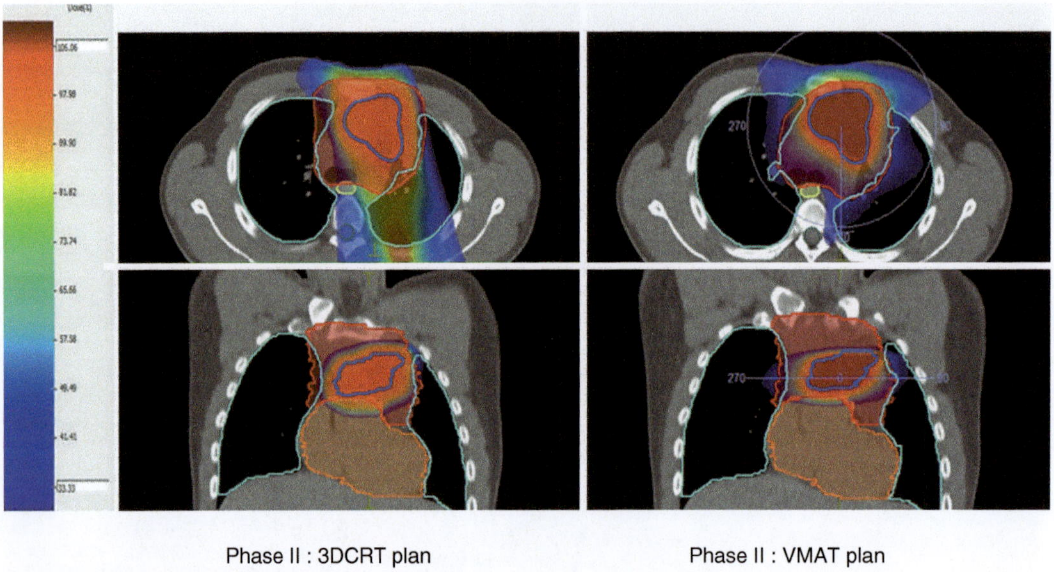

Fig. 5.5 Dose distribution with 3D and VMAT planning technique for Phase II

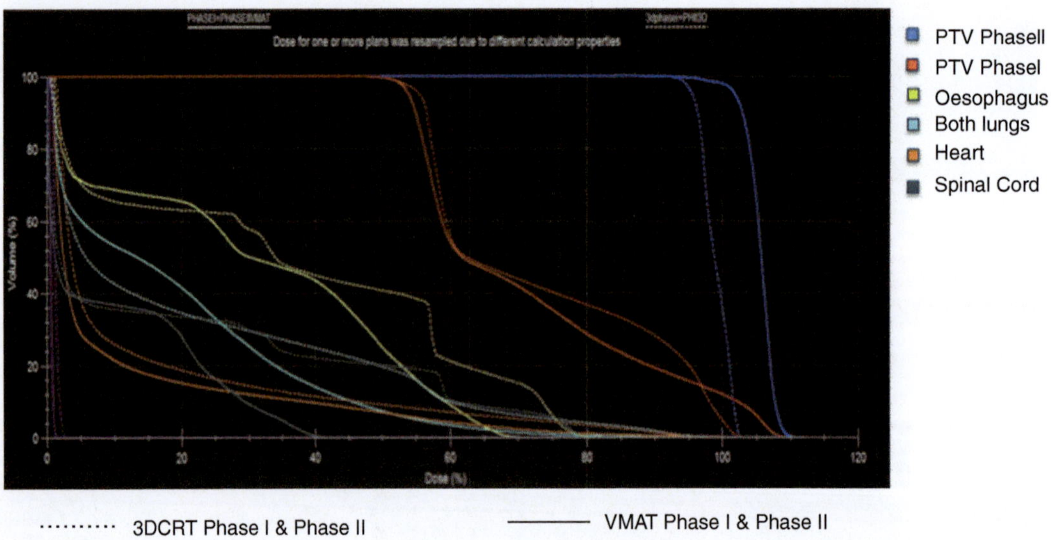

Fig. 5.6 Dose-volume histogram (DVH) comparison for 3D and VMAT planning technique

References

1. National Comprehensive Cancer Network (2015) NCCN clinical practice guidelines in oncology: Hodgkin Lymphoma Version 2
2. Meyer M, Gospodarowicz M, Connors J et al (2005) Randomized comparison of ABVD chemotherapy with a strategy that includes radiation therapy in patients with limited stage Hodgkin's lymphoma: National Cancer Institute of Canada Clinical Trial Group and the Easter Cooperative Oncology Group. J Clin Oncol 23:4634–4642
3. Diehl V, Brillant C, Engert A et al (2005) HD10: investigating reduction of combined modality treatment intensity in early stage Hodgkin's lymphoma. Interim analysis of a randomized trial of the German Hodgkin Study Group (GHSG) [abstract]. J Clin Oncol 23:Abstract 6506
4. Katsochi D, Sandilos P, Paraskevopoulou C (2014) Imaging in radiation therapy. Imag Clin Oncol. 27–41 Springer
5. Robertson VL, Anderson CS, Keller FG et al (2011) Role of FDG-PET in the definition of involved field radiation therapy and management of pediatric Hodgkin's lymphoma. Int J Radiat Oncol Biol Phys 80(2):324–332
6. ICRU: International Commission on Radiation Units and Measurements (1999) ICRU report 62: prescribing, recording, and reporting Photon Beam Therapy
7. IAEA International Atomic Energy Agency (2008) The role of PET/CT in radiation treatment planning for cancer patients. IAEA-TECDOC-1603
8. Grégoire V et al (2007) PET-based treatment planning in radiotherapy: a new standard? J Nucl Med 48(1):6 8S–77S
9. Hicks RJ et al (2001) (18)FDG-FDG PET provides high-impact and powerful prognostic stratification in staging newly diagnosed non-small cell lung cancer. J Nucl Med 42(11):1596–1604
10. Oelfke U et al (2006) Linac intergrated kV-cone beam CT: technical features and first applications. Med Dosim 31(1):62–70
11. Morin O et al (2006) Megavoltage cone-beam CT: system description and clinical applications. Med Dosim 31(1):51–61
12. Hansen EK et al (2006) Repeat CT imaging and replanning during the course of IMRT for head-and-neck cancer. Int J Radiat Oncol Biol Phys 64(2):355–362
13. Chang J, Cox J (2010) Improving radiation conformality in the treatment of non–small cell lung cancer. Semin Radiat Oncol 20(3):171–177
14. Ling CC et al (2000) Towards multidimensional radiotherapy (MD-CRT): biological imaging and biological conformality. Int J Radiat Oncol Biol Phys 47:551–560

Part II

PET/CT in Hodgkin Lymphoma

PET/CT in Hodgkin Lymphoma

6

Theodoros P. Vassilakopoulos,
Phoivi Rondogianni, Sofia N. Chatziioannou,
Effimia P. Vrakidou, Vasileios I. Telonis,
Roxani D. Efthymiadou, John A. Andreou,
and Vassilios K. Prassopoulos

6.1 Introduction

Hodgkin lymphoma (HL) is the most firmly established indication for the use of positron emission tomography with integrated computed tomography (PET/CT) in the field of malignant lymphomas. In routine clinical practice, PET/CT is increasingly used for initial staging and final response assessment as well as in early interim (mid-treatment) response assessment. PET/CT is the standard of care, being strongly recommended for baseline staging and final response assessment by the recently published 2014 guidelines [1, 2]. In contrast, the use of PET/CT for the interim evaluation is not recommended yet, despite its strong prognostic significance in intermediate and advanced stages, because data on effective treatment modification are still insufficient [1–4]. Routine follow-up with PET/CT is not recommended in patients who have achieved a PET-negative status after first-line chemotherapy, due to the high false-positive rate [1–4].

T.P. Vassilakopoulos, MD (✉) • V.I. Telonis, MD
Department of Haematology, National and Kapodistrian University of Athens, School of Medicine, Laikon General Hospital, Athens, Greece
e-mail: tvassilak@med.uoa.gr; vasilis.telonis@yahoo.com

P. Rondogianni, MD, FENMB
Department of Nuclear Medicine and PET/CT, Evangelismos General Hospital, Athens, Greece
e-mail: phrontog@yahoo.gr

S.N. Chatziioannou, MD
Centre for Clinical and Translational Research, Biomedical Research Foundation of the Academy of Athens, Athens, Greece
e-mail: sofiac@bcm.tmc.edu

E.P. Vrakidou, MD
Department of Hematology, HYGEIA Hospital, Athens, Greece
e-mail: evrakidou@gmail.com

R.D. Efthymiadou, MD
Director of PET/CT Department, "HYGEIA" Hospital, Erythrou Stavrou 4 and Kifissias, Maroussi 15123, Greece
e-mail: r.efthimiadi@hygeia.gr

J.A. Andreou, MD • V.K. Prassopoulos, MD
Department of Nuclear Medicine and PET/CT, HYGEIA Hospital, Athens, Greece
e-mail: j.andreou1@gmail.com; vprasso@otenet.gr

J.A. Andreou et al. (eds.), *PET/CT in Lymphomas: A Case-Based Atlas*,
DOI 10.1007/978-3-319-27380-8_6

6.2 PET/CT in Initial Staging

6.2.1 General Considerations

PET/CT is more accurate than conventional imaging in the initial staging of HL due to its superior performance in detecting disease in normal-sized lymph nodes and extranodal sites [1–4]. Additionally, baseline PET/CT review may facilitate the interpretation of posttreatment findings in individual cases [1–4]. Along these lines, upstaging is observed by PET/CT in ~20 % of the cases, while ~5 % are downstaged, for an overall stage shift in 1 out of 4 patients [2–4]. The impact on treatment selection is less pronounced, since treatment strategy is modified in only 10–15 % of the patients; however, changes in radiotherapy (RT) planning are much more common [3]. Despite the undoubtful contribution of PET/CT in the initial staging of HL, our current knowledge on decision-making is still based on conventional staging in the absence of formal evidence for the impact of PET/CT.

6.2.2 PET in the Assessment of Bone Marrow Involvement

A major and proven practical consequence of the application of baseline PET/CT in HL is the elimination of the need of bone marrow biopsy (BMb) according to current recommendations [1, 2]. This is because PET/CT is more sensitive than BMb and treatment decisions are not typically affected in the rare cases of positive – but biopsy-negative – PET/CT. It should be noted that PET/CT is suggestive of BM involvement only in the presence of focal lesions (bone marrow scores 4 and 5; see below), while diffuse increased uptake (with intensity > liver) is typically the result of reactive BM changes caused by the cytokine milieu present in HL and should not be confused with BM involvement [5, 6].

Patterns and grading [6] of bone marrow 18-FDG uptake can be classified as follows: no increased uptake in the bone marrow (score 1) (Fig. 6.1a), diffusely increased 18-FDG uptake but less than or equal to the uptake of the liver (score 2) (Fig. 6.1b, c), diffusely increased 18-FDG uptake exceeding the uptake of the liver (score 3) (Fig. 6.1d), unifocal 18-FDG uptake (score 4) with no associated CT finding (Fig. 6.1e), and multifocal 18-FDG uptake in the bone marrow (score 5) (Fig. 6.1f).

In a study conducted by El-Galaly et al. [5], among 454 HL patients staged by both PET/CT and BMb, only 6 % had BM involvement by

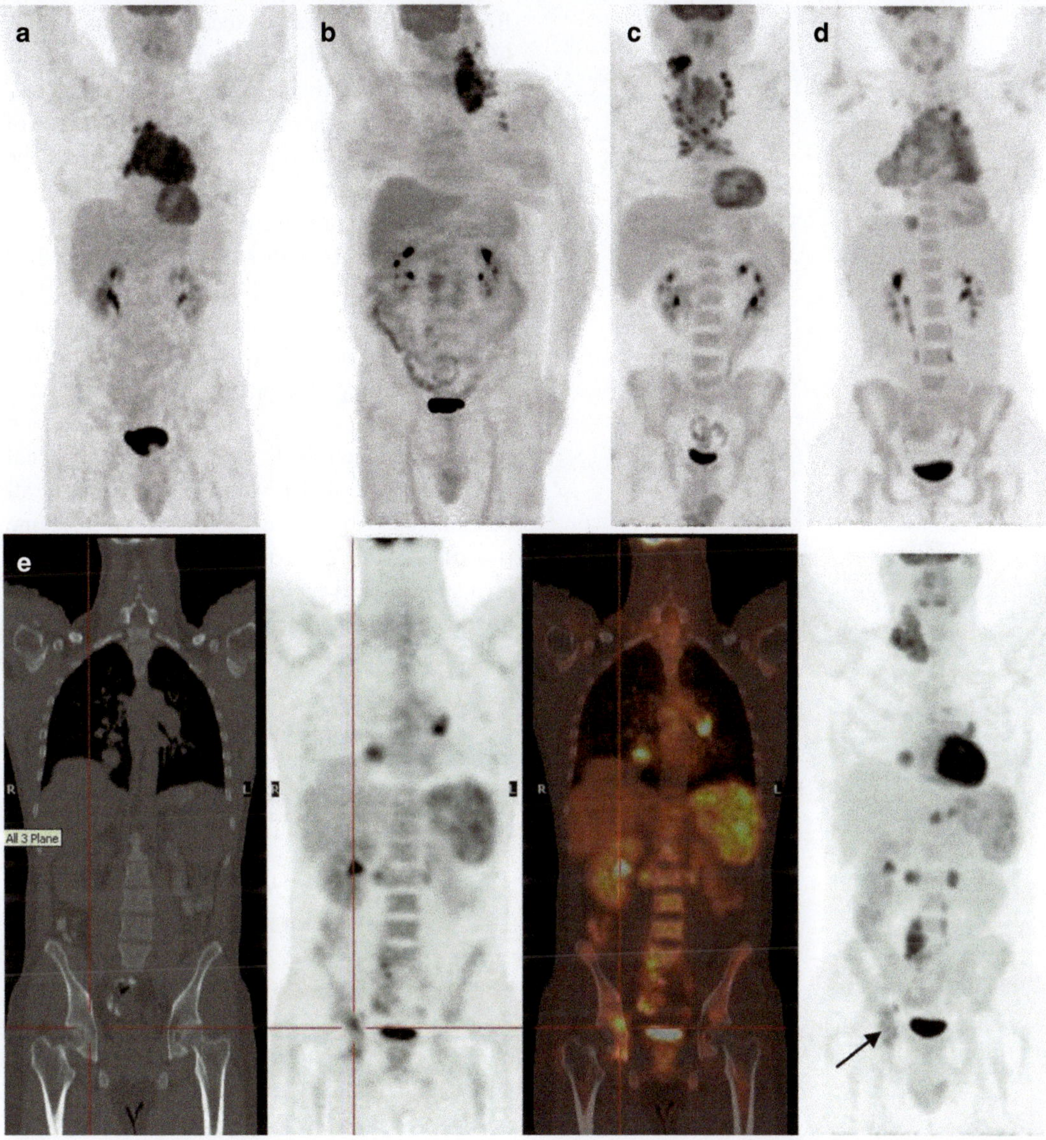

Fig. 6.1 Patterns and grading of bone marrow 18-FDG uptake. (**a**) No increased bone marrow 18-FDG uptake in the bone marrow (score 1). (**b**) Diffusely increased bone marrow 18-FDG uptake but less than the uptake of the liver (score 2). (**c**) Diffusely increased bone marrow 18-FDG uptake equal to the uptake of the liver (score 2). (**d**) Diffusely increased bone marrow 18-FDG uptake exceeding the uptake of the liver (score 3). (**e**) Unifocal 18-FDG uptake (score 4) at the right iliac bone with no associated CT finding (From *left* to *right*: Coronal CT, PET and Fused images (*red cross*) and MIP PET image (*black arrow*). (**f**) Multifocal 18-FDG uptake in the bone marrow (score 5) (*black arrows*). *Comment*: Only scores 4 and 5 suggest the presence of bone/bone marrow involvement [1, 2, 5, 6]. Focal increased uptake in the absence of bone lesions in the CT portion of PET/CT is considered as true bone marrow involvement. Scores 2 and 3 are not suggestive of bone marrow involvement. They rather reflect the increased cytokine activity, which is observed in HL, leading to "acute phase reaction" and reactive bone marrow changes (leukocytosis, thrombocytosis, anemia, elevated ESR and CRP, B-symptoms) [5, 6]

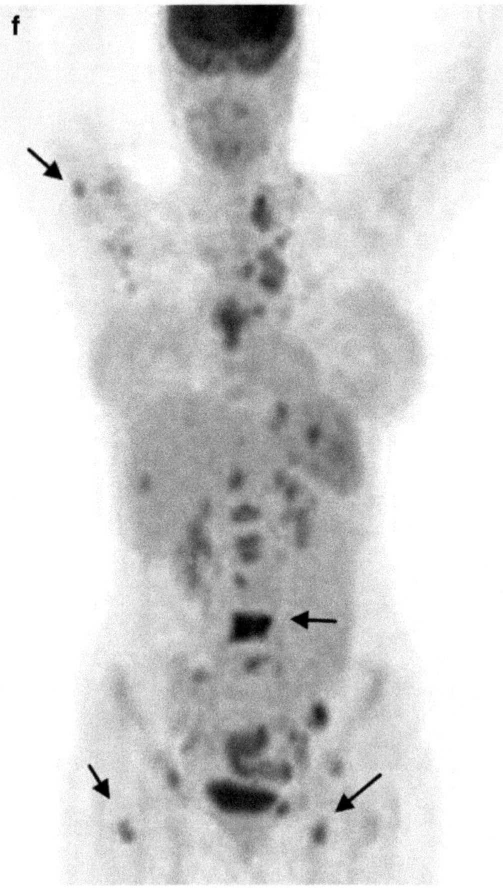

Fig. 6.1 (continued)

BMb, but more than twice (13 %) had PET/CT-positive bone lesions and a negative BMb. Less than 1 % of the patients (4/454) had a positive BMb in the absence of PET/CT evidence of BM disease, and all 4 patients already had stage III, i.e., advanced disease. Therefore, there was no effect on treatment design. Similarly, only 1.1 % of patients with HL and a negative BM PET/CT had a positive BMb in a meta-analysis of 955 patients, including the previously mentioned study [7]. Our experience, based on 172 patients, is very similar, further demonstrating that there is not even a small high-risk subgroup [6, 8], in which BMb could offer additional information, so that BMb can be omitted in all PET-staged patients, regardless of the baseline risk of BM involvement [6]. The above studies also suggest that the outcomes of patients with positive BMb and those with multifocal PET/CT BM lesions but negative BMb are equally poor [5, 6]. Thus, in HL, the biological and prognostic significance of BM involvement detected by means of PET/CT only appears to be similar to that of histologically proven BM disease [5, 6].

6.2.3 Potential Prognostic Role of Baseline PET/CT

The true tumor burden might be better estimated by baseline PET/CT compared to conventional methods with the calculation of total metabolic tumor volume (TMTV) [9], which was independently associated with prognosis in small- or medium-sized series of patients with HL [10, 11].

6.3 PET/CT in Response Assessment After Completion of Therapy

6.3.1 Criteria for Response Assessment and Definitions of PET Positivity

Following the completion of therapy, the contribution of PET/CT is based on its ability to effectively discriminate between residual CT findings containing viable lymphoma or necrotic/fibrotic tissue. PET was first incorporated in the revised criteria of response in malignant lymphomas in 2007 [12, 13], eliminating the previously described completed remission unconfirmed (CRu) category. In the absence of progressive disease, a negative PET became compatible with CR irrespectively of the depth of the conventional radiographic response. In that set of criteria, the reference level for the definition of PET positivity was linked to the size of the residual mass [12]: Positivity required FDG uptake exceeding the background for residual lesions <2 cm or normal-sized nodes, but a mild uptake above the background, not exceeding the uptake of the mediastinal blood pool, was still considered negative for residual abnormalities measuring ≥2 cm. Special mention was also made to the definition of positivity in the cases of lung, splenic, liver, and bone marrow lesions. The Deauville 5-point scale (D5-PS), a simpler means to classify the degree of FDG uptake, was initially described for the evaluation of interim PET. According to the latest recommendations, the D5-PS has now been adopted for end-of-treatment PET (ePET) [1, 2], using the definitions described in Table 6.1. A detailed description of current criteria of staging and response assessment (final and interim) is provided in the Appendix.

6.3.2 Clinical Results

The positive and negative predictive value (PPV and NPV) of ePET depends on the intensity of the applied chemotherapy regimen (BEACOPP-escalated versus ABVD), the use of radiotherapy (RT), and the *a priori* probability of relapse, as reflected by clinical stage or other prognostic factors.

Table 6.1 Five-point scale for the evaluation of interim and end-of-treatment PET/CT scan in patients with malignant lymphomas (Deauville criteria)

1.	No abnormal FDG uptake
2.	FDG uptake ≤ mediastinum
3.	Mediastinum < FDG uptake ≤ liver
4.	FDG uptake moderately increased above the liver at any site
5.	FDG uptake markedly increased above the liver at any site and/or new sites of disease

Interim PET scans graded as 1, 2, or 3 are considered negative. Scores 4 and 5 define positive interim PET scans. The same classification has been adopted for end-of-treatment PET/CT scan as well. However, handling of score 3 may be flexible, depending on whether treatment reduction or escalation is planned [1–3]. A detailed description of current criteria of staging and response assessment (final and interim) is provided in the Appendix.

6.3.2.1 Outcome of Patients with Negative PET Following Chemotherapy

In early-stage HL, i.e. stage I/II, the 5-year relapse-free survival (RFS) rate for patients who achieve a negative ePET with ABVD is approximately 95 % [14–17]. These figures mainly apply for patients who receive further RT, a typical standard approach in this setting [14, 15, 17]. If RT is omitted, this rate is falling down to <90 % even for patients with a favorable baseline profile (no B-symptoms, no bulky disease) [15].

In contrast, in stage III/IV disease, the 5-year RFS rate is ~80 %, but it should be kept in mind that only few of these patients are irradiated [14]. Under more aggressive chemotherapy with BEACOPP-escalated, the NPV appears to be higher in patients with advanced-stage HL: For patients with a residual mass >2.5 cm and a negative ePET, 5-year RFS is approximately 90 % without RT [18]. This outcome was almost identical with that of patients with CR or residual masses <2.5 cm, who did not undergo PET/CT [18].

6.3.2.2 Outcome of Patients with Positive PET Following Chemotherapy

In early-stage HL, a positive PET/CT after ABVD is associated with a rather poor 5-year RFS of 40–65 % despite additional RT [15, 17, 19, 20]. Prognosis might be further stratified according to the degree of 18 FDG uptake, but this should be further evaluated [20, 21]. In an analysis of the RAPID trial, D5-PS score 5 predicted for inferior disease control and increased HL-related mortality following additional RT compared with scores 3 and 4, which were prognostically similar, in patients with non-bulky, stage IA/IIA HL [15, 21].

After ABVD, advanced-stage patients who remain ePET-positive have similar outcomes with ePET-positive early-stage patients. However, following intensive chemotherapy with BEACOPP-escalated, RT in >2.5 cm PET-positive residuals may provide very high disease control rates with long-term RFS >80 % [18]. The degree of conventional radiographic response appears to correlate with disease control after BEACOPP-escalated and RT, since prognosis is worse for patients with residual masses reduced by <40 % compared with their baseline diameter [22].

6.3.3 Is PET-Guided Omission of Radiotherapy Feasible?

Although the most firmly established use of ePET in HL is final response assessment after initial treatment, randomized trials evaluating PET-guided treatment decisions, especially the omission of RT in ePET-negative patients, are very limited.

Currently, there is no evidence that RT could be omitted in patients with HL and bulky disease (even if loosely defined as any mass ≥5 cm), who have residual radiographic abnormalities after an adequate response (>75 %) to conventional chemotherapy of standard intensity [23]. The scenario appears to be different if response has been achieved with intensive chemotherapy, such as BEACOPP-escalated or similar regimens. Although there is no randomized evidence, there are strong data to support that RT can be omitted irrespectively of the initial bulk in advanced HL patients who have achieved a substantial response with BEACOPP: Patients with CR or those with residual lesions <2.5 cm (no PET evaluation performed in these subgroups), as well as those with >2.5 cm residual mass but a negative ePET, have a 5-year RFS of approximately 90 % without additional RT [18].

The omission of RT in early-stage HL in case of PET negativity after ABVD x2 or x3 was evaluated in 2 recent randomized trials, namely, the H10 [24] and the RAPID trial [15]. However, PET was handled as an interim evaluation, rather than ePET. The message derived from both trials is in fact the same: RT cannot be omitted without an increase in the relapse risk even in non-bulky, favorable early-stage HL with a negative PET/CT (D5-PS 1 or 2) after ABVD x2–3. Despite differences in disease control, the impact of this difference on long-term overall survival is very doubtful and should be prospectively assessed with much longer follow-up against the long-term consequences of RT.

6.4 Interim Response Assessment

6.4.1 Scientific Basis and Prognostic Significance

A considerably accurate early prediction of response to chemotherapy can be obtained on the basis of the observation that functional (PET) changes precede anatomic tumor shrinkage in malignant lymphomas. This observation may guide effective treatment modifications. PET/CT-based early response assessment after 2 or even after a single cycle of chemotherapy (interim PET – iPET) has provided important prognostic information for patients with intermediate- and advanced-stage HL [25–27]. However, current recommendations do not propose the use of iPET to guide treatment decisions, because no relevant evidence of survival benefit from randomized trials has become available yet [1, 2].

The D5-PS is the standard tool for the evaluation of iPET in HL. Any positivity in previously involved sites with 18-FDG uptake up to that of the liver is acceptable as a favorable interim response, so that scores 1–3 and 4–5 are considered negative and positive, respectively. Recent data suggest that an approach based on SUVmax reduction between baseline and iPET (ΔSUVmax at a cutoff of 71 %) may provide even better discrimination [28], similarly to what is observed in DLBCL (see relevant chapter).

The applicability of D5-PS was verified in the international validation study under ABVD chemotherapy, where 3-year PFS rates of 95 % and 28 % were observed for patients with early unfavorable and advanced HL and a negative or positive iPET, respectively [29]. Reproducibility of iPET negativity or positivity according to the D5-PS definitions was substantial to almost perfect among pairs of 6 expert reviewers [30]. It should be underlined that central review of PET studies was crucial for the achievement of this very efficient discrimination, since local interpretation was associated with a much lower difference between cases with negative and positive iPET (3-year PFS 94 % vs. 54 %) [30]. However, in low risk patients, those with localized disease and no adverse factors, especially bulky disease (who roughly constitute the early favorable group), the outcome of iPET-positive group may be much better than the ~30 % reported above [17, 21, 24, 25, 31–34], i.e., the PPV of iPET is rather low in early-stage patients without risk factors.

Under more intensive treatment with BEACOPP-escalated, the NPV of iPET is also >90 %; nevertheless, the PPV is much lower compared with ABVD-treated patients, since the long-term PFS of iPET-positive patients may be up to 50–70 % [35] or even higher [36].

6.4.2 Can Treatment Be Modified in Response to Interim PET Results?

Two conditions must be met if iPET is to be used to guide treatment decisions: First, an effective alternative therapy should exist in order to improve the outcome of iPET-positive patients. Second, the NPV should be sufficiently high to avoid relapses in the majority of patients, who achieve an iPET-negative status.

Regarding the first condition, accumulating data suggest that treatment intensification with BEACOPP-escalated is highly effective in overcoming the adverse impact of a positive iPET after ABVD x2 in advanced- or even intermediate (early unfavorable)-stage HL, providing long-term PFS rates of 60–65 % vs. an expected rate of ~30 % based on historical data [37–39]. In contrast, if first-line therapy includes BEACOPP-escalated instead of ABVD, the long-term PFS of iPET-positive patients may be 50–70 %, or even higher, as stated above [35, 36]. In this setting, improvement of the outcome of iPET-positive patients appears difficult. For example, the addition of rituximab was not successful in improving the outcome of iPET+ patients after BEACOPP-escalated x2, in the GHSG HD18 [36]. Finally, it is important to underline that the preliminary results of the H10 trial, reported at the 2015 ICML Lugano Meeting, provide the first evidence that switch to 2 cycles of BEACOPP-escalated may improve PFS of patients with stage I/II (non-advanced) HL, who remain PET-positive after ABVD x2. Indeed, the 5-year PFS was 91 % versus 77 % for patients who continued with ABVD (p = 0.002), while the 5-year overall survival was marginally improved, being 96 % versus 89 % (p = 0.062) (data presented by John Raemaekers but not published yet).

Although the first condition for success appears to be fulfilled with the acceptable salvageability rate with BEACOPP-escalated for patients who still remain iPET+ after ABVD x2 [37–39], the second condition now becomes equally interesting and important: As data mature, it becomes more clear that the NPV of iPET may not be so perfect as initially thought in patients with truly advanced HL: In the US S0816 trial, the 2-year PFS of 277 patients with stage III/IV HL treated with ABVD x6 was ~80 % and did not differ according to the D5-PS score (81 %, 80 %, and 78 % for scores 1,2, and 3, respectively) [38]. Smaller studies also provided similar results [32, 40, 41]. The a priori risk of failure as reflected by stage IV (or extranodal involvement) or other prognostic factors may affect the NPV of iPET and should be further investigated [40, 42]. Thus, in the RATHL trial, patients with a negative iPET had a ~85 % PFS rate at 3 years and the risk of failure was predicted by stage and IPS [39, 43]. Biological prognostic factors may also be relevant (Bologna study) [44]; a study of clinical and biological factors will be shortly implemented to address this crucial issue.

Overall, although iPET-adapted therapy appears attractive, randomized trials are not yet mature enough to examine the presence of a potential survival benefit over ABVD. More importantly, iPET-adapted strategies have not been compared with intensive chemotherapy approaches, such as the frontline use of BEACOPP-escalated x6 and BEACOPP-escalated x2 plus ABVD x2 plus RT in advanced- and intermediate-stage HL, respectively [18, 45, 46]. Conversely, the non-inferiority of iPET-adapted therapy compared to the invariable use of BEACOPP-escalated in these HL subgroups should also be addressed in randomized trials. The AHL 2011 trial (NCT01358747) is currently addressing a similar question: Advanced stage patients receive 6 cycles of BEACOPP-escalated versus an iPET adapted strategy including 2 initial cycles of BEACOPP-escalated and ABVD x4 in case of iPET negativity or BEACOPP-escalated x4 if iPET is positive. Initial data suggest comparable efficacy of the two arms [47].

Conclusions

The use of PET/CT is now considered mandatory for baseline staging, providing more accurate information and obviating the need of BMb in HL. PET/CT has been the long-standing "gold standard" for final response assessment. Early iPET evaluation provides valuable prognostic information in HL, and treatment intensification with BEACOPP-escalated can improve disease control in patients with persistent PET positivity after 2 cycles of ABVD. However, no randomized evidence of survival benefit exists yet, and such strategies have not been compared with frontline intensive chemotherapy approaches. Therefore, we do not know whether iPET-based chemotherapy intensification is ultimately better than ABVD in terms of overall survival (but data of marginal significance do exist for intermediate stages) or if it could be equivalent (non-inferior) with the frontline use of BEACOPP-escalated x6 or BEACOPP-escalated x2 plus ABVD x2 plus RT in advanced and intermediate-stage HL, which constitutes the standard of care in many centers. The same is true for iPET-driven treatment de-escalation after 2 cycles of BEACOPP-escalated, although there is some relevant preliminary evidence [47]. The exact role of PET/CT in guiding treatment decisions needs to be defined by randomized trials; evidence-based approaches are expected to become available in the near future.

Hodgkin Lymphoma: Case 1

A 65-year-old male with a history of renal cell carcinoma 15 years ago presented with dry cough, prolonged low-grade fever, drenching night sweats, >10 % weight loss within the last month, and generalized pruritus. Initial evaluation revealed palpable splenomegaly 3 cm blcm with no other physical findings. Whole-body CT scan revealed hepatosplenomegaly with heterogeneity of splenic parenchyma; multiple retrocrural, retroperitoneal, abdominal, and pelvic enlarged lymph nodes up to 3 cm; and multiple mediastinal and right hilar nodes up to 4 cm. A bone marrow biopsy was negative. Under local anesthesia, surgical excision of a small (<1 cm), deeply lying, left supraclavicular node, which was seen on CT review, revealed mixed-cellularity classical HL. A staging PET/CT confirmed the presence of extensive, highly hypermetabolic (SUVmax 15) lymphadenopathy both above and below the diaphragm (Fig. 6.2a – open arrows); highly increased, heterogeneous, and patchy 18-FDG uptake in the spleen as well as a focal lesion in the liver (Fig. 6.2a, b – thick black and white arrows); and

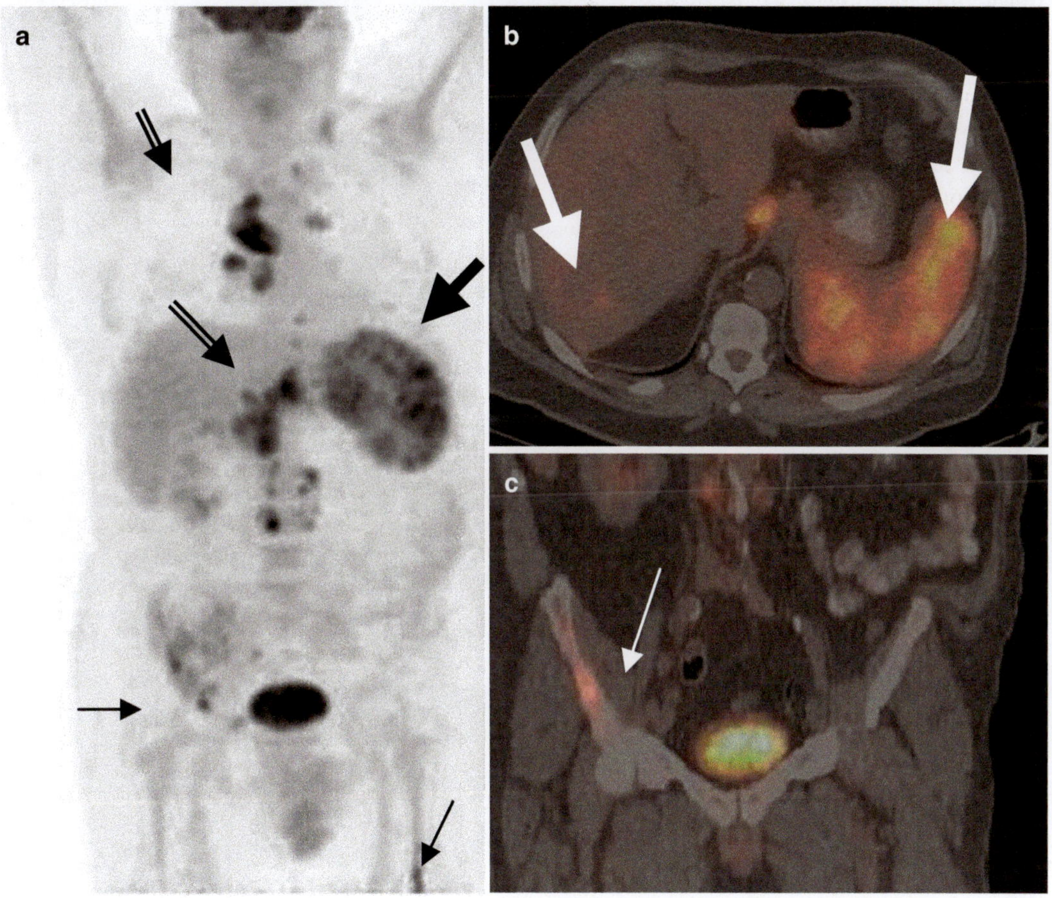

Fig. 6.2 (**a**–**c**) A staging PET/CT confirmed the presence of extensive, highly hypermetabolic (SUVmax 15) lymphadenopathy both above and below the diaphragm (**a** – *open arrows*); highly increased, heterogeneous, and patchy 18-FDG uptake in the spleen as well as a focal lesion in the liver (**a**, **b** – *thick black* and *white arrows*); and hypermetabolic foci in the right iliac bone and left femur with no associated CT findings, consistent with bone marrow involvement (**a**, **c** – *thin black* and *white arrows*)

hypermetabolic foci in the right iliac bone and left femur with no associated CT findings, consistent with bone marrow involvement (Fig. 6.2a, c – thin black and white arrows).

Clinical stage was IIIB but was upgraded to IVB by PET/CT. The patient also had anemia, mild leukocytosis without lymphocytopenia, normal serum albumin levels, elevated ESR (88 mm/h) and CRP, and elevated LDH (1.6×) and β2-microglobulin levels. The value of IPS, based on conventional staging, was 3. The patient received 8 cycles of ABVD combination chemotherapy and achieved a complete remission, which was confirmed by a normal end-of-treatment PET/CT (Fig. 6.3).

Discussion: PET/CT upstages approximately 20 % of patients with HL [2–4]. In this case, upstaging was due to demonstration of disease in the liver and bone marrow. PET/CT reveals >2 times more cases of bone marrow involvement, as in this case, in which bone marrow biopsy was negative [5, 6]. Even if interim PET were an established standard practice, the age of the patient precluded treatment intensification to BEACOPP-escalated due to the high treatment-related mortality observed in patients 60–65 years old [48], and this was the reason of omitting interim PET in this case. However, the RATHL trial is currently evaluating the omission of bleomycin in patients with negative interim PET in order to avoid pulmonary toxicity, which may be lethal, especially in older patients [43]. The interim results are encouraging, making iPET useful in this setting as well.

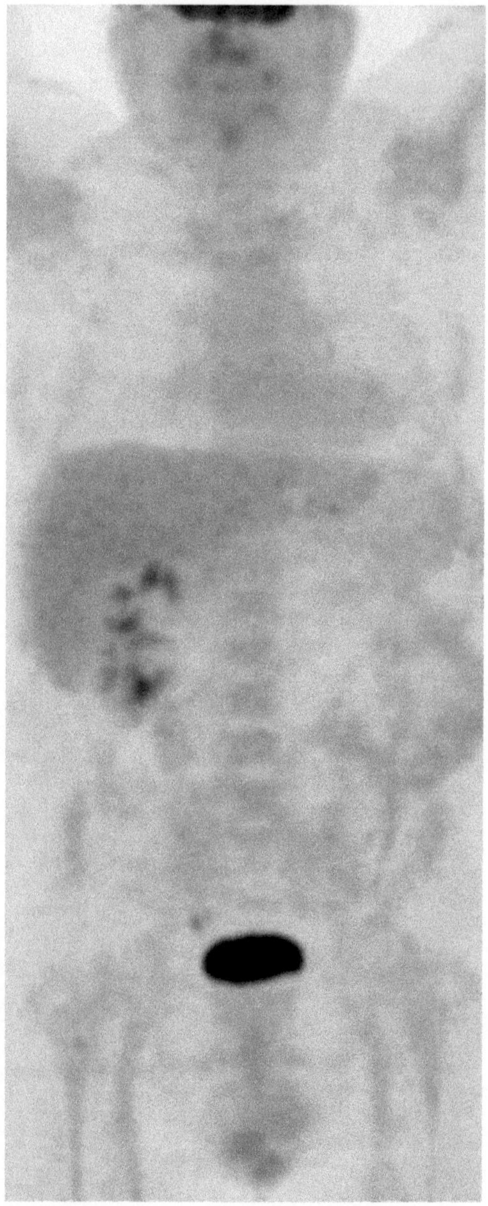

Fig. 6.3 Normal end-of-treatment PET/CT

Hodgkin Lymphoma: Case 2

A 28-year-old man presented due to an otherwise asymptomatic left submandibular swelling, which proved to be nodular sclerosing Hodgkin's lymphoma. Full CT staging revealed multiple bilateral cervical nodes up to 5 cm and a single node at the hepatogastric junction with a short axis of 1.2 cm. A bone marrow biopsy was negative. PET/CT staging further revealed left axillary lymphadenopathy and demonstrated the borderline abdominal finding (Fig. 6.4a, b) confirming that clinical stage was IIIA with minimal infradiaphragmatic involvement. The patient had mild leukocytosis with severe lymphocytopenia (<8 %), reduced serum albumin levels, a normal ESR (19 mm/h) with mildly elevated CRP, elevated LDH (1.3x), and normal β_2-microglobulin levels. The value of IPS was 3. An interim PET evaluation was completely negative (D5-PS score 1) (Fig. 6.5a, b). Thus, he continued with 4 further cycles of ABVD chemotherapy (for a total of 6 cycles) and converted to PET-negative despite the presence of residual cervical and mediastinal lymph nodes measuring 1.6–2.0 cm. Finally, he received involved-field RT, excluding the solitary small focus of infradiaphragmatic disease. He remains in complete remission 2.5 years later.

Discussion: In this case, PET/CT confirmed the presence of disease in a borderline, solitary lymph node located at the hepatogastric junction, which was the only potential infradiaphragmatic localization, thus confirming the classification as stage IIIA. A negative interim PET/CT is associated with a favorable long-term remission rate with continued ABVD chemotherapy [29, 32, 37–41, 43, 49]. This was further supported by the negative final PET/CT and further follow-up.

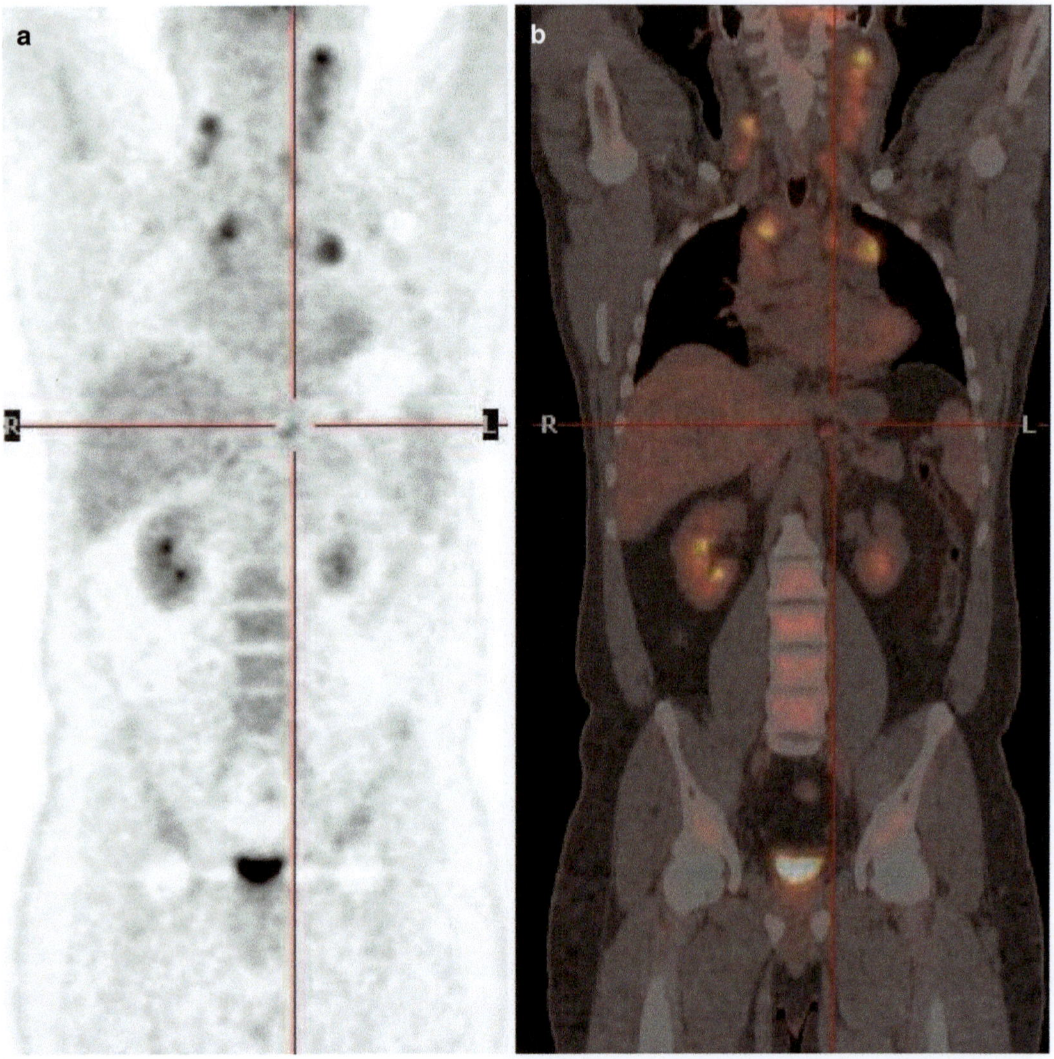

Fig. 6.4 (**a**, **b**) PET/CT primary staging demonstrated a borderline-sized hypermetabolic abdominal finding

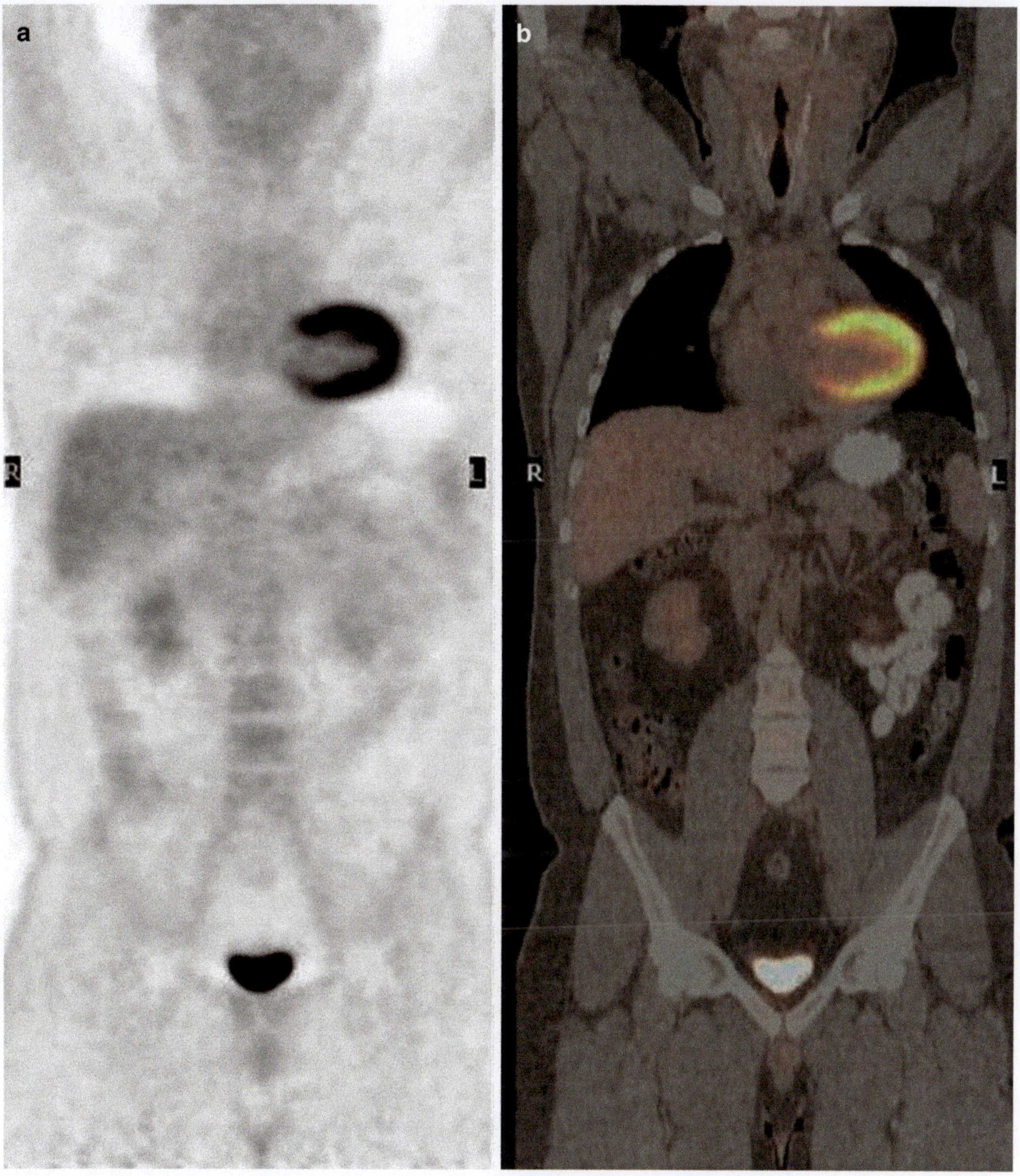

Fig. 6.5 Interim PET/CT evaluation was completely negative (D5- PS score1)

Hodgkin Lymphoma: Case 3

A 46-year-old male patient presented with left iliac lymphadenopathy. Lymph node biopsy revealed: Hodgkin's lymphoma, mixed cellularity. Conventional staging revealed nodal disease below the diaphragm (left iliac lymphadenopathy). Bone marrow biopsy showed no infiltration. Thus the patient had early-stage IA favorable Hodgkin's lymphoma. Baseline PET/CT confirmed the presence of left iliac lymphadenopathy (lymph nodes along the left common and external iliac arteries, SUVmax 3.1 and 2.4, respectively) (Fig. 6.6).

The patient received ABVD chemotherapy, and an iPET/CT was performed after two cycles showing complete resolution of the FDG uptake (Fig. 6.7). The patient continued two more ABVD cycles followed by involved-site RT. At the end of chemotherapy, the patient remained in complete remission, with negative PET/CT, and remains in CR with no further treatment for 3 years after the diagnosis (Fig. 6.8).

Discussion: In this case, PET/CT confirmed the staging classification of the conventional staging. The negative iPET signifies a favorable prognosis [15, 24], which is further supported by the negative ePET and follow-up.

There is still no clear evidence that HL patients benefit from having treatment adapted according to the results of iPET. More than 90 % of early-stage HL patients are cured with standard therapy. However, these patients still have a reduced life expectancy due to treatment-related illnesses including second cancers and cardiopulmonary disease. A substantial number of early-stage HL patients are subjected to some amount of overtreatment, and this is an argument for using iPET to identify good-risk, early-stage patients eligible for less intensive treatment. Recent trials have investigated such PET response-adapted therapy in early-stage HL [15, 24].

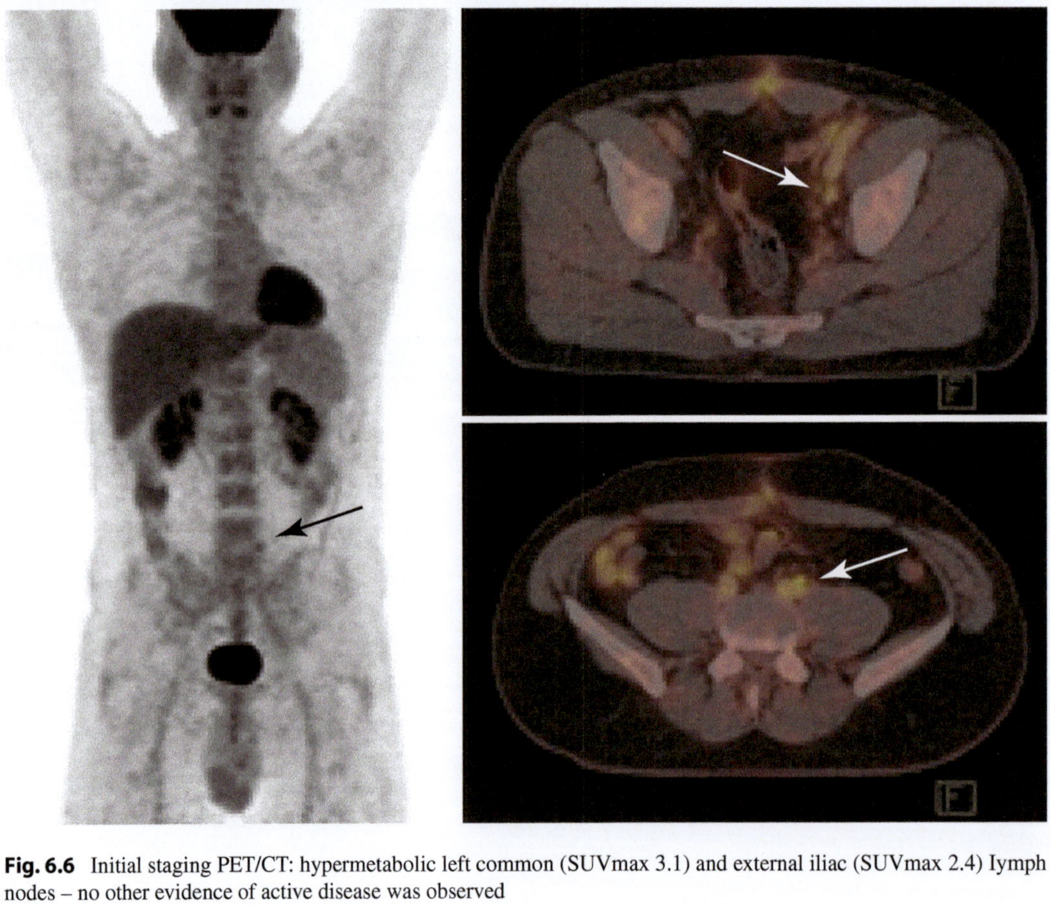

Fig. 6.6 Initial staging PET/CT: hypermetabolic left common (SUVmax 3.1) and external iliac (SUVmax 2.4) lymph nodes – no other evidence of active disease was observed

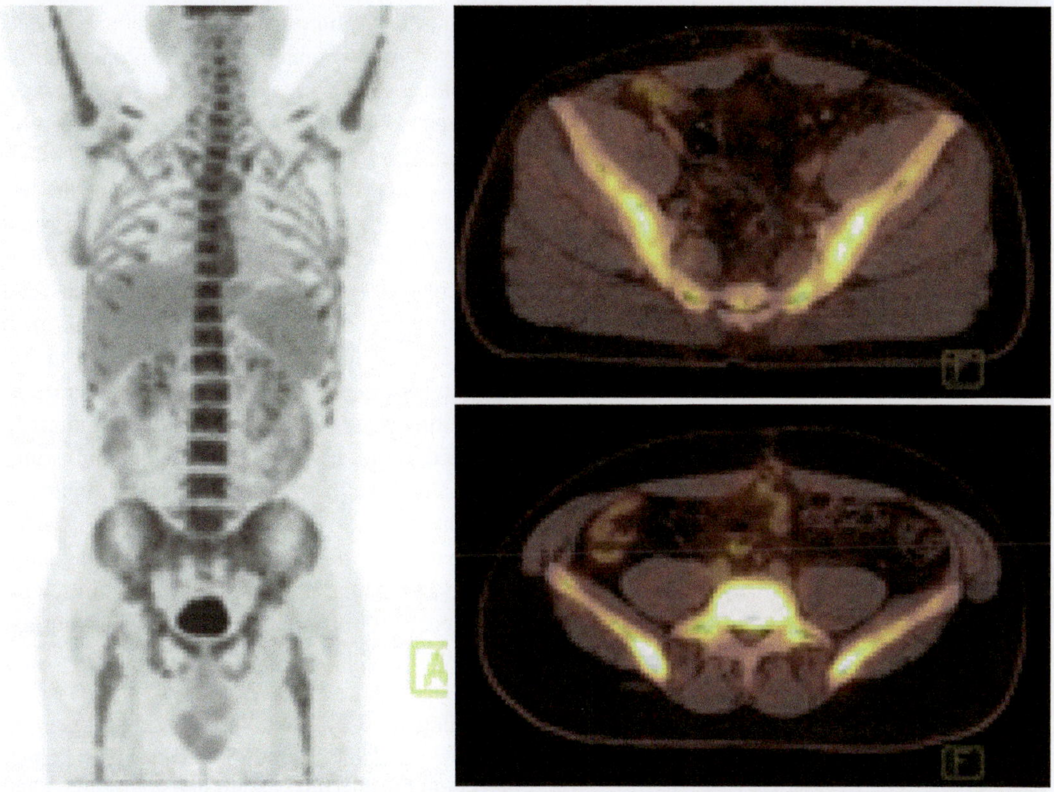

Fig. 6.7 Interim PET/CT: no increased FDG activity at the sites of prior disease. Notice the diffuse increased FDG uptake at the bone marrow attributed to granulocyte colony-stimulating factor (G-CSF) administration, which should be avoided in this setting

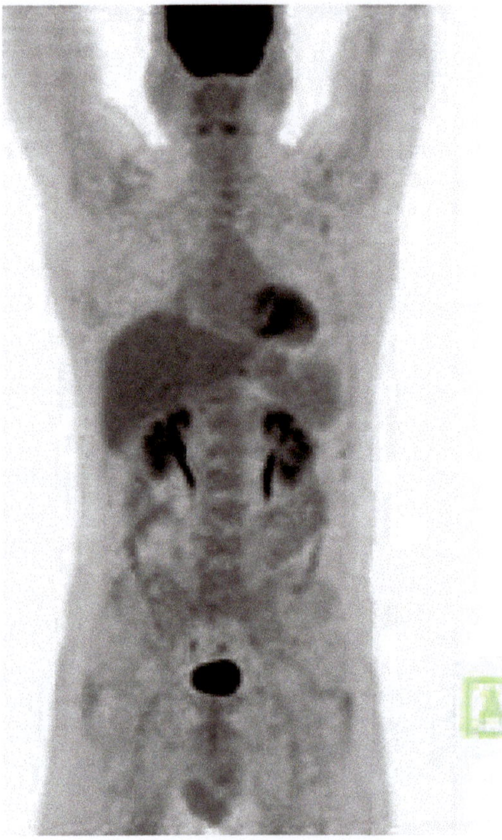

Fig. 6.8 End-of-treatment PET/CT: no evidence of active disease

Hodgkin Lymphoma: Case 4

A 40-year-old woman presented with a long history of nephrotic syndrome under steroid therapy, subsequent erythema nodosum, and left supraclavicular lymphadenopathy of 1 month duration. She also reported alcohol-related pain of the left shoulder during the last 6 months. Excisional biopsy revealed nodular sclerosing classical HL. Full conventional staging additionally revealed mediastinal lymphadenopathy, left pleural effusion, a small lung nodule, and a solitary 3 cm splenic lesion. A bone marrow biopsy was negative. Clinical stage was IIIASE. PET/CT staging revealed additional disease sites including right cervical, left axillary, and splenic hilar lymphadenopathy, without, however, stage shift (Fig. 6.9). The patient also had mild leukocytosis without lymphocytopenia, normal serum albumin levels, elevated ESR (60 mm/h) and CRP, and normal LDH and β_2-microglobulin levels. The value of IPS was 0.

Following 2 cycles of the ABVD regimen, an iPET revealed low-grade 18-FDG uptake (SUVmax 2.6) in the mediastinal lymph nodes just above the mediastinal blood pool activity, but lower than that of the liver, corresponding to a D-5PS score 3, which is interpreted as negative (Fig. 6.10a–c). ABVD chemotherapy was continued up to a total of 6 cycles. A repeated PET/CT after the end of chemotherapy was completely negative (Fig. 6.11a–c). She remains in complete remission 9 months after the completion of chemotherapy.

Discussion: Interim PET was considered negative corresponding to D5-PS score 3. The patient continued on ABVD with a favorable final outcome. According to the Deauville and the recent Lugano criteria, a mild residual positivity with an intensity not exceeding that of the liver is acceptable as a favorable response in the interim (as well as at the end-of-treatment) setting, especially if treatment escalation is intended in response to a positive interim result.

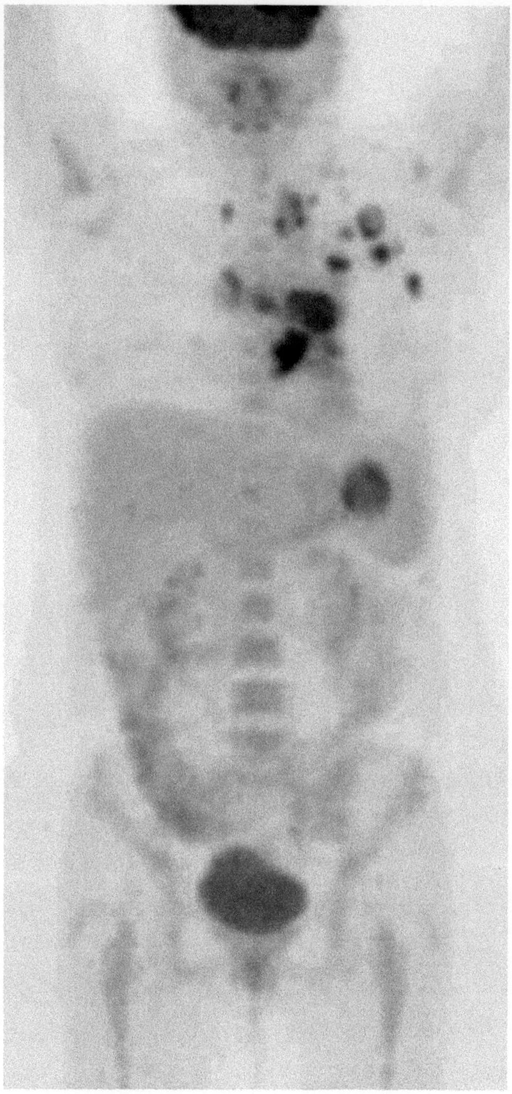

Fig. 6.9 Primary staging with PET/CT revealed additional disease sites (right supraclavicular, left axillary, and splenic hilar nodes)

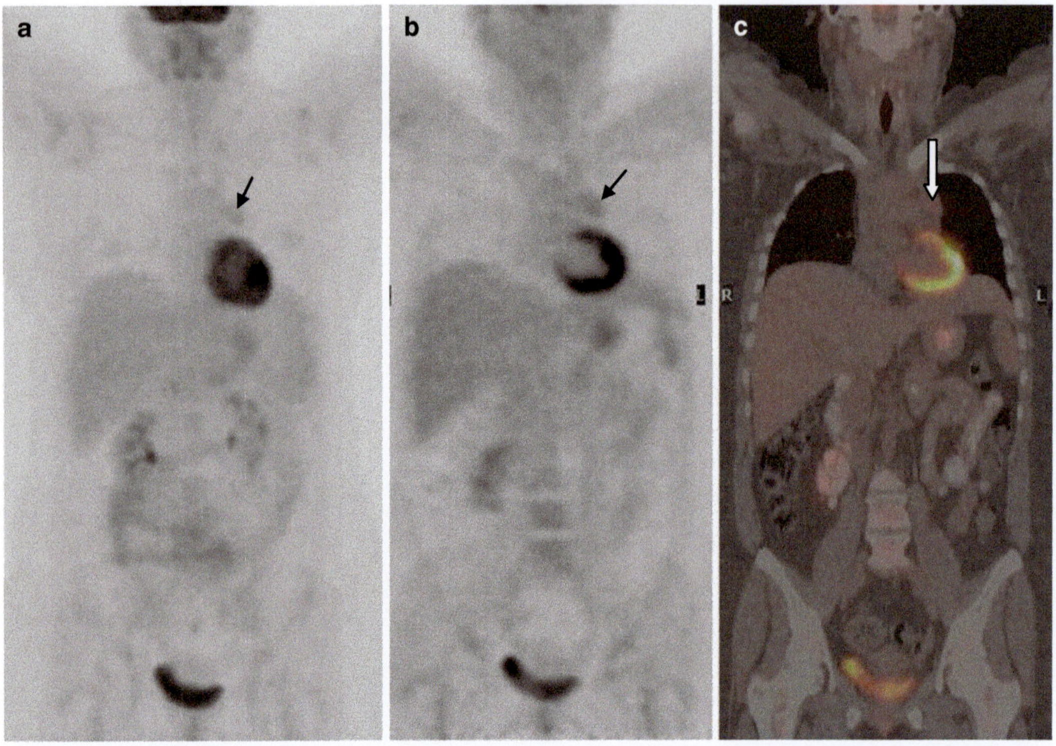

Fig. 6.10 (**a**–**c**) Interim PET/CT revealed low-grade 18-FDG uptake (SUVmax 2.6) corresponding to a D-5PS score 3

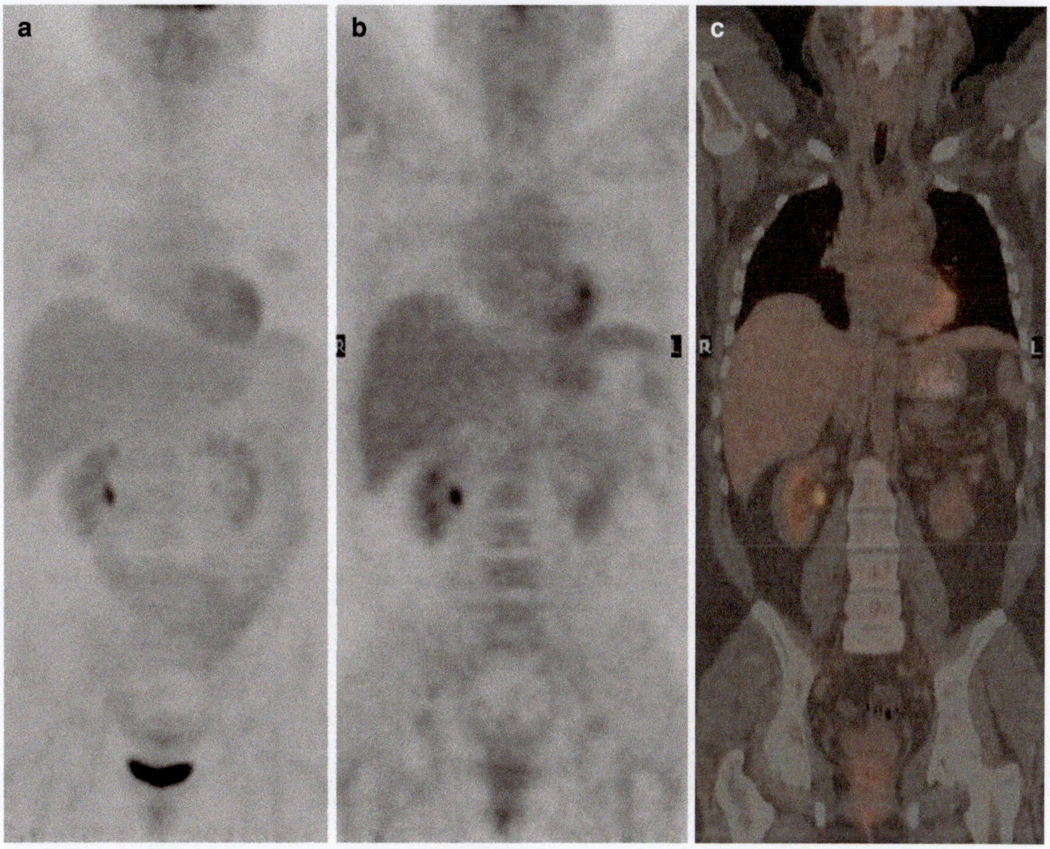

Fig. 6.11 (**a**–**c**) PET/CT after the end of chemotherapy was completely negative

Hodgkin Lymphoma: Case 5

A 39-year-old female patient presented with left cervical lymphadenopathy, pruritus and a mild weight loss of 2 kg. Her lymph node biopsy showed: Hodgkin lymphoma, nodular sclerosis.

Conventional staging revealed nodal disease above of the diaphragm (left supraclavicular and mediastinal lymphadenopathy) stage IIA (or IIβ due to the mild weight loss). The value of IPS was 0 (39 years old, female, stage IIB, Hb 13.1 g/dL, serum albumin 4.6 g/dL, WBC 5200/μL, lymphocytes 25 %). Bone marrow biopsy showed no infiltration. The patient had early-stage favorable HL.

Baseline PET/CT confirmed the presence of left supraclavicular (SUVmax 8.8) and mediastinal disease (SUVmax 4) (Fig. 6.12).

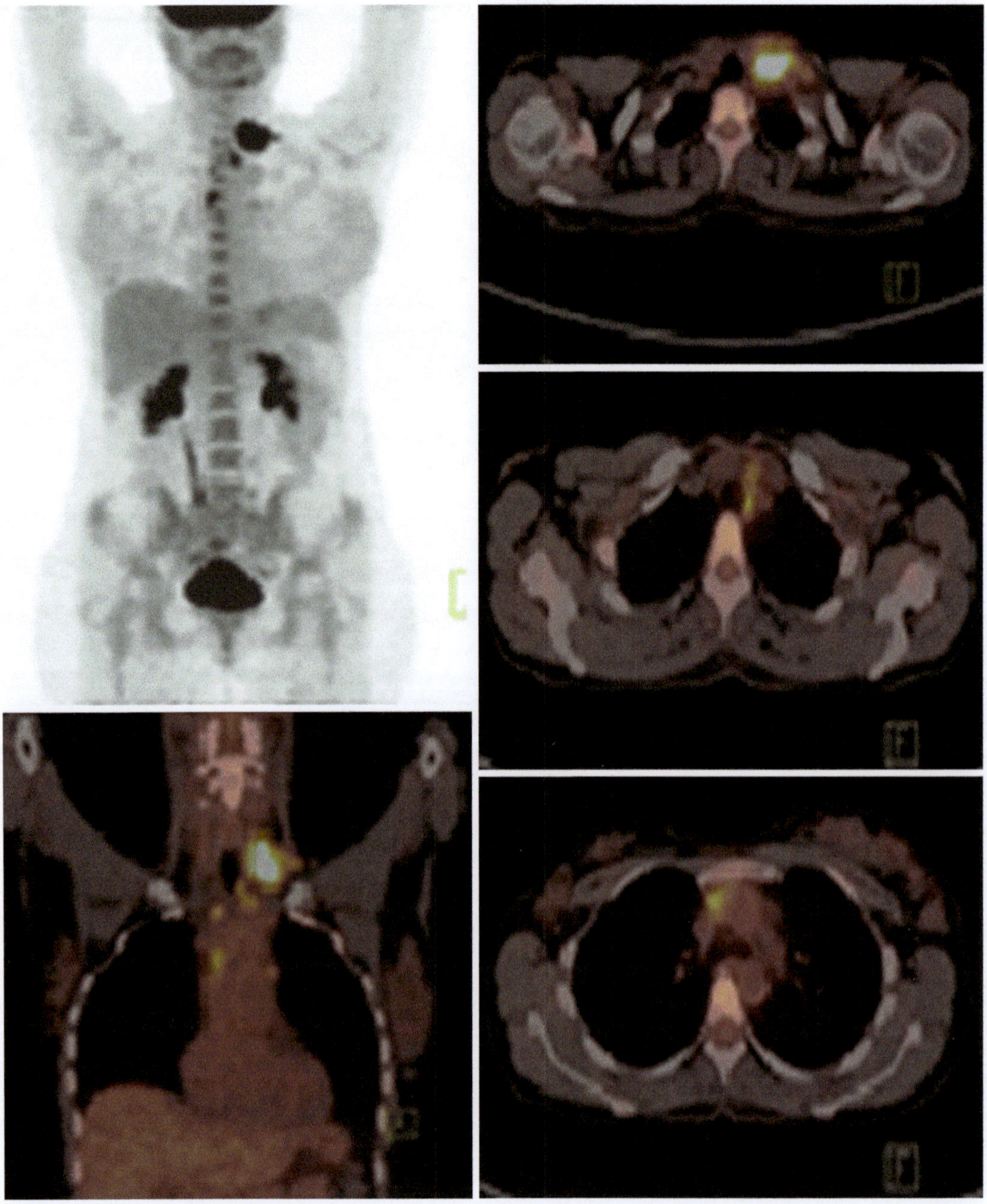

Fig. 6.12 Initial staging PET/CT: hypermetabolic lesions at the left supraclavicular area (SUVmax 8.8) and the upper anterior mediastinum (SUVmax 4)

The patient received ABVD chemotherapy, and a follow-up PET/CT was performed after two cycles showing complete resolution of the FDG uptake (Fig. 6.13).

Following the negative PET/CT result, the patient continued with 4 more ABVD cycles and involved-site RT. At the end of treatment, the patient remained in complete remission with a negative PET/CT scan (Fig. 6.14).

The patient remains in CR with no further treatment for 2 years after the initial diagnosis.

Discussion: In this case, PET/CT confirmed conventional staging classification. The negative iPET/CT signifies better prognosis and is associated with very favorable long-term remission rates with continuing ABVD regimen in early-stage disease. The negative ePET/CT supports this further (Fig. 6.14).

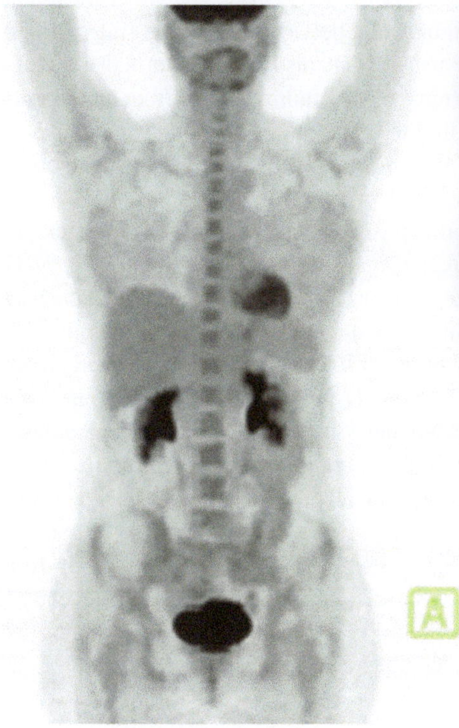

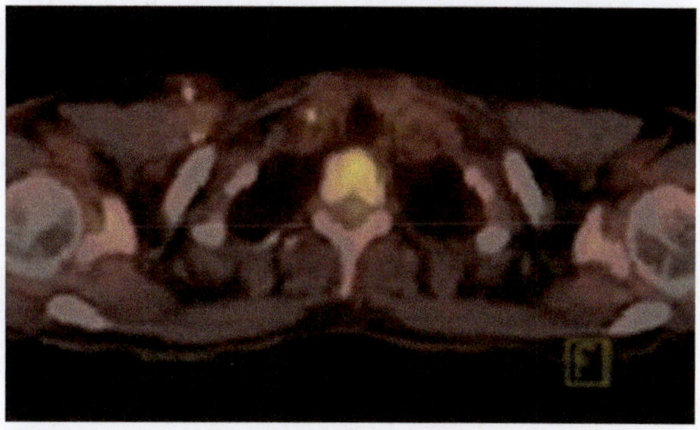

Fig. 6.13 Interim PET/CT (after two cycles of ABVD chemotherapy): no hypermetabolic lesions are observed – complete remission

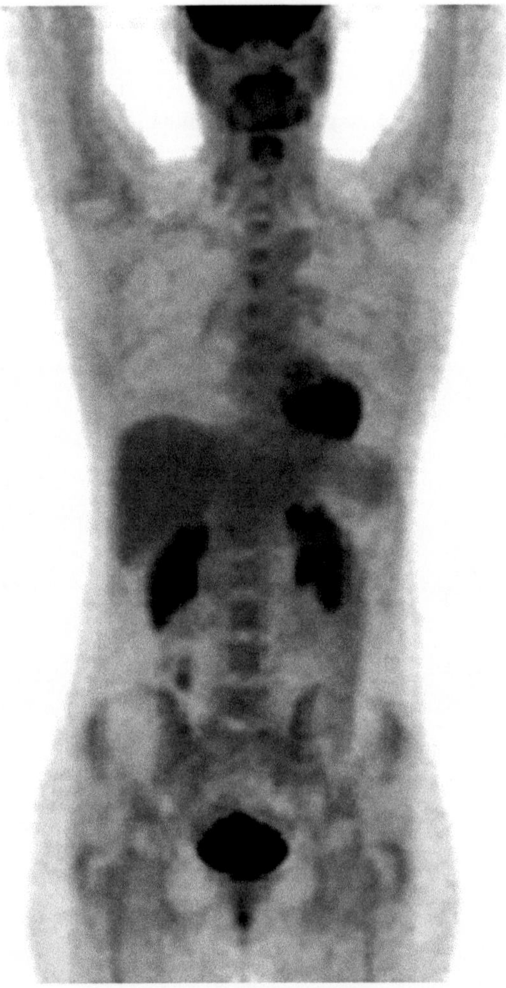

Fig. 6.14 End-of-treatment PET/CT reveals no hypermetabolic lesions

Hodgkin Lymphoma: Case 6

A 39-year-old man presented due to a right inguinofemoral mass associated with fever, which proved to be mixed-cellularity classical HL. Conventional staging revealed extensive infradiaphragmatic disease with a maximal diameter of 4 cm, and a bone marrow biopsy demonstrated infiltration by HL with associated granulomatous lesions. Clinical stage was IVB. Staging PET/CT demonstrated mild 18-FDG uptake (SUVmax 3.5) in mediastinal, abdominal, and pelvic lymph nodes (Fig. 6.15a – open arrows) but also mild abnormal 18 FDG (SUVmax 3) in multiple bone foci not corresponding to CT findings, being thus indicative of bone marrow involvement (Fig. 6.15a – black arrows, b–d).

Following 2 cycles of the ABVD regimen, an iPET/CT revealed low-grade symmetric 18-FDG uptake in lung hili (SUVmax 2). The uptake was just higher than the uptake of the mediastinal blood pool but lower than that of the liver, corresponding to a D-5PS score 3, which was in favor of adequate interim metabolic response. Furthermore, lung hilar nodes were not involved at baseline and all other disease sites had resolved (Fig. 6.16).

ABVD chemotherapy was continued up to a total of 8 cycles. A new PET/CT after the end of chemotherapy revealed low-grade, abnormal 18-FDG uptake (SUVmax 3) in bilateral hilar

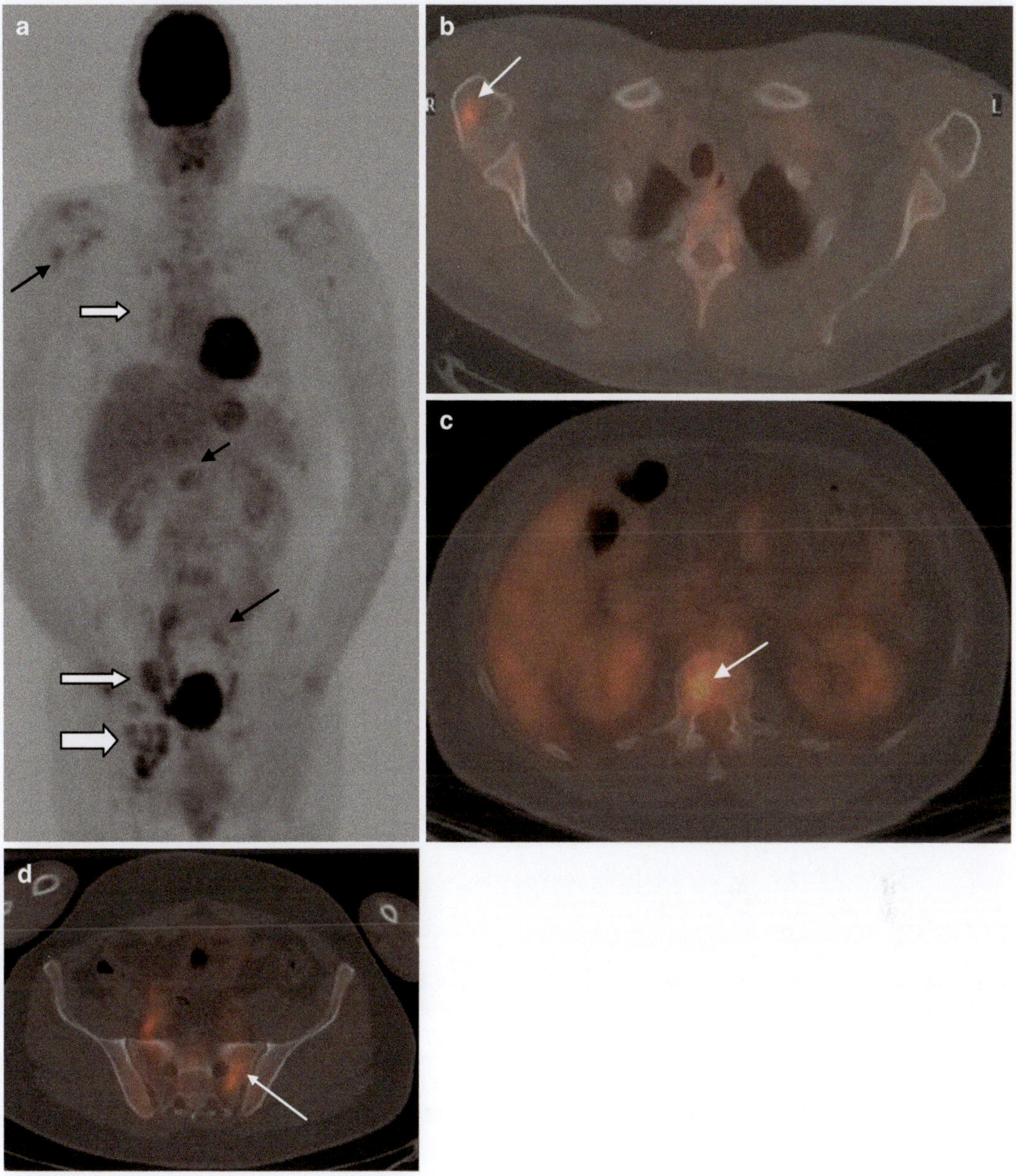

Fig. 6.15 Staging PET/CT (**a–d**). Mild 18-FDG uptake (SUVmax 3.5) in mediastinal, abdominal, and pelvic lymph nodes (**a** – *open arrows*) but also mild abnormal 18-FDG uptake (SUVmax 3) in multiple bone foci not corresponding to CT findings, being thus indicative of bone marrow involvement (**a** – *black arrows*, **b–d**)

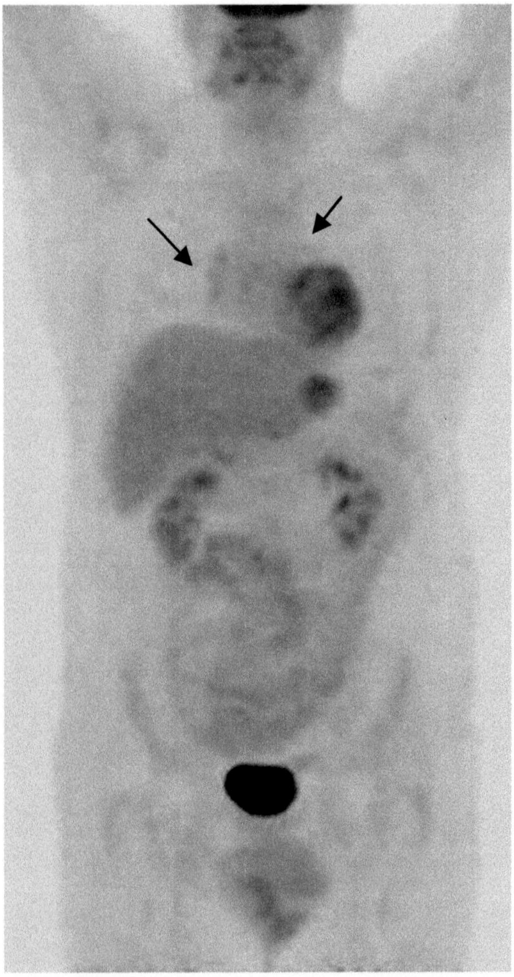

Fig. 6.16 Interim PET/CT corresponding to a D5-PS score 3. Low-grade, symmetric FDG uptake in lung hili (arrows) just higher than that of the mediastinal blood pool but lower than the liver. Note also that hilar lymphadenopathy had not been detected at baseline PET/CT and all disease sites had resolved in the interim study

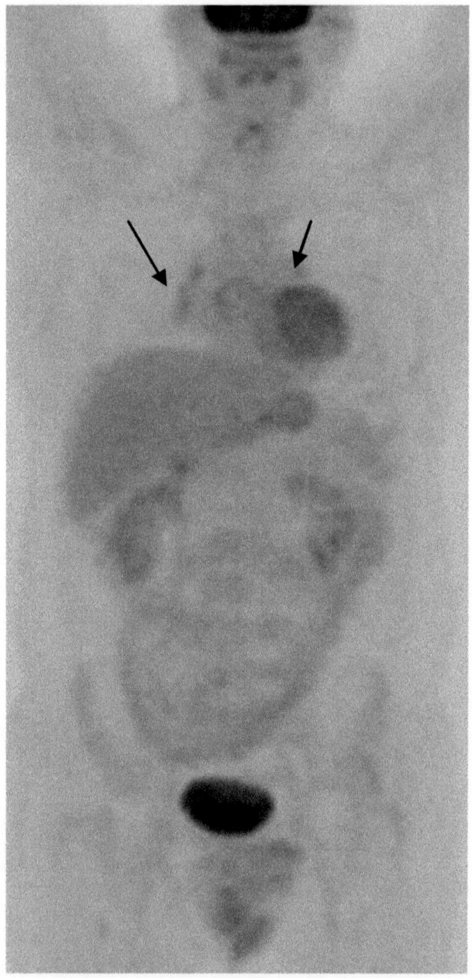

Fig. 6.17 PET/CT after the end of chemotherapy. Low-grade, abnormal 18-FDG uptake (SUVmax 3) in bilateral hilar and peribronchial as well as right paratracheal and subcarinal lymph nodes (*arrows*). The uptake was equal to that of the liver corresponding to a D5-PS score 3

and peribronchial as well as right paratracheal and subcarinal lymph nodes. The uptake was equal to that of the liver corresponding to a D5-PS score 3 (Fig. 6.17). Notably, conventional restaging including a repeated bone marrow biopsy was compatible with CR. A sarcoid-like condition was suspected based on the anatomic localization of lymphadenopathy and the findings of the initial bone marrow biopsy. However, lymphadenopathy anatomically progressed 7 months later, and recurrent HL was histologically confirmed.

After salvage chemotherapy with IGEVx3, PET/CT revealed faint, symmetric 18-FDG uptake (SUV max 2.5) in both lung hili (Fig. 6.18). Subsequently the patient received high-dose therapy with BEAM and ASCT. A new PET/CT, performed 3 months after ASCT, revealed increased abnormal 18-FDG uptake (SUVmax 6) in multiple mediastinal lymph nodes (Fig. 6.19a – thin black arrow, b) but also in abdominal lymph nodes around the porta hepatis and pancreas (Fig. 6.19a, thick black arrow, c). The disease remained initially stable (clinical complete remission), but finally the patient developed progressive disease by the conventional definition 7 months after the ASCT.

Discussion: A negative iPET may have lower-than-expected negative predictive value in patients with extranodal or stage IV HL or patients with high IPS, although this remains to be formally proved [40, 42, 43]. Despite a negative iPET (D5-PS score 3), this patient converted to PET/CT-positive by the end of ABVD based on the IHP (but not the D5-PS) criteria and developed clinical progression 7 months later (false-negative interim result). A positive PET/CT prior to ASCT does not preclude a favorable outcome if there is no progressive disease by conventional staging [50], but the optimal cutoff to define positivity in this setting has not been defined yet. Disease relapse post-ASCT carries a poor prognosis. Brentuximab vedotin can be the next treatment option based on its official indication [51]. Interestingly, the AETHERA trial recently demonstrated that consolidation with brentuximab vedotin, given shortly after ASCT, can improve PFS in patients deemed at high risk of subsequent relapse/progression [52].

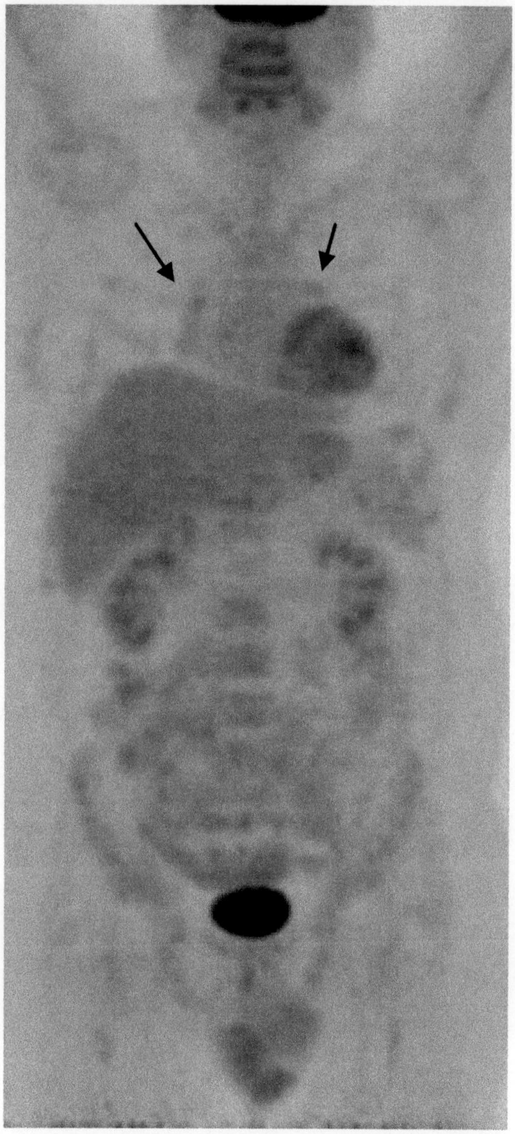

Fig. 6.18 PET/CT after salvage chemotherapy. Faint, symmetric 18-FDG uptake (SUV max 2.5) in both lung hili (*arrows*)

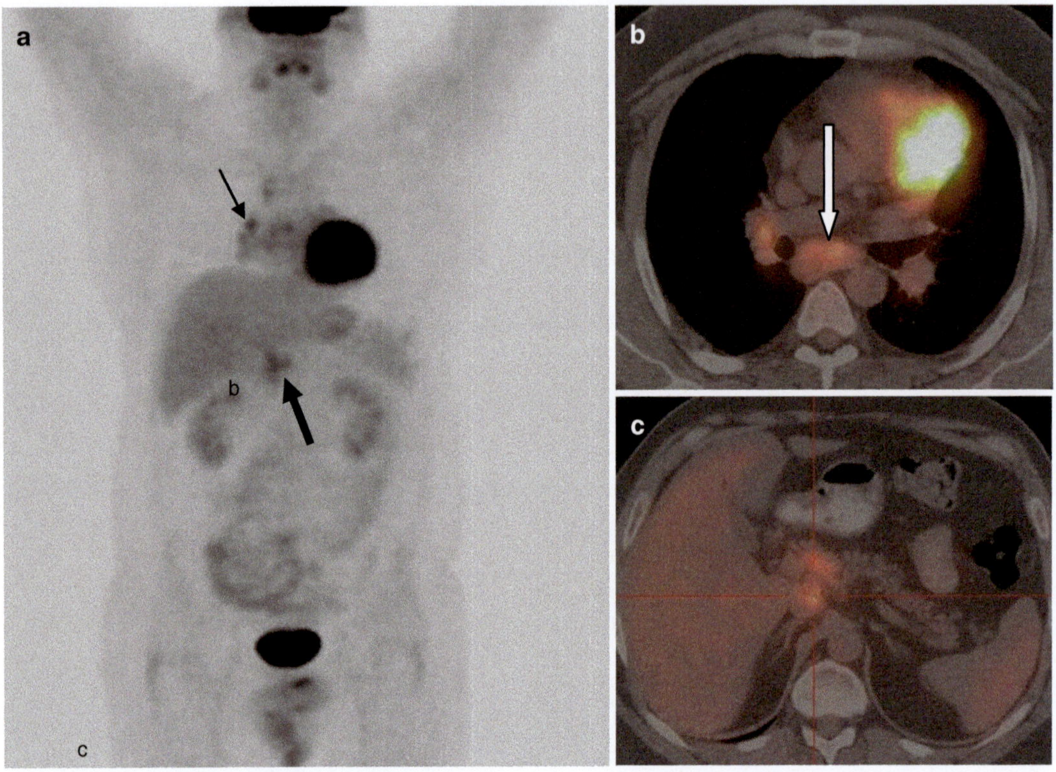

Fig. 6.19 (**a**–**c**) A new PET/CT, performed 3 months after ASCT. Increased abnormal 18-FDG uptake (SUVmax 6) in multiple mediastinal lymph nodes (**a**, *thin black arrow*; **b**, *white arrow*) but also in abdominal lymph nodes around the porta hepatis and pancreas (**a**, *thick black arrow*; **c**, *red cross*)

Hodgkin Lymphoma: Case 7

A 33-year-old man sought medical advice due to an incidentally discovered left supraclavicular swelling. Biopsy revealed mixed-cellularity classical HL. Physical examination and complete CT staging revealed bilateral cervical/supraclavicular, mediastinal, right hilar, and para-aortic lymphadenopathy up to 3 cm, multiple focal splenic lesions measuring 4–8 cm, and a right upper lobe lung lesion. Clinical stage was IVSA. PET/CT confirmed the above findings (Fig. 6.20a) and additionally revealed a right adrenal hypermetabolic lesion (Fig. 6.20b, c – arrows). The patient also had anemia, mild leukocytosis without lymphocytopenia, normal serum albumin levels, elevated ESR (93 mm/h) and CRP (99.7 mg/L), and elevated LDH and β_2-microglobulin levels. The value of IPS was 2.

Following 2 cycles of the ABVD regimen, an iPET was interpreted as negative, since residual FDG uptake was thought to be no greater than that of the liver, corresponding to D-5PS score 3 (Fig. 6.21). The patient received 6 further ABVD cycles with adequate mid-treatment conventional radiographic response but developed early progression by CT at final reevaluation. PET/CT assessment at that point showed increased 18-FDG uptake (SUVmax 13) in mediastinal lymph nodes and a 2 cm lung nodule in the right upper lobe (Fig. 6.22).

Subsequently, the patient was treated with 4 cycles of IGEV salvage chemotherapy with stable disease by conventional restaging. PET/CT remained positive (Fig. 6.23). The disease remained also stable after 3 cycles of ESHAP salvage chemotherapy. Subsequently, the patient underwent high-dose therapy with TEAM as conditioning regimen and autologous stem cell support. Interestingly PET/CT was normal 3 months after ASCT despite stability of the size of residual lesions on CT (Fig. 6.24) and continued to be negative following subsequent radiotherapy (Fig. 6.25). He remains in remission 3 years later.

Discussion: A negative iPET is associated with favourable outcomes with continued ABVD chemotherapy in intermediate and advanced stage HL [29, 32, 37–41, 43, 49]. In stage III/IV patients, PFS may be ~80 % [38]. In the present case iPET proved to be false negative. This is probably more likely in patients with stage IV or extranodal disease [40, 42, 43], as was the case here, or those with high IPS [43]. Finally, PET/CT positivity prior to ASCT is an adverse prognostic factor but does not preclude a favorable outcome, since approximately 40 % of these patients are finally cured [50].

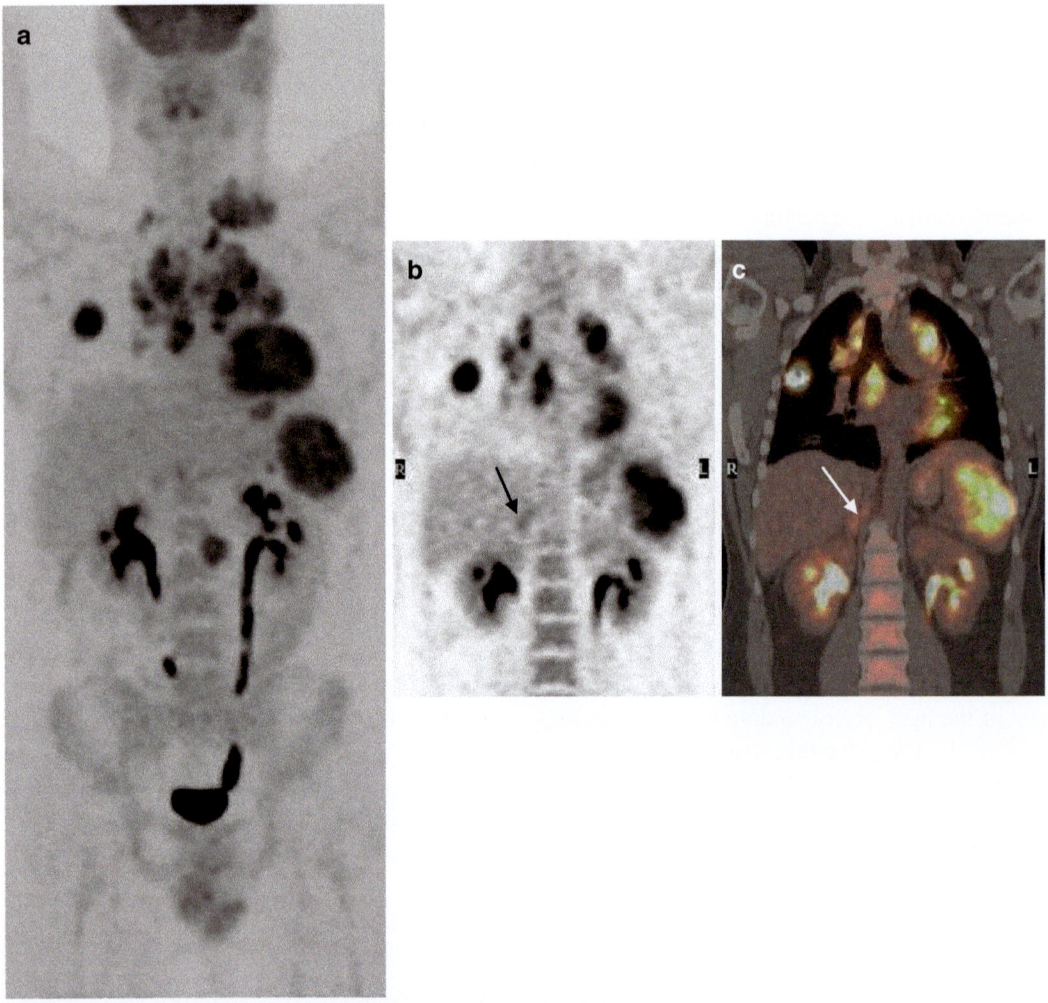

Fig. 6.20 (**a**–**c**) PET/CT staging revealed bilateral cervical/supraclavicular, mediastinal, right hilar, and para-aortic lymphadenopathy, multiple focal splenic lesions measuring 4–8 cm, and a right upper lobe lung lesion. (**a**) The right adrenal hypermetabolic lesion (**b**, **c** – *arrows*) was not evident in initial CT

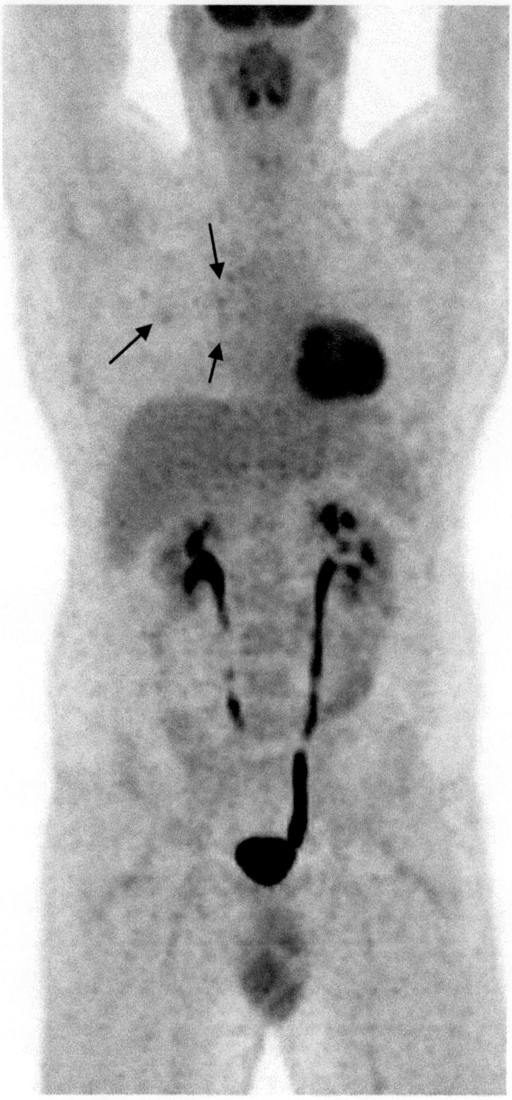

Fig. 6.21 Interim PET/CT was interpreted as negative, since residual FDG uptake was thought to be no greater than that of the liver, corresponding to D-5PS score 3 (*arrows*)

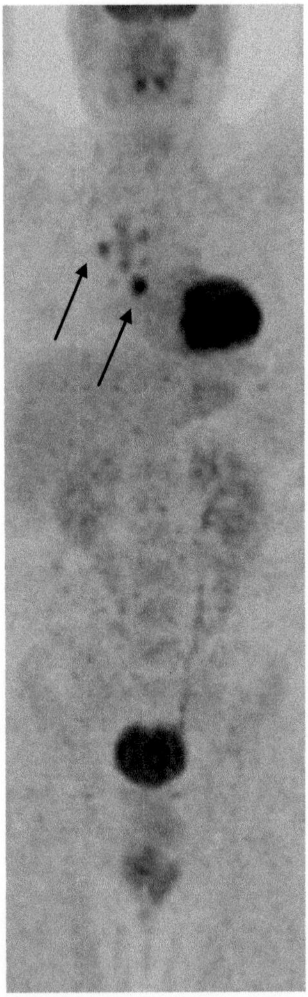

Fig. 6.22 PET/CT after ABVD therapy. PET/CT assessment at that point showed increased 18-FDG uptake (SUVmax 13) in mediastinal lymph nodes and a lung nodule of 2 cm diameter in the right upper lobe (*arrows*). The findings were graded as score 5 according to the D5-PS and the patient had progressive disease according to CT findings

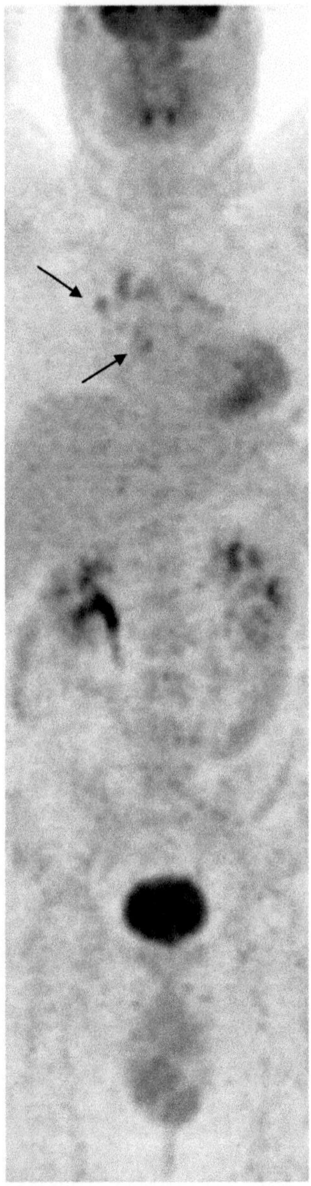

Fig. 6.23 PET/CT remained positive after IGEV salvage chemotherapy

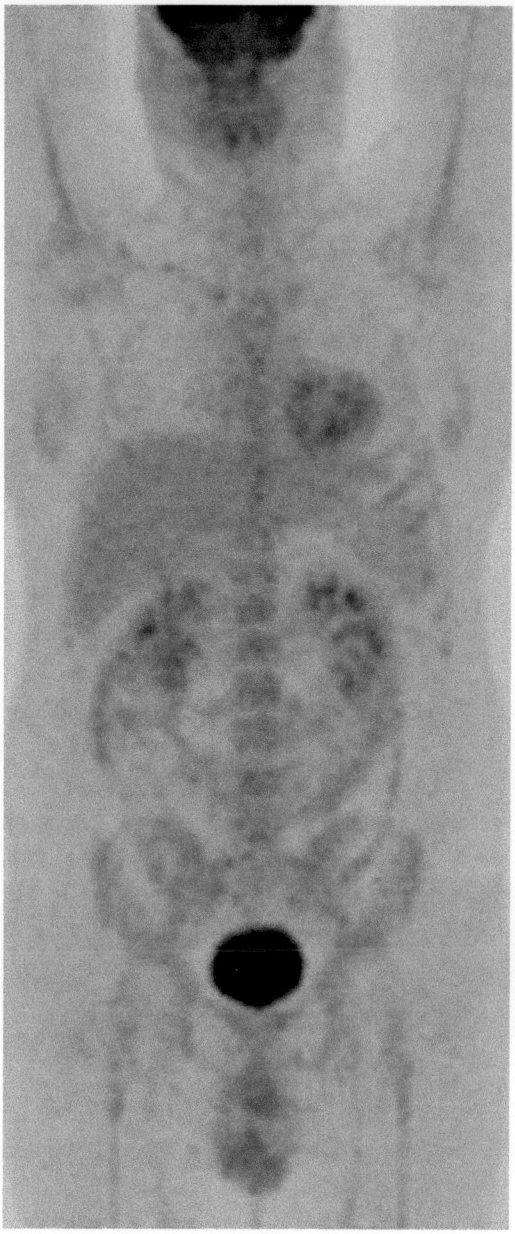

Fig. 6.24 PET/CT was normal 3 months after ASCT

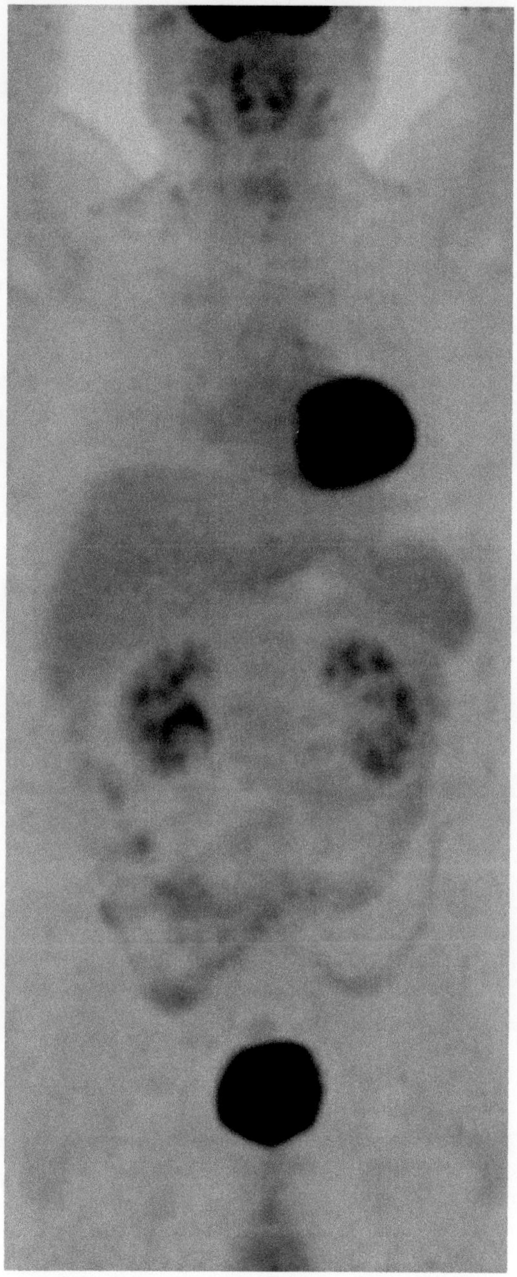

Fig. 6.25 PET/CT remained negative following subsequent RT

Hodgkin Lymphoma: Case 8

A 58-year-old man presented with extensive but small-sized (up to 2 cm) lymphadenopathy at the para-aortic and retrocrural area, porta hepatis, and hepatogastric junction, as well as mediastinal, bilateral hilar, and bilateral axillary lymphadenopathy up to 3 cm, and a focal right-sided pleural lesion discovered during medical evaluation for a short episode of fever. Left axillary lymph node biopsy revealed nodular sclerosing classical HL. Conventional clinical stage was IIIA. PET/CT staging confirmed the presence of hypermetabolic (SUVmax 14) lymphadenopathy above and below the diaphragm. It further revealed cervical and left external iliac lymphadenopathy (Fig. 6.26a – thin black arrows) as well as a single hypermetabolic focus (SUVmax 3) at the left iliac bone (anterior iliac crest) with no associated CT finding, consistent with bone marrow involvement (Fig. 6.26a–c – thick black and white arrows). The patient also had mild leukocytosis without lymphocytopenia, decreased serum albumin levels, elevated ESR (90 mm/h) and CRP, and normal LDH and β_2-microglobulin levels. The value of IPS was 3 (or 4 by PET staging).

Following 2 cycles of the ABVD regimen, an iPET/CT revealed an impressive response; however, persistent, abnormal 18-FDG uptake (SUVmax 4.5) was noted in a residual left axillary node. The uptake exceeded that of the liver corresponding to a Deauville 5-point scale score 4 (Fig. 6.27a, b). In response to this finding, chemotherapy was intensified to BEACOPP-escalated. After 6 cycles of intensive therapy, ePET converted to negative. The patient remains in complete remission 4 months later.

Discussion: In this case, PET/CT revealed a single focus of bone marrow involvement, which was not uncovered by trephine biopsy performed in the same iliac crest, since it was located at the anterior iliac crest, while bone marrow biopsies are obtained from the posterior one. A single focus is a rare pattern of PET/CT-detected bone marrow involvement [5, 6]. Following a positive interim PET, treatment was switched to BEACOPP-escalated, since there are data suggesting better outcomes with this approach compared with continued ABVD [37–39, 40, 43]. It should be noted that the decision for treatment intensification was made due to a single D-5PS score 4 finding and despite the turnoff of all other extensive lesions. In clinical practice, such impressive but not complete responses are frequently associated with reluctance of the treating physicians to change the chemotherapy regimen.

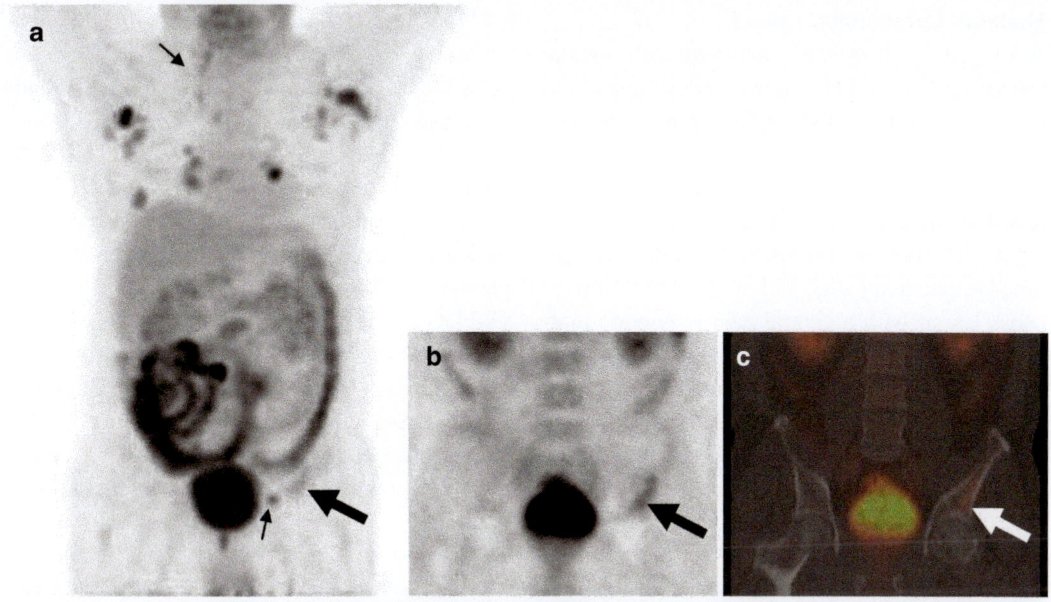

Fig. 6.26 (**a**–**c**) PET/CT staging confirmed the presence of hypermetabolic (SUVmax 14) lymphadenopathy above and below the diaphragm. Cervical and left external iliac lymphadenopathy, which had not been detected at conventional staging (**a** – *thin black arrows*) and a single hypermetabolic focus (SUVmax 3) at the left iliac bone (anterior iliac crest) with no associated CT finding, consistent with bone marrow involvement (**a**–**c** – *thick black* and *white arrows*) are further noted

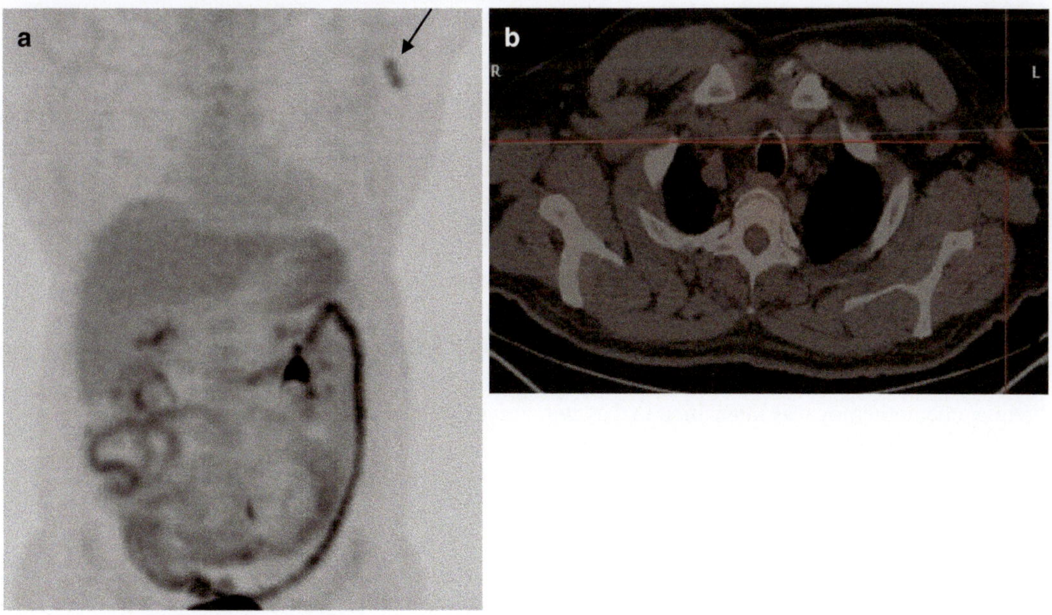

Fig. 6.27 (**a**, **b**) Interim PET/CT. Abnormal 18-FDG uptake (SUVmax 4.5) was noted in a residual left axillary node. The uptake exceeded that of the liver corresponding to a Deauville 5-point scale score 4

Hodgkin Lymphoma: Case 9

A 44-year-old man was diagnosed with nodular sclerosing classical HL after a right submandibular lymph node biopsy, which was performed during the evaluation of "psoas abscess" and prolonged fever. Full CT and MRI staging also revealed mediastinal lymphadenopathy, including a paraesophageal mass, para-aortic and right iliac lymphadenopathy, and an 8.2×5.0 cm right psoas lesion with a central cavity. A bone marrow biopsy was negative. Conventional clinical stage was IIIEA. PET/CT staging demonstrated even more extensive lymphadenopathy with abnormal 18-FDG uptake (SUVmax 12), confirmed the increased metabolic activity of the psoas lesion (SUVmax 8.7) in extension of right iliac lymph nodes (Fig. 6.28a, b), and also revealed a 1.3 cm hypermetabolic subcutaneous nodule of the right lower anterior pelvic wall (Fig. 6.28a – black arrow, c). PET resulted to upstage to stage IVB. The patient also had anemia, marked leukocytosis and lymphocytopenia (<8 %), markedly decreased serum albumin levels, highly elevated ESR (124 mm/h) and CRP (328 mg/L), and elevated LDH and β_2-microglobulin levels. The value of IPS based on conventional staging was 5.

Following 2 cycles of the ABVD regimen, an iPET/CT revealed persistent, abnormal 18-FDG uptake at two sites: the right psoas lesion, even more marked compared to baseline (SUVmax 10.7 vs. 8.7), and the paraesophageal lymph node with reduced intensity compared to baseline (SUVmax 5.3 vs. 12.3). Both markedly exceeded liver uptake, corresponding to a Deauville 5-point scale score 5 (Fig. 6.29a–c). In response to this finding, chemotherapy was intensified to 6 cycles of BEACOPP-escalated.

Final response assessment revealed a partial remission by conventional imaging with an 6.3×3.0 cm residual psoas lesion and persistently abnormal 18-FDG uptake on PET/CT (SUVmax 3.5) corresponding to D5-PS score 4 (Fig. 6.30a, b). At that point he received RT at a dose of 4800 cGy to the residual psoas lesion and right iliac and inguinal nodes. Approximately 3 months after the completion of RT a repeated PET/CT revealed faint 18-FDG uptake at the right psoas (SUVmax 2) just above the surrounding tissues (background), but not exceeding the uptake of the mediastinum (Fig. 6.31a–c). Psoas lesion also resolved on MRI performed 3 additional months later. The patient remains in remission 20 months after the completion of RT.

Discussion: A positive iPET/CT after ABVD x2 (D5-PS 4 or 5) predicts for a poor tumor control of only 30 % if ABVD is continued [29, 32]. Switch to BEACOPP-escalated may provide tumor control rates of 60–70 % in this setting [37–39, 40, 43]. Similar results can also be achieved by early IGEV salvage chemotherapy and ASCT [54]. Despite the acceptable tumor control with early treatment intensification, there is still no randomized evidence of survival benefit for this strategy. The present patient remained PET/CT-positive after BEACOPP-escalated as well with a single focus of D5-PS score 4, measuring >2.5 cm, having achieved a conventional PR. Such patients are effectively managed by RT if BEACOPP-escalated is the primary therapy, with tumor control rates >80 % [18]. This strategy was followed in this particular case, although the patient under consideration potentially had a less favorable prognosis, because he had been negatively selected for BEACOPP-escalated following iPET positivity after ABVD x2.

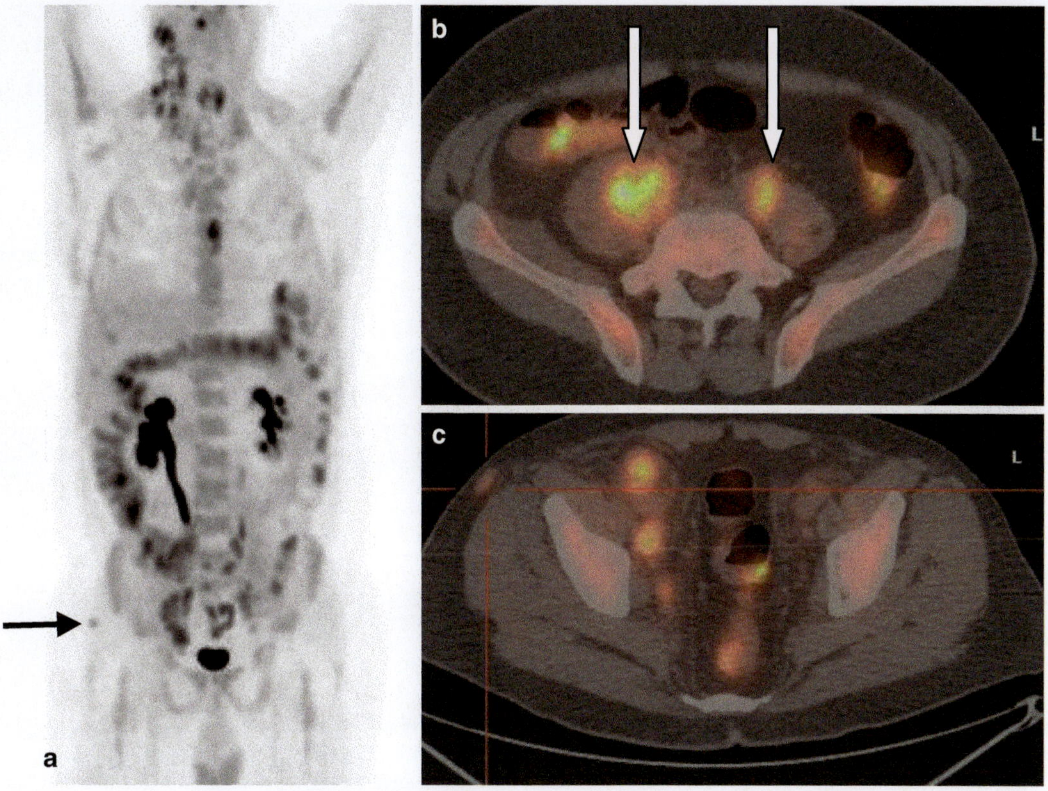

Fig. 6.28 (**a**–**c**) PET/CT staging demonstrated extensive lymphadenopathy with abnormal 18-FDG uptake (SUVmax 12) and increased metabolic activity of the psoas lesion (SUVmax 8.7) in extension of right iliac lymph nodes (**b** – *white arrows*). It also revealed a 1.3 cm hypermetabolic subcutaneous nodule of the right lower anterior pelvic wall (**a**, *black arrow*; **c**, *red cross*)

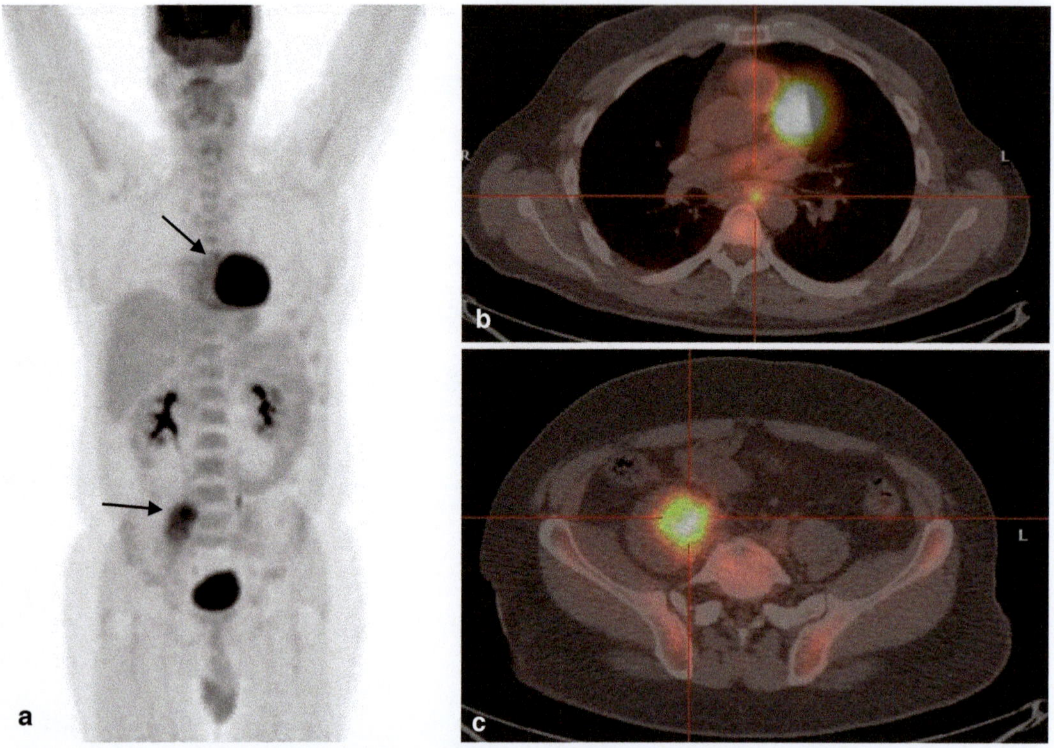

Fig. 6.29 (**a**–**c**) Interim PET/CT revealed persistent, abnormal 18-FDG uptake at two sites: the right psoas lesion, even more marked compared to baseline (SUVmax 10.7 vs 8.7) (**a**, *lower black arrow*, and **c**, *red cross*), and the paraesophageal lymph node with reduced intensity compared to baseline (SUVmax 5.3 vs. 12.3) (**a**, *black arrow,* and **b**, *red cross*)

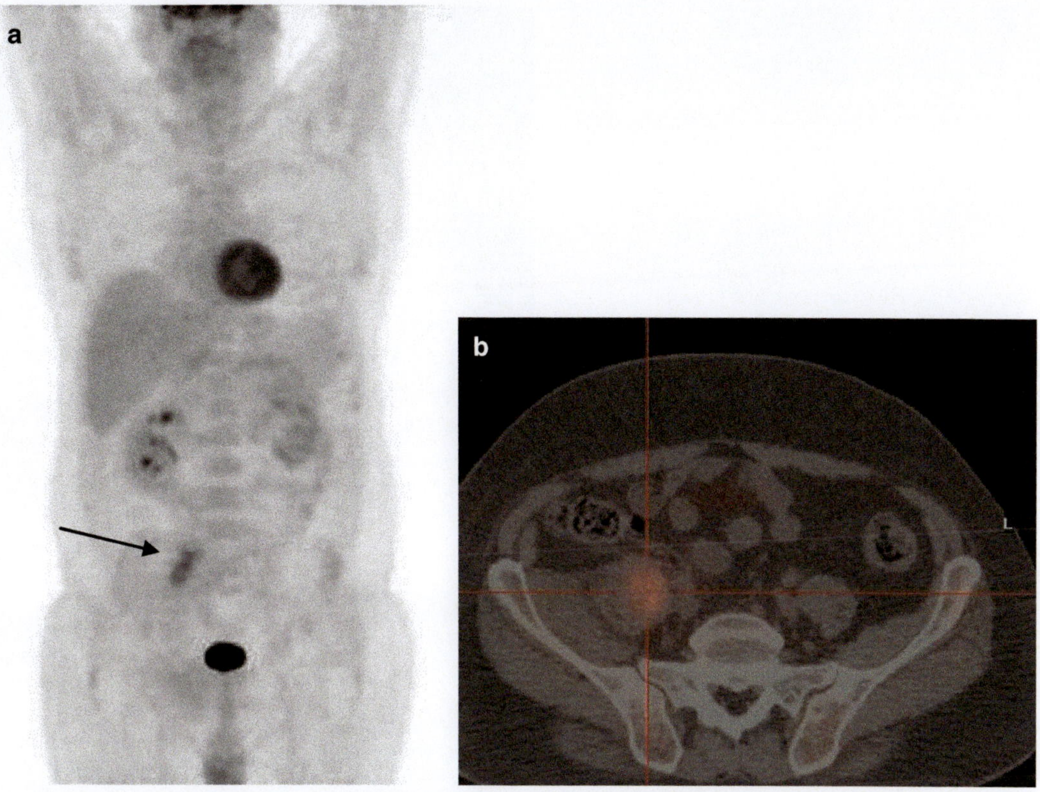

Fig. 6.30 (**a**, **b**) PET/CT final response assessment revealed a partial remission by conventional imaging with a 6.3 × 3.0 cm residual psoas lesion and persistently abnormal 18-FDG uptake on PET/CT (SUVmax 3.5) corresponding to D5-PS score 4

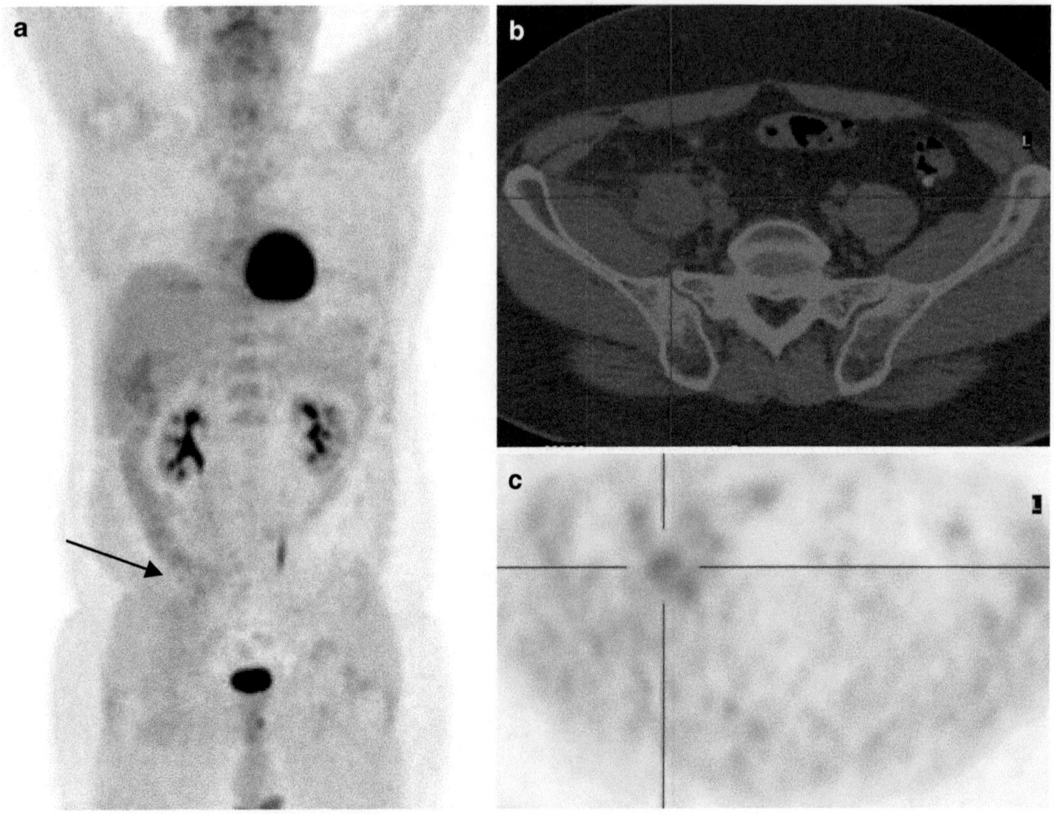

Fig. 6.31 (**a**–**c**) PET/CT approximately 3 months after the completion of RT revealed faint 18-FDG uptake at the right psoas (SUVmax 2) just above the surrounding tissues (background), but not exceeding the uptake of the mediastinum, corresponding to a D5-PS score of 2 (**a**–**c**)

Hodgkin Lymphoma: Case 10

A 20-year-old woman presented with fever up to 39.5 °C, drenching night sweats, and a very bulky (15 cm) mediastinal mass associated with pericardial thickening. A 2 cm right epiphrenic node and an 1.5 cm right lung nodule were also evident on CT. Biopsy of a small supraclavicular node revealed nodular sclerosing classical HL. A bone marrow biopsy was negative. Clinical stage was IIXEB, and the patient was classified as advanced stage based on the German Hodgkin Study Group scheme. PET/CT staging confirmed the above findings, revealing increased 18-FDG uptake (SUVmax 9) in the already known lesions, including mediastinal and right epiphrenic nodes (Fig. 6.32a) as well as the right lung nodule (SUVmax 4) (Fig. 6.32b). The patient had also severe anemia and lymphocytopenia (<8 %), markedly decreased serum albumin levels, highly elevated ESR (151 mm/h) and CRP (305 mg/L), and normal LDH and β_2-microglobulin levels. The value of IPS was 3.

Following 2 cycles of the ABVD regimen, an iPET/CT revealed persistently increased 18-FDG uptake (SUVmax 5) in the residual 11 cm mediastinal mass. The uptake moderately exceeded that of the liver, corresponding to a Deauville 5-point scale score 4 (Fig. 6.33). In response to this finding, chemotherapy was intensified to 6 cycles of BEACOPP-escalated. Final response assessment revealed a partial remission by conventional imaging with a 7 cm residual mediastinal lesion and persistently abnormal 18-FDG uptake (SUV max 5) on PET/CT corresponding to a D5-PS score 4 (Fig. 6.34). At that point she received involved-field RT at a dose of 4320 cGy. Despite further shrinkage of the irradiated lesions, the patient progressed 3 months after the completion of RT.

A new PET/CT revealed new multiple hypermetabolic lung nodules (SUVmax 4) and a left paracardial-epiphrenic mass (SUVmax 7), while the uptake at the residual original mediastinal mass was milder (SUVmax 4) (Fig. 6.35a–c). Subsequently, the patient received IGEV and ESHAP salvage chemotherapy without any benefit (progressive disease). Fortunately, she responded partially to 3 cycles of brentuximab vedotin and was forwarded to BEAM high-dose therapy and ASCT. Three months later she developed again progressive disease with new lung nodules and new findings in right hilar and left peribronchial nodes (Fig. 6.36a–c). She received again brentuximab vedotin with a good response. After 7 cycles, a very good partial remission has been achieved with only a single lung nodule. The patient is evaluated for potential allogeneic stem cell transplant from an unrelated donor.

Discussion: Following a positive iPET/CT after ABVD x2 (D5-PS 4 or 5), switch to BEACOPP-escalated may provide tumor control rates of 60–70 % [37–39, 40, 43]. Unfortunately, 30–40 % still develop progressive disease even after early intensification, as occurred in this case. The patient proved totally refractory to RT and 2 lines of salvage chemotherapy but responded to brentuximab vedotin [51, 52], so that ASCT became feasible. Persistent PET positivity prior to ASCT is associated with worse outcomes in chemosensitive patients, but does not render ASCT futile, since long-term remission rates up to 40–45 % can still be achieved [50]. However, in this case, further progression developed soon after ASCT, but responded again to brentuximab vedotin.

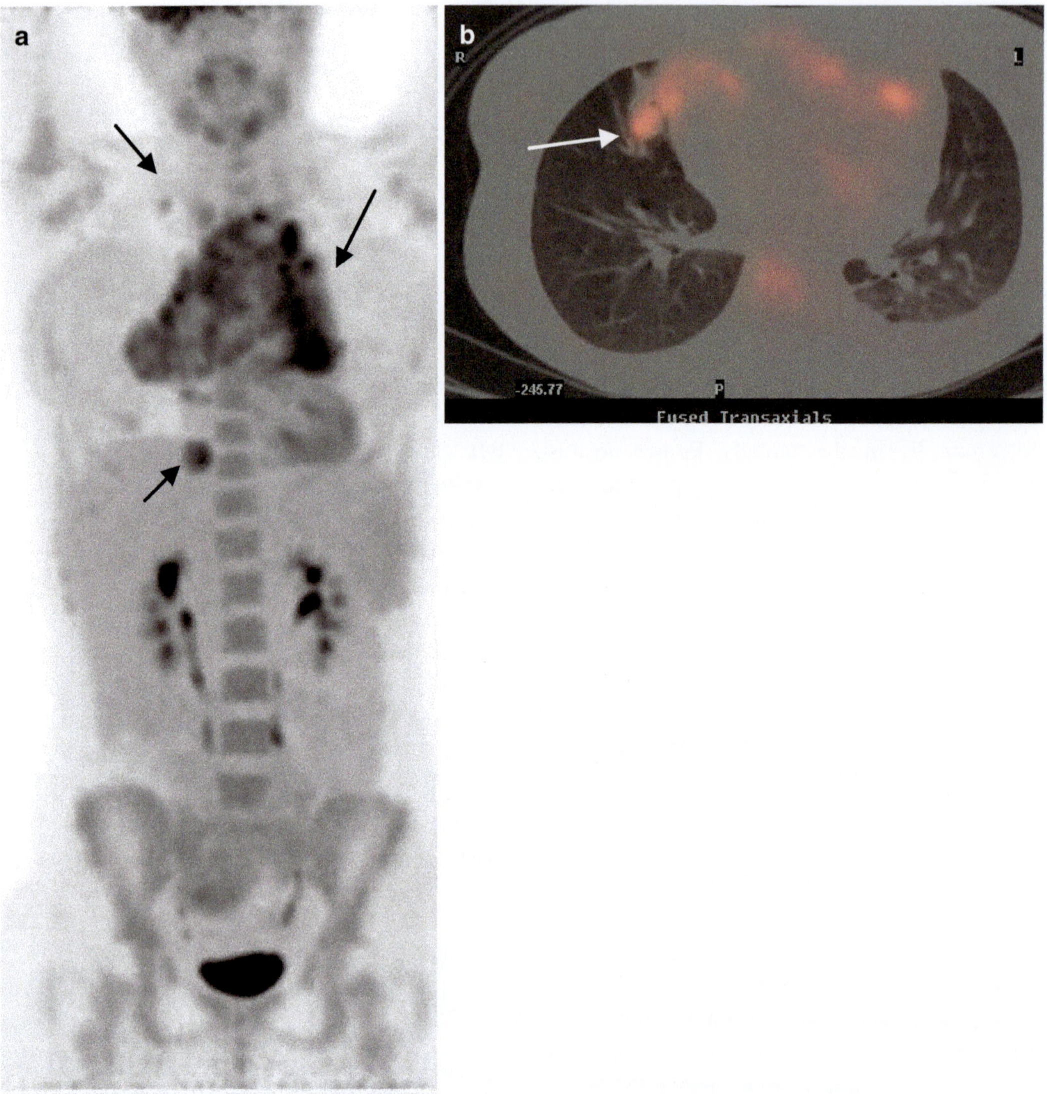

Fig. 6.32 (**a**, **b**) PET/CT staging revealed increased 18-FDG uptake (SUVmax 9) at the mediastinum and right epiphrenic area (**a** – *black arrows*) but also demonstrated abnormal 18-FDG uptake (SUVmax 4) in a 1.5 cm lung nodule at the right middle lobe (**b** – *white arrow*)

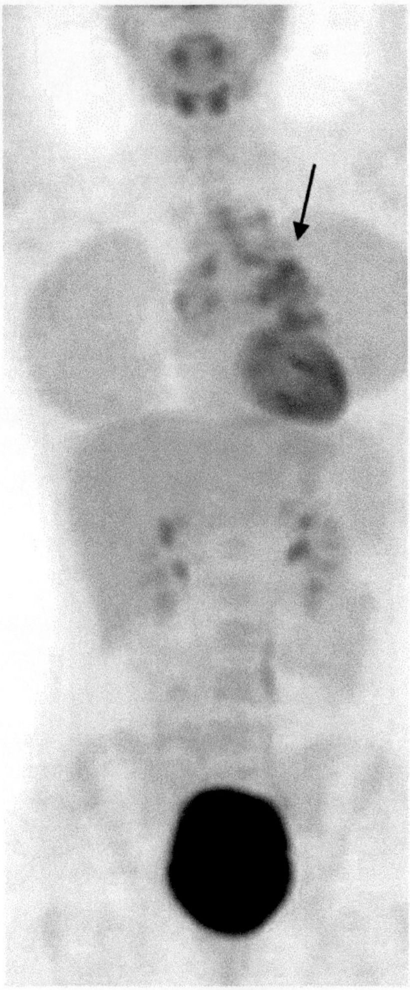

Fig. 6.33 Interim PET/CT revealed persistently increased 18-FDG uptake (SUVmax 5) in the residual 11 cm mediastinal mass. The uptake moderately exceeded that of the liver, corresponding to a D5-PS score 4

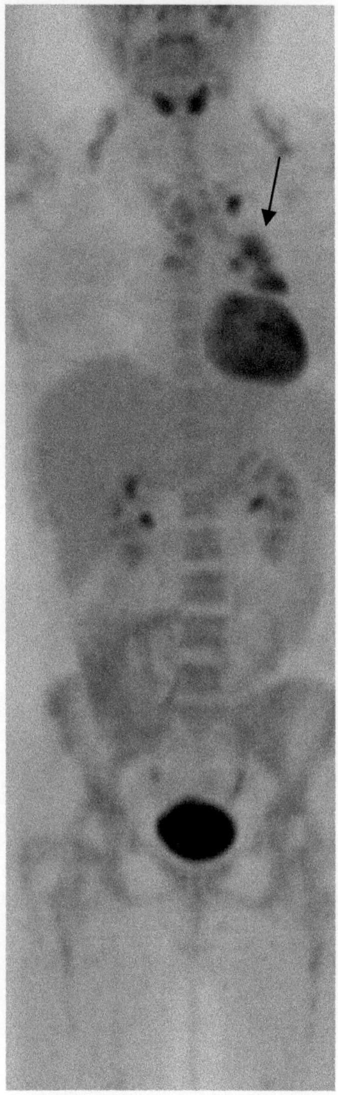

Fig. 6.34 PET/CT after 6 cycles of BEACOPP-escalated. Final response assessment revealed a 7 cm residual mediastinal lesion with persistent abnormal 18-FDG uptake (SUV max 5) on PET/CT, corresponding to a D5-PS score 4

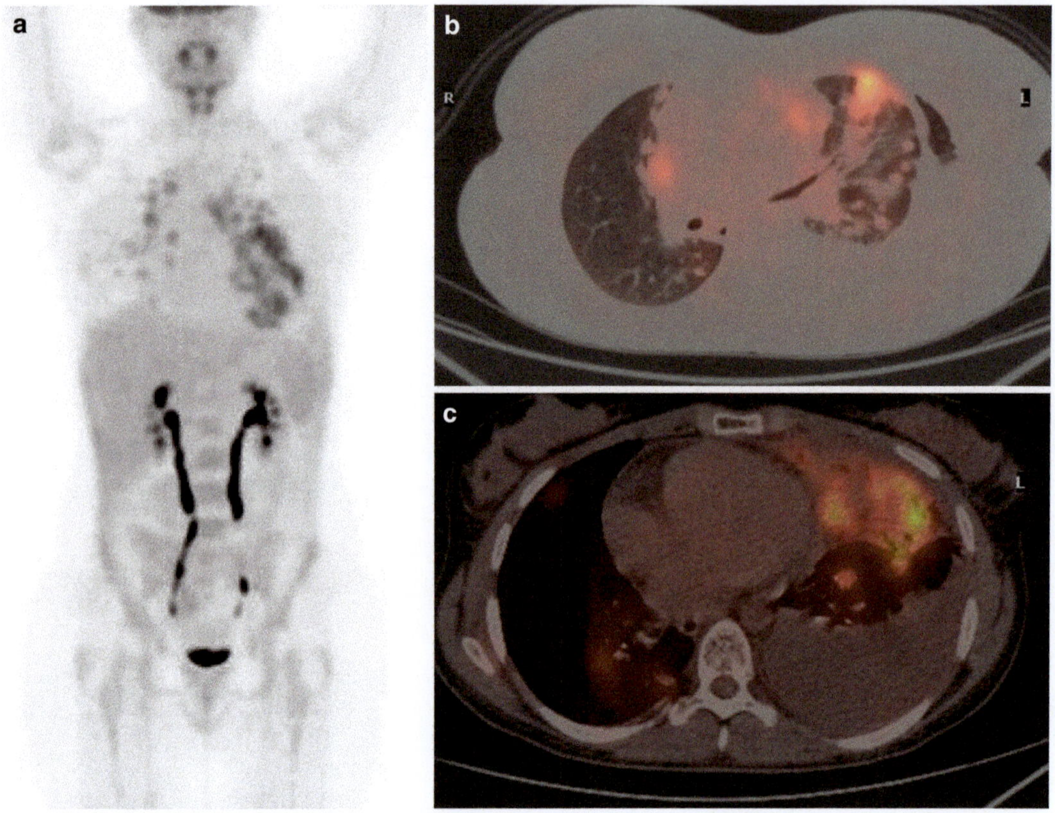

Fig. 6.35 (**a**–**c**) PET/CT 3 months after the completion of RT revealed new multiple hypermetabolic lung nodules bilaterally (SUVmax 4) (**a** and **b**) and a left paracardial-epiphrenic mass (SUVmax 7) (**c**), while the uptake at the residual original mediastinal mass was milder (SUVmax 4) (**a**)

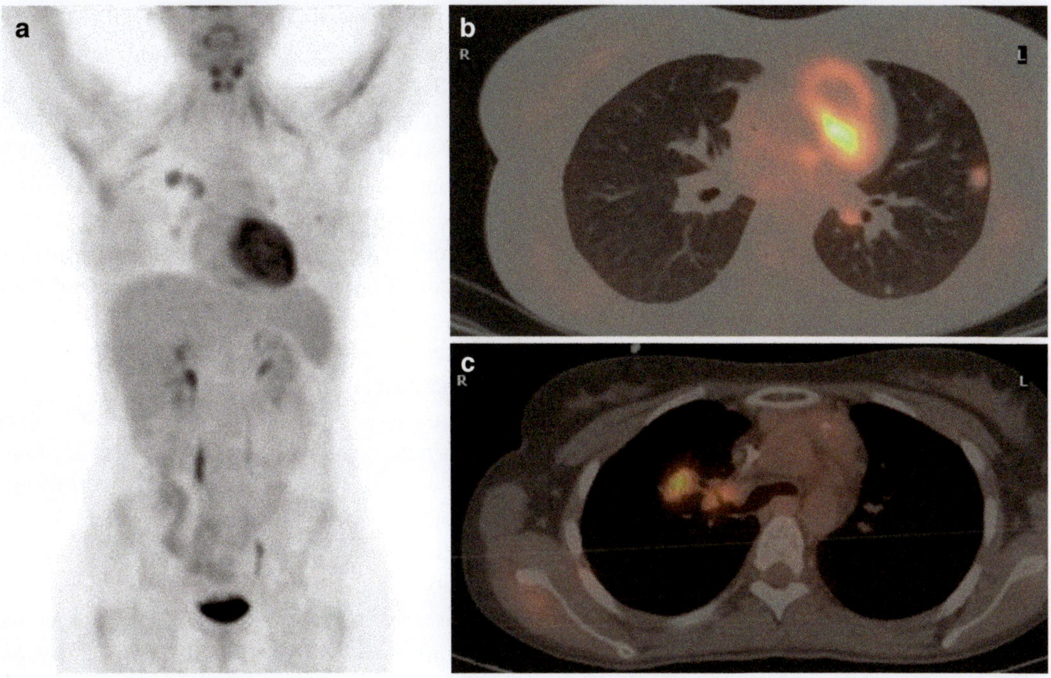

Fig. 6.36 (**a**–**c**) PET/CT three months later after BEAM high-dose therapy and ASCT revealed progressive disease with new lung nodules and new findings in right hilar and left peribronchial nodes (**a**–**c**)

Hodgkin Lymphoma: Case 11

A 27-year-old male patient presented with night sweats, fever, and bilateral supraclavicular lymphadenopathy. Lymph node biopsy showed: Hodgkin lymphoma, nodular sclerosis.

Conventional staging showed supraclavicular and mediastinal lymphadenopathy (nodal disease above the diaphragm): stage IIB.

The value of the IPS was 1 (27 years old, male, stage IIB, Hb 16.1 g/dL, serum albumin 4 g/dL, WBC 14,320/μL lymphocytes 10 %, absolute lymphocyte count 1432/μL).

Bone marrow biopsy showed no infiltration. Thus, the patient had early-stage HL with unfavourable prognostic factors (IIB plus ≥ 3 sites).

Baseline PET/CT showed extensive mediastinal (SUVmax 11), supraclavicular, and infraclavicular nodal disease (SUVmax 8) and hypermetabolic nodes along the right internal mammary vessels (SUVmax 6.2) (Fig. 6.37).

The patient received 2 cycles of ABVD chemotherapy, and an iPET/CT was performed showing complete resolution of the FDG uptake by all nodes except two retrosternal lymph nodes in the upper mediastinum having SUVmax 4.6 (versus of 9 at baseline PET/CT) and 2.4 (D5-PS score 4) (Fig. 6.38).

The patient received 2 additional ABVD cycles. A follow-up PET/CT was performed showing persistence of the FDG uptake by the same two mediastinal lymph nodes with SUVmax 3.4 instead of 4.6 and 2.9 instead of 2.4 with D5-PS score 4 (Fig. 6.39).

In response to the above findings, the patient received intensive chemotherapy with BEACOPP-escalated. After one cycle the patient developed severe chest pain and elevation of cardiac enzymes. Treatment was withheld until his cardiac condition was stabilized (the diffential diagnosis included coronary spasm that led to myocardial ischemia vs. myocarditis). A PET/CT was performed after his stabilization and prior to initiating therapy revealing increased FDG uptake by a single lymph node in front of the ascending aorta with SUVmax 3.4 (Deauville 4), together with a hypermetabolic focus in the left 3rd rib (SUVmax 4.8) (Fig. 6.40). Further evaluation of the thoracic wall by CT scan and MRI revealed no disease infiltration, and the increase in the FDG uptake by the focus in the rib was attributed to G-CSF (hypermetabolic bone marrow).

With a positive PET/CT scan, 5-PS 4, and cardiac toxicity, de-escalation of therapy was performed, and the patient received 2 cycles of BEACOPP-baseline. A new PET/CT was performed showing persistence of the hypermatabolic lymph node in front of the ascending aorta, albeit at a lower level (D5-PS score 3) and disappearance of the hypermetabolic bone focus in the rib.

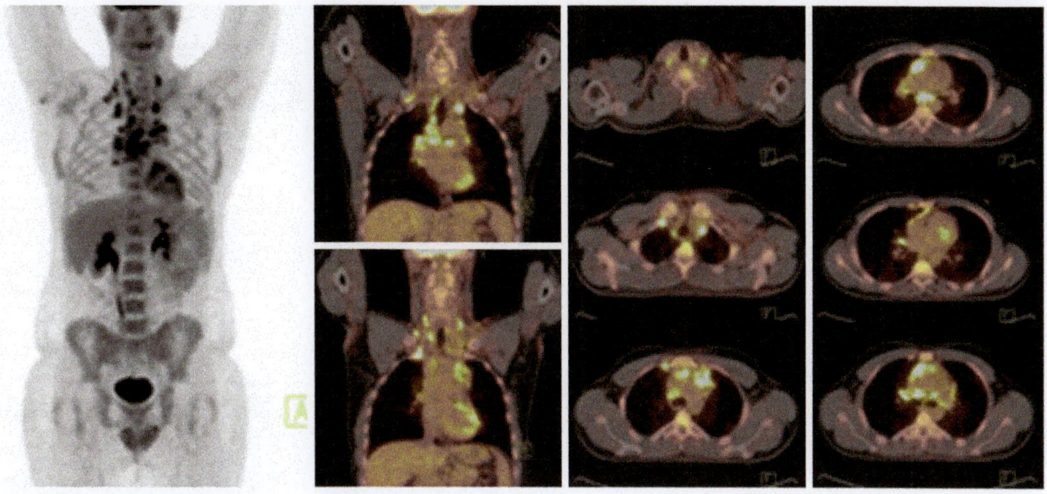

Fig. 6.37 Initial staging PET/CT: hypermetabolic lymph nodes at the supraclavicular area; at the paratracheal, prevascular, precarinal, and infracarinal space; at the right pulmonary hilum; and along the right internal mammary vessels (SUVmax 11)

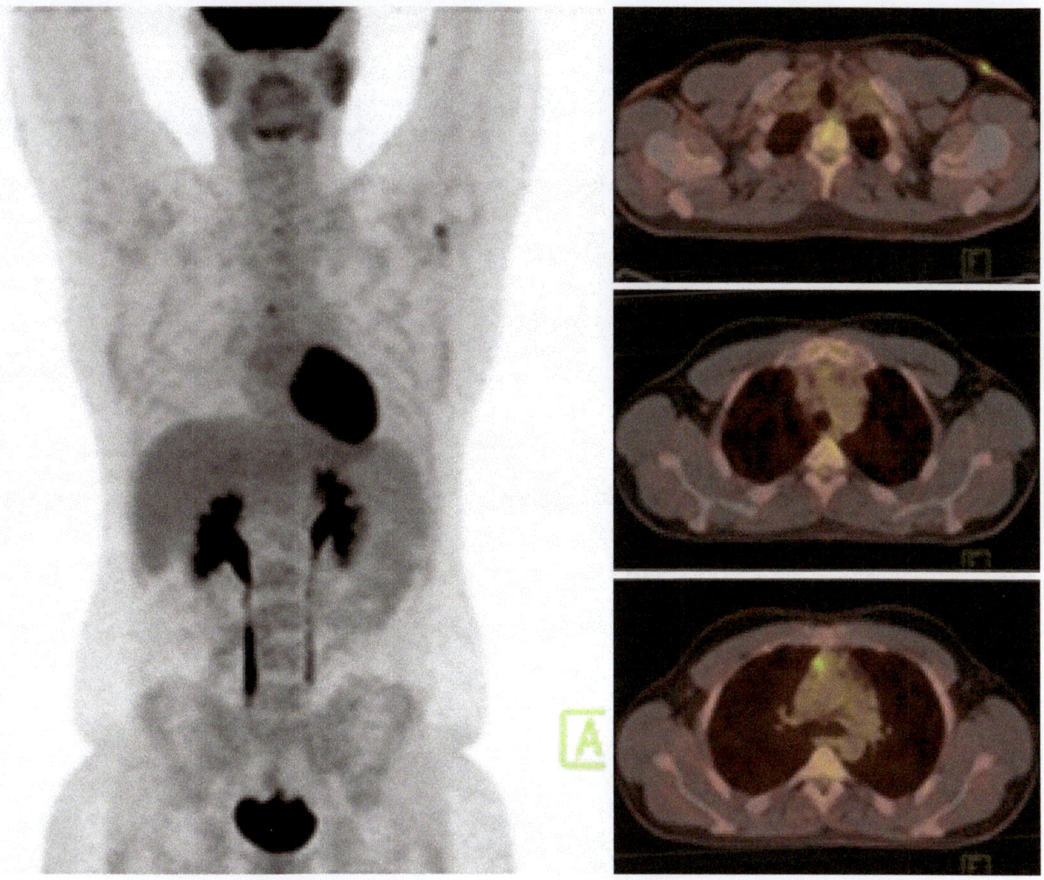

Fig. 6.38 Interim PET/CT: after 2 cycles of ABVD major improvement was achieved, without however a complete metabolic response. Residual hypermetabolic lymph node at the mediastinum (SUVmax 4.6) corresponding to a D5-PS score of 4. Note the finding located at the left axilla (*left figure*), which appears to be a cutaneous lesion (*right, upper figure*) not related to lymphoma

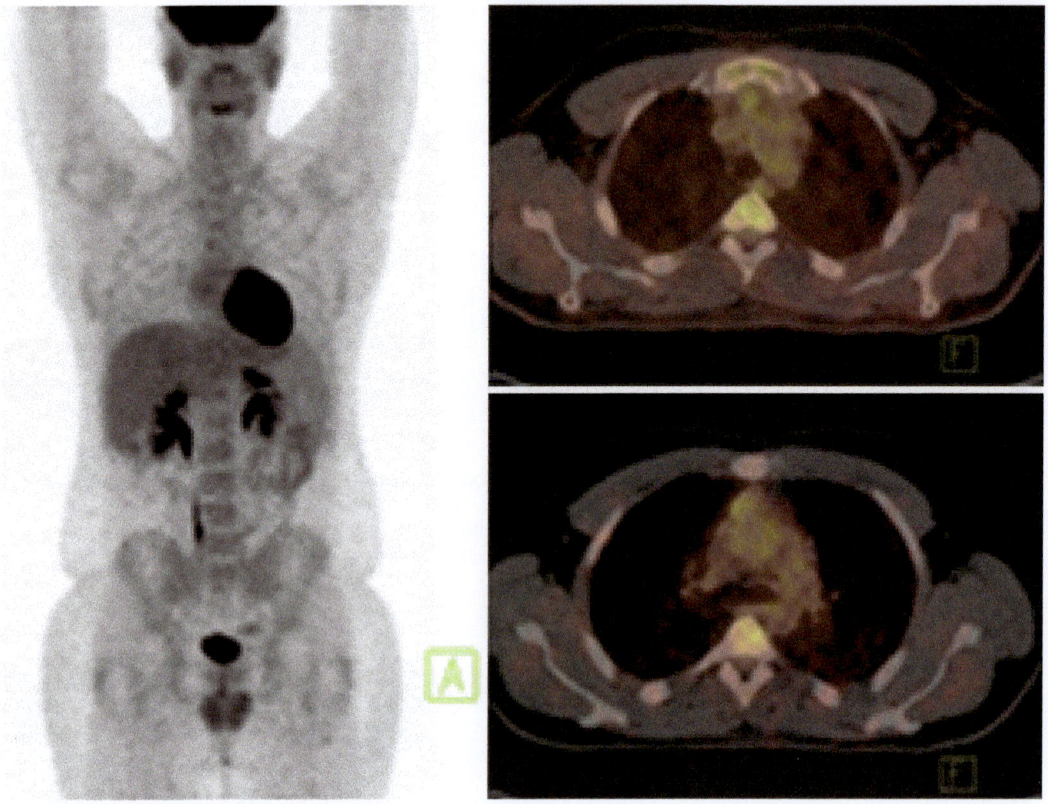

Fig. 6.39 Follow-up PET/CT: two residual hypermetabolic lymph nodes at the upper mediastinum (SUVmax 2.9 and 3.4, respectively), interpreted as D5-PS score 4)

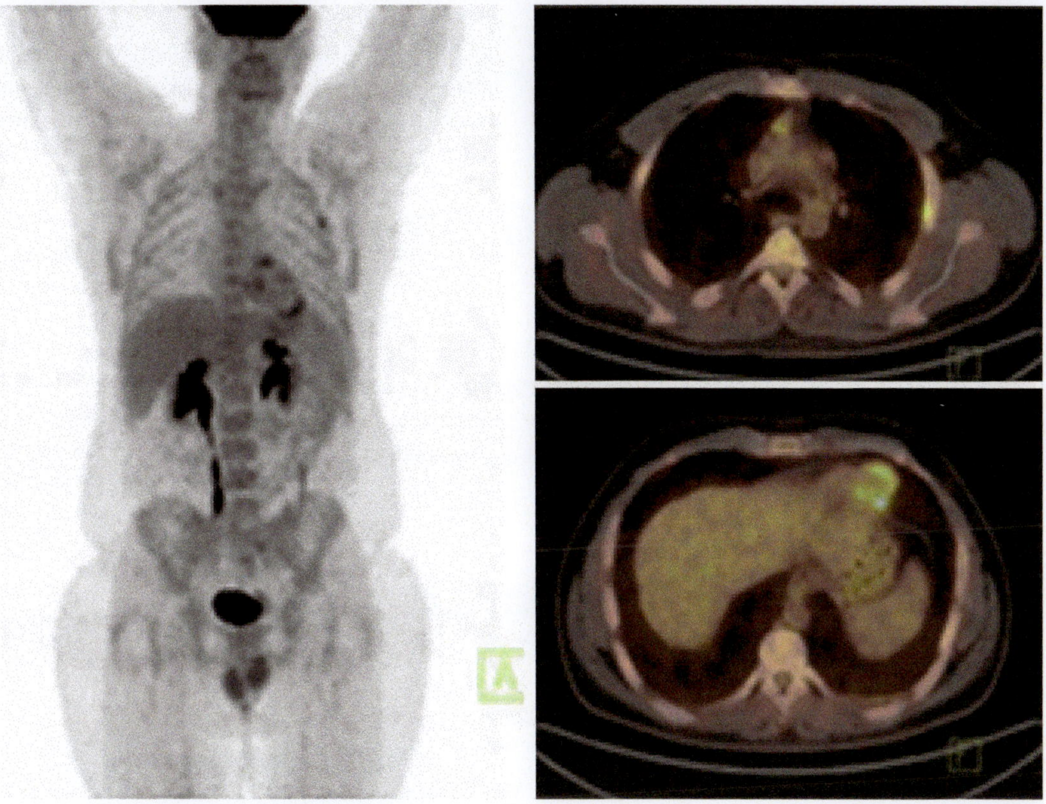

Fig. 6.40 PET/CT post one cycle of BEACOPP-escalated: residual node at the upper mediastinum (D5-PS score 4) and focal increase in FDG uptake at the left 3rd rib

As his cardiac condition was stable with no scarring of the myocardium, and as the patient was not deemed eligible for IFRT, the patient received 1 more cycle of BEACOPP-baseline and 2 cycles of BEACOPP-escalated.

A final PET/CT was done showing no residual disease and complete resolution of the FDG uptake by all lymph nodes.

Discussion: In this case, iPET was positive with a D5-PS score 4. ABVD chemotherapy was continued for 2 additional cycles. A repeated PET/CT was performed after the 4th ABVD cycle, in which positivity persisted with a D5-PS 4. At that point, treatment intensification based on BEACOPP was decided. After 6 cycles, the patient achieved a complete metabolic response.

As stated in the recent response evaluation recommendations, published by Cheson et al [1], a D5-PS score of 4 or 5 at interim PET is classified as partial metabolic response, suggesting chemosensitive (responding) disease, provided that FDG uptake has reduced from baseline. At the end of treatment, a D5-PS score of 4 or 5 with residual masses of any size is again classified as partial metabolic response, but suggests treatment failure, indicating the presence of residual disease, even if FDG uptake has reduced from baseline. If the D5-PS is 4 or 5 and the intensity of FDG uptake has not changed from baseline or has increased and/or new foci compatible with lymphoma have appeared, the case is classified as treatment failure (stable disease and progressive disease respectively), both at the interim and the end-of-treatment setting.

In patients with partial metabolic response after ABVD x2, BEACOPP-based approaches provide very good PFS rates both in localized (mainly intermediate stages; unpublished data from the H10 EORTC trial, presented in the 2015 ICML Lugano Meeting), and advanced stages (also including some intermediate ones) [37, 43, 55], as occurred in this patient.

Hodgkin Lymphoma: Case 12

A 32-year-old patient with HL, nodular sclerosis, stage II was referred for PET/CT examination for initial staging. FDG-PET/CT revealed hypermetabolic lymph nodes at the neck, supra- and infraclavicular area, and mediastinum (Fig. 6.41). The patient was referred for interim FDG-PET/CT examination, after 2 cycles of ABVD, which was negative for residual disease at the above described sites. The patient received 4 additional cycles of ABVD, as well as RT of the neck, clavicular region, and mediastinum, and was referred for end-of-treatment FDG-PET/CT examination. FDG-PET/CT examination was negative for hypermetabolic supradiaphragmatic lesions (Fig. 6.42). However, a small focal uptake at the dolichosigmoid was noted (Fig. 6.42) both in standard (1 h after FDG administration, SUVmax 6.53) and delayed acquisition (2 h after FDG administration, SUVmax 10). Therefore further endoscopic evaluation was recommended. Colonoscopy revealed a polypoid lesion which was excised. Biopsy was consistent with adenocarcinoma of the sigmoid.

Discussion: FDG uptake at the large and -in a lesser degree- in the small intestine is a common finding, usually diffuse and often nonspecific. It is commonly attributed to physiological radiopharmaceutical concentration and excretion through the gastrointestinal system. Attention should be paid when FDG concentration at the intestine is focal. Incidental colonic focal FDG uptake during PET/CT examination for other non-colon-related diseases occurs in 1.3–3.4 % of patients [56]. It has been reported that ~61 % of focal FDG uptake at the colon actually corresponds to finding in colonoscopy [57], with a PPV of colon cancer of ~42 % [58]. Correlation of FDG avidity with malignancy is reported higher, and colonoscopy should not be delayed when SUV is higher than 11 [56]. Delayed acquisition may be helpful in order to both discriminate if focal FDG uptake is due to physiological excretion or inflammation and to direct for further clinical and laboratory assessment.

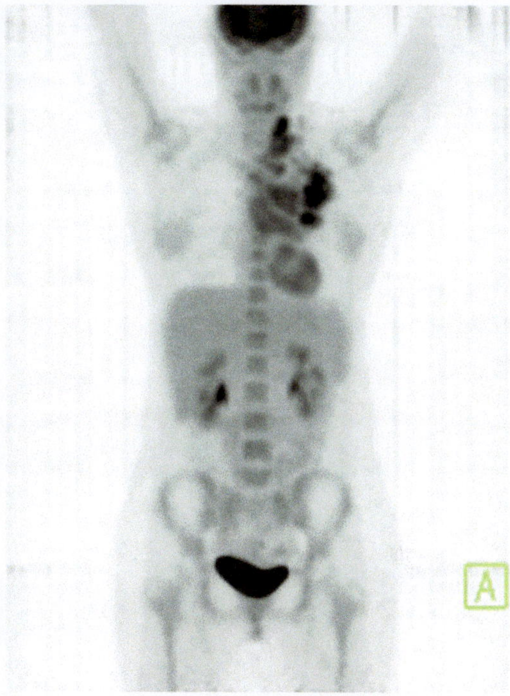

Fig. 6.41 Initial staging PET/CT: hypermetabolic supradiaphragmatic lymph nodes

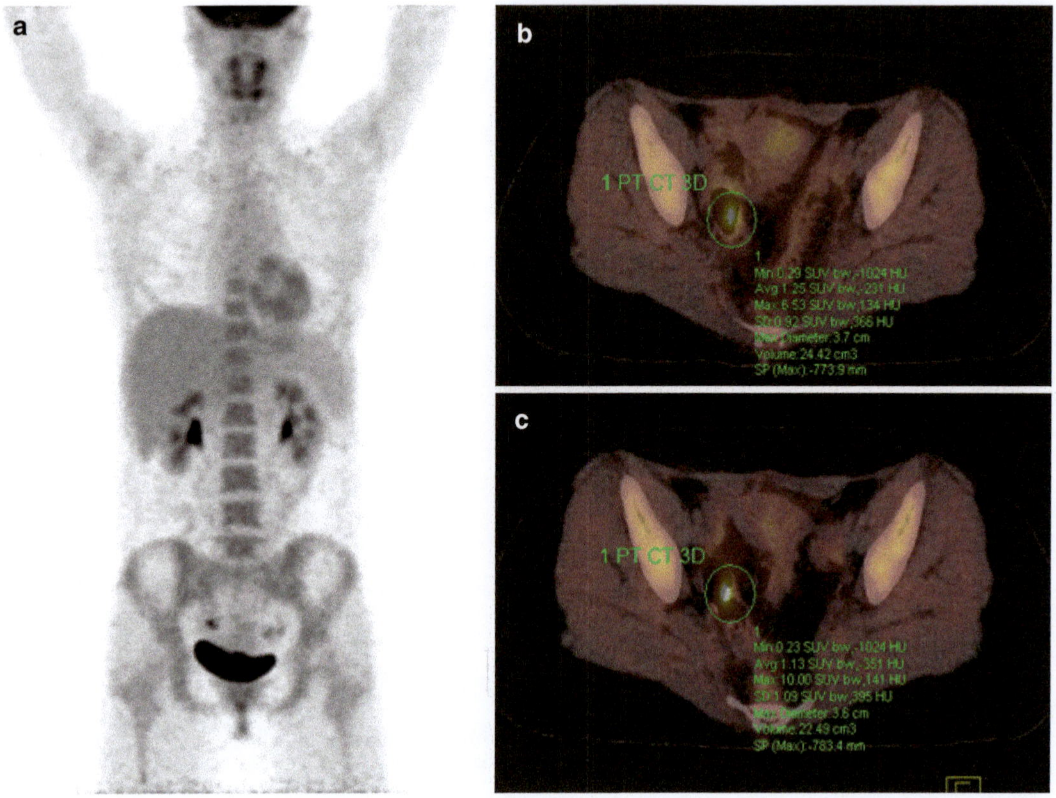

Fig. 6.42 MIP-PET (**a**), PET/CT standard (**b**), and delayed (**c**) acquisition reveal hypermetabolic focus at the dolichosigmoid. SUVmax further increases in delayed acquisition

Hodgkin Lymphoma: Case 13

A 38-year-old woman presented with a 2.5 cm left supraclavicular enlargement. Nodular sclerosing HL was diagnosed after excisional biopsy. Full CT staging also revealed a 2.8×1.5 cm mediastinal lymph node. Full blood counts and serum chemistry were within normal limits and a bone marrow biopsy was negative. Conventional clinical stage was IIA without risk factors, falling into the early favorable subgroup. PET/CT staging, performed after the initial biopsy, was positive at the mediastinum and left lung hilum (SUVmax 6.8) (Fig. 6.43a, b) but also revealed increased FDG uptake at splenic hilar nodes (SUVmax 3.2) and three vertebrae (T7, T11, L3 with SUVmax 3.2) without relevant CT findings (Fig. 6.43c, d).

Following 2 cycles of the ABVD regimen, an iPET/CT was negative, with mild uptake in the mediastinum (D-5PS score 3; Fig. 6.44). However, after 6 cycles of ABVD, final PET assessment converted to positive at the mediastinum (Fig. 6.45). Progressive disease was confirmed by CT, since the mediastinal lesion increased in size compared to mid-treatment nadir.

The patient received 44Gy salvage RT. Upon restaging, 3 months later, the patient achieved a radiographic complete remission, but mild new findings emerged on PET/CT, including a left lung hilar node, a deeply lying right inguinal node, and a left femur bone lesion, all with SUVmax of 2.6–3.4 (Fig. 6.46a, b).

One year later, the patient developed new supraclavicular nodes, and relapsing disease was histologically confirmed. She was treated with IGEV salvage chemotherapy with conventional radiographic CR but persistence of low- to moderate-grade PET positivity at subcarinal and right hilar nodes (SUVmax 2.2 and 3.5 and 7.4; Fig. 6.47). The patient underwent high-dose therapy with BEAM as conditioning regimen and autologous stem cell support. She denied further PET-based evaluation and remains in clinical and conventional radiographic remission 22 months post-ASCT.

Discussion: PET/CT upstages ~20 % of patients with HL [1–4]. In this case, upstaging was totally unexpected, since the patient appeared to have early favorable supradiaphragmatic disease, but PET/CT demonstrated latent disease at splenic hilar nodes and 3 spinal bone marrow foci. PET/CT reveals >2 times more cases of bone marrow involvement, as in this case, in which bone marrow biopsy was negative, since the iliac crests were spared [5, 6]. However, the prognosis of patients with PET-based or histologically confirmed bone marrow involvement appears to be similar, being inferior to other cases without involved bone marrow [5, 6]. Interestingly, interim PET provided a false-negative result in this case, which might be partially justified by the baseline stage IV classification due to extranodal disease, which could probably be associated with a lower negative predictive value [38, 40, 42, 43]. Finally, a positive PET/CT prior to ASCT does not preclude a favorable outcome if there is no progressive disease by conventional staging [50], although the rather short follow-up cannot exclude a future relapse in this specific case.

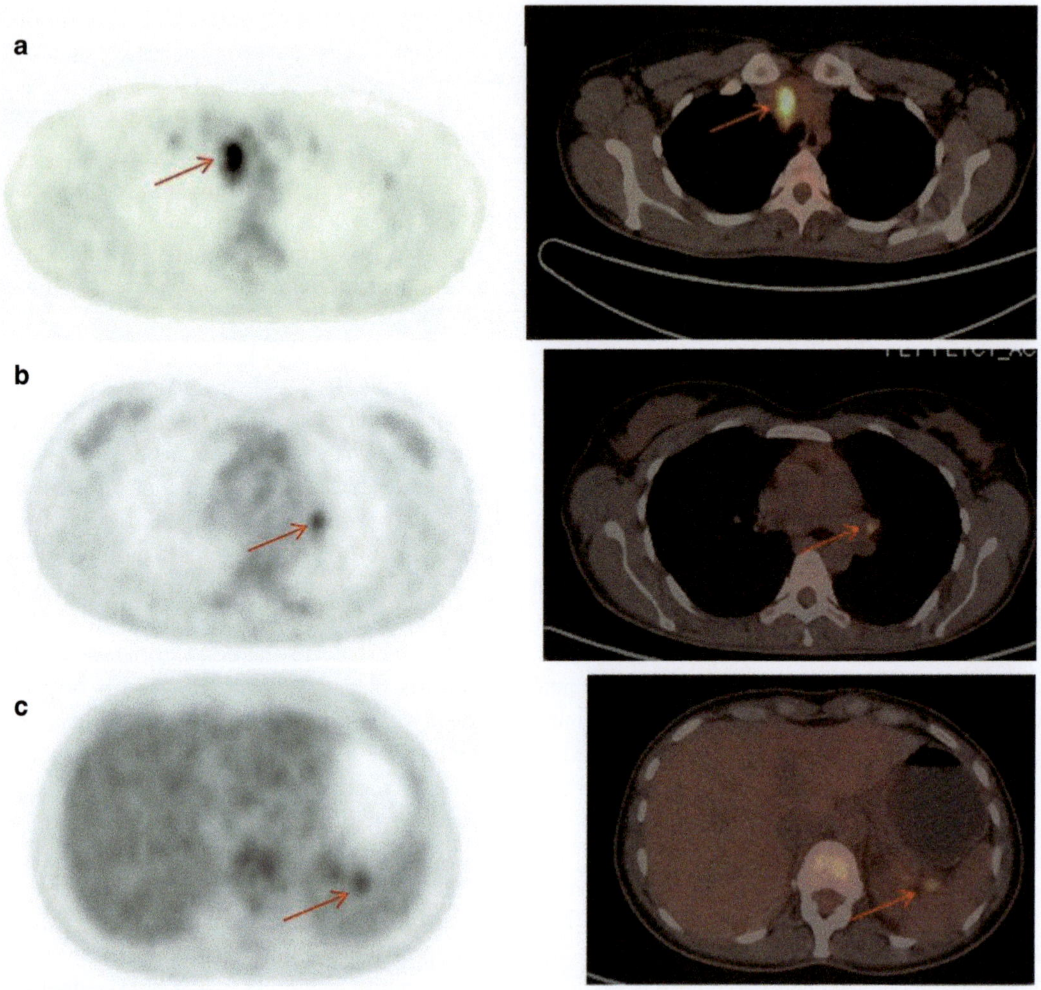

Fig. 6.43 (**a–d**) PET/CT staging. Hypermetabolic lesions at the anterior mediastinum (**a**), left hilar lymph node (**b**), splenic hilar nodes (**c**), T11 vertebra (**d**)

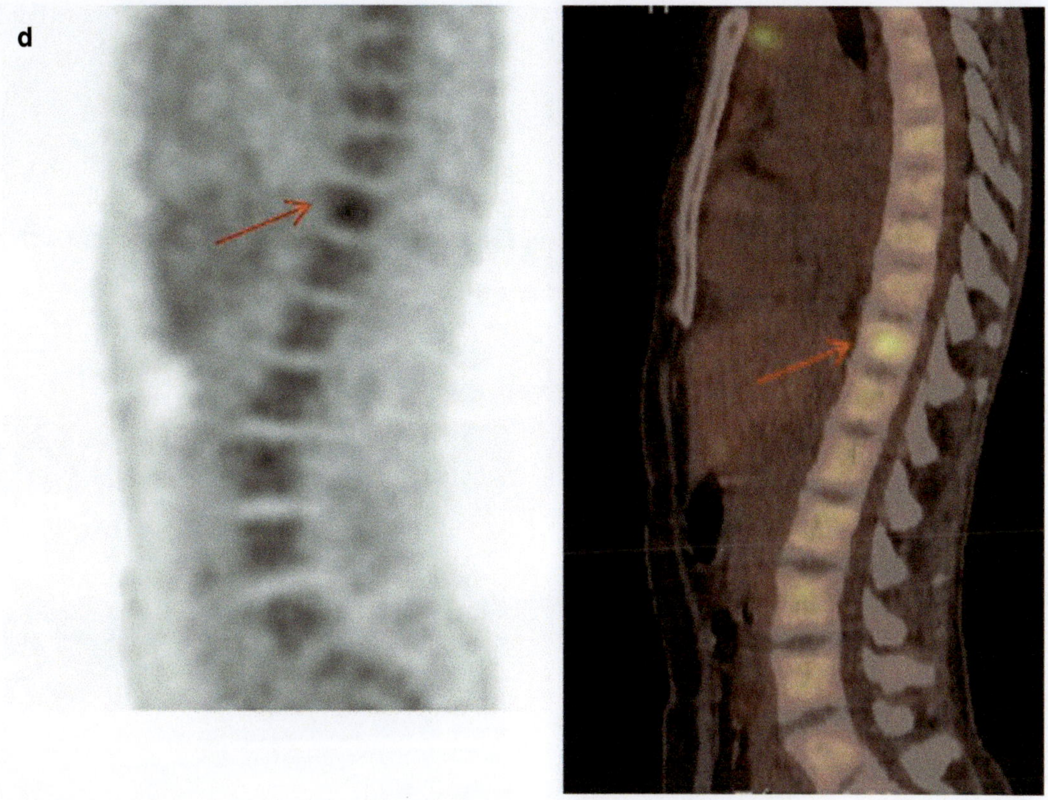

Fig. 6.43 (continued)

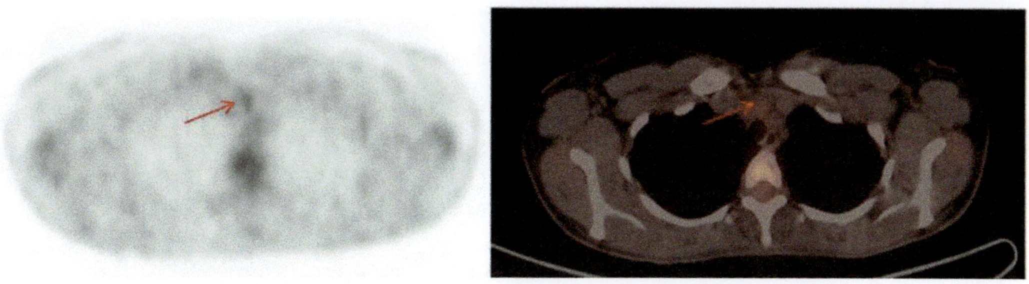

Fig. 6.44 Interim PET/CT: mild hypermetabolism at the anterior mediastinum (D-5PS score 3)

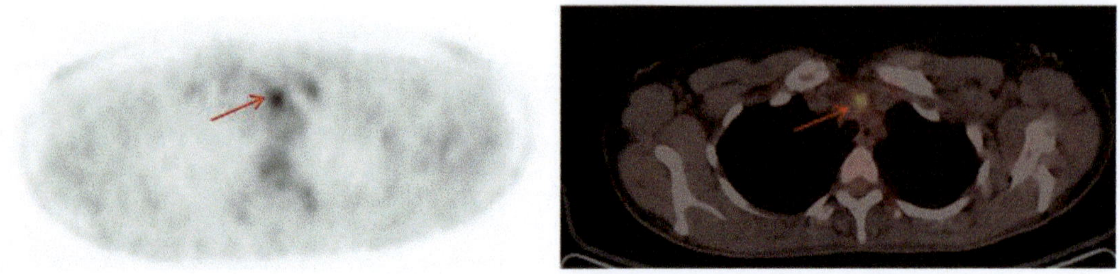

Fig. 6.45 PET/CT after the end of ABVD therapy. Hypermetabolism at the anterior mediastinum

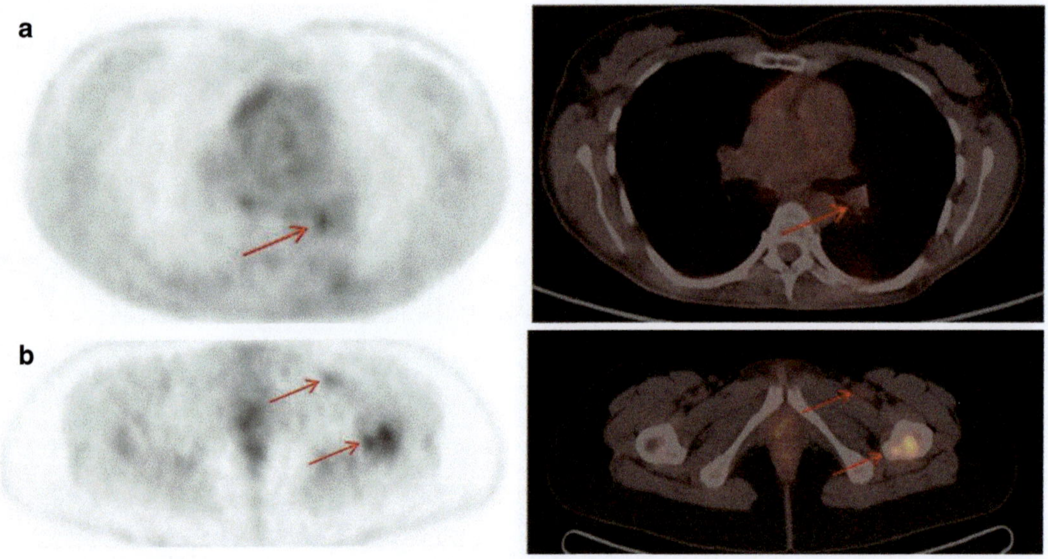

Fig. 6.46 (**a**, **b**) PET/CT restaging. Mild hypermetabolism at a left hilar lymph node (**a**), at a deep left inguinal node, and at the left femur (**b**)

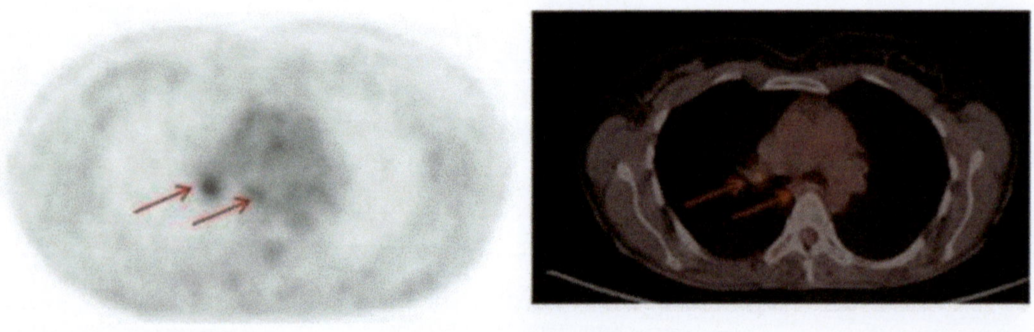

Fig. 6.47 PET/CT after IGEV salvage chemotherapy. Mild hypermetabolism at subcarinal and right hilar lymph nodes

References

1. Cheson BD, Fisher RI, Barrington SF, Cavalli F, Schwartz LH, Lister TA et al (2014) Recommendations for the initial evaluation, staging, and response assessment of Hodgkin and non-Hodgkin lymphoma: the Lugano classification. J Clin Oncol 32:3059–3067
2. Barrington SF, Mikhaeel GN, Kostakoglu L, Meignan M, Hutchings M, Müeller SP et al (2014) Role of imaging in the staging and response assessment of lymphoma: consensus of the International Conference on Malignant Lymphomas Imaging Working Group. J Clin Oncol 32:3048–3058
3. Vassilakopoulos TP, Prassopoulos V, Rondogianni P, Chatziioannou S, Konstantopoulos K, Angelopoulou MK (2015) Role of FDG-PET/CT in staging and first-line treatment of Hodgkin and aggressive B-cell lymphomas. MEMO 8:105–114
4. Hutchings M (2012) How does PET/CT help in selecting therapy for patients with Hodgkin lymphoma? Hematology Am Soc Hematol Educ Programm Book 2012:322–327
5. El-Galaly TC, d'Amore F, Mylam KJ et al (2012) Routine bone marrow biopsy has little or no therapeutic consequence for positron emission tomography/computed tomography-staged treatment-naïve patients with Hodgkin lymphoma. J Clin Oncol 30:4508–4514
6. Vassilakopoulos TP, Rondogianni P, Prassopoulos V, Chatziioannou S, Moschogiannis M, Poziopoulos C et al (2014) Comparative assessment of bone marrow involvement (BMI) by bone marrow biopsy (BMB) or positron emission tomography/computed tomography (PET/CT) in Hodgkin lymphoma (HL). Haematologica/The Hematology J 99(Suppl 1):401 (abstract 1050)
7. Adams HJ, Kwee TC, de Keizer B, Fijnheer R, de Klerk JM, Littooij AS et al (2014) Systematic review and meta-analysis on the diagnostic performance of FDG-PET/CT in detecting bone marrow involvement in newly diagnosed Hodgkin lymphoma: is bone marrow biopsy still necessary? Ann Oncol 25:921–927
8. Vassilakopoulos TP, Angelopoulou MK, Constantinou N et al (2005) Development and validation of a clinical prediction rule for bone marrow involvement in patients with Hodgkin lymphoma. Blood 105:1875–1880
9. Meignan M, Itti E, Gallamini A, Younes A (2015) FDG PET/CT imaging as a biomarker in lymphoma. Eur J Nucl Med Mol Imaging 42:623–633
10. Kanoun S, Rossi C, Berriolo-Riedinger A, Dygai-Cochet I, Cochet A, Humbert O et al (2014) Baseline metabolic tumor volume is an independent prognostic factor in Hodgkin lymphoma. Eur J Nucl Med Mol Imaging 41:1735–1743
11. Song MK, Chung JS, Lee JJ, Jeong SY, Lee SM, Hong JS et al (2013) Metabolic tumor volume by positron emission tomography/computed tomography as a clinical parameter to determine therapeutic modality for early stage Hodgkin's lymphoma. Cancer Sci 104:1656–1661
12. Cheson BD, Pfistner B, Juweid ME et al (2007) Revised response criteria for malignant lymphoma. J Clin Oncol 25:579–586
13. Juweid ME, Stroobants S, Hoekstra OS et al (2007) Use of positron emission tomography for response assessment of lymphoma: consensus of the Imaging Subcommittee of International Harmonization Project in Lymphoma. J Clin Oncol 25:571–578
14. Vassilakopoulos TP, Pangalis GA, Boutsikas G et al (2012) Prognostic factors in patients with Hodgkin lymphoma (HL) and a negative PET/CT after ABVD chemotherapy: potential applications for the design of follow-up strategies. Haematologica/The Hematology J 97(Suppl 1):87 (abstract 218)
15. Radford J, Illidge T, Counsell L et al (2015) Results of a trial of PET-directed therapy for early-stage Hodgkin's lymphoma. N Engl J Med 372:1598–1607
16. Hartridge-Lambert SK, Schoder H, Lim RC, Maragulia JC, Portlock CS (2013) ABVD alone and a PET scan complete remission negates the need for radiologic surveillance in early-stage, nonbulky Hodgkin lymphoma. Cancer 119:1203–1209
17. Sher DJ, Mauch PM, van den Abbeele A, LaCasce AS, Czerminski J, Ng AK (2009) Prognostic significance of mid- and post-ABVD PET imaging in Hodgkin's lymphoma: the importance of involved field radiotherapy. Ann Oncol 20:1848–1853
18. Engert A, Haverkamp H, Kobe C et al (2012) Reduced-intensity chemotherapy and PET-guided radiotherapy in patients with advanced stage Hodgkin's lymphoma (HD15 trial): a randomised, open-label, phase 3 non-inferiority trial. Lancet 379:1791–1799
19. Barnes JA, LaCasce AS, Zukotynski K et al (2011) End-of-treatment but not interim PET scan predicts outcome in nonbulky limited stage Hodgkin's lymphoma. Ann Oncol 22:910–915
20. Vassilakopoulos TP, Rontogianni P, Pangalis GA et al (2012) Outcome and prognostic factors in patients with Hodgkin lymphoma (HL) who remain PET/CT-positive after ABVD combination chemotherapy: potential applications for the design of subsequent treatment. Haematologica/The Hematology J 97(Suppl 1):562 (abstract 1404)
21. Radford J, Illidge T, Counsell N, Hancock B, Pettengell R, Johnson P et al (2015) PET score following 3 cycles ABVD has greater prognostic value than pre-treatment risk stratification in the RAPID trial in early stage Hodgkin lymphoma (HL). Hematol Oncol 33(S1):144 (abstract 082)
22. Kobe C, Kuhnert G, Kahraman D, Haverkamp H, Eich HT, Franke M et al (2014) Assessment of tumor size reduction improves outcome prediction of positron emission tomography/computed tomography after chemotherapy in advanced-stage Hodgkin lymphoma. J Clin Oncol 32:1776–1781
23. Picardi M, De Renzo A, Pane F et al (2007) Randomized comparison of consolidation radiation versus observation in bulky Hodgkin's lymphoma

with post-chemotherapy negative positron emission tomography scans. Leuk Lymphoma 48:1721–1727
24. Raemaekers JM, André MP, Federico M, Girinsky T, Oumedaly R, Brusamolino E et al (2014) Omitting radiotherapy in early positron emission tomography-negative stage I/II Hodgkin lymphoma is associated with an increased risk of early relapse: clinical results of the preplanned interim analysis of the randomized EORTC/LYSA/FIL H10 trial. J Clin Oncol 32:1188–1194
25. Hutchings M, Loft A, Hansen M et al (2006) FDG-PET after two cycles of chemotherapy predicts treatment failure and progression-free survival in Hodgkin lymphoma. Blood 107:52–59
26. Gallamini A, Hutchings M, Rigacci L et al (2007) Early interim 2-[18F]fluoro-2-deoxy-D-glucose positron emission tomography is prognostically superior to international prognostic score in advanced-stage Hodgkin's lymphoma: a report from a joint Italian-Danish study. J Clin Oncol 25:3746–3752
27. Hutchings M, Kostakoglou L, Zaucha AM et al (2014) In vivo treatment sensitivity testing with positron emission tomography/computed tomography after one cycle of chemotherapy for Hodgkin lymphoma. J Clin Oncol 32:2705–2711
28. Rossi C, Kanoun S, Berriolo-Riedinger A, Dygai-Cochet I, Humbert O, Legouge C et al (2014) Interim 18F-FDG PET SUVmax reduction is superior to visual analysis in predicting outcome early in Hodgkin lymphoma patients. J Nucl Med 55:569–573
29. Gallamini A, Barrington SF, Biggi A, Chauvie S, Kostakoglou L, Gregianin M et al (2014) The predictive role of interim positron emission tomography for Hodgkin lymphoma treatment outcome is confirmed using the interpretation criteria of the Deauville five-point scale. Haematologica 99:1107–1113
30. Biggi A, Gallamini A, Chauvie S, Hutchings M, Kostakoglu L, Gregianin M et al (2013) International validation study for interim PET in ABVD-treated, advanced-stage Hodgkin lymphoma: interpretation criteria and concordance rate among reviewers. J Nucl Med 54:683–690
31. Kostakoglu L, Schoder H, Johnson JL et al (2012) Interim FDG PET imaging in stage I/II non bulky Hodgkin lymphoma: would using combined PET and CT criteria better predict response than each test alone? Leuk Lymphoma 53:2143–2150
32. Oki Y, Chuang H, Chasen B, Jessop A, Pan T, Fanale M et al (2014) The prognostic value of interim positron emission tomography scan in patients with classical Hodgkin lymphoma. Br J Haematol 165:112–116
33. Rigacci L, Puccini B, Zinzani PL, Biggi A, Castagnoli A, Merli F et al (2015) The prognostic value of positron emission tomography performed after two courses (interim-pet) of standard therapy on treatment outcome in early stage Hodgkin lymphoma. A multicentric study by the Fondazione Italiana Linfomi (FIL). Am J Hematol 90:499–503
34. Simontacchi G, Filippi AR, Ciammella P, Buglione M, Saieva C, Magrini SM et al (2015) Interim PET after two ABVD cycles in Early-Stage Hodgkin Lymphoma: outcomes following the continuation of chemotherapy plus radiotherapy. Int J Radiat Oncol Biol Phys 92(5):1077–83. doi:10.1016/j.ijrobp.2015.04.021
35. Markova J, Kobe C, Skopalova M et al (2009) FDG-PET for assessment of early treatment response after four cycles of chemotherapy in patients with advanced stage Hodgkin's lymphoma has a high negative predictive value. Ann Oncol 20:1270–1274
36. Borchmann P, Haverkamp H, Lohri A, Kreissl S, Greil R, Markova J et al (2014) Addition of rituximab to $BEACOPP_{escalated}$ to improve the outcome of early interim PET positive advanced stage Hodgkin lymphoma patients: second planned interim analysis of the HD18 study. Blood (ASH Annual Meeting Abstracts) 124:Abstract 500
37. Gallamini A, Patti C, Viviani S et al (2011) Early chemotherapy intensification with BEACOPP in advanced-stage Hodgkin lymphoma patients with a interim-PET positive after two ABVD courses. Br J Haematol 152:551–560
38. Press O, Li H, Schoder H, LeBlanc M, Rimsza L, Friedberg JW et al (2013) Response-adapted therapy of stage III-IV Hodgkin lymphoma based on interim FDG-PET imaging: Early results of US Intergroup S0816. Haematologica 98(S2):36 (abstract T108)
39. Johnson P, Federico M, Fossa A, O'Doherty M, Roberts T, Stevens L et al (2013) Responses and chemotherapy dose adjustment determined by PET-CT imaging: first results from the international Response Adapted Therapy in advanced Hodgkin lymphoma (RATHL) study. Hematol Oncol 31(S1):138 (abstract 126)
40. Vassilakopoulos TP, Angelopoulou MK, Rondogianni P et al (2011) Interim PET-Scan for early response assessment and potential modification of treatment plan after 2 ABVD cycles in advanced stage Hodgkin Lymphoma (HL). Haematologica/Hematol J 96(Suppl 2):Abstract 322
41. Ganesan P, Rajentranath R, Kannan K, Radhakrishnan V, Ganesan TS, Udupa K et al (2015) Phase II study of interim PET-CT-guided response-adapted therapy in advanced Hodgkin's lymphoma. Ann Oncol 26:1170–1174
42. Cimino G, Zaucha JM, Cirillo S, Saviolo C, Hutchings M, El-Galaly TC et al (2014) The complementary prognostic role of baseline and interim PET in predicting treatment outcome in advanced-stage Hodgkin lymphoma Blood. (ASH Annual Meeting Abstracts) 124:Abstract 4405
43. Johnson PW, Federico M, Fossa A, O'Doherty M, Roberts T, Stevens L et al (2015) Response-adapted therapy based on interim FDG-PET scans in advanced Hodgkin lymphoma: first analysis of the safety of de-escalation and efficacy of escalation in

the international RATHL study (CRUK/07/033). Hematol Oncol 33(S1):102 (abstract 008)
44. Agostinelli C (2014) A clinical-pathological algorithm based on the combination of interim PET with biological markers in classical Hodgkin lymphoma. Presented at the Fifth International Workshop on PET in Lymphoma, Menton, 19–20 Sept 2014. http://eitti.free.fr
45. Engert A, Diehl V, Franklin J et al (2009) Escalated-dose BEACOPP in the treatment of patients with advanced-stage Hodgkin's lymphoma: 10 years of follow-up of the GHSG HD9 study. J Clin Oncol 20:4548–4554
46. von Tresckow B, Plütschow A, Fuchs M et al (2012) Dose-intensification in early unfavorable Hodgkin's lymphoma: final analysis of the German Hodgkin Study Group HD14 trial. J Clin Oncol 30:907–913
47. Casasnovas O, Brice P, Bouabdallah R et al (2015) Randomized phase III study comparing an early PET driven treatment de-escalation to a not PET-monitored strategy in patients with advanced stages Hodgkin lymphoma: Interim analysis of the AHL2011 Lysa study. Blood 126:577 (abstract)
48. Wongso D, Fuchs M, Plutschow A et al (2013) Treatment-related mortality in patients with advanced-stage Hodgkin lymphoma: an analysis of the German Hodgkin Study Group. J Clin Oncol 31:2819–1824
49. Vassilakopoulos TP, Johnson PWM. Treatment of advanced-stage Hodgkin lymphoma: Who really needs BEACOPP? Semin Hematol 2016 (in press)
50. Angelopoulou MK, Moschogiannis M, Rondogianni P et al (2013) PET/CT in the setting of autologous stem cell transplantation (ASCT) for relapsed/refractory Hodgkin lymphoma (HL): performance of various interpretation systems. Haematologica 98(S2):41 (abstract P119)
51. Vassilakopoulos TP, Angelopoulou MK (2013) Advanced and relapsed/refractory Hodgkin lymphoma: what has been achieved during the last 50 years. Semin Hematol 50:4–14
52. Younes A, Gopal AK, Smith SC et al (2012) Results of a pivotal phase II study of brentuximab vedotin for patients with relapsed or refractory Hodgkin's lymphoma. J Clin Oncol 30:2183–2189
53. Moskowitz CH, Nademanee A, Masszi T et al (2015) Brentuximab vedotin as consolidation therapy after autologous stem-cell transplantation in patients with Hodgkin's lymphoma at risk of relapse or progression (AETHERA): A randomized, double-blind, placeb-controlled, phase 3 trial. Lancet 385 (9980):1853–1862
54. Zinzani PL, Broccoli A, Gioia D et al (2015) Interim PET response-adapted therapy in advanced-stage Hodgkin's lymphoma: final results of the phase II part of the Fondazione Italiana Linfomi (FIL) HD0801 study. Hematol Oncol 33(S1):164 (abstract 119)
55. Gallamini A, Rossi A, Patti C et al (2015) Interim PET-adapted chemotherapy in advanced Hodgkin lymphoma (HL). Results of the second interim analysis of the Italian GITIL/FIL DH0607 trial. Hematol Oncol 33(S1):163 (abstract 118)
56. van Hoeij FB, Keijsers RG, Loffeld BC et al (2015) Incidental colonic focal FDG uptake on PET/CT: can the maximum standardized uptake value (SUVmax) guide us in the timing of colonoscopy? Eur J Nucl Med Mol Imaging 42:66–71
57. Keyzer C, Dhaene B, Blocklet D et al (2015) Colonoscopic findings in patients with incidental colonic focal FDG uptake. AJR Am J Roentgenol 204(5):W586–W591
58. Liu T, Behr S, Khan S et al (2015) Focal colonic FDG activity with PET/CT: guidelines for recommendation of colonoscopy. World J Nucl Med 14(1):25–30

Part III

PET/CT in Non-Hodgkin's Lymphomas

Aggressive B-Cell Lymphomas 7

Theodoros P. Vassilakopoulos,
Vassilios K. Prassopoulos, Phoivi Rondogianni,
Sofia N. Chatziioannou, Vasileios I. Telonis,
and Effimia P. Vrakidou

7.1 Introduction

Aggressive B-cell lymphomas include diffuse large B-cell lymphomas not otherwise specified (DLBCL NOS), other subtypes of DLBCL [T-cell/histiocyte-rich LBCL, DLBCL leg type, primary DLBCL of the central nervous system (CNS), and Epstein-Barr virus (EBV+) DLBCL of the elderly], "other neoplasms of large B cells," mainly including primary mediastinal large B-cell lymphoma (PMLBCL) and several other very uncommon entities (see Chap. 4), and cases with borderline features between DLBCL and Hodgkin lymphoma (HL) or DLBCL and Burkitt lymphoma, the so-called gray-zone lymphomas. This chapter is focused to DLBCL NOS and other subtypes of DLBCL (except of primary CNS, which is covered in Chap. 13) as well as to PMLBCL, i.e., the most frequent entities classified in aggressive B-cell lymphomas.

As already stated in the chapter devoted to HL, the recently published 2014 recommendations [1, 2] suggest the use of PET/CT for baseline staging and final response assessment in all FDG-avid lymphoma subtypes. Interim evaluation is not recommended for the time being in DLBCL and related disorders outside clinical trials. Routine follow-up with PET/CT after the achievement of a PET-negative status with first-line treatment is definitely not recommended, because of the high risk of false-positives leading to many unnecessary invasive procedures.

7.2 PET/CT in Initial Staging

7.2.1 General Considerations

The use of PET/CT for the initial staging of aggressive B-cell lymphomas is currently recommended, because it is more accurate than conventional staging in detecting disease in

T.P. Vassilakopoulos, MD (✉) • V.I. Telonis, MD
Department of Haematology,
National and Kapodistrian University of Athens,
School of Medicine, Laikon General Hospital,
17, Agiou Thoma street, Goudi, Athens 11527, Greece
e-mail: tvassilak@med.uoa.gr;
vasilis.telonis@yahoo.com

V.K. Prassopoulos, MD • E.P. Vrakidou
Department of Nuclear Medicine and PET/CT,
HYGEIA Hospital, Athens, Kifissias and Erythrou
Staurou 4, Maroussi 15123, Greece
e-mail: vprasso@otenet.gr

P. Rondogianni, MD, FENMB
Department of Nuclear Medicine and PET/CT,
Evangelismos General Hospital, Athens, 45-47
Ipsilantou Street, Athens 11576, Greece
e-mail: phrontog@yahoo.gr

S.N. Chatziioannou, MD
Centre for Clinical and Translational Research,
Biomedical Research Foundation of the Academy
of Athens, 4 Soranou Ephessiou Street,
Athens 11527, Greece
e-mail: sofiac@bcm.tmc.edu

J.A. Andreou et al. (eds.), *PET/CT in Lymphomas: A Case-Based Atlas*,
DOI 10.1007/978-3-319-27380-8_7

normal-sized lymph nodes and provides a better evaluation of extranodal sites. Furthermore, it may facilitate the interpretation of posttreatment PET/CT [1–3]. Upstaging is much more frequent than downstaging, but designing treatment based on PET/CT results rather than conventional staging has not been adequately evaluated so far. Furthermore, the effect of PET/CT-based treatment modifications may not be so relevant in DLBCL and PMLBCL compared to HL, because the duration of standard rituximab-based chemoimmunotherapy is not strongly depended on the extent of the disease, especially in centers which have not adopted abbreviated immunochemotherapy plus RT for limited stages. Furthermore, the detection of subclinical disease sites may not affect the design of subsequent RT, if applicable [3–6].

7.2.2 PET in the Assessment of Bone Marrow Involvement

The introduction of PET/CT in the initial staging virtually eliminated the need for a bone marrow biopsy (BMb) in HL [1–3]. According to current recommendations, a BMb is still indicated for the detection of discordant histology in DLBCL, if this is relevant for patient management or required by a clinical trial [1, 2]. However, the topic still remains debatable and the scientific basis for these recommendations is analyzed below. The recommendations for DLBCL apply also to PMLBCL, in the absence of any more specific reference. However, the baseline probability of bone marrow involvement in this entity is very low (almost zero), and it would be reasonable to omit BMb in the absence of relevant findings in PET/CT, especially because a positive result would not alter treatment strategy [7, 8]. In the above entities, PET/CT is suggestive of BM involvement only if focal lesions with increased uptake are present.

The frequency of BM involvement in DLBCL is approximately 15 %. Cellular infiltration can be concordant (large cell) or discordant (small cell) with an almost equal frequency [9]. Quite frequently, discordant histology may not be demonstrated by PET/CT [10], but may affect patients' outcome. Similarly to HL, PET/CT reveals on average twice more cases of BM involvement than BMb does in DLBCL [11–15]. However, in contrast to HL, approximately one-third of patients with positive BMb (range, 14–50 %) have a negative PET/CT, accounting for 1.5–8 % of the total DLBCL population in various studies [11–15]. Consequently, several cases of BM involvement may be overlooked if BMb is omitted, but most of them bear already features of advanced disease and management is not affected. However, there are now data demonstrating that PET+/BMb- cases may have a better prognosis than BMb+cases, i.e., that BM involvement is a poor prognostic factor only if detected at the histologic level [11–13, 15]. Thus, although recent recommendations [1, 2] state that "… PET/CT is more sensitive than BMb, but it is reported to miss low-volume diffuse involvement of 10–20 % of the marrow. … If the scan is negative, a BMB is indicated to identify involvement by discordant histology if relevant for a clinical trial or patient management," in contrast to HL, the exact role of BMB in DLBCL remains to be further investigated, based on the above considerations [3, 16].

7.2.3 Potential Prognostic Role of Baseline PET/CT

Total metabolic tumor volume (TMTV) as determined by PET/CT may be a more precise estimation of the true tumor burden than the conventionally calculated one. Total lesion glycolysis (TLG) represents a combined evaluation of both TMTV and intensity of metabolic activity (SUV mean of each lesion) [17]. Preliminary results in small- or medium-sized series suggest that both higher MTV [18, 19] and high TLG [20] may be independently associated with worse prognosis in DLBCL.

Similar results were recently published regarding PMLBCL, based on 103 patients from the IELSG26 study, who were treated predominantly with R-MACOP-B (84 %) or R-CHOP (16 %), both followed by RT [21]. All three baseline PET/CT parameters (SUVmax, MTV, and TLG determined exclusively for mediastinal disease) were associated with outcome, but only high TLG was independently associated with prognosis, overcoming the role of the remaining two PET parameters, bulky disease and other conventional prognostic factors. At 5 years, progression-free survival (PFS) was 99 % versus 64 % for patients with low (2/3 of the total population) versus high TLG (1/3 of the total population) ($p < 0.0001$), while 5-year OS was 100 % versus 80 %, respectively, ($p = 0.0001$) [21].

Although interesting, this information deserves further prospective evaluation along with many established prognostic factors before implemented in clinical practice.

7.3 PET/CT in Response Assessment After Completion of Therapy

PET/CT provides the most effective means to differentiate between viable lymphoma and necrotic or fibrotic tissue on CT in patients with aggressive B-cell lymphomas. A more detailed discussion regarding the gradual change of the criteria of response in the PET era is provided in Chap. 6. The Deauville 5-point scale (D5-PS), initially described for the evaluation of interim PET, has been now adopted for end-of-treatment PET (ePET), as proposed by the latest recommendations [1, 2]. The 5-PS is shown in detail in Chap. 6, Table 1. A detailed description of current criteria of staging and response is provided in the Appendix.

7.3.1 Diffuse Large B-Cell Lymphoma (DLBCL)

Despite the widespread use of PET/CT for the evaluation of response in DLBCL, published data regarding the role of ePET are rather limited [4, 22–27]. The negative predictive value of PET/CT after R-CHOP is lower compared with HL after chemotherapy, with long-term event-free survival (EFS) rates in the range of 70–85 % [4, 22–27]. The probability of failure may depend on baseline relapse risk, as reflected by the International Prognostic Index (IPI) or its components [24], as well as on conventional radiologic response (complete versus partial remission) or the size of residual mass [4, 23]. Patients with DLBCL who remain PET/CT positive after R-CHOP have a <40–50 % probability to remain disease-free [4, 22–27]. However, false-positive findings are not infrequent. Furthermore, the chance of salvaging patients with a localized PET positivity by RT may be as high as 80 % [4], although such figures highly depend on patient selection and should be further confirmed.

7.3.2 Primary Mediastinal Large B-Cell Lymphoma

The negative predictive value of PET/CT in PMLBCL after immunochemotherapy is very high: Cure rates exceed 95 % for patients with negative PET/CT after R-CHOP, R-MACOP-B, or R-da-EPOCH, especially if subsequently irradiated, but also even if RT is omitted in many patients [8, 28, 29]. Conversely, if RT is to follow, PET/CT-positive residual masses are associated with rather low progression rates, being effectively controlled in 65–70 % of cases [8, 28]. The paradigm of PMLBCL provides strong support to the decision to adopt D5-PS for the final evaluation of response to treatment and set a flexible cutoff permitting score of 3 to be considered as "negative": Indeed, following RT, the prognosis of patients with D5-PS score of 3 is extremely favorable [8, 28, 30]. These patients enjoy cure rates even 100 %, with all progressions restricted to patients with D5-PS scores of 4–5. These findings have been reproduced by multiple published studies [8, 28–30].

The next question raised is also important: Since PFS of PET/CT-positive patients is 65–70 % after additional RT, which patients are at highest risk of progression? It appears that not only D5-PS 3 but also D5-PS 4 patients with "low" FDG uptake have equally favorable outcomes with long-term PFS >90 %, while patients with higher SUVmax (e.g., ≥5) probably have significantly inferior outcomes [28, 29]. However, even those patients with marked 18FDG uptake have a long-term PFS of approximately 50 % and can be salvaged with RT irrespectively of the degree of FDG uptake [28, 31]. Since the majority of patients who remain PET positive after immunochemotherapy will be cured with RT, patients with PMLBCL should not be referred for high-dose therapy and autologous transplantation solely based on a positive PET/CT [31, 32]. This is even more applicable if uptake is not marked. Conversely, whether RT could be safely omitted or not in PET-negative patients is currently evaluated by the IELSG-37 randomized trial [33].

7.4 Interim Response Assessment

Early response assessment has provided a major prognostic clue for patients with DLBCL [34], while the results are controversial in PMLBCL [35–37]. However, current recommendations do not propose the use of interim PET (iPET) to guide treatment decisions, because there is still no proven salvage therapy capable to improve the outcome of patients with DLBCL and a positive iPET, while the NPV of iPET is rather low [1, 2]. As discussed below, D5-PS is not the optimal tool for early interim response assessment in DLBCL and has been replaced by the evaluation of SUVmax alterations in this setting.

7.4.1 Diffuse Large B-Cell Lymphoma

7.4.1.1 Scientific Basis and Prognostic Significance

Interim PET is a strong prognostic factor of the outcome after R-CHOP or similar regimens in DLBCL, but the differences between negative and positive cases are less pronounced compared to advanced HL. Importantly, the reproducibility of the D5-PS is moderate in DLBCL [26, 38–40]. In the NHL International Validation Study [41], 120 DLBCL patients were treated with R-CHOP-21 or intensified R-CHOP-14 or R-ACVBP-14, and treatment was not modified in response to iPET performed after two cycles of immunochemotherapy. The concordance among three reviewers regarding whether iPET was negative or positive (visual analysis, D5-PS) was substantial (Fleiss' $\kappa=0.66$) if the liver – the optimal cutoff- was used as reference (scores of 4, 5 positive). When a semiquantitative approach based on SUVmax reduction between baseline and iPET (ΔSUVmax at a cutoff of 66 %) was adopted, concordance was upgraded to almost perfect (Fleiss' $\kappa=0.81$). The 3-year PFS was approximately 79 % versus 44 % in patients with ΔSUVmax of >66 % and ≤66 %, while 3-year PFS was 81 % versus 59 % using the D5-PS (scores of 4, 5 positive) [41]. Thus, the semiquantitative ΔSUVmax criterion was more reproducible and prognostically superior than the D5-PS. In the LNH-2007-3B trial, higher-risk, young DLBCL patients were randomized to receive R-CHOP-14 or R-ACVBP-14 and underwent iPET after two and four cycles. Treatment was modified according to iPET results. The cutoff for ΔSUVmax was set at 66 % for PET-2 and 70 % for PET-4. At 2 years, PFS was 77 % versus 57 % and 83 % versus 40 % according to the results of PET-2 and PET-4 despite treatment intensification in case of iPET positivity [42]. Visual analysis based on D5-PS was again less accurate than the semiquantitative ΔSUVmax approach.

7.4.1.2 Can Treatment Be Modified in Response to Interim PET Results?

In the PETAL trial [43], 853 patients with aggressive lymphomas, including 757 with CD20+ aggressive B-cell lymphomas (80 % DLBCL), received R-CHOPx2 and underwent iPET. Using the criterion of ΔSUVmax <66 % to define positivity, 13 % remained positive and were randomized between six further R-CHOP cycles versus intensive immunochemotherapy with a protocol designed for Burkitt lymphoma. Although previous observations were confirmed and iPET positivity was an independent adverse prognostic factor along with IPI, treatment intensification failed to improve disease control and overall survival compared to R-CHOP. This was applicable to the DLBCL subgroup as well [43]. Furthermore, in the majority of patients who achieved an iPET-negative status, the negative predictive value was rather low, since the long-term failure rate exceeded 20–30 %. Similar conclusions were derived from the ECOG E3404 study, in which treatment modification to R-ICE ×4 was planned in response to a positive iPET after R-CHOP×3. The 2-year PFS was 42 %, failing to reach the predefined level of efficacy in patients with DLBCL, which had been set at 45 % [44]. The negative predictive value was again rather low with a 4-year failure rate of 29 % for iPET-negative patients. In contrast, the negative predictive value was improved and the 2-year PFS reached 91 % in a phase 2 trial of advanced stage aggressive B-cell lymphoma patients from British Columbia, in which iPET negativity was defined more strictly (according to the IHP criteria corresponding to D5-PS 1 or 2) and iPET was performed later, after four cycles of R-CHOP [45].

According to the above data, iPET-based treatment intensification in DLBCL is not currently justified outside the setting of trials.

7.4.2 Primary Mediastinal Large B-Cell Lymphoma

No clear evidence exists so far as to whether iPET is a strong predictor of the outcome of PMLBCL, since data are conflicting [35–37]. In a study from Memorial Sloan Kettering Cancer Center, 51 patients with PMLBCL received four cycles of accelerated R-C_{1000}HOP-14 and underwent iPET, which was negative in 53 % of them [35, 37]. All patients subsequently received non-cross-resistant therapy with three cycles of ICE with or without rituximab and no additional RT. No difference in PFS emerged according to iPET result irrespective of the criterion used to define positivity. In a retrospective study of 30 patients from Israel, the initial treatment regimen (19 R-VACOP-B and 11 R-CHOP) was continued irrespective of iPET result, and RT was not given [36]. A positive iPET was observed in 14/30 patients (47 %) and the 3-year PFS was 94 % versus 57 % for iPET- and iPET+ cases ($p=0.015$).

According to these limited data, iPET cannot be recommended for interim response assessment in PMLBCL, and iPET-based treatment modification cannot be proposed. However, data on iPET under R-CHOP-21 in PMLBCL are almost absent.

Conclusions

PET/CT is now considered mandatory for baseline staging aggressive B-cell lymphomas, providing more accurate information. Furthermore, PET/CT has been the longstanding "gold standard" for final response assessment. Regimens effective in overcoming the adverse impact of persistent interim PET positivity have not yet been described in DLBCL, where the use of iPET remains much more controversial than in HL and is not recommended by current guidelines.

Aggressive B-Cell Lymphomas: DLBCL – Case 1

A 66-year-old man presented with prolonged fever up to 39 °C, weight loss, and multiple subcutaneous nodules located at the left eyelid, the anterior thoracic and abdominal wall, and the back. Biopsy of a subcutaneous nodule revealed a DLBCL of non-germinal center cell origin. CT imaging was completely negative except of a 2 cm right adrenal lesion. A bone marrow biopsy was negative. Clinical stage was IVB. IPI value was "3," i.e., high-intermediate risk, due to advanced age and stage and elevated LDH levels (3.39×). Pretreatment PET/CT demonstrated the above described as well as other, diffusely distributed subcutaneous nodules (SUVmax of 2.0) (Fig. 7.1a) and the adrenal lesion (SUVmax of 2.5) (Fig. 7.1c), but also revealed left inguinal lymphadenopathy (SUVmax of 6.5), which was not felt on clinical examination neither shown on CTs (Fig. 7.1b). He received eight cycles of the R-CHOP regimen and achieved a clinical and radiographic complete remission except of the right adrenal lesion, which remained stable in size. A repeated PET/CT was completely negative. The patient remains in sustained remission 5 years later.

Discussion: This is a very unusual DLBCL case. The readily assessable tumor burden was too low to justify the prominent B-symptoms experienced by the patient. Interestingly, even PET/CT failed to uncover a much higher, subclinical disease burden, which might explain the clinical symptoms. Furthermore, it demonstrated a focus of latent nodal disease, without however, changing clinical stage or IPI. SUVmax was also low compared with the usually observed values in DLBCL. Although the mild FDG uptake of the adrenal lesion disappeared, its size remained stable. Therefore, it was considered as adenoma.

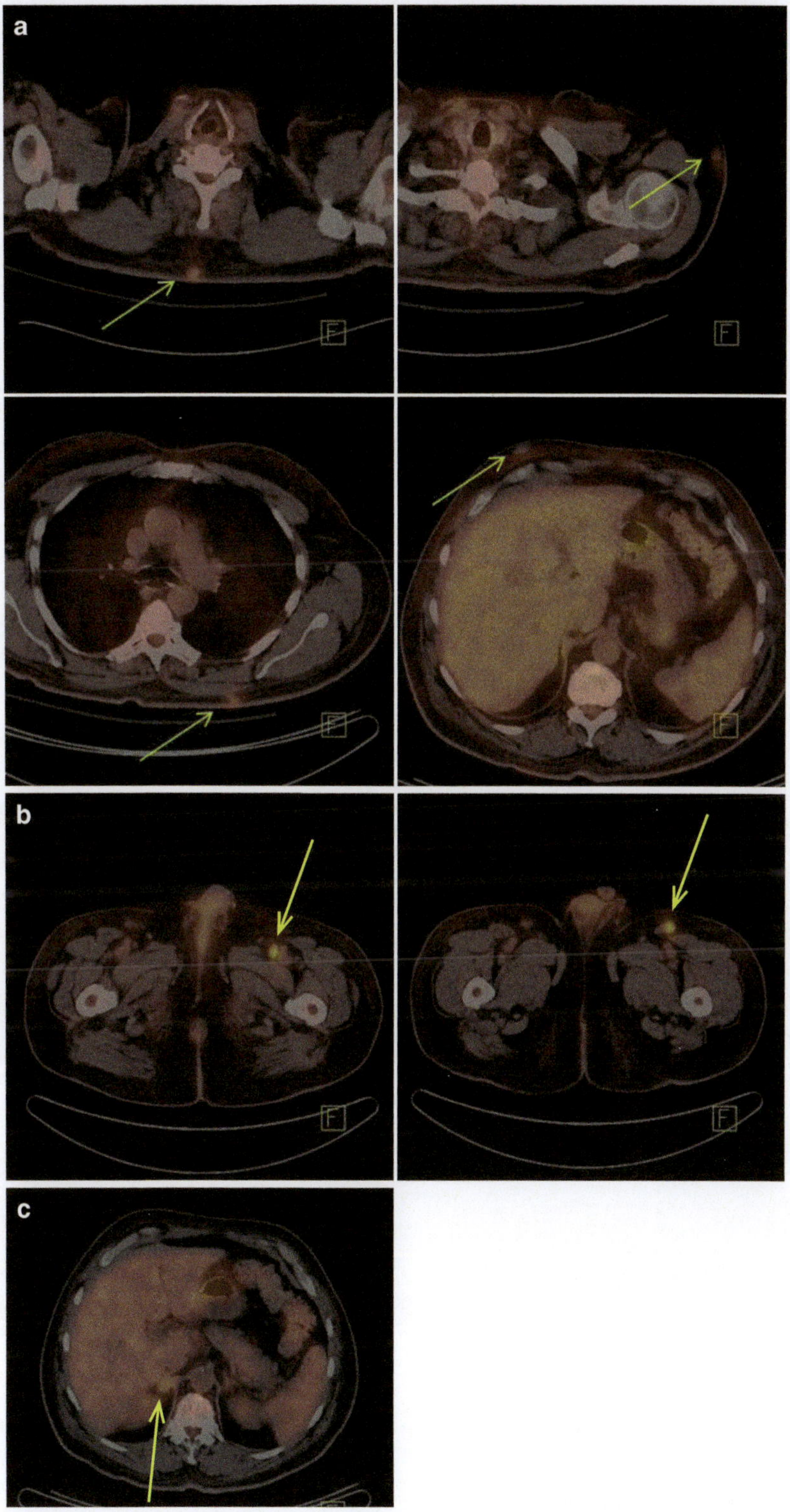

Fig. 7.1 Initial staging fused PET/CT images. (**a**) Small subcutaneous nodules (*arrows*) at the thorax and abdomen with increased metabolic activity (SUVmax of 2.0). (**b**) Hypermetabolic left inguinal lymph nodes (SUVmax of 6.5). (**c**) Small enlargement of the right adrenal gland with mildly increased uptake of the radiopharmaceutical (SUVmax of 2.5)

Aggressive B-Cell Lymphomas: DLBCL – Case 2

A 41-year-old man was diagnosed with DLBCL of germinal center cell origin following a biopsy of a 5.5×3.2 cm right arm mass. He was otherwise asymptomatic. A complete CT staging demonstrated nodular lesions in the peritoneal fat and a liver lesion with nonspecific radiologic features. PET/CT confirmed the above localizations (Fig. 7.2a, g, h) and further revealed abnormal FDG uptake in a nodular lesion within the right gluteal muscle (Fig. 7.2b), in the right rectus abdominis (Fig. 7.2c, d), the right iliac bone and the small bowel, mainly the jejunum (Fig. 7.2c, e, f). A bone marrow biopsy was negative. The clinical stage was IVA. IPI value was "2," i.e., low-intermediate risk, due to advanced stage and multiple extranodal sites (aaIPI "1," also low intermediate). The patient received eight cycles of R-CHOP. Restaging after immunochemotherapy revealed CR and PET/CT was negative, with all of the above lesions having completely disappeared (Fig. 7.3). He remains in complete remission 15 months after the final reevaluation.

Discussion: Conventional staging revealed a nonspecific liver lesion and nodular lesions in the peritoneal fat without nodal sites affected. This is a very unusual scenario for an otherwise stage IEA DLBCL. PET/CT was very helpful in clarifying the nature of these lesions and confidently establishes that disease stage was indeed IVA. Furthermore, PET/CT revealed additional peculiar extranodal sites. The lymphomatous nature of all these extranodal lesions is supported by their complete disappearance following R-CHOP. Lymph nodes were indeed spared in this extremely unusual case even when assessed by PET/CT. The negative predictive value of ePET in this scenario is expected to be rather high due to the low-intermediate aaIPI and the absence of measurable disease at the conclusion of therapy [23, 24] , as well as the complete absence of abnormal 18FDG-uptake [45].

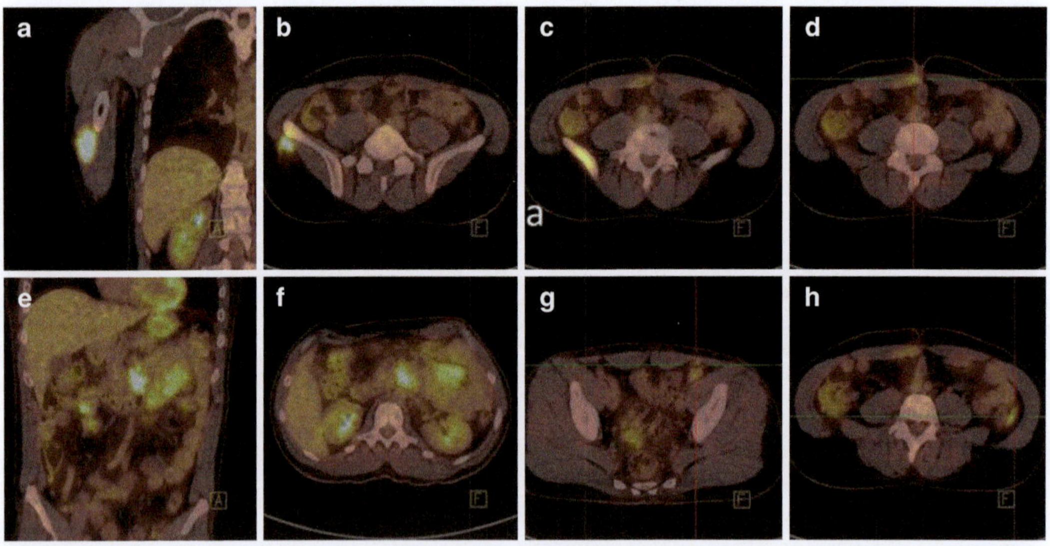

Fig. 7.2 Fused PET/CT images (**a**–**h**). Hypermetabolic lesion in the soft tissue of the anterolateral surface of the right arm (**a**), at the gluteal muscle (**b**), and at the right rectus abdominis (**c**, **d**). Hypermetabolic visualization of small intestine helices and lesions with increased uptake of the radiopharmaceutical adjacent to the descending colon and the iliac vessels, corresponding to peritoneal fat (**e**–**h**)

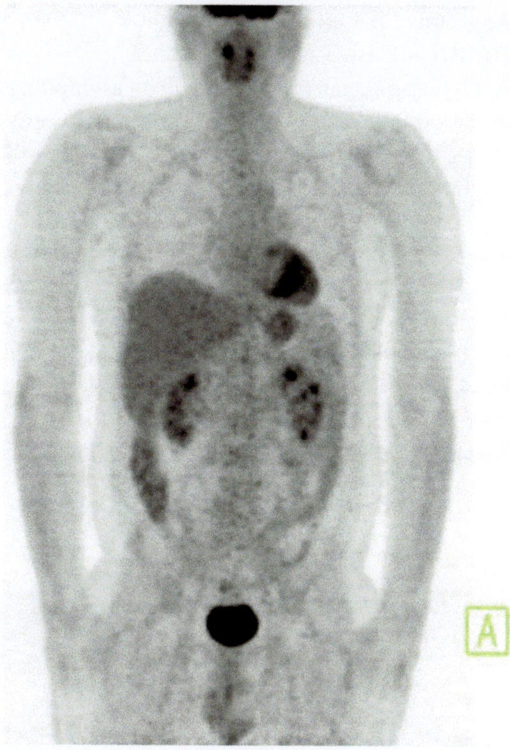

Fig. 7.3 MIP-PET: Elimination of the hypermetabolic lesions at all the previous described sites

Aggressive B-Cell Lymphomas: DLBCL – Case 3

A 48-year-old man presented with an asymptomatic 4 cm left neck swelling. Excisional biopsy revealed a DLBCL of non-germinal center cell origin. Whole-body CT evaluation and bone marrow biopsy were negative. IPI value was "1," i.e., low risk, due to elevated LDH levels (1.25×), but aaIPI was low-intermediate. PET/CT revealed highly increased 18FDG uptake with SUV max of 31 in a left middle internal jugular lymph node block (Fig. 7.4a, b). After six cycles of R-CHOP, the patient achieved a radiographic CR. PET/CT converted to completely negative (Fig. 7.5a, b)

Discussion: In this case, conventional staging and PET/CT provided the same stage classification. The highly increased SUVmax of 31 is consistent with an aggressive lymphoma, such as DLBCL. A negative PET/CT after R-CHOP is associated with a 70–85 % probability of cure [4, 22–27]. Due to the lower baseline risk of relapse/failure (aaIPI = 1, relapse risk 15–27 %, varying according to the use of RT) [5, 46], the elimination of the risk of primary progression, the complete radiographic response with no residual lesion, and the complete metabolic response with absolutely no FDG uptake [45], the individualized probability of cure in this case is high.

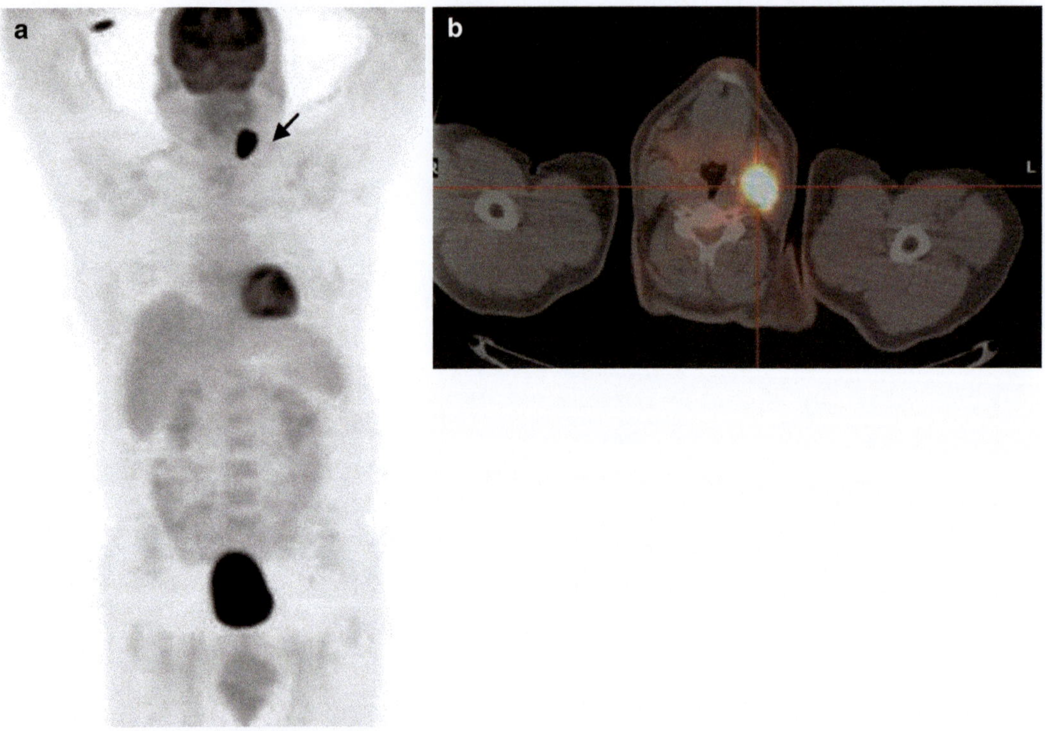

Fig. 7.4 (**a**, **b**) MIP-PET and fused PET/CT examination – initial staging: Highly increased 18FDG uptake in a left middle internal jugular lymph node block (*arrow*)

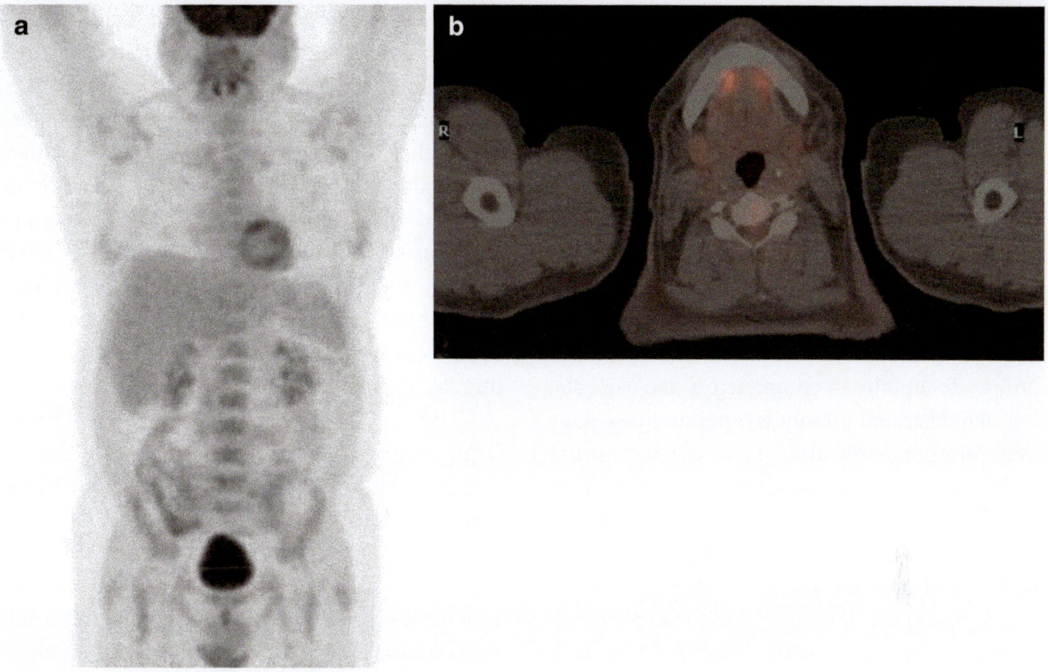

Fig. 7.5 (**a**, **b**) MIP-PET and fused PET/CT examination – end of treatment: Negative for abnormal hypermetabolic lesions

Aggressive B-Cell Lymphomas: DLBCL – Case 4

An 80-year-old woman presented to our Department with a diagnosis of DLBCL. She had experienced deep venous thrombosis of the left lower limb and pulmonary embolism, due to compressive effect of a left-sided pelvic mass, also causing ureter obstruction, which was initially thought to be a gynecologic cancer. She had no B-symptoms, but her general condition was impaired with a PS of "3." She had no peripheral lymphadenopathy. A complete CT and MRI staging demonstrated a large left pelvic mass with a cystic portion, measuring 11×9 cm and infiltrating the uterus as well as paraortic lymphadenopathy with nodes up to 1.8 cm. A bone marrow biopsy was negative. The clinical stage was IIEXA. IPI and aaIPI values were "3" and "2," i.e., high-intermediate risk, due to advanced age, impaired PS of 3, and elevated LDH levels (1.90×). PET/CT confirmed the above findings (Fig. 7.6a): The left pelvic mass beared a photopenic area at its anterior portion and was highly hypermetabolic (SUVmax of 29.9), as were the multiple para-aortic nodes (SUVmax of 34.4). PET/CT also revealed increased uptake at the interior area of the right psoas (SUVmax of 10.2) and bilateral inguinal nodes (SUVmax of 4.5). Additionally, PET/CT revealed supradiaphragmatic disease at paracardial, bilateral axillary, and bilateral cervical/supraclavicular lymph nodes (heterogeneous SUVmax up to 15.0), resulting to a PET-based stage of IIIEXA (Fig. 7.6b–d). The significance of a small, right lower lobe, subpleural nodule with very mild uptake (SUVmax of 1.5) was considered indeterminate. The patient received six cycles of reduced R-CHOP and achieved a PR with persistence of a large residual mass measuring 5×5 cm. A repeated end-of-treatment PET/CT was completely negative. She remains in continuous remission 2.5 years later.

Discussion: Although PET/CT resulted to a shift from stage II to stage III, resulting also to an IPI upgrade to high risk, this had not any effect on treatment strategy. Even in the presence of large residual masses, a negative PET/CT is consistent with complete remission in DLBCL, as shown by the long remission interval achieved in this case.

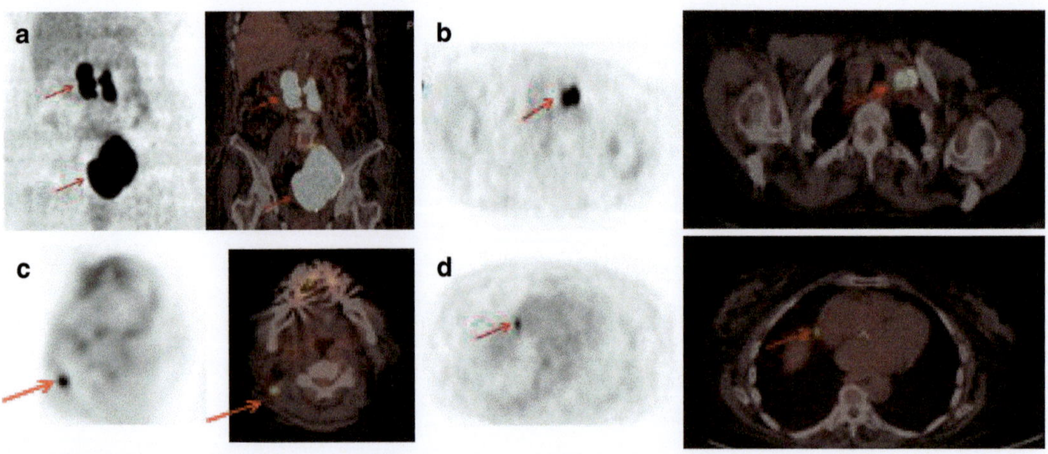

Fig. 7.6 Initial staging PET and fused PET/CT images: Significant hypermetabolism in a left-sided pelvic mass and in para-aortic lymph nodes bilaterally (**a**), hypermetabolic left supraclavicular lymph nodes (**b**), right cervical lymph nodes (**c**), and right paracardial lymph node (**d**) (hypermetabolic lesions are indicated with *red arrows*)

Aggressive B-Cell Lymphomas: DLBCL – Case 5

A 66-year-old male patient presented with difficulty in swallowing.

CT scans of the neck, chest, and abdomen revealed small left cervical lymphadenopathy <1.5 cm. Neck CT scan also demonstrated soft tissue swelling of the oropharynx and tonsils, which could not be accurately evaluated due to artifacts caused by teeth implants.

Lymph node biopsy showed DLBCL. Bone marrow biopsy showed no infiltration by the disease. Thus by conventional staging, the patient was most probably stage IIEA (or IA if the oropharyngeal findings were not taken into account). The IPI score was 1 due to the advanced age of the patient.

Baseline PET/CT confirmed the presence of cervical lymphadenopathy but also showed supraclavicular and infraclavicular lymphadenopathy with high metabolic activity (SUVmax of 22.7). In addition, it revealed enlargement of the left lateral and posterolateral wall of the pharynx with very high metabolic activity (SUVmax of 18.8) (Fig. 7.7).

The patient received the R-CHOP regimen. An interim PET/CT was performed after the completion of two cycles showing complete resolution of the FDG uptake by the cervical, supraclavicular, and infraclavicular lymph nodes and by the soft tissues of the pharynx. However, a new finding was the increased FDG uptake by the marrow of the shaft of the right humerus (SUVmax of 3.1) (Fig. 7.8). In the baseline PET/CT, the FDG uptake at that site was slightly increased in comparison to the left (SUVmax <1.9).

A bone biopsy of the above described lesion was performed showing no infiltration by the DLBCL.

The patient received four more cycles of R-CHOP and involved site RT. A follow-up PET/CT showed only increase of the FDG uptake by the marrow of the shaft of the right humerus with SUVmax only 1.7 (Fig. 7.9).

The patient remains in CR with no further treatment for 2 years after the diagnosis.

Discussion: In this case, PET/CT confirmed that stage was IIEA and also revealed supraclavicular and infraclavicular lymphadenopathy. Although by conventional staging all lymph nodes detected were less than 1.5 cm in diameter, PET/CT showed involvement of more sites and very high metabolic activity. Also, the swelling of the oropharynx and tonsils, which could not be accurately evaluated by conventional methods, proved to have a high FDG uptake by PET/CT.

PET-CT using FDG is more accurate than CT for staging in NHL with increased sensitivity, particularly for small-sized nodes and extranodal disease. Upstaging occurs more often than downstaging and may result to management alterations in some patients.

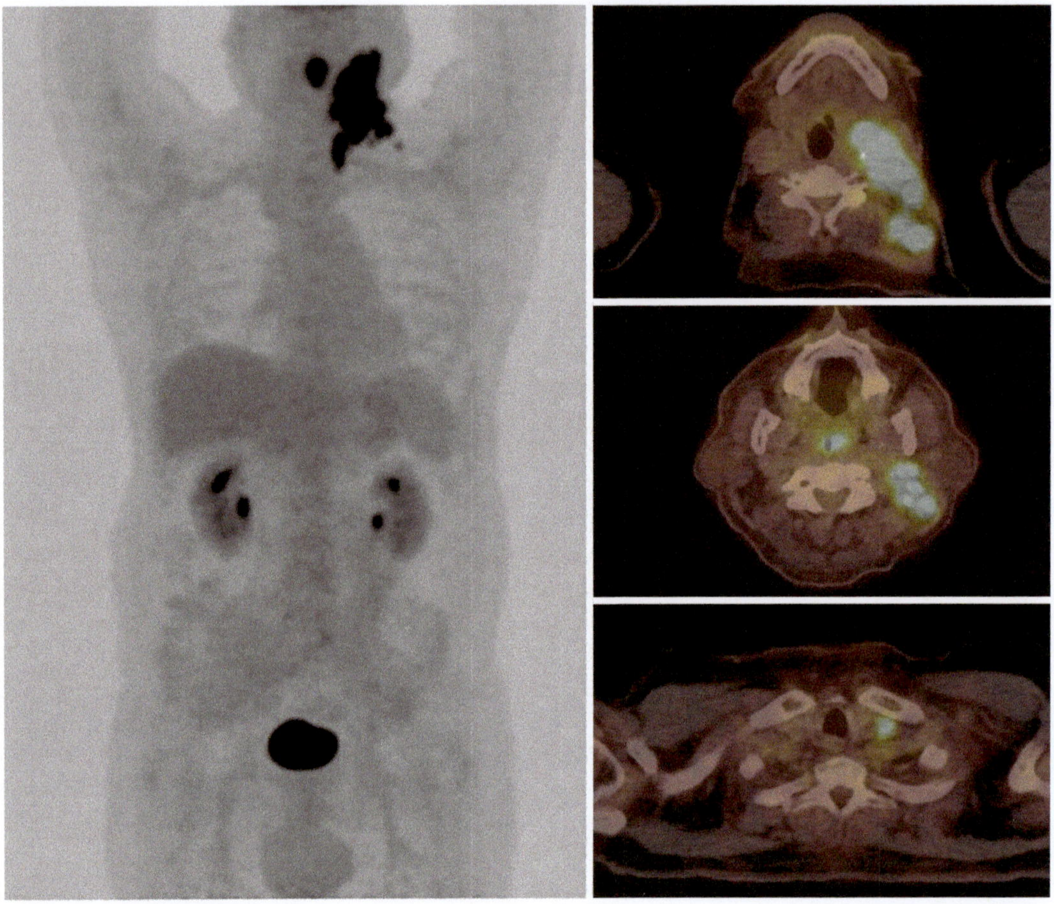

Fig. 7.7 MIP-PET and fused PET/CT – initial staging: FDG PET shows increased metabolic activity in the pharynx, enlarged left-sided neck, supra- and infraclavicular lymph nodes

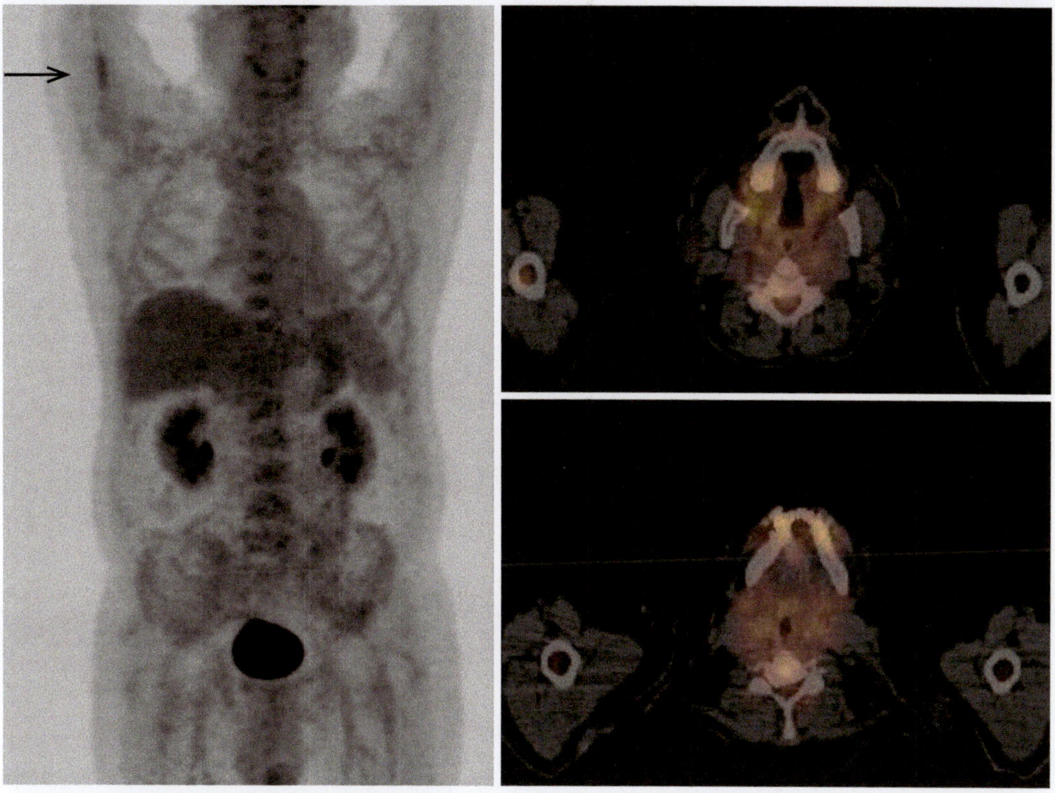

Fig. 7.8 MIP-PET and fused PET/CT – interim PET: No abnormal FDG uptake is shown in the neck. A small focus with mildly increased metabolic activity is observed in the shaft of the right humerus (*arrow*)

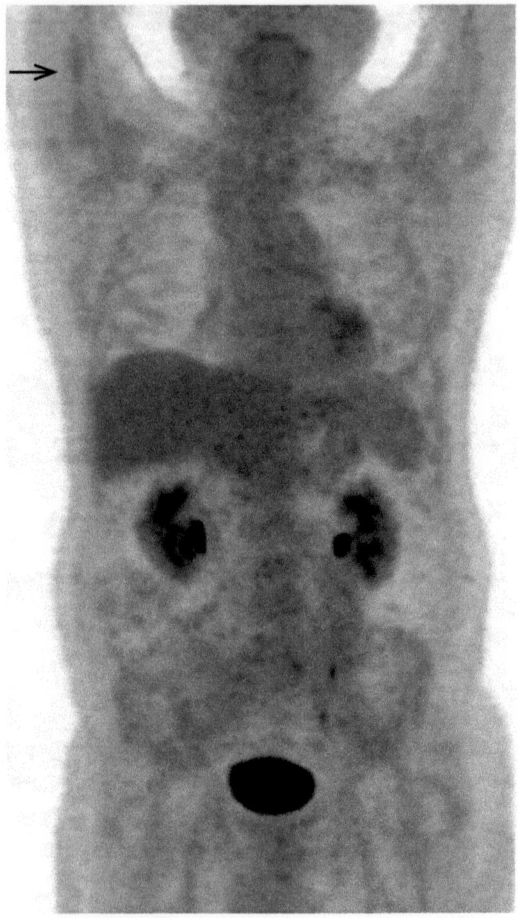

Fig. 7.9 MIP-PET – follow-up: FDG uptake in the shaft of the right humerus (*arrow*) is lower than the previous scan

Aggressive B-Cell Lymphomas: DLBCL – Case 6

A 79-year-old female patient presented with bone pain (especially of the lower right ribs and lumbar spine) with a history of methotrexate administration due to scleroderma. MRI of the lumbar spine and pelvis showed multiple bone lesions in all lumbar and lower thoracic vertebrae as well as in the right side of the sacrum and right iliac bone, indicative of malignancy. A right iliac bone biopsy was performed showing infiltration by DLBCL, while bone marrow biopsy showed no infiltration.

Baseline PET/CT revealed multiple hypermetabolic lesions (SUVmax of 13.5) in C5 and C6, in multiple thoracic (T6, T7, T8, T9, T11, T12) and in all lumbar vertebrae. Increased FDG uptake was also evident by several bone lesions in the sternum, ribs, and pelvic bones. Small hypermetabolic lymph nodes were identified in the right posterior cervical triangle, in the right supra- and infraclavicular areas, among the muscles of the right upper anterior thoracic wall (SUVmax of 4.6), and at the right lower retrocrural space (SUVmax of 5.9). Below the diaphragm there were small hypermetabolic lymph nodes along the right external iliac vessels and right inguinal area (SUVmax of 3.8) (Fig. 7.10).

Thus, the patient had Ann Arbor stage IVA DLBCL with an IPI score of 3 (age >60, increased LDH, stage IV; high -intermediate).

The patient received chemotherapy with the R-CHOP regimen (with modified doses according to her age), and an interim PET/CT was performed after 3 cycles showing complete resolution of the FDG uptake by all the affected lymph nodes. In addition, there was decrease in the extent and the degree of the metabolic activity of the bone lesions. There was persistence of the FDG uptake but to a lesser extent by the vertebrae and pelvic bones (SUVmax of 5.5 – ΔSUVmax −59 %) (Fig. 7.11).

The patient received 3 additional R-CHOP cycles. A follow-up PET/CT was performed after the completion of the 6th cycle showing further improvement with further decrease in the metabolic activity of the above described affected bones (SUVmax of 3.8 instead of 5.5) (Fig. 7.12).

The patient received involved site RT, and a PET/CT was performed 6 months after the completion of the treatment showing complete resolution of the FDG uptake by all involved areas (Fig. 7.13).

The patient remains in CR for 1½ year after the diagnosis.

Discussion: In this patient with stage VIA DLBCL, the interim PET-CT showed partial response. The end-of-treatment PET/CT showed a complete response.

In real life, interim PET imaging is frequently performed in clinical practice, and its purpose is to ensure the effectiveness of the treatment and exclude the possibility of progression. PET-CT shows metabolic response earlier than anatomic response and has the potential to replace CT. Studies have shown that iPET is a strong prognostic indicator in NHL. However, in the absence of proven effective therapy for iPET-positive patients, the use of iPET is not currently recommended for DLBCL in routine clinical practice.

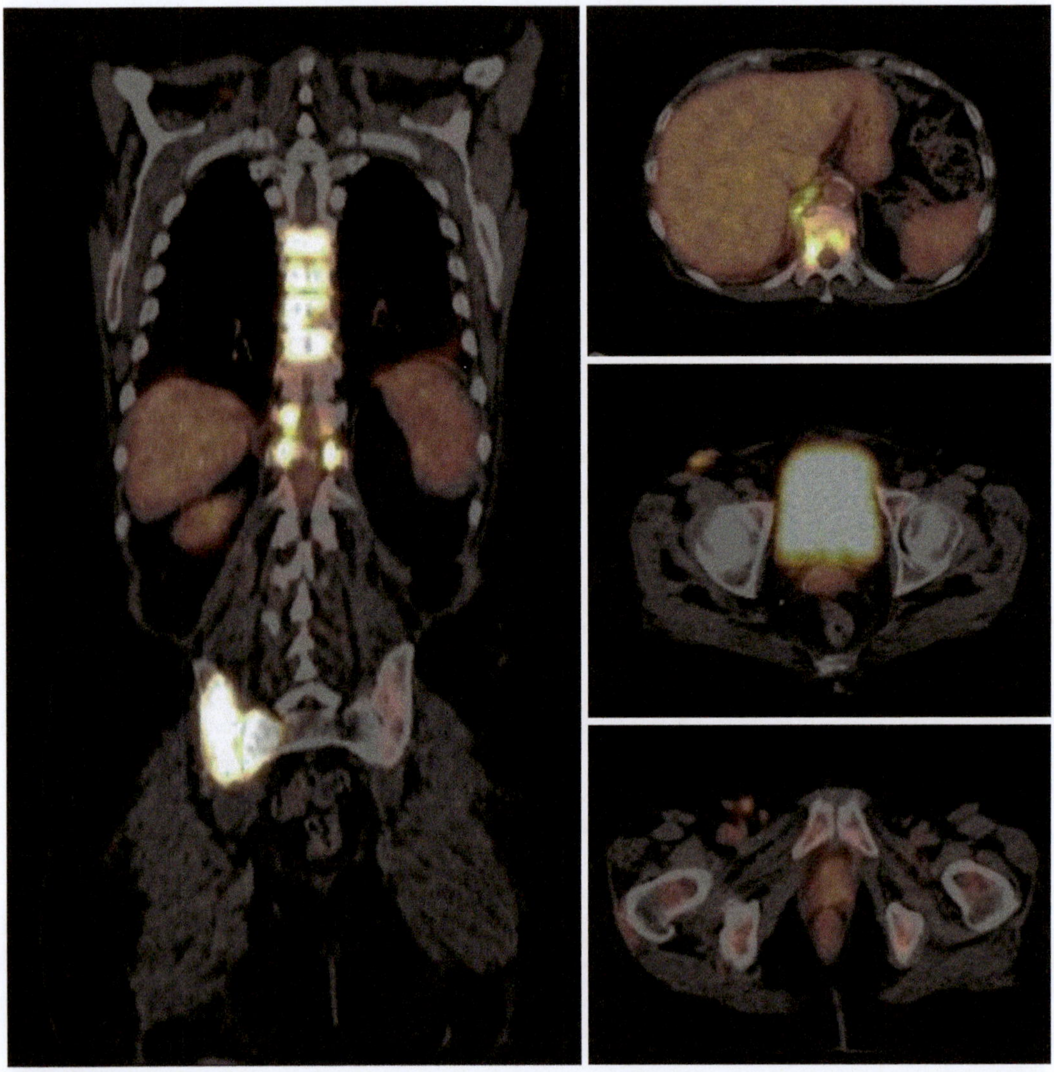

Fig. 7.10 FDG PET/CT – baseline: Increased metabolic activity in multiple lymph nodes (*right panel*), and in multiple vertebrae of the thoracic and lumbar spine as well as the right iliac bone and sacrum (*left panel*)

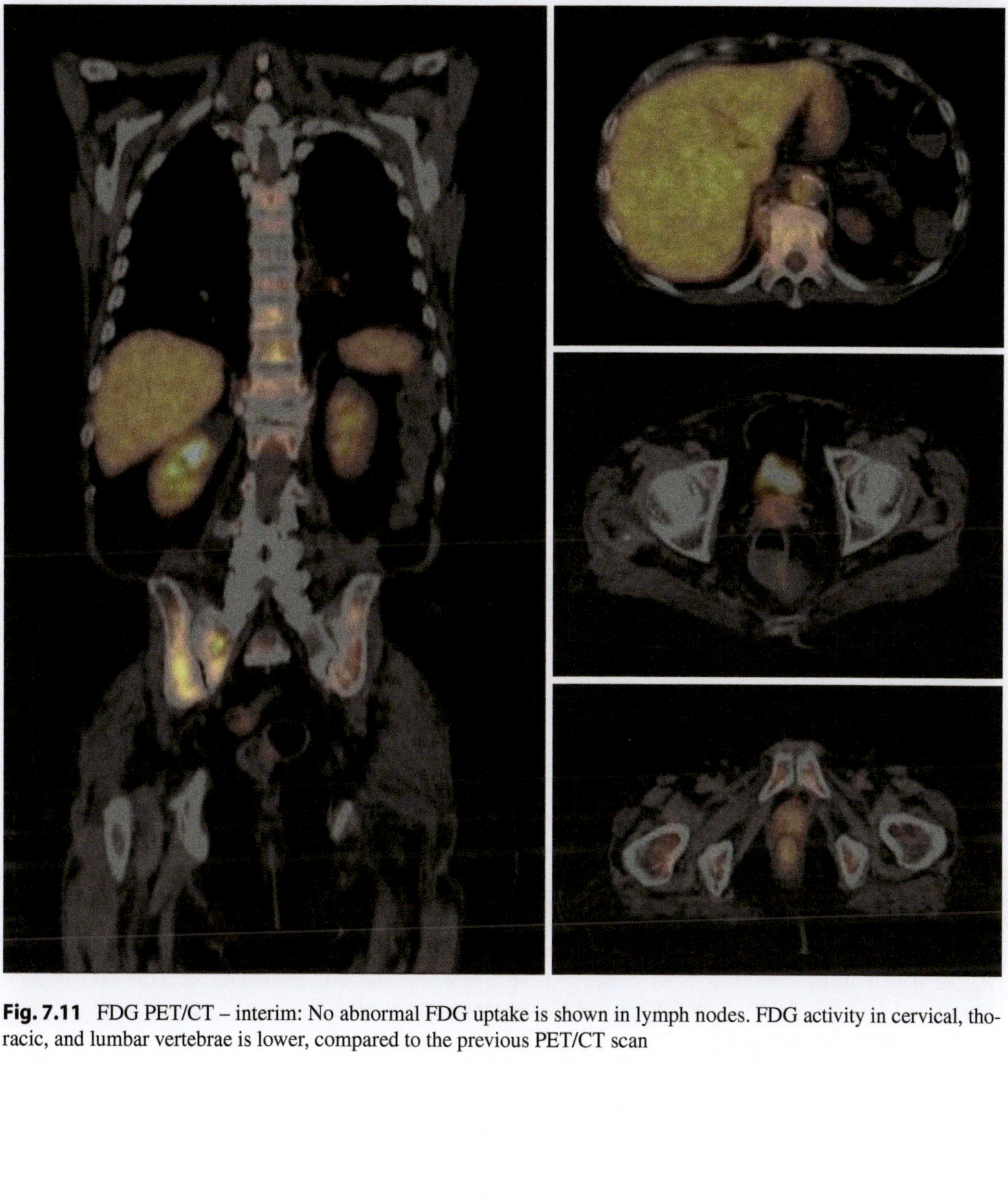

Fig. 7.11 FDG PET/CT – interim: No abnormal FDG uptake is shown in lymph nodes. FDG activity in cervical, thoracic, and lumbar vertebrae is lower, compared to the previous PET/CT scan

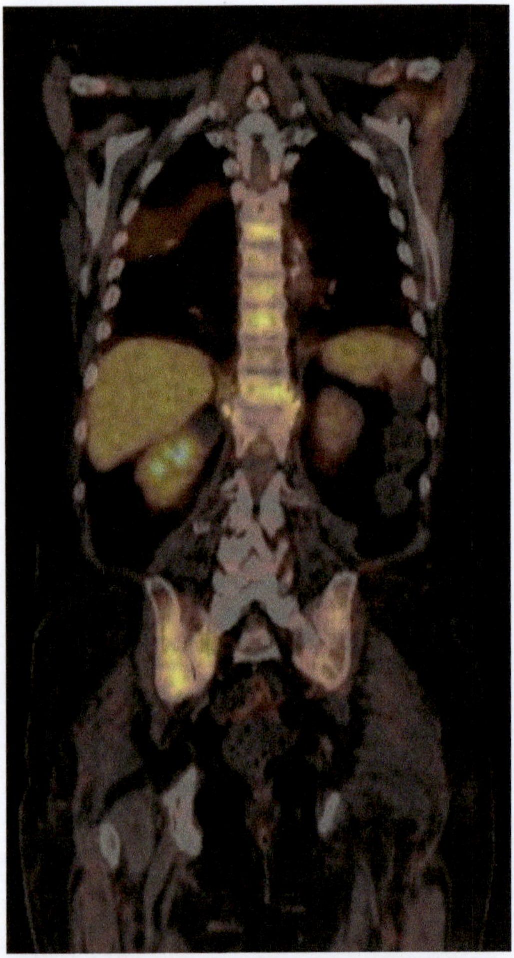

Fig. 7.12 FDG PET/CT at the end of chemotherapy: Further improvement, with lower FDG uptake in bone structures compared to the previous scan

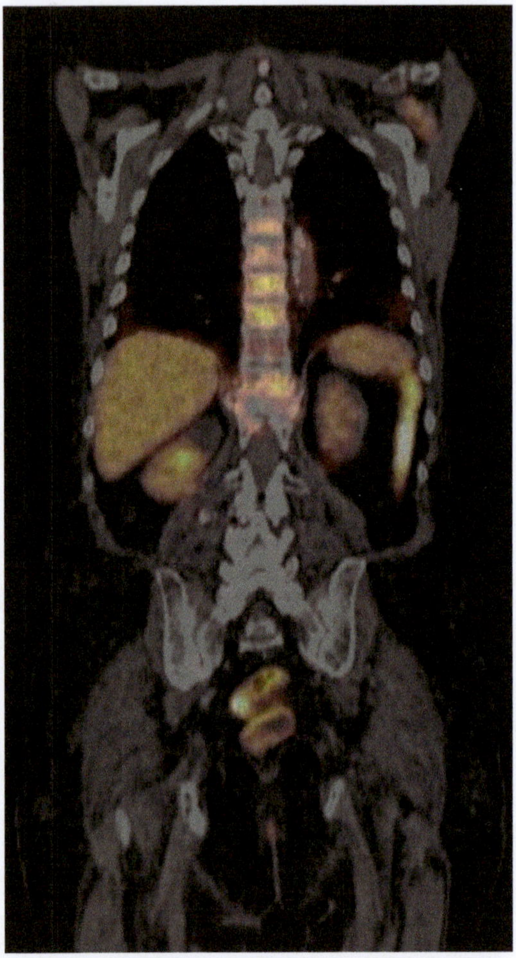

Fig. 7.13 FDG PET/CT 6 months after the completion of treatment: Normal distribution of FDG uptake. Bones appear normal

Aggressive B-Cell Lymphomas: DLBCL – Case 7

A 57-year-old female patient presented to us with abdominal colicky pain, not relieved by analgesics. A CT of the abdomen showed a huge nodular abdominal mass surrounding the abdominal aorta extending from the origin of the celiac artery to the orifices of the renal vessels. This mass engulfed the celiac artery and the initial parts of its branches (common hepatic and splenic), the upper mesenteric artery, and the left renal artery and vein. Nevertheless all the above vessels were patent. There were also nodular paraortic masses (left and right and along the length of the common iliac arteries, as well) and several enlarged mesenteric lymph nodes. CT of the chest and neck showed no lymph node involvement.

An open biopsy of the mass was performed showing infiltration by DLBCL.

A baseline PET/CT was performed showing a huge lymph node block in the upper abdomen mainly on the left side extending from the origin of the celiac artery to the bifurcation of the aorta with increased FDG uptake (SUVmax of 4.3).

Thus the patient had DLBCL stage IIA with a low-risk IPI score of 1 (increased serum LDH) (Fig. 7.14). She received chemotherapy with R-CHOP regimen.

An interim PET/CT was performed after 3 cycles showing complete resolution of the FDG uptake (Fig. 7.15).

The patient continued 3 additional cycles of R-CHOP and the follow-up PET/CT was negative.

The patient remains in CR for 3 years after the initial diagnosis.

Discussion: In this case, conventional staging and PET/CT provided the same stage classification. A interim PET/CT under R-CHOP is associated with better prognosis. The negative end-of-treatment PET/CT with the low IPI score signifies low risk of relapse, confirmed by the excellent subsequent course.

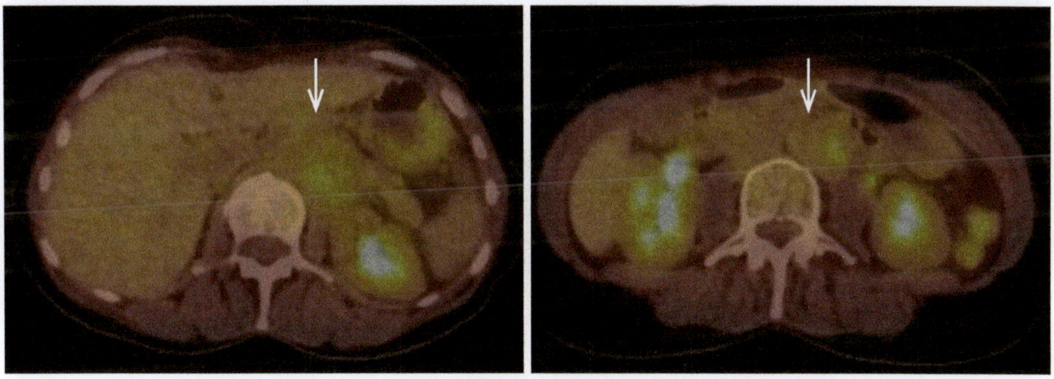

Fig. 7.14 Fused PET/CT – initial staging: Increased FDG uptake is shown in lymph nodes in the abdomen (*arrows*)

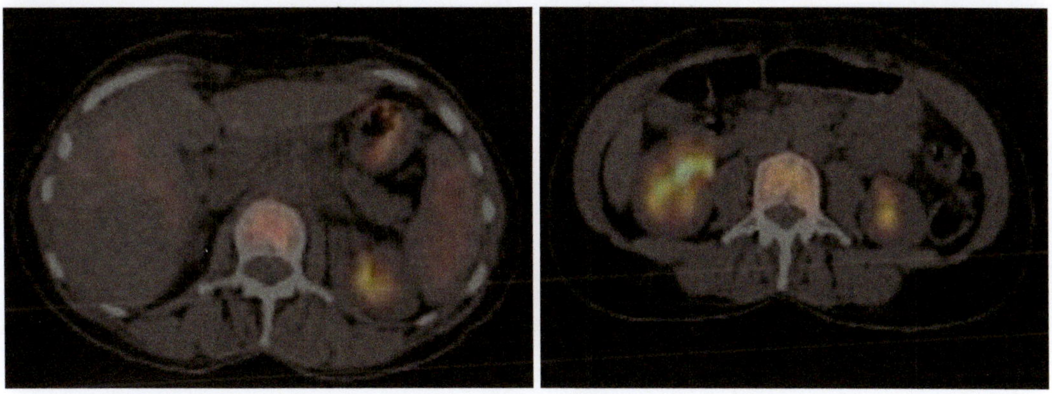

Fig. 7.15 Fused PET/CT – interim: No enlarged lymph nodes or abnormal FDG uptake is noted in the abdomen

Aggressive B-Cell Lymphomas: DLBCL – Case 8

A 62-year-old male patient presented with shortness of breath, weakness, fever, night sweats, difficulty in swallowing, and appetite loss.

Chest CT scan showed bilateral pleural effusions, more prominent on the right side, pericardial effusion, mediastinal lymphadenopathy, bilateral supraclavicular lymphadenopathy, and significant compression of the superior vena cava and the right pulmonary artery. Abdominal CT showed multiple enlarged mesenteric (up to 4 cm), and left paraortic lymph nodes as well as enlarged nodes around the celiac trunk. Neck CT showed multiple enlarged cervical and supraclavicular nodes (up to 5.8 cm) compressing the large vessels mainly at the level of the hyoid bone. Lymph node biopsy revealed DLBCL while bone marrow biopsy showed no infiltration.

As showed in figure 7.16, PET/CT showed multiple hypermetabolic lymphatic masses in the neck (bilateral cervical, supraclavicular, infraclavicular with SUVmax of 17.3) and the mediastinum (prevascular, aortopulmonary, subcarinal, pretracheal, and paratracheal with SUVmax of 15.6). There were also hypermetabolic hilar and axillary lymph nodes. In the abdomen and pelvis, there were multiple lymph nodes with increased FDG uptake involving the peripancreatic, hepatogastric, and gastrosplenic areas (SUVmax of 12.2) as well as involving the paraortic, mesenteric and inguinal lymph nodes. PET/CT also showed a hypermetabolic lesion in the right anterior lateral thoracic wall in proximity to the sternum and multiple, hypermetabolic implants in the left perirenal area and in the upper part of the left iliac muscle (SUVmax of 5.4).

Thus the patient had an Ann Arbor stage IVB DLBCL, with a high-risk IPI score of 5 (age >60, increased LDH, ECOG performance status 2, stage IV, ≥2 extranodal sites).

He received 2 cycles of the HyperCVAD regimen. An interim PET/CT following the second cycle showed complete resolution of the FDG uptake in all areas (Fig. 7.17).

Due to lack of patient compliance and his refusal to continue with intensive chemotherapy, the patient received one more R-HyperCVAD cycle and three cycles of R-CHOP. A follow-up PET/CT following these cycles of therapy showed reappearance of hypermetabolic lymph nodes in the mediastinum (Fig. 7.18).

The patient received two cycles of R-ICE. A new PET/CT was done showing complete resolution of the FDG uptake in all regions (Fig. 7.19).

Discussion: In this case, the negative interim PET/CT was not associated with a favorable final response, most probably because of the lack of compliance and de-escalation of treatment. Additional factors to this might have been the high IPI score.

Nevertheless, the patient was effectively salvaged with 2 cycles of R-ICE achieving a PET-negative status.

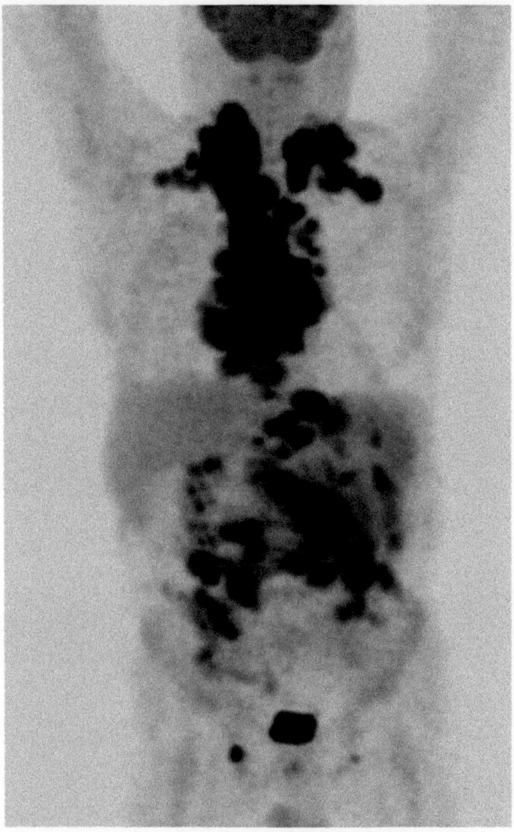

Fig. 7.16 Multiple hypermetabolic lesions are seen in the neck, thorax, abdomen, and pelvis

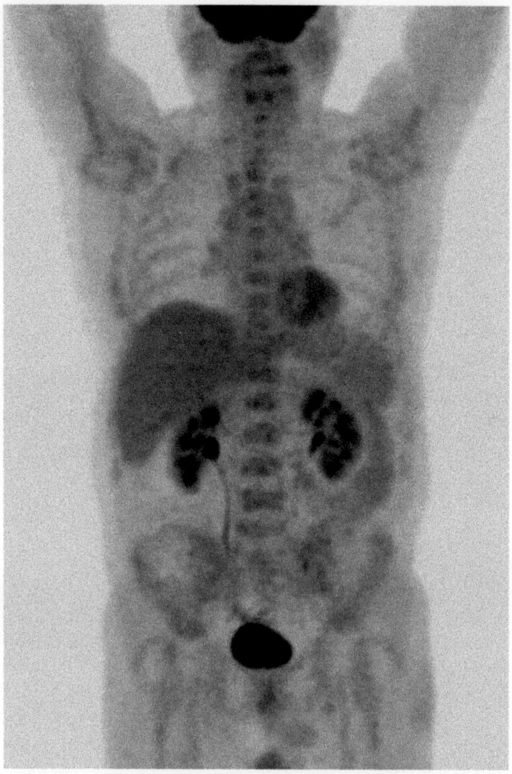

Fig. 7.17 No residual mass or abnormal FDG uptake is shown in the neck, mediastinum, and mesentery

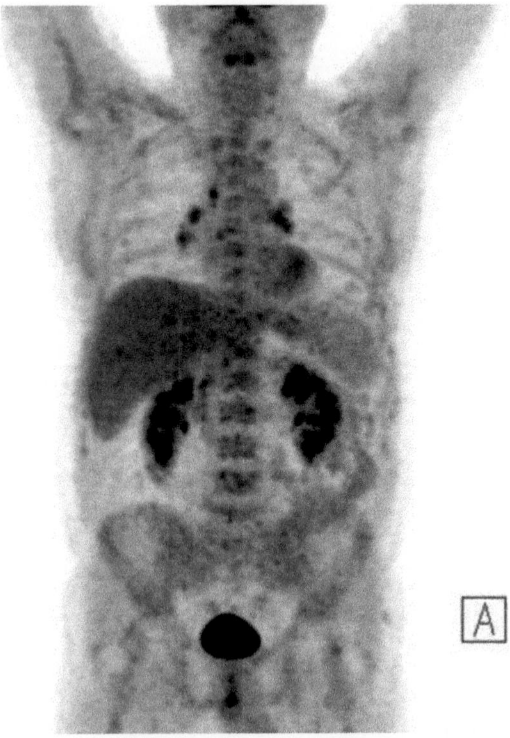

Fig. 7.18 PET/CT shows increased FDG uptake in mediastinal and hilar lymph nodes, new findings compared to the previous PET/CT

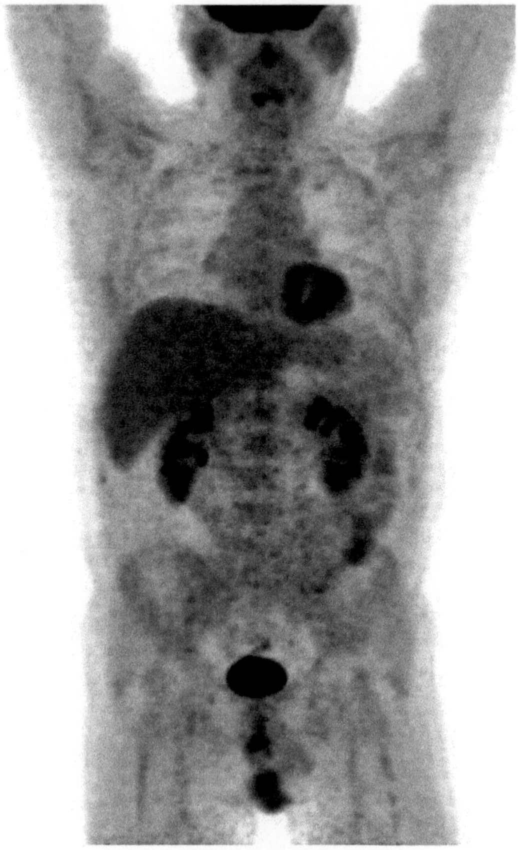

Fig. 7.19 No abnormally increased FDG uptake is shown. The mediastinum and hila appear normal

Aggressive B-Cell Lymphomas: DLBCL – Case 9

An otherwise asymptomatic 81-year-old man presented with right cervical and right axillary lymphadenopathy of 8 cm and 10 cm maximal diameter, respectively. An axillary lymph node revealed a DLBCL of non-germinal center cell origin. A complete CT staging additionally demonstrated left axillary (2 cm) and right hilar lymphadenopathy and a 2.5 cm focal splenic lesion. A bone marrow biopsy was negative. The clinical stage was IIISA. IPI and aaIPI values were "3" and "2," respectively, i.e., high-intermediate risk, due to advanced age and stage and elevated LDH levels (1.64×). Baseline PET/CT revealed a significantly increased FDG uptake (maximum SUVmax of 16.9) in all of the above anatomic sites (Fig. 7.20a–f) as well as in the right tonsil (Fig. 7.20a) and a left inguinal lymph node. The patient received 6 cycles of "reduced" R-CHOP according to his age and 2 additional rituximab infusions. A complete radiographic CR was achieved by CT with a residual axillary node of 1.4 cm. A repeated end-of-treatment PET/CT was completely negative (Fig. 7.21). Thereafter, he remains in complete remission 32 months after final reevaluation.

Discussion: Despite the identification of more disease sites in this case, PET/CT did not change neither clinical stage nor IPI. The completely negative ePET and the absence of measurable residual lesions are compatible with the excellent subsequent clinical course of this patient, obscuring the potential adverse significance of the high-intermediate IPI and aaIPI classification.

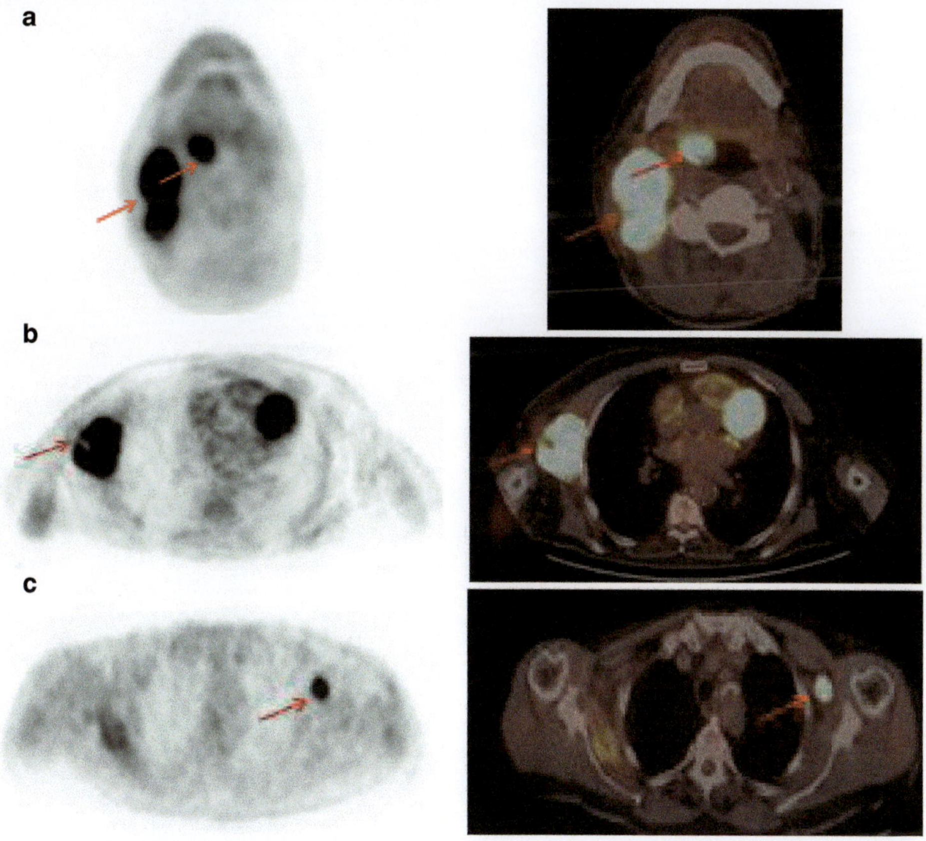

Fig. 7.20 PET and fused PET/CT – initial staging: Hypermetabolic lesions in *right* cervical nodal mass and tonsil (**a**), axillary lymph nodes (**b**, **c**), *right* pulmonary hilum (**d**), spleen (**e**), and *left* inguinal lymph node (**f**) (hypermetabolic lesions are indicated with *red arrows*)

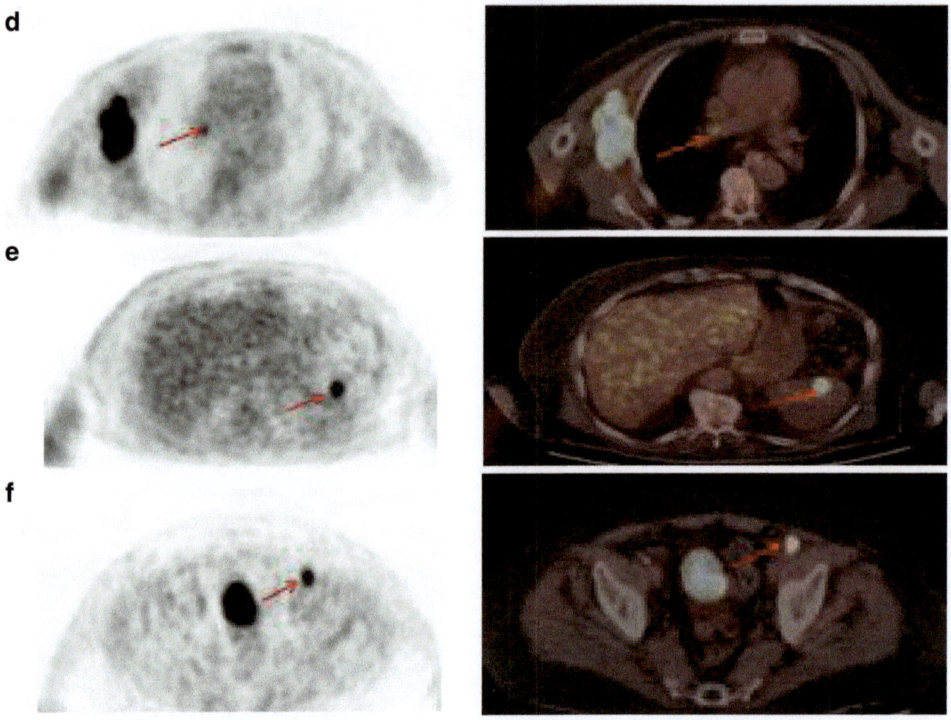

Fig. 7.20 (continued)

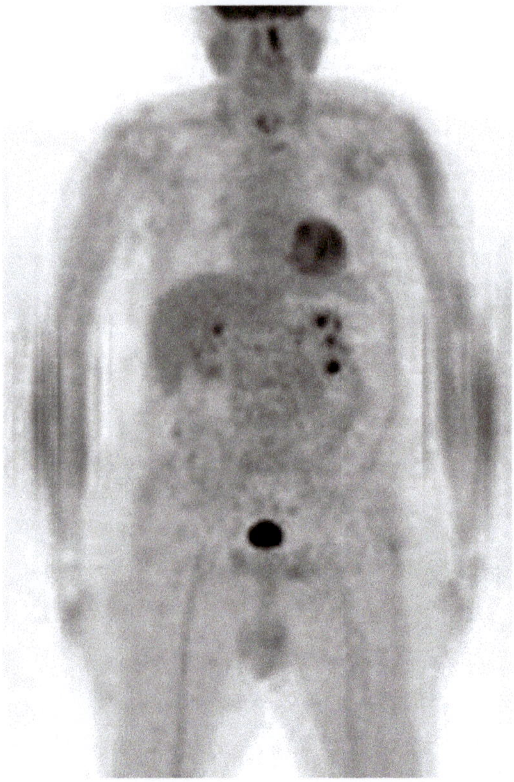

Fig. 7.21 MIP-PET – end of treatment: Negative for abnormal hypermetabolic lesions

Aggressive B-Cell Lymphomas: DLBCL – Case 10

A 66-year-old woman presented with prolonged fever. Physical examination revealed a 2 cm left supraclavicular lymph node, extensive para-aortic, retrocrural, and celiac lymphadenopathy up to 5.5 cm, smaller pelvic nodes, and multiple splenic lesions up to 7 cm. A DLBCL of non-germinal center cell origin was diagnosed following a supraclavicular lymph node biopsy. A bone marrow biopsy was negative. Clinical stage was IIISB, while IPI was 3, i.e., "high-intermediate" due to advanced age and stage and elevated serum LDH levels (3.14×). She received 8 cycles of the R-CHOP regimen and achieved a complete remission with a completely negative PET/CT (Fig. 7.22), albeit multiple residual splenic lesions up to 2.5 cm still persisted. Routine follow-up CTs were performed 4 months later and revealed mediastinal, subcarinal, and bilateral hilar lymphadenopathy up to 3 cm with associated multiple, small lung nodules bilaterally. A PET/CT performed 1 month later confirmed the above findings (including small supraclavicular lymphadenopathy), which had highly increased metabolic activity (SUVmax of 14.5), and additionally demonstrated a moderately hypermetabolic node at the hepatogastric space (SUVmax of 5.3) (Fig. 7.23). Based on PET findings, an excisional biopsy of a 1.5 cm, deeply lying, non-palpable supraclavicular node was performed by an experienced thoracic surgeon under local anesthesia according to Daniels' procedure. Histologic examination revealed granulomatous lymphadenopathy consistent with sarcoidosis. The diagnosis was confirmed by bronchoscopy and TBNA. The radiographic findings remained stable 1 month after biopsy but began to decrease in size 2 months later. Spontaneous complete resolution was observed 6 months after their first appearance without any treatment. She remains in complete remission 2 years after the resolution of this granulomatous reaction.

Discussion: The negative PET in this case was still associated with a considerable risk of relapse, because of the high-intermediate baseline IPI and, probably, the persistence of residual lesions >2 cm by conventional radiology [4, 22–27]. Despite this, the very rapid reappearance of lymphadenopathy within 4 months from PET negativity and its distribution (bilateral hilar nodes involved) suggested that an alternative etiology should be excluded. In any case, histologic confirmation of relapse is highly desirable and is recommended to perform, if technically feasible. A repeated PET/CT revealed highly hypermetabolic lymphadenopathy, which could easily be confused with DLBCL, but ultimately proved to be a sarcoid-like reaction. Furthermore, PET/CT revealed an otherwise disregarded supraclavicular node, the excisional biopsy of which was crucial to establish the diagnosis in an "easy" way, obviating the need for an extensive surgical intervention. Sarcoid-like reactions are rather rare, but should be considered in the differential diagnosis of "suspected relapse" in patient with malignant lymphomas [49].

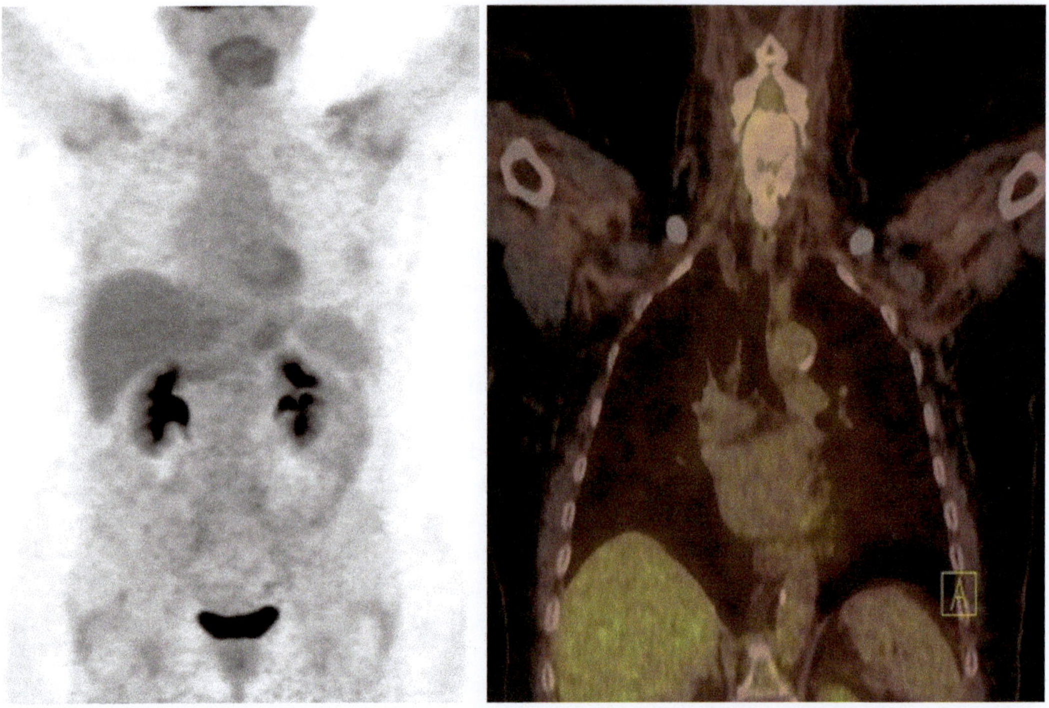

Fig. 7.22 MIP-PET and fused PET/CT images: No lesions of increased uptake of the radiopharmaceutical are observed

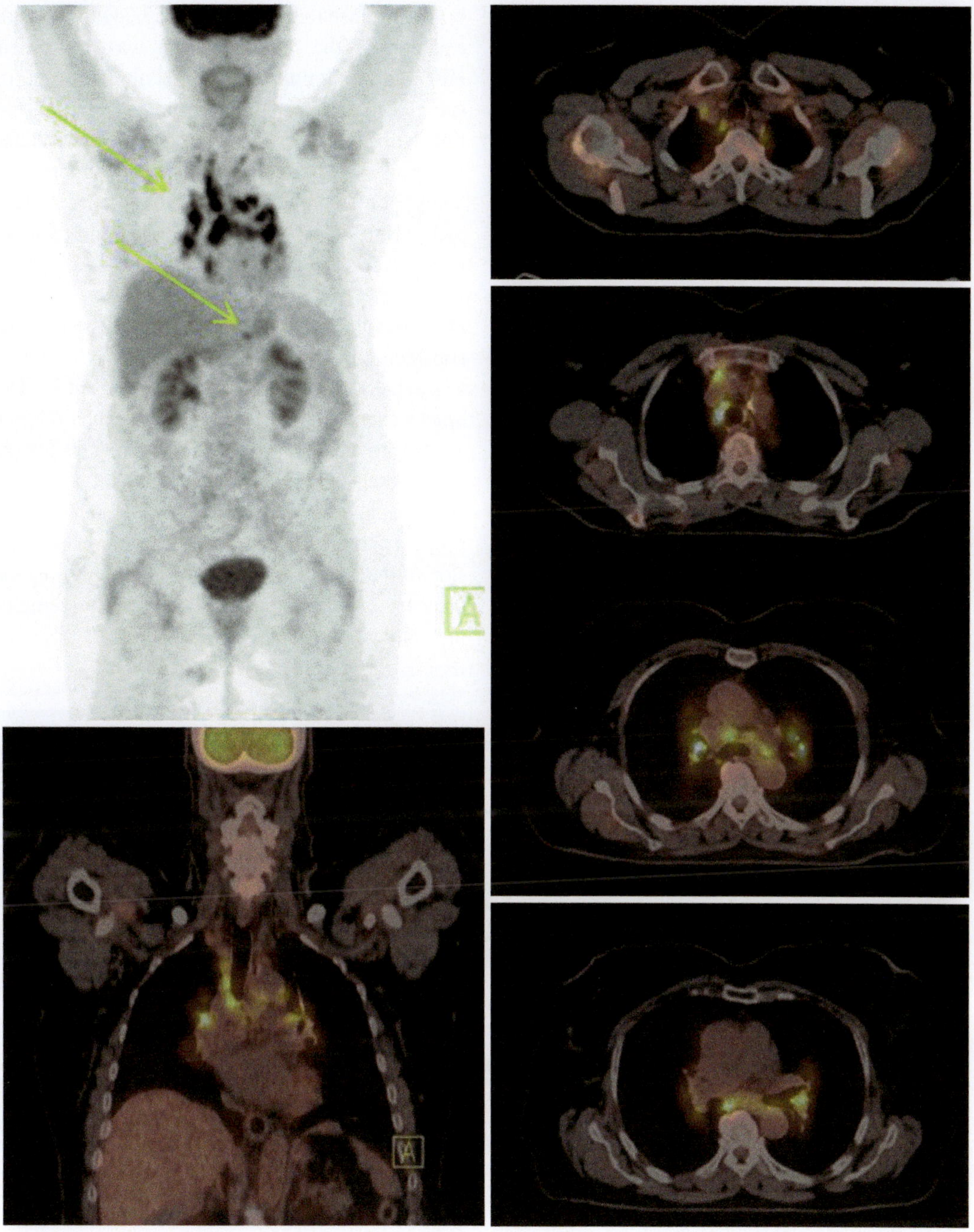

Fig. 7.23 MIP-PET and fused PET/CT images: Multiple hypermetabolic lesions are observed at the mediastinum (at the entrance of the thorax, the prevascular space, right paratracheal, the aorta-pulmonary region, infra-carinal area, the pulmonary hilum bilaterally) suggestive of active disease (SUVmax of 14.5), as well as at the hepatogastric space (SUVmax of 5.3) (*arrows* in the MIP image). Interestingly, these lesions were due to a sarcoid-like reaction (see text)

Aggressive B-Cell Lymphomas: DLBCL – Case 11

A 45-year-old woman presented with a large soft tissue subcutaneous mass of 12 cm diameter in the internal surface of the right thigh. Excisional biopsy demonstrated a DLBCL NOS of germinal center cell origin. CT and MRI staging revealed right inguinal and right external iliac lymphadenopathy up to 2 cm. A bone marrow biopsy was negative. Clinical stage was IIEXA. The IPI value was "1," i.e., low risk, due to elevated LDH levels (1.12×), but aaIPI was low-intermediate risk ("1"). She received 8 cycles of R-CHOP combination chemotherapy and achieved a >75 % reduction of the dominant mass, although a ~4 cm residual abnormality still persisted. PET/CT demonstrated mildly increased 18FDG uptake (SUVmax of 2) in the right inguinofemoral residual lesion. The uptake was higher than that of the mediastinum but lower than that of the liver parenchyma corresponding to D5-PS score of 3, consistent of metabolic response to treatment (Fig. 7.24a, b). A wide excision of the residual lesion was performed. Histologic examination revealed fibroadiposal tissue and moderately thick, reactive T-cell infiltration with no evidence of lymphoma. A repeated PET/CT performed 3 months after surgery was completely negative. The patient remains in complete remission 22 months after the end-of-treatment PET/CT examination.

Discussion: End-of-treatment PET/CT would be considered positive based on the IHP criteria [47, 48], which were used until mid-2014, since FDG uptake exceeded that of the mediastinal blood pool in a >2 cm residual mass. Not exceeding the uptake of the liver, D5-PS score was 3, which is considered negative according to the recently adopted Lugano classification [1, 2]. Indeed, complete excision of the residual tissue failed to demonstrate the presence of lymphoma, and the patient still remains in complete remission ~2 years later.

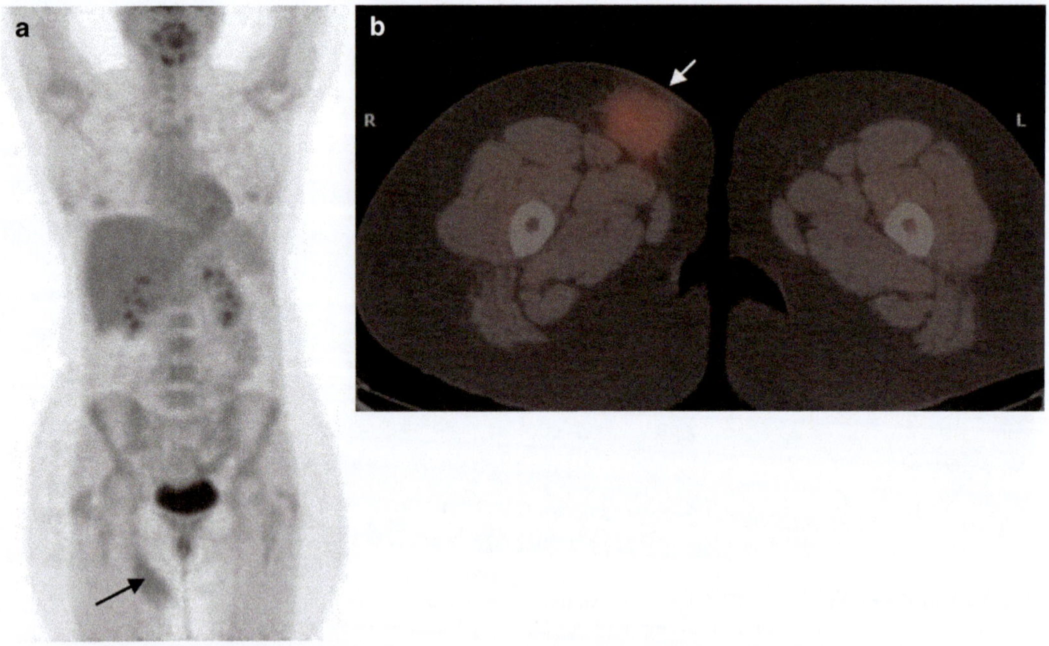

Fig. 7.24 (**a**, **b**) MIP-PET and fused PET/CT post-chemotherapy: Mildly increased 18FDG uptake (SUVmax of 2, higher than that of the mediastinum but lower than that of the liver parenchyma) in the right inguinofemoral residual lesion (*black arrow* in MIP and *white arrow* in the fused images)

Aggressive B-Cell Lymphomas: DLBCL – Case 12

A 49-year-old man presented with a rapidly increasing 8 cm left inguinal swelling and pruritus. A lymph node biopsy established the diagnosis of DLBCL of non-germinal center cell origin. Complete CT staging also revealed left iliac lymphadenopathy up to 3.2 cm. A bone marrow biopsy was negative. Clinical stage was IIA. The IPI value was "1," i.e., low risk (aaIPI "1" or low-intermediate risk), due to the elevated LDH levels (1.21×). After 3 cycles of R-CHOP immunochemotherapy, a >80 % disease reduction was achieved. Further response was obtained following 6 R-CHOP cycles, after which a 2.4 cm left inguinal residual lesion was present. PET/CT revealed very mild 18FDG uptake (SUVmax of 1.5), lower than that of the mediastinal blood pool, in the left inguinal nodal residue, corresponding to a D5-PS score of 2 (Fig. 7.25a, b). No further treatment was administered, and the patient remains in clinical remission 14 months after the final PET/CT, while the size of the residual mass has been decreasing up to 1.6 cm.

Discussion: End-of-treatment PET/CT would be considered negative based on the IHP criteria [47, 48], since FDG uptake did not exceed that of the mediastinal blood pool in a >2 cm residual lesion. D5-PS score was 2, which is also considered negative according to the recently adopted Lugano classification [1, 2]. The lack of clinical significance for this mild uptake is supported in this case by the ongoing shrinkage of the residual abnormality and the uneventful follow-up.

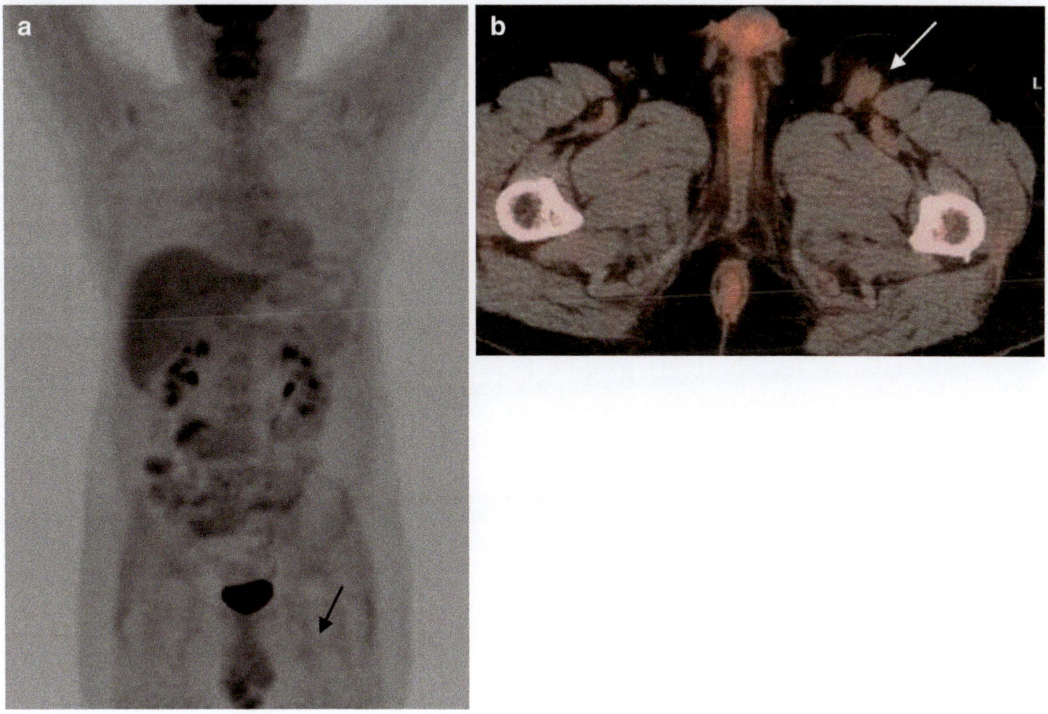

Fig. 7.25 (**a**, **b**) MIP-PET and fused PET/CT – end of treatment: Mild (lower than the mediastinum) FDG uptake at a *left* inguinal nodal residue (*black arrow* in MIP and *white arrow* in the fused images)

Aggressive B-Cell Lymphomas: DLBCL – Case 13

A 48-year-old man presented with pain at the left gluteal region for a period of 3 months. He was otherwise asymptomatic and had a long-standing history of mild renal insufficiency. A focus of abnormal signal was detected within the left iliac bone in close proximity to the ilio-sacral joint on MRI. There was an associated 3 cm soft tissue mass and gluteal muscle edema as well as similar bone findings within the right iliac (1 cm) and sacral bone (2 cm). A left iliac bone biopsy led to the diagnosis of a DLBCL-NOS of germinal center cell origin. A bone marrow biopsy was negative. Clinical stage was IVA. The IPI value "1," i.e., low risk, due to the advanced stage, but aaIPI was classified as low-intermediate risk ("1"). He received 6 cycles of R-CHOP combination chemotherapy: All other disease sites disappeared with the exception of the left iliac bone lesion, which remained stable in size, but the abnormal signal became more heterogeneous. On PET/CT, this lesion was not photopenic ("cold"), but had mild 18FDG uptake (SUVmax of 2.5) lower than that of the mediastinum and corresponding to D5-PS score of 2 (Fig. 7.26a, b). No further treatment was recommended. A repeated PET/CT performed 5 months later due to "new" local findings on MRI was completely negative. The patient remains in complete remission 6 months after the end-of-treatment PET/CT examination.

Discussion: End-of-treatment PET/CT would be considered negative based on the IHP criteria [47, 48], since FDG uptake did not exceed that of the mediastinal blood pool in a >2 cm residual lesion, although bone lesions are recommended to be characterized as negative on PET/CT when they are completely photopenic. D5-PS score was 2, which is also considered negative according to the recently adopted Lugano classification [1, 2]. The lack of clinical significance for this mild uptake is supported in this case by the spontaneous conversion of PET/CT to negative 5 months later.

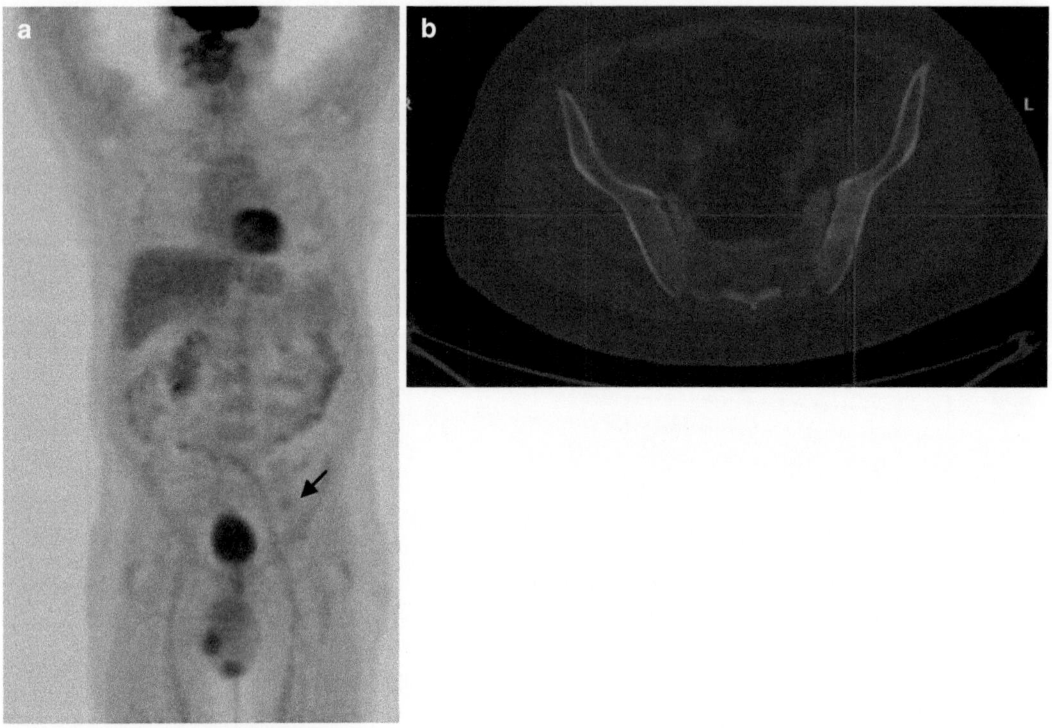

Fig. 7.26 (**a**, **b**) MIP-PET and fused PET/CT – end of treatment: Mild 18FDG uptake at the *left* iliac bone, lower than that of the mediastinum (*black arrow* in the MIP image)

Aggressive B-Cell Lymphomas: DLBCL – Case 14

A 50-year-old patient sought for a medical advice due to very bulky inguinal lymphadenopathy, accompanied by vomiting and weight loss. Histological examination led to the diagnosis of a DLBCL of non-germinal center cell origin. CT imaging revealed heterogeneity of the right liver lobe, splenomegaly, para-aortic lymphadenopathy up to 2.6 cm, left iliac lymphadenopathy forming a 9 cm confluent mass, and a similar 12 cm left inguinal mass. A bone marrow biopsy was negative. The clinical stage was IVXB. Both IPI and aaIPI value was "2," i.e., low-intermediate and high-intermediate risk, respectively, due to advanced stage and elevated LDH levels (1.48×). The patient received 8 cycles of R-CHOP combination immunochemotherapy. Conventional restaging revealed a PR. A huge, clinically palpable residual left inguinal mass still persisted measuring ~8 cm by physical examination. A residual liver lesion of 3.2 cm also persisted. PET/CT demonstrated mildly increased 18FDG uptake (SUVmax of 2) in the left inguinal lymph node enlargement, which was higher than that of the mediastinal blood pool but lower than the liver, corresponding to D5-PS score of 3 (Fig. 7.27a, b). As the lesion was greater than 2 cm, the PET/CT was interpreted as positive according to the IHP criteria, indicating metabolically active residual disease, but would be considered negative according to D5-PS criteria. A complete excision and histologic examination of the residual inguinal mass was performed: No evidence of disease was found. The patient remains in complete remission 18 months after that biopsy.

Discussion: Although the left inguinal residual mass was extremely bulky and ePET was positive according to the IHP criteria, it is considered negative based on the recently established Lugano criteria [1, 2]. The absence of lymphoma was substantiated by a negative histologic examination after complete resection and the uneventful follow-up.

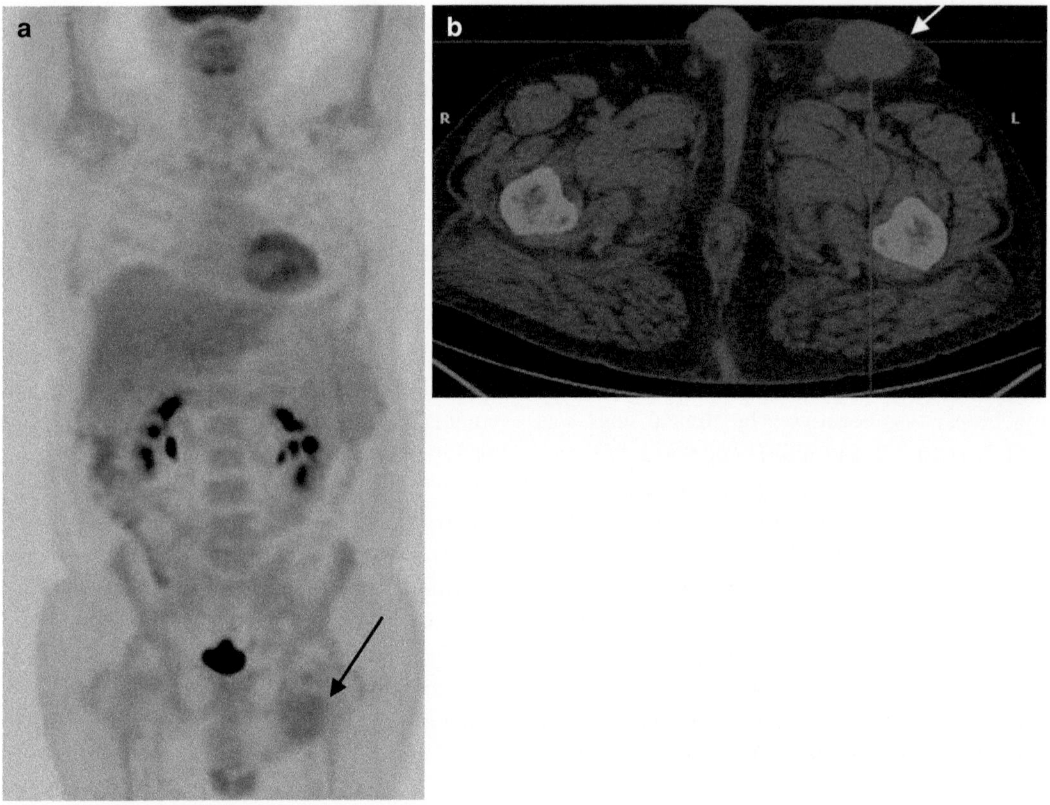

Fig. 7.27 (**a**, **b**) MIP-PET and fused PET/CT – end of treatment: Mild FDG uptake (higher than the mediastinum, lower than the liver) at the *left* inguinal mass (*black arrow* in MIP and *white arrow* in the fused images)

Aggressive B-Cell Lymphomas: DLBCL – Case 15

A 64-year-old patient presented with scrotal and right lower limb edema as well as right inguinofemoral lymphadenopathy up to 5.5 cm. A right inguinal lymph node excisional biopsy revealed a DLBCL of the anaplastic morphologic subtype. CT staging revealed para-aortic, bilateral iliac, and bilateral inguinal lymphadenopathy (max diameter 5.5 cm). A bone marrow biopsy was negative. The clinical stage was IIA. The IPI was "2" and aaIPI was "1," i.e., both low-intermediate risk, due to advanced age and elevated serum LDH levels (1.04×). The patient received 8 cycles of R-CHOP combination immunochemotherapy. A CRu was achieved with a 1.8 cm residual lesion at the right inguinal area. A PET/CT demonstrated mild residual 18FDG uptake (SUVmax of 2) at the right inguinal area, exceeding that of the mediastinum but not the liver, thus corresponding to a D5-PS score of 3 (Fig. 7.28a, b). Subsequently, he underwent RT at a dose of 4400 cGy at the right inguinofemoral and iliac area. A repeated PET/CT, performed 4 months later, was negative (D5-PS score of 1). At the follow-up, 8 months later, CT imaging demonstrated an increasing in size 1.5 cm left iliac node, and a new PET/CT was positive for hypermetabolic left iliac and para-aortic lymphadenopathy. Salvage immunochemotherapy with the R-ESHAP regimen was instituted. After a PET-negative CR achievement, the patient underwent BEAM high dose therapy and autologous stem cell transplantation.

Discussion: After R-CHOP, PET/CT remained positive with a D5-PS score of 3. This was positive according to the IHP criteria [47, 48], but is now considered negative, based on the recent Lugano classification [1, 2]. Treatment with RT was decided based on the IHP-based PET positivity. A PET-negative complete remission was achieved with this strategy. However, 8 months later, disease relapse developed in a previously involved, but not irradiated area. Although RT has led to satisfactory results in patients who respond to R-CHOP but remain PET positive, the risk of relapse is at least 20 % even when the most optimistic data are taken into account [4, 22–27].

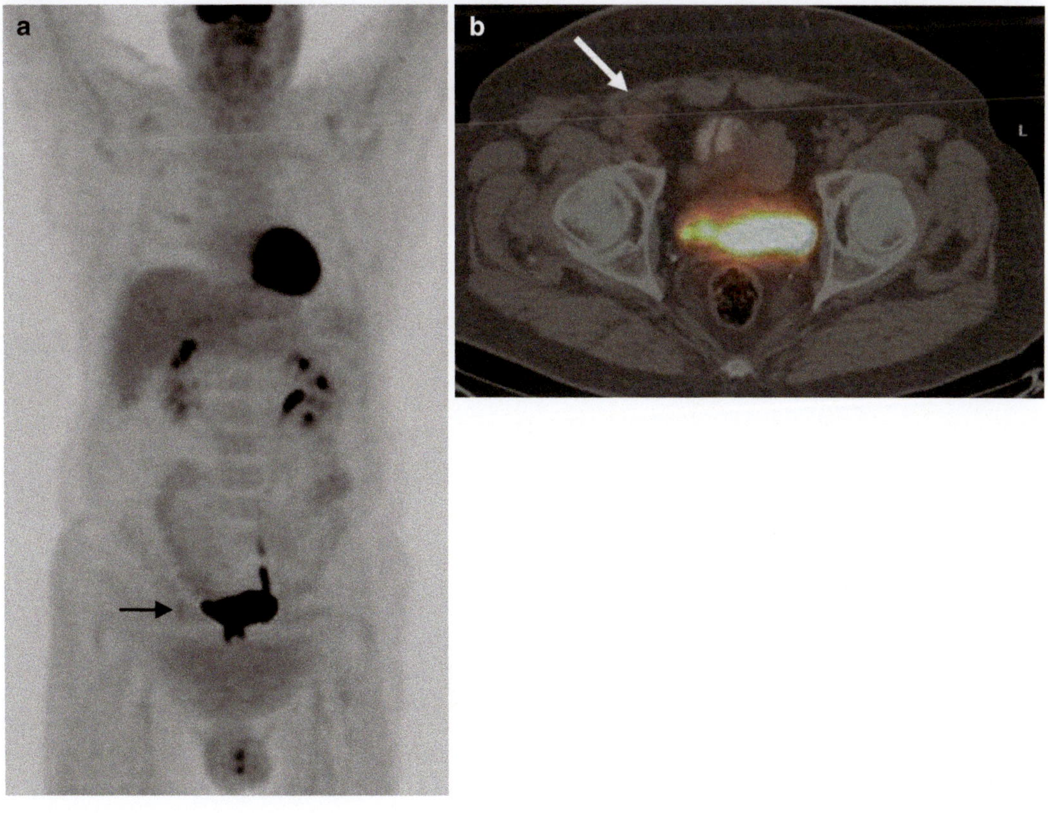

Fig. 7.28 (**a**, **b**) MIP-PET and fused PET/CT – end of chemoimmunotherapy: Mild FDG uptake at a *right* inguinal lymph node (*arrows*), not exceeding the uptake of the liver (D5-PS score 3)

Aggressive B-Cell Lymphomas: DLBCL – Case 16

A 33-year-old man presented with left upper quadrant pain due to a large splenic focal lesion and para-aortic lymphadenopathy. CT-guided biopsy demonstrated a DLBCL NOS of non-germinal center cell origin. A bone marrow biopsy was negative. Clinical stage was IISA. IPI and aaIPI value was "1," i.e., low- and low-intermediate risk, respectively, due to elevated LDH levels (1.12×). He received 8 cycles of R-CHOP combination chemotherapy and achieved a >75 % reduction of the dominant splenic mass, although residual abnormality and para-aortic nodes up to 2 cm still persisted. PET/CT demonstrated mildly increased 18FDG uptake (SUVmax of 3.7) around the splenic residual mass not exceeding the uptake of liver, corresponding to a D5-PS score of 3. Paraortic lymph nodes were negative (Fig. 7.29a–c). A new PET/CT, 3 months later, demonstrated an increase in 18FDG uptake of the splenic mass (SUVmax of 6.5). The uptake was higher than that of the liver and, thus, upgraded to a D5-PS score of 4 (Fig. 7.30a–c). A splenectomy was performed, since this was the sole abnormal focus. Histologic examination of the whole spleen and the residual lesion demonstrated necrosis, with no clear evidence of residual lymphoma. A PET/CT performed 3 months after splenectomy revealed two new nodules with mildly increased 18FDG uptake at the left paracolic area in contact with the omentum (SUVmax of 4). The findings were probably of inflammatory postsurgical origin or due to splenosis (Fig. 7.31a–c) and were confirmed on a subsequent MRI. After 3 months, a new MRI demonstrated a slight decrease of the nodules. Without additional treatment, the patient remains in remission 17 months after the end-of-treatment PET/CT examination.

Discussion: After R-CHOP, PET/CT remained positive with a D5-PS score of 3, which progressed to 4 after 3 months. However, no clear evidence of disease was found on subsequent splenectomy. Although new findings emerged following splenectomy, their lymphomatous nature has not been proved. A post-surgery inflammatory etiology or splenosis cannot be excluded, and the PET-positive nodules do not increase, but rather decrease in size with time. In the absence of progressive disease, histologic confirmation of residual disease post-chemotherapy is highly desirable prior to proceeding to salvage chemotherapy and ASCT, because false-positives are not so rare [4, 24].

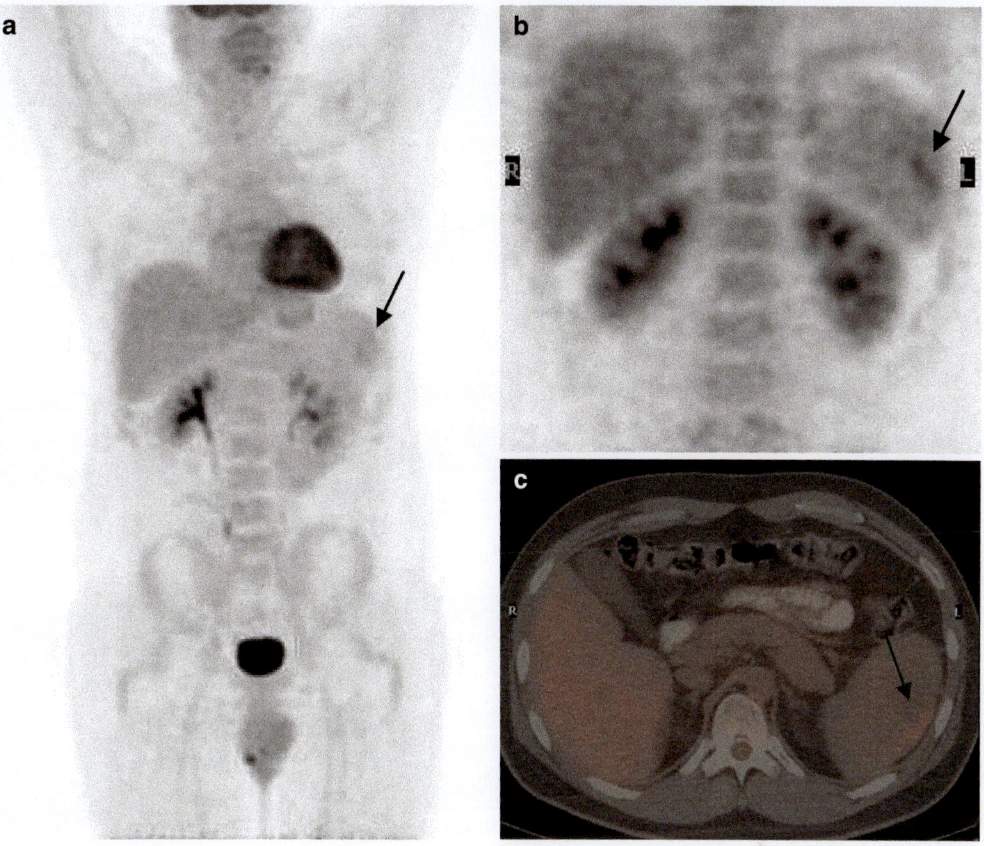

Fig. 7.29 (**a–c**) MIP-PET and fused PET/CT- end of chemotherapy: Mild FDG uptake at a spleen lesion (*arrows*)

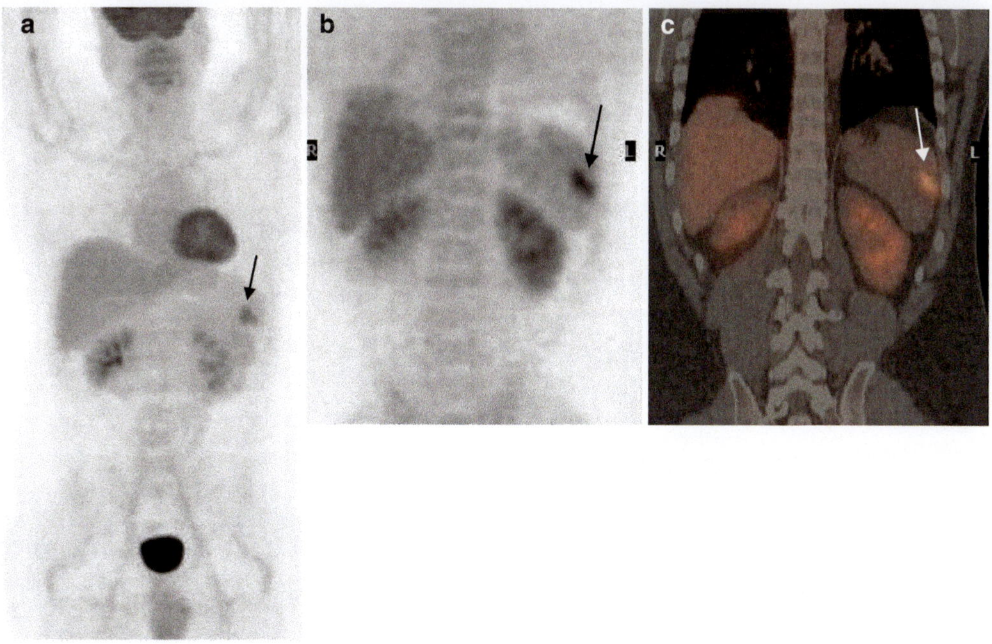

Fig. 7.30 (**a–c**) MIP-PET and fused PET/CT – follow-up: Hypermetabolic lesion at the spleen (*arrows*)

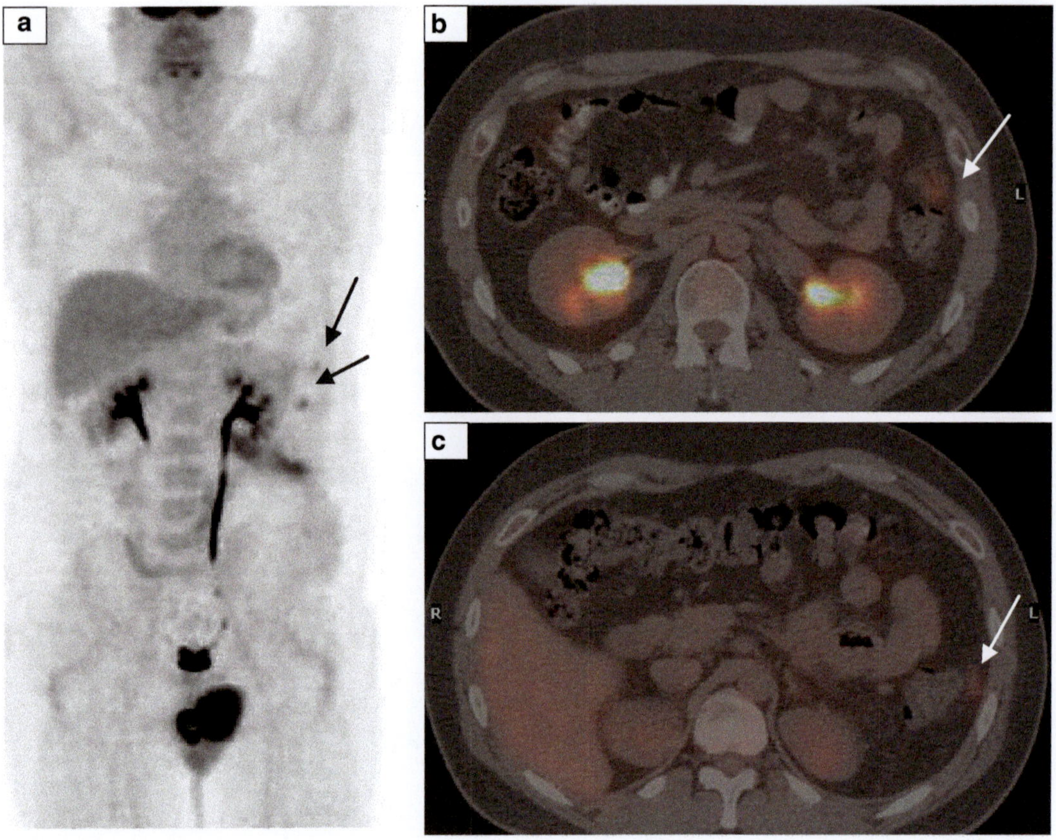

Fig. 7.31 (**a–c**) MIP-PET and fused PET/CT post splenectomy: Two nodules (*arrows*) with mildly increased uptake of the radiopharmaceutical at the left paracolic area in contact with the omentum

Aggressive B-Cell Lymphomas: DLBCL – Case 17

A 76-year-old woman presented with a slowly growing right submandibular. Excisional biopsy revealed a DLBCL of germinal center cell origin (by immunohistochemical criteria), which could have arisen from a preexisting marginal zone lymphoma. Staging CT imaging demonstrated a 7×4 cm right submandibular lymph node, mediastinal lymphadenopathy up to 2.5 cm, and celiac nodes up to 2 cm. The bone marrow biopsy was negative. Clinical stage was IIIA. The IPI and aaIPI values were "2" and "1," respectively – both low-intermediate risk – due to advanced age and stage. She received 6 cycles of the R-CHOP regimen. Except of the already completely resected submandibular mass, the remaining low-volume nodal disease was not significantly reduced (stable disease). PET/CT revealed multiple hypermetabolic foci above and below the diaphragm with 18FDG uptake higher than that of the liver parenchyma (SUVmax of 4.5), corresponding to a D5-PS score of 4, i.e., indicative of metabolically active residual disease (Fig. 7.32 – black arrows). No further treatment was administered. Interestingly, the anatomic findings still remain stable for 2 years, as concluded by serial CT reevaluations.

Discussion: After R-CHOP, PET/CT remained positive with a D5-PS score of 4. However, disease progression has not still occurred, 2 years after the positive PET/CT. This is rather unusual for an aggressive lymphoma. Two explanations may apply in this case: Either mediastinal and celiac FDG uptake represent false-positive findings, or it is due to the persistence of an underlying low-grade (marginal zone?) component, the presence of which could be hypothesized on the basis of the baseline pathology report. If a baseline PET was available, this could facilitate the interpretation of the post-chemotherapy PET/CT. In a British Columbia study, a positive PET/CT (including D5-PS score of 3) following R-CHOP with findings not amenable to curative radiotherapy (or not selected for radiotherapy) was associated with a low, but still measurable 4-year PFS of 33 % [4], thus suggesting the false-positives are not extremely unusual.

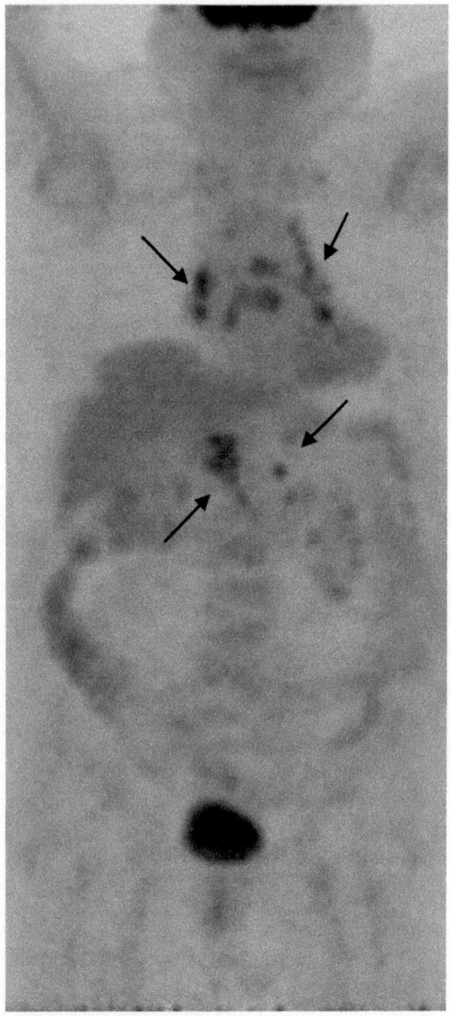

Fig. 7.32 MIP-PET: Multiple hypermetabolic lesions above and below the diaphragm (SUVmax of 4.5) (*arrows*) after 6 cycles of R-CHOP

Aggressive B-Cell Lymphomas: DLBCL – Case 18

A 52-year-old man presented with local pain, due to a bulky, rapidly growing soft tissue mass, located at the lower, right posterior thoracic wall (level T9-T12), which was also extending into the peritoneal cavity. He was otherwise asymptomatic. An excisional biopsy demonstrated a DLBCL NOS of non-germinal center cell origin. A bone marrow biopsy was negative. Clinical stage was IXA. IPI value was "1," i.e., low risk, and aaIPI was also "1" (low-intermediate risk) due to elevated LDH levels (1.55×). He received 8 cycles of R-CHOP combination chemotherapy. Interim and final MRI restaging demonstrated a gradual decrease in the size of the mass from a baseline of 13.5×12.5 cm to 6.2×3.6 cm and 1.9×1.2 cm, respectively. A PET/CT scan was performed 7 days after the final MRI. It demonstrated a highly hypermetabolic (SUVmax of 18.5) residual lesion in the left posterolateral thoracic wall between the 11th and 12th rib (Fig. 7.33a, b). The 18FDG uptake of the lesion was markedly higher than that of the liver parenchyma corresponding to a D5-PS score of 5, indicative of persistent disease. Meanwhile, the patient experienced local pain again. A new MRI performed 20 days after PET/CT revealed progressive disease with an increase in mass size to 3.5×2.9 cm and emergence of a smaller, new satellite lesion. The patient is currently receiving salvage therapy with R-ESHAP.

Discussion: End-of-treatment PET/CT is considered mandatory in DLBCL for the evaluation of response to immunochemotherapy. D5-PS is the standard tool for the evaluation of ePET, with scores 4 and 5 considered positive. Despite the marked FDG uptake observed in this case, the size of the mass was rather small, and local RT could be considered as an option. However, in the presence of so high uptake, it would be reasonable to exclude the scenario of a very rapid, early progression. Indeed, the size of the residual mass increased within 27 days, confirming that the patient had not a PR, as suggested by MRI restaging 7 days prior to PET/CT, but actually had primary progressive disease. In this case, RT was postponed, and the patient was forwarded to salvage immunochemotherapy with the intention of high-dose therapy and ASCT.

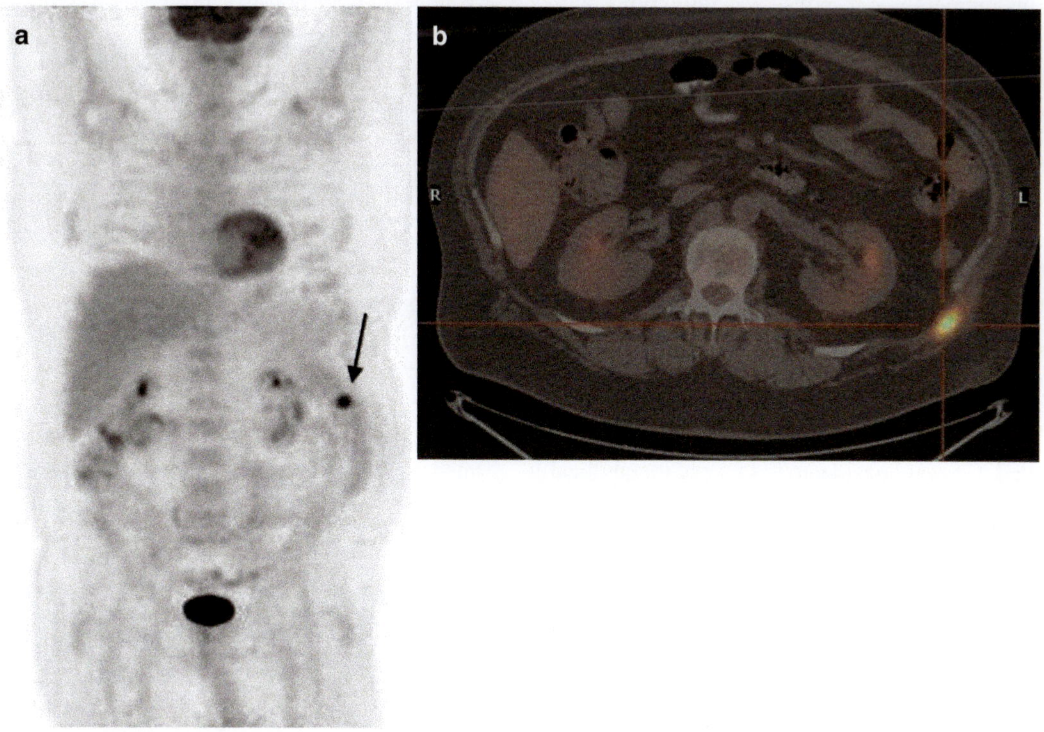

Fig. 7.33 (**a**, **b**) MIP-PET and fused PET/CT – end of treatment: Highly hypermetabolic (SUVmax of 18.5) residual lesion in the *left* posterolateral thoracic wall between the 11th and 12th rib (*arrow* in the MIP image)

Aggressive B-Cell Lymphomas: PMLBCL – Case 19

A 28-year-old woman, suffering from spina bifida and paraparesis, sought a medical advice because of atypical chest complaints, fever, and night sweats. Pericardial effusion and a large mediastinal mass causing superior vena cava syndrome were detected. Complete CT staging revealed mediastinal lymphadenopathy 11×9 cm in size, pleural effusion, bilateral multiple lung nodules, and a left supraclavicular nodal mass. After a nondiagnostic supraclavicular lymph node biopsy, the diagnosis of PMLBCL was established by a CT-guided biopsy of the mediastinal mass. The bone marrow biopsy was negative. The clinical stage was IVA, while aaIPI was classified as high risk due to advanced stage, elevated LDH (4.35×), and poor performance status.

Baseline PET/CT showed highly abnormal 18FDG uptake in the mediastinal mass and supraclavicular lymph nodes bilaterally (SUVmax of 18) but no uptake in one nodule of 1.3 cm diameter at the apicoposterior segment of the left upper lung lobe (Fig. 7.34a–c). After 3 cycles of R-CHOP combination immunochemotherapy, the radiographic response was only minor with a 2 cm reduction in the diameter of the mediastinal mass and reduction of the pleural effusion but concomitant worsening of the pericardial effusion. Salvage immunochemotherapy was instituted with the R-ESHAP regimen without a notable response after two cycles (mediastinal mass 9×8 cm). R-IGEV was then administered with achievement of adequate response (from 9.0×8.0 to 6.5×2.8 cm). A new PET/CT showed moderate 18FDG uptake in the residual mediastinal mass exceeding the uptake of the mediastinal pool but not that of the liver parenchyma and corresponding to a D5-PS score of 3 (Fig. 7.35a, b). PET/CT was considered in favor of metabolically active residual disease according to the IHP criteria – as the mass diameter was greater than 2 cm and the 18FDG uptake higher than that of the mediastinal blood pool – but it would be considered negative according to the D5-PS criteria. Subsequently, she received BEAM high-dose therapy and ASCT.

The size of the mediastinal mass remained stable. A new PET/CT 2 months after ASCT still showed moderate 18FDG uptake (SUVmax of 4.5) at the mediastinum, while mild uptake in a right inguinal node was considered unrelated to the disease (Fig. 7.36a, b).

Mediastinal RT was administered at a total dose of 36 Gy. On restaging, 3 months later, a mediastinal residual mass of 4.8 cm still persisted. PET/CT still showed mildly increased 18FDG uptake by the residual mass slightly exceeding that of the mediastinal blood pool (D5-PS score of 3; Fig. 7.37a, b). The patient remains in remission compatible with cure 4 years post-ASCT with further shrinkage of the mediastinal residual lesion to 3.1 cm.

Discussion: This patient had a poor response to R-CHOP without however progression while on treatment. Further salvage chemotherapy resulted to a better disease control with a borderline residual 18FDG uptake, which was considered positive according to the IHP criteria held at that time [47, 48], but negative according to the recent Lugano criteria [1, 2]. Even high-dose therapy and ASCT and subsequent radiotherapy did not eliminate this uptake, which proved to be compatible with cure. As discussed in the first-line treatment of PMLBCL, RT is extremely effective in controlling residual masses with relatively mild FDG uptake (SUVmax up to 5) with success rates even >90 % [8, 28, 30], but this has not been confirmed in the post-ASCT setting.

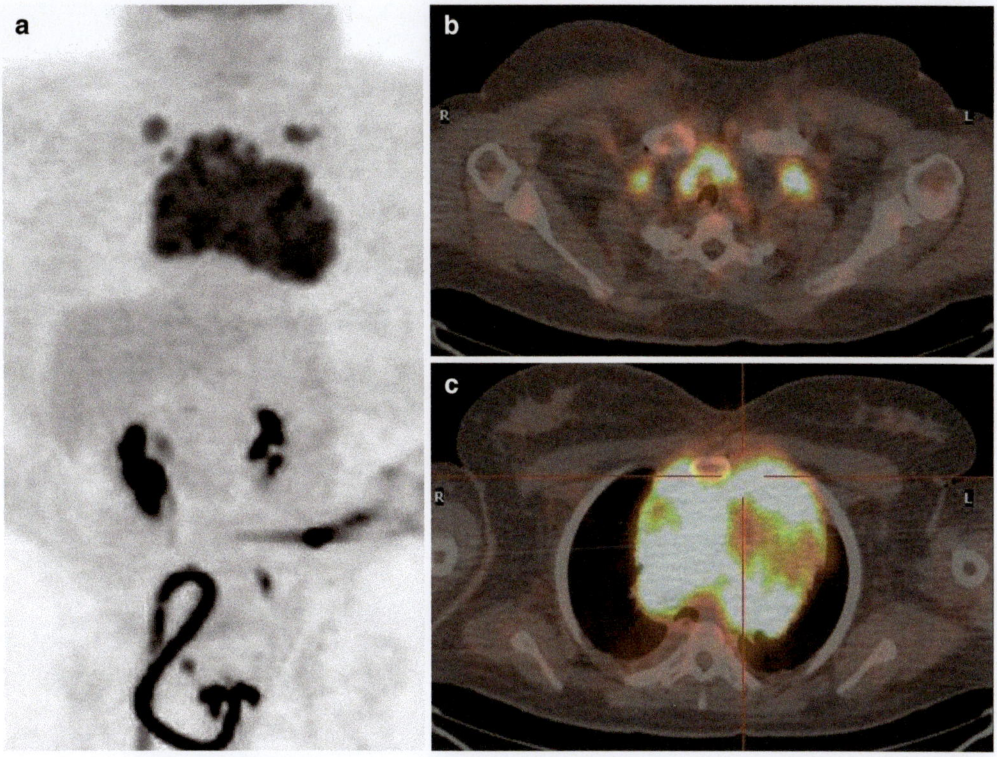

Fig. 7.34 (**a–c**) MIP-PET and fused PET/CT- initial staging: highly abnormal 18FDG uptake at a mediastinal mass and supraclavicular lymph nodes bilaterally

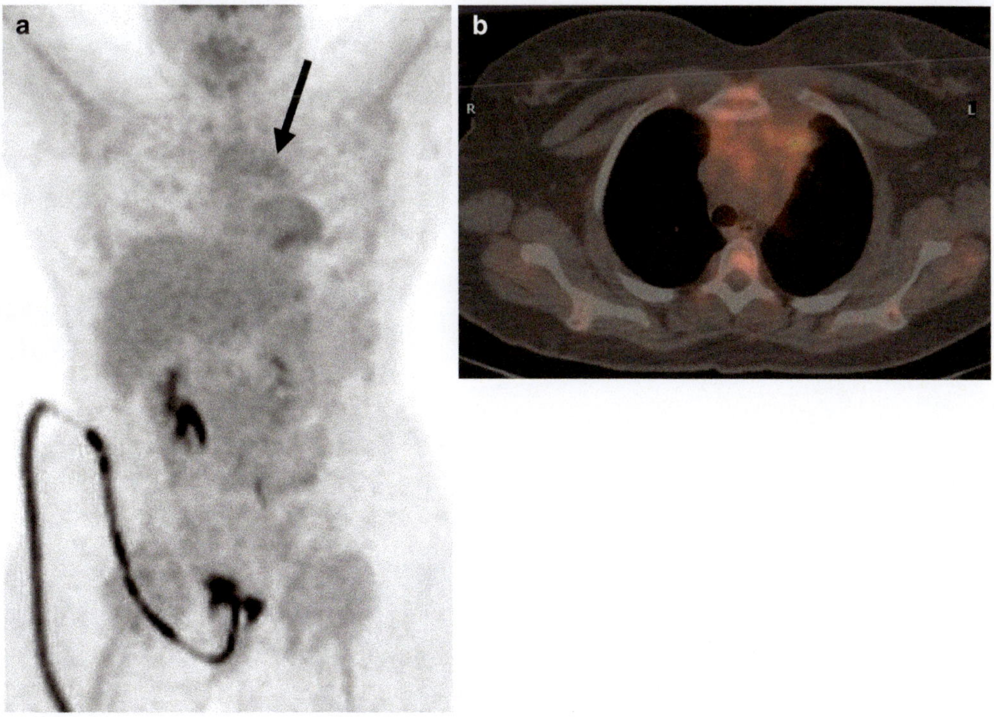

Fig. 7.35 (**a**, **b**) MIP-PET and fused PET/CT restaging after immunochemotherapy: moderate 18FDG uptake in the residual mediastinal mass exceeding the uptake of the mediastinal pool but not that of the liver parenchyma (*arrow* in the MIP image) (D5-PS score 3)

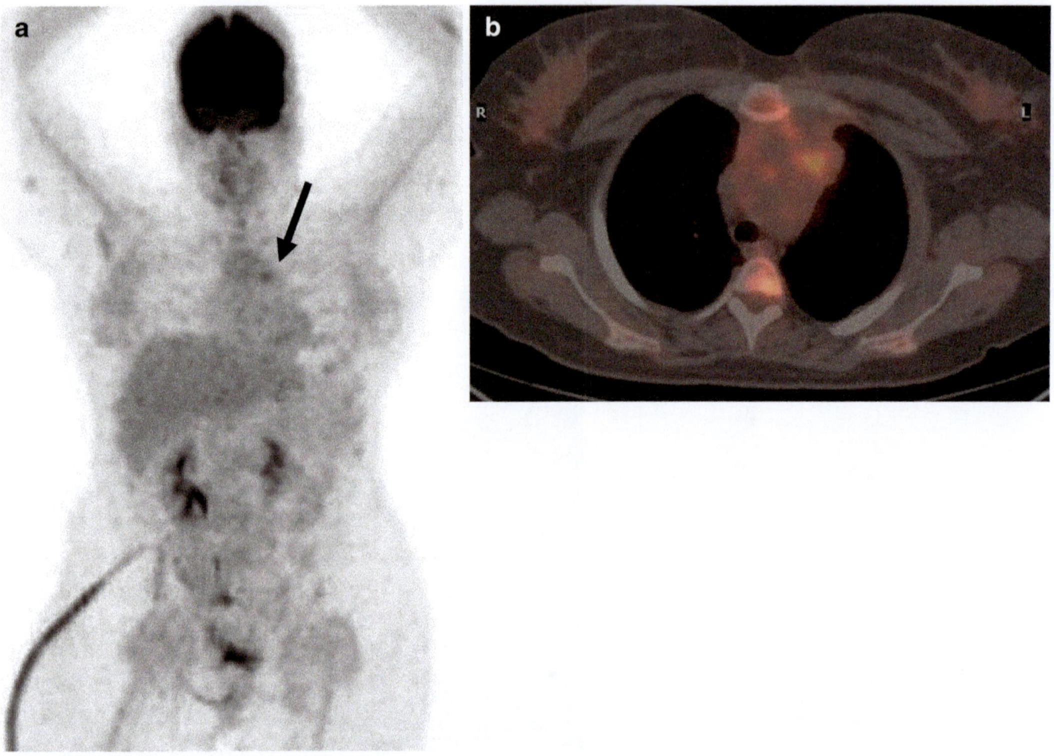

Fig. 7.36 (**a**, **b**) MIP-PET and fused PET/CT post autologous transplantation: moderate 18FDG uptake at the residual mediastinal mass (*arrow* in the MIP image) (SUVmax 4.5)

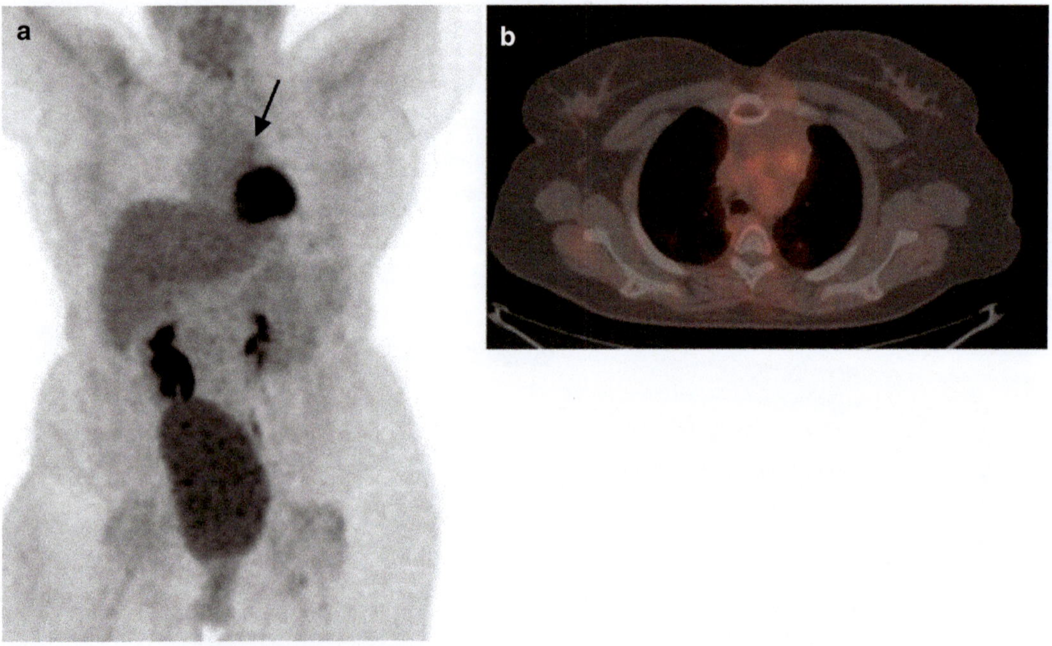

Fig. 7.37 (**a**, **b**) MIP-PET and fused PET/CT after mediastinal RT: mildly increased 18FDG uptake at the residual mass (*arrow* in the MIP image) slightly exceeding that of the mediastinal blood pool

Aggressive B-Cell Lymphomas: PMLBCL – Case 20

A 36-year-old woman presented with upper gastrointestinal hemorrhage due to a malignant gastric ulcer of lymphomatous origin. Complete CT staging revealed a large, 10 cm mediastinal mass and paracardial lymphadenopathy, a significant pericardial and a small left pleural effusion, retropancreatic lymphadenopathy, and enlargement of the right kidney. The whole anatomic distribution of the disease was compatible to PMLBCL. This diagnosis was confirmed by a review and appropriated immunohistochemical evaluation of gastric biopsy material [50]. A bone marrow biopsy was negative. The clinical stage was IVA and the value of the aaIPI was "2," i.e., high intermediate, due to advanced stage and elevated LDH levels (2.27×).

The patient received 8 cycles of R-CHOP immunochemotherapy: A 3.5×3.0 cm residual mediastinal mass persisted, which had increased 18FDG uptake on PET/CT (SUVmax of 4.6) higher than that of the mediastinal blood pool and the liver corresponding to a D5-PS score of 4. The findings were in favor of metabolically active residual disease according either to the IHP or to the D5-PS criteria (Fig. 7.38a, b). RT was administered at a dose of 4000 cGy. The size of the residual lesion was further reduced, but PET/CT performed 3 months later still demonstrated mildly increased FDG uptake (SUVmax of 3.6) slightly higher than that of the mediastinum but lower than that of the liver, corresponding to a D5-PS score of 3. This uptake would be considered abnormal according to the IHP criteria but not according to the D5-PS criteria (Fig. 7.39a, b). No further PET evaluation was performed. The size of the residual mass gradually decreased until normalization. The patient remains in continuous remission 6 years after the completion of RT.

Discussion: Gastric involvement is a rare event in PMLBCL, always indicating disseminated, stage IV disease [50]. Following R-CHOP, this patient remained with a 3.5×3.0 cm residual mass and a locally positive PET/CT with D5-PS score of 4 and a SUVmax of 4.6. This was considered as a very good radiographic response, but PET/CT was positive based either on the IHP [47, 48] or the Lugano criteria [1, 2]. However, this level of PET positivity is associated with a >50 % chance of cure with radiotherapy [8, 28, 30], and preliminary data suggest that this figure may be even >90 % if SUVmax is <5, as was the case here [28].

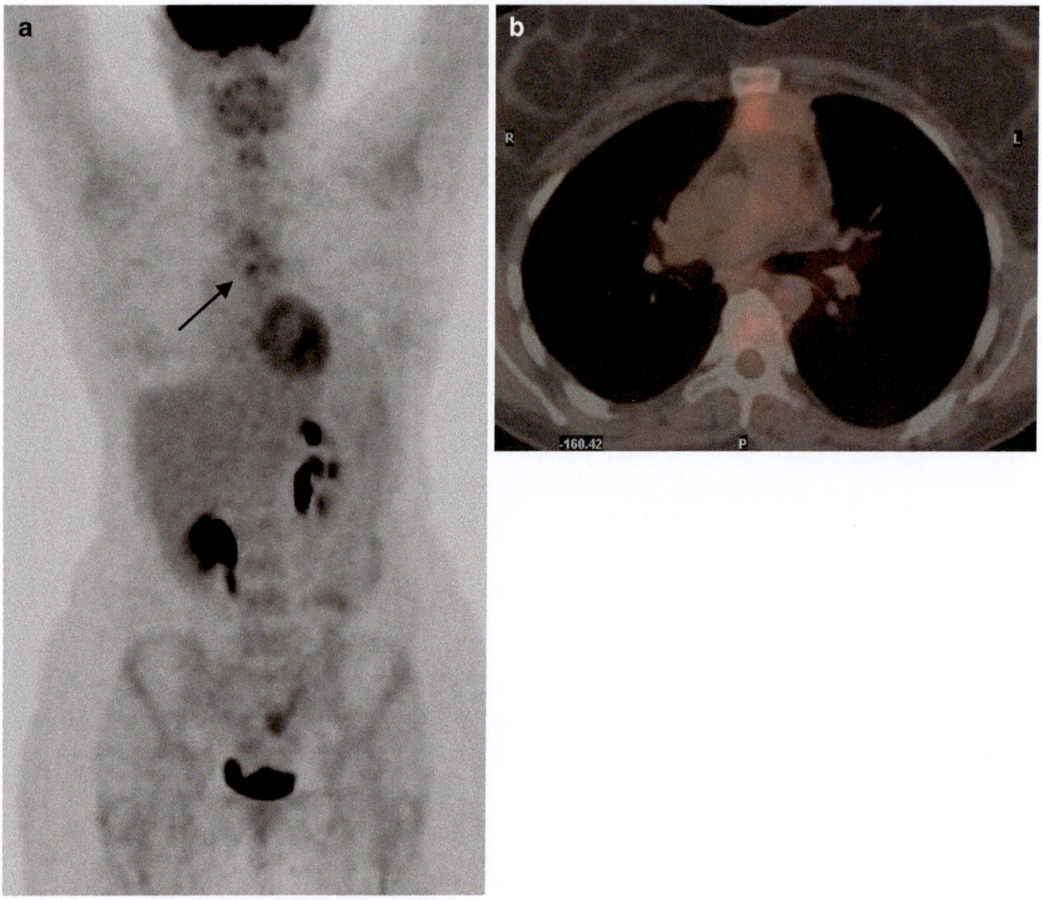

Fig. 7.38 (**a**, **b**) MIP-PET and fused PET/CT post immunochemotherapy with R-CHOP: Residual hypermetabolic mediastinal mass (*arrow* in the MIP image) with uptake exceeding that of the liver (D5-PS score 4)

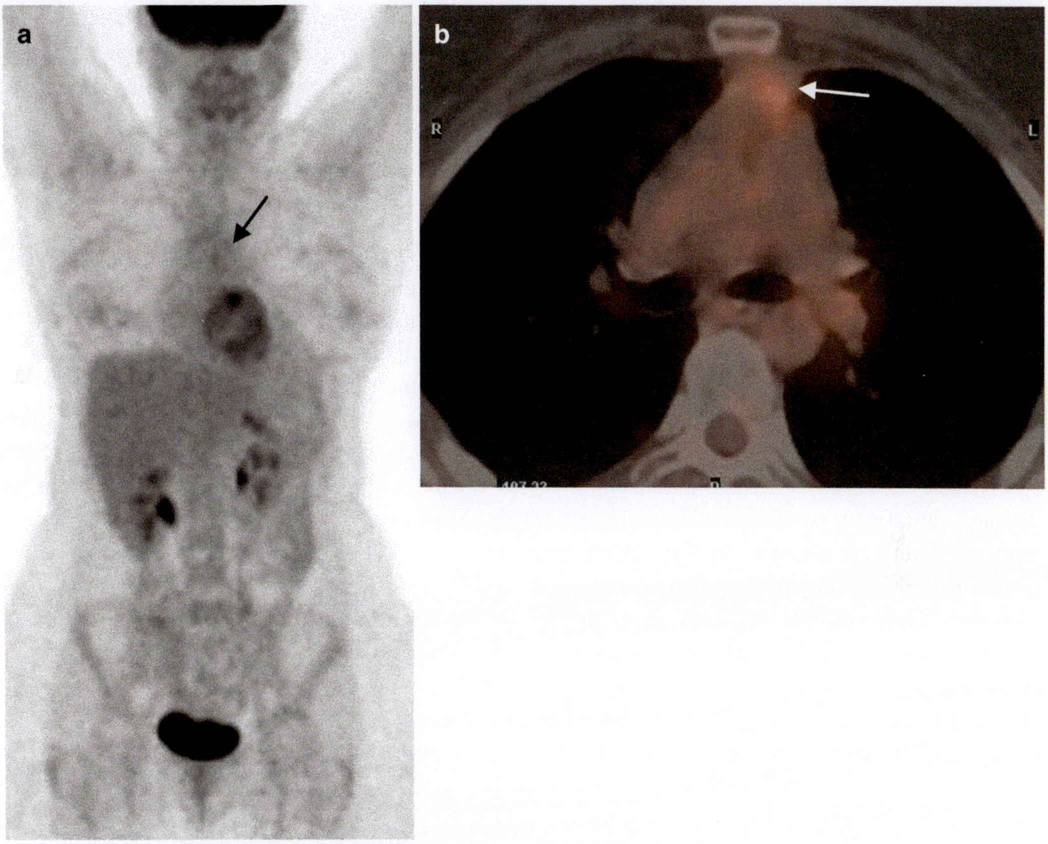

Fig. 7.39 (**a**, **b**) MIP-PET and fused PET/CT post RT: Mildly increased FDG uptake (*arrows*), slightly higher than that of the mediastinum but lower than that of the liver (D5-PS score 3)

Aggressive B-Cell Lymphomas: PMLBCL – Case 21

A 21-year-old man presented with generalized pruritus and a history of recent acute pericarditis. A 10.0×9.5 cm mediastinal mass was present. On histologic examination a primary mediastinal large B-cell lymphoma was diagnosed, which was also contiguously extended to the pleura, lung, and fatty tissue. A bone marrow biopsy was negative. Clinical stage was IIEXA, since all extranodal sites were contiguously involved adjacently to the mediastinal mass. The age-adjusted IPI was "1" (low-intermediate risk) due to an elevated serum LDH level (2.37×). The patient received 6 cycles of R-CHOP immunochemotherapy and achieved a good radiographic response with a residual mediastinal mass, which had further improved compared with mid-treatment restaging. However, PET/CT revealed intense 18FDG uptake at the residual mediastinal mass (SUVmax of 20), corresponding to D5-PS score of 5 and indicating persistent disease according both to the IHP and D5-PS criteria (Fig. 7.40a, b). Subsequently, he received involved-field radiotherapy at a dose of 4600 cGy. A repeated PET/CT performed 3 months later was completely negative (Fig. 7.41). The patient remains in continuous complete remission 28 months after the negative PET/CT.

Discussion: After response to R-CHOP, PET/CT remains positive according IHP criteria in at least 40 % of the patients [8, 28–30]. Even patients with the highest FDG uptake, as was the case in this patient, may convert to negative and be eventually cured with radiotherapy, provided that they have not developed progressive disease compared with the nadir of the mass size obtained at the mid-treatment evaluation [28, 32]. If a response has been achieved with immunochemotherapy, PET/CT positivity is not an indication to proceed to salvage chemotherapy and ASCT in the absence of conventionally defined disease progression [32]. However, not infrequently, such a strategy is followed by many physicians in clinical practice, especially when residual FDG uptake is high.

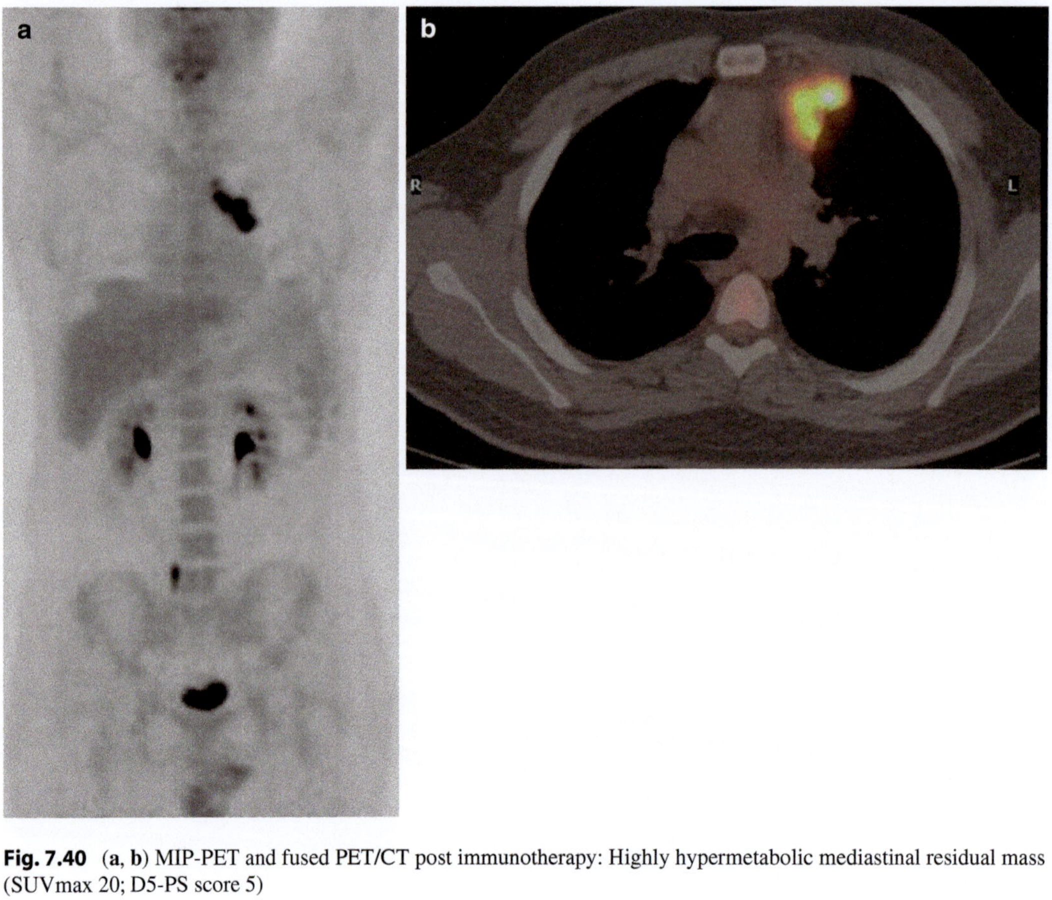

Fig. 7.40 (**a**, **b**) MIP-PET and fused PET/CT post immunotherapy: Highly hypermetabolic mediastinal residual mass (SUVmax 20; D5-PS score 5)

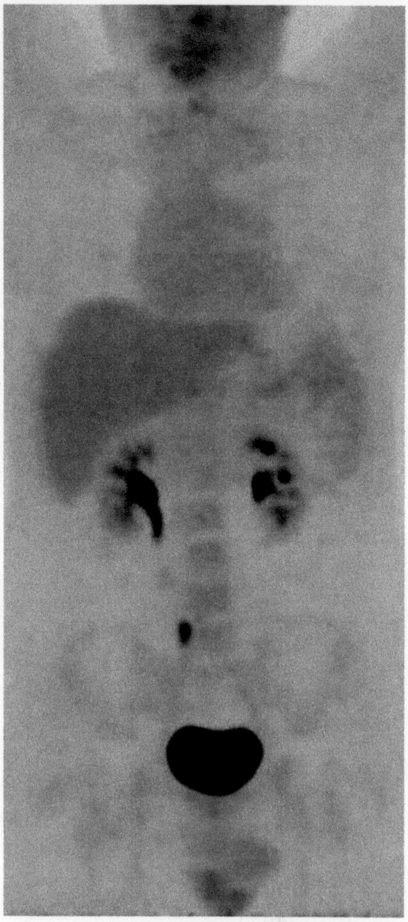

Fig. 7.41 MIP-PET post radiotherapy: No hypermetabolic lesions are observed

Aggressive B-Cell Lymphomas: PMLBCL – Case 22

A 28-year-old woman presented with a mediastinal mass and a small left supraclavicular lymph node, discovered during evaluation of left-sided chest pain, productive cough, and hemoptysis. A lymph node biopsy revealed primary mediastinal large B-cell lymphoma. CT imaging revealed a 12 cm mediastinal mass extending to and infiltrating the thoracic wall, a left upper lung lobe opacification, a small left pleural and pericardial effusion, and left supraclavicular lymphadenopathy. A bone marrow biopsy was negative. Baseline PET/CT confirmed the above findings (SUVmax of 22) and further revealed other sites of mediastinal and left axillary lymphadenopathy (Fig. 7.42a, b). The clinical stage was IVA and the value of the aaIPI was "2," i.e., high intermediate, due to advanced stage and elevated LDH levels (1.26×). The patient received eight cycles of R-CHOP immunochemotherapy and a complete radiographic remission was achieved. However, PET/CT-based evaluation of response uncovered the presence of small but clearly hypermetabolic mediastinal nodes (SUVmax of 7.7; D5-PS score 5) as well as two residual hypermetabolic (SUVmax of 5.2) nodules at the left upper lung lobe (Fig. 7.43a, b). Subsequently, she underwent 30Gy involved-field radiotherapy; the dose was increased to 44 Gy at the sites of PET positivity. Despite CT stability at 1.5 month after restaging PET/CT, progressive disease was observed at 3 months by both conventional CT and PET/CT, which revealed an 6×4 cm, highly hypermetabolic lesion of the right lower lung lobe (SUVmax of 29), and a small right peribronchial node (SUVmax of 11) (Fig. 7.44a–c). She underwent salvage chemotherapy with the R-ESHAP regimen, but disease progression developed after the second cycle. Further salvage chemotherapy with rituximab and high doses of methotrexate and cytarabine was administered with minor tumor reduction compatible with "stable disease." Subsequently, the patient received TEAM high-dose therapy and ASCT but developed again progressive disease 3.5 months later. Multiple further salvage attempts were unsuccessful and the patient succumbed to the disease 21 months after the initial diagnosis.

Discussion: Following R-CHOP, this patient virtually achieved a complete conventional radiographic response. However, three distinct subcentimeter lesions were detected by PET/CT, which demonstrated significant hypermetabolism with SUVmax up to 7.7. Since all lesions could be encompassed within a RT field and the anticipated success rate could be >50%, the patient received RT [8, 28, 30]. However, disease progression occurred 3 months later and the patient failed to attain any clinically meaningful, sustained response with multiple salvage approaches, including high-dose therapy and ASCT.

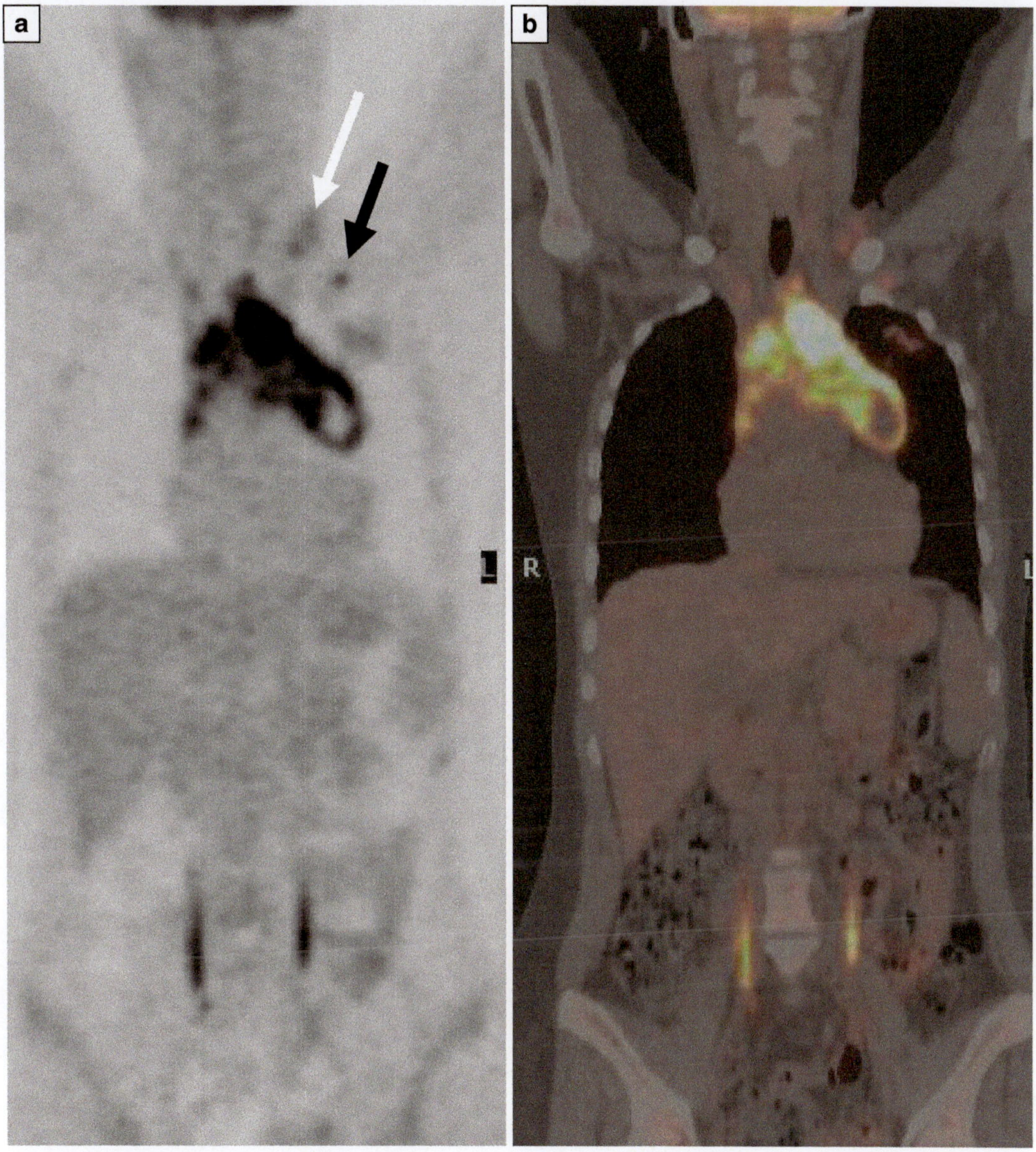

Fig. 7.42 (**a**, **b**) PET and fused PET/CT – initial staging: Mediastinal hypermetabolic mass, *left* supraclavicular lymphadenopathy (*white arrow*) and further revealed other sites of mediastinal and *left* axillary lymphadenopathy (*black arrow*)

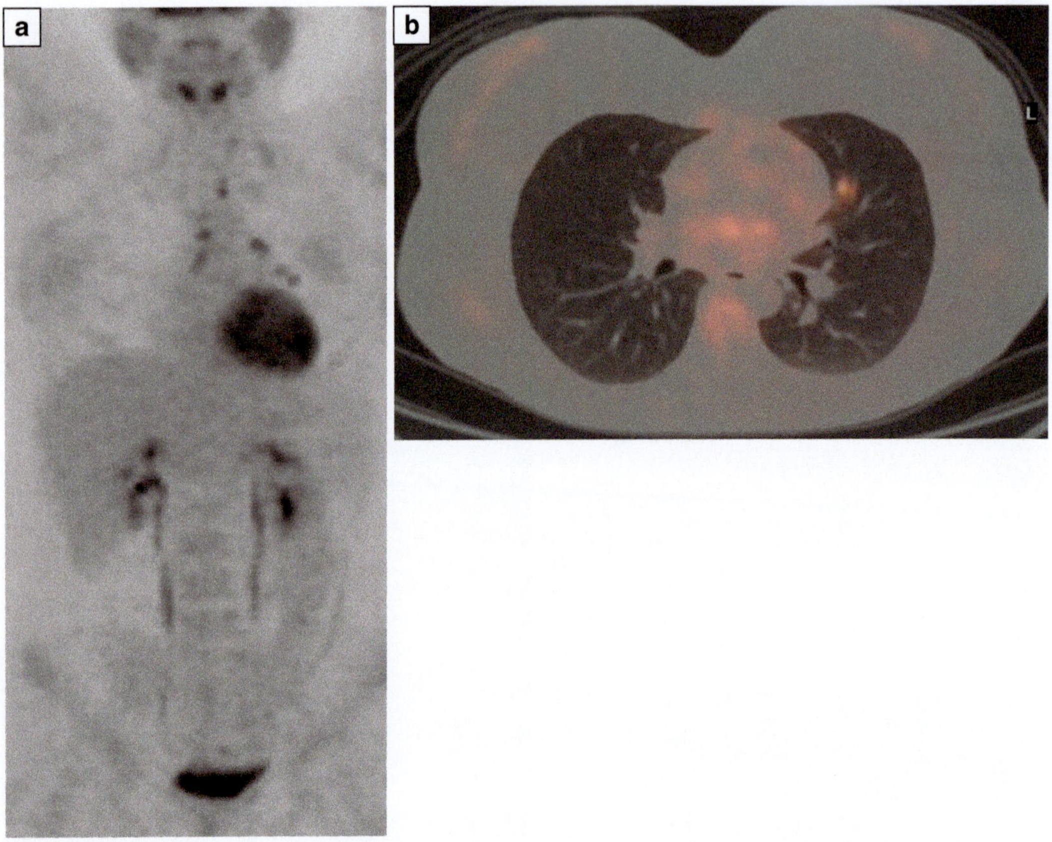

Fig. 7.43 (**a**, **b**) MIP-PET and fused PET/CT – after immunochemotherapy with R-CHOP: Small, highl hypermetabolic mediastinal lymph nodes (D5-PS score 5) (**a**) and hypermetabolic nodule at the left upper lung lobe (**b**)

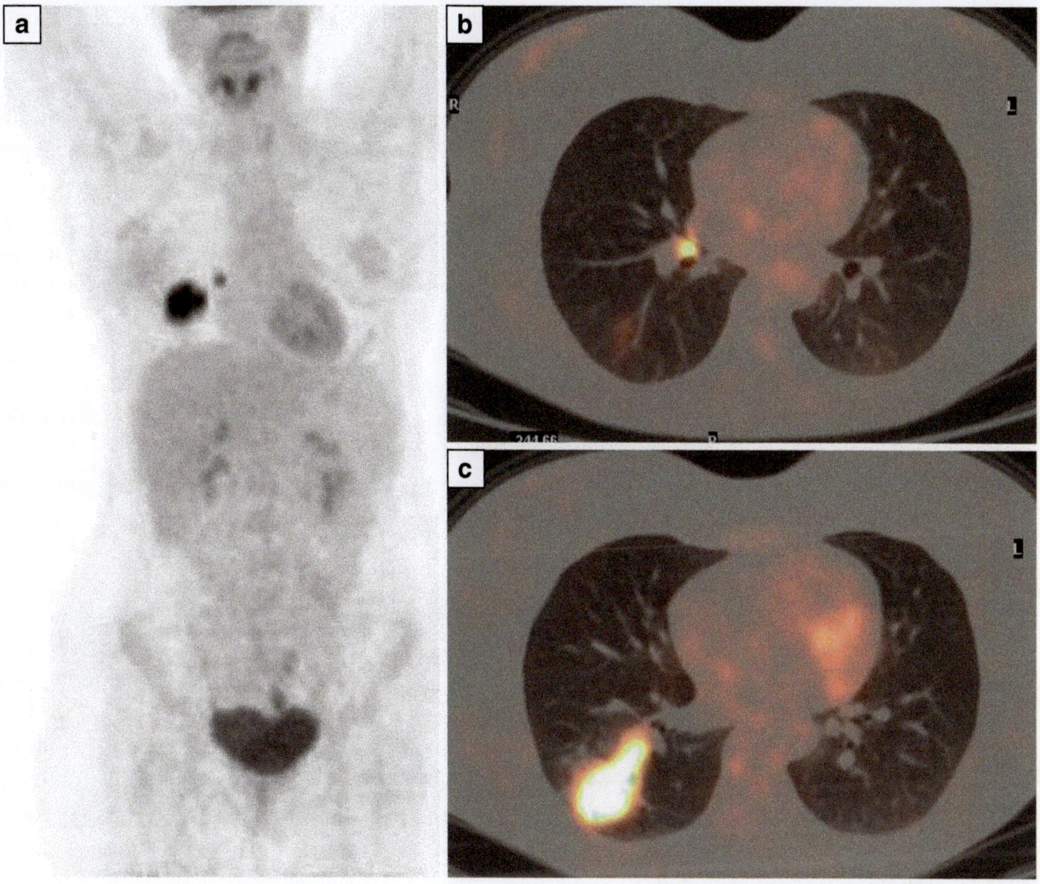

Fig. 7.44 (**a**–**c**) MIP-PET and fused PET/CT – after radiotherapy: Small *right* peribronchial lymph node (**a**, **b**) and highly hypermetabolic lesion of the right lower lung lobe (**a**, **c**)

Aggressive B-Cell Lymphomas: PMLBCL – Case 23

A 24-year-old woman presented with disseminated pruritus, night sweats, mild dry cough, and tachycardia. A mediastinal mass was found. Biopsy of the mediastinal mass revealed primary mediastinal large B-cell lymphoma. Complete staging revealed a small but clearly abnormal right supraclavicular lymph node, a 15 cm mediastinal mass, and a left lung lesion located at the lingula. The clinical stage was IIXEB and the value of the aaIPI was "1," i.e., low intermediate, due to elevated LDH levels (1.37×). The patient received eight cycles of R-CHOP immunochemotherapy: A 4.0×1.8 cm residual mediastinal mass and a 2.1×2.1 cm left lung nodule still persisted. Both of them were highly hypermetabolic on PET/CT (SUVmax of 10.5 and 16.5, respectively) corresponding to D5-PS score of 5. There were also multiple hypermetabolic foci in the neck bilaterally due to activation of brown fat (Fig. 7.45a, b). She underwent salvage chemotherapy with the R-ESHAP regimen with a borderline response (47 % reduction of the lesions to 3.2×1.4 cm and 1.2×1.4 cm, respectively) after the second cycle. Subsequently, the patient received BEAM high-dose therapy and ASCT. PET/CT performed 1.5 months after ASCT revealed persistent, highly intense 18FDG uptake (SUVmax of 16) at the already known areas, although there was no increase in the size of the lesions. There was again increased 18FDG uptake in the neck bilaterally corresponding to sites of activated brown fat (Fig. 7.46a, b). Involved field RT with the dose increased to 50 Gy at the sites of PET positivity was administered starting 1.5 month after ASCT. At 3.5 months following ASCT, CT restaging was stable but the patient developed neurologic symptoms and a brain lesion was discovered on MRI. The patient also developed intense pain and swelling of the left lower mandible resembling to a dental abscess. Surprisingly, a PET/CT performed 1 week after the "stable" CT evaluation revealed extensive mediastinal and abdominal lymphadenopathy and bilateral lung, adrenal, and renal disease, confirmed CNS disease and the lymphomatous nature of the mandibular lesion, and revealed sites of bone marrow involvement (Fig. 7.47). Some of these findings became evident by conventional imaging performed one additional week later. The patient succumbed to the disease soon thereafter, 13 months after the initial diagnosis after failure to respond to subsequent salvage chemotherapy.

Discussion: Following R-CHOP, this patient achieved a very satisfactory conventional radiographic response with two distinct residual lesions measuring 4 and 2 cm. However, PET/CT still remained highly positive with SUVmax >10 and up to 16.4 at both sites (D5-PS score of 5). Although even such very high uptake may be controlled with RT in at least 50 % of cases in the absence of documented progressive disease [8, 28, 30], the "empiric" decision made in this case was to proceed with salvage immunochemotherapy and ASCT. Unfortunately, neither this aggressive approach nor subsequent salvage radiotherapy resulted to sufficient disease control.

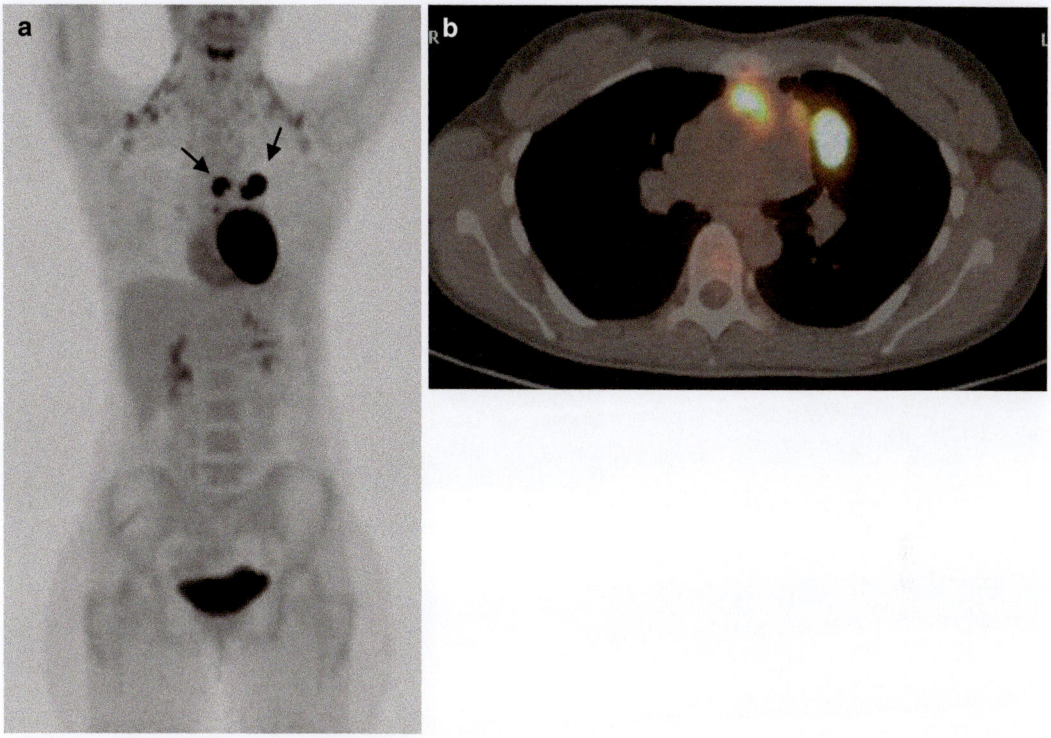

Fig. 7.45 (**a**, **b**) MIP-PET and fused PET/CT after immunochemotherapy: Residual hypermetabolic mediastinal mass and hypermetabolic left lung nodule (*arrows* in the MIP image). Bilaterally increased 18FDG uptake in the neck corresponded to sites of activated brown fat

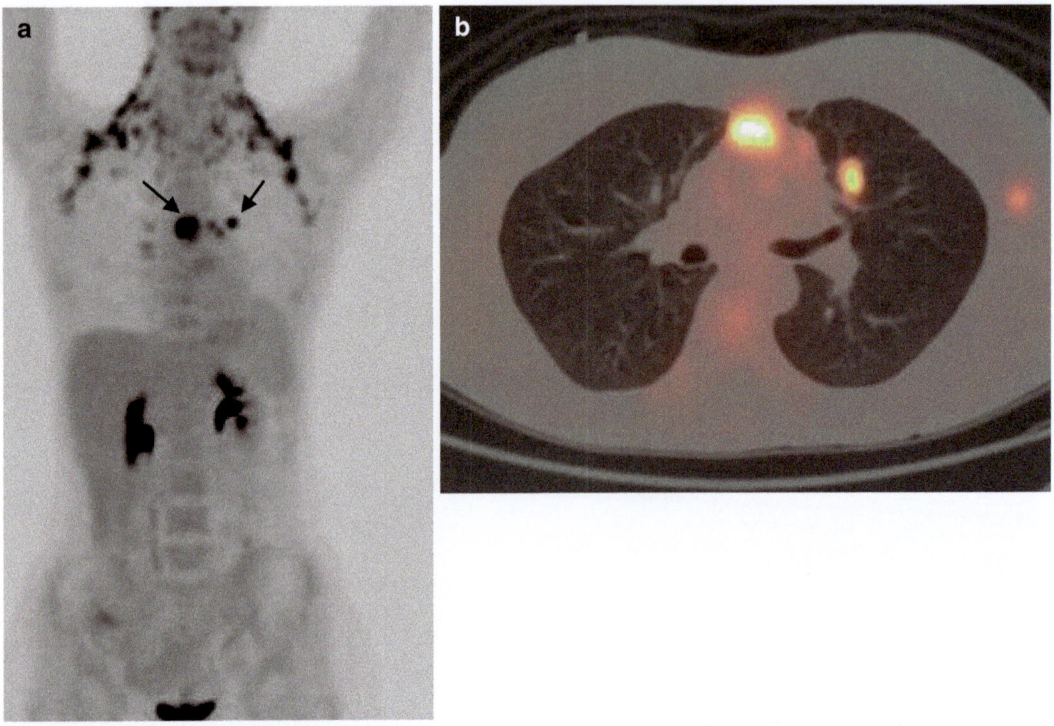

Fig. 7.46 (**a**, **b**) MIP-PET and fused PET/CT after ASCT: Intense 18FDG uptake at the already known areas (mediastinum and *left* lung) (*arrows* in the MIP image). Increased 18FDG uptake in the neck bilaterally corresponding to sites of activated brown fat

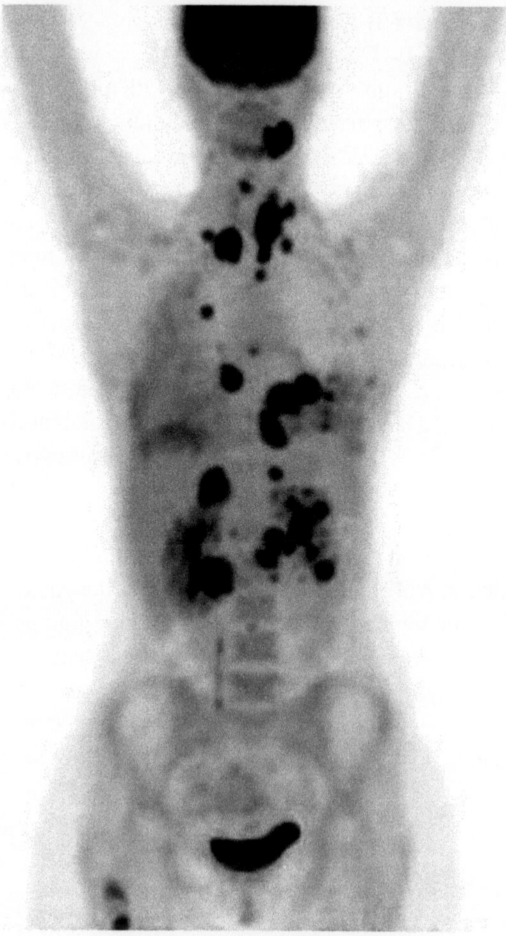

Fig. 7.47 MIP-PET post radiotherapy: Extensive hypermetabolic mediastinal and abdominal lymphadenopathy, a left lower mandible lesion, bilateral lung, adrenal, and renal lesions, as well as osseous foci indicating bone marrow involvement

Aggressive B-Cell Lymphomas: PMLBCL – Case 24

A 34-year-old woman presented with a mediastinal mass discovered due to disseminated pruritus and dyspnea. Biopsy of the mediastinal mass revealed primary mediastinal large B-cell lymphoma. Complete staging revealed a 7×8 cm mediastinal mass extending to the right lung, paracardial lymphadenopathy, and pericardial thickening with moderate pericardial effusion. The clinical stage was IIEA and the value of the aaIPI was "1," i.e., low intermediate, due to elevated LDH levels (1.21×). After a good mid-treatment PR, the patient developed progressive disease at the mediastinum following the 7th cycle of R-CHOP immunochemotherapy with increase in the size of some residual lymph nodes. A 3 cm lesion was also seen at the gastrosplenic region. PET/CT confirmed these findings demonstrating highly hypermetabolic mediastinal lymphadenopathy (SUVmax of 30) (Fig. 7.48a) corresponding to a D5-PS score of 5 and indicative of progressive disease. The uptake of the abdominal finding was mild (SUVmax of 3.6) (Fig. 7.48a, b). The patient failed to respond to any subsequent salvage therapy and succumbed to the disease 5 months later.

Discussion: Following R-CHOP, this patient remained highly positive on PET/CT with SUVmax ≫10. However, conventional evaluation revealed that the disease had increased in size compared to the mid-treatment assessment. This is a crucial information, because the >50 % salvageability rates, even for residual masses with very high FDG uptake, reliably apply only if the patient is classified as a responder [28]. In contrast, conventionally documented disease progression is another common scenario in patients with very high SUXmax after R-CHOP, in which salvage chemotherapy and ASCT are indicated instead of additional RT. Unfortunately, many of these patients do not respond to any subsequent chemotherapy and are unable to be forwarded to ASCT, as was the case here.

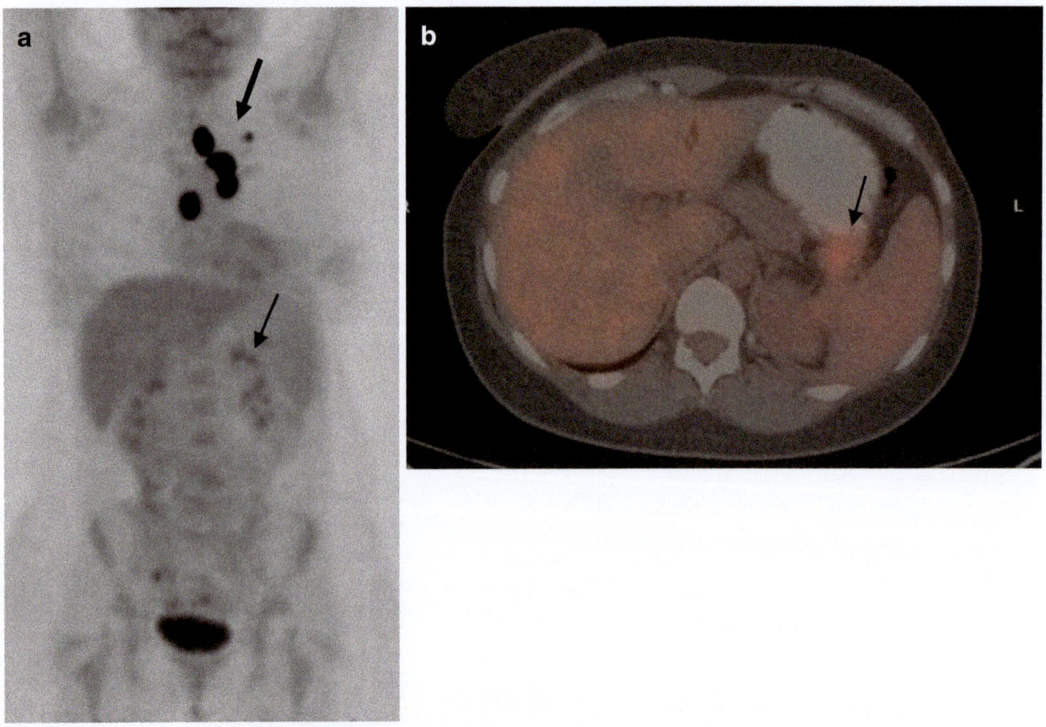

Fig. 7.48 (**a**, **b**) MIP-PET and PET/CT post immunochemotherapy: Increased FDG uptake at mediastinal lymph nodes (**a** – *thick arrow*), as well as at a lymph node of the gastrosplenic space (**a**, **b** – *thin arrow*)

References

1. Cheson BD, Fisher RI, Barrington SF, Cavalli F, Schwartz LH, Lister TA et al (2014) Recommendations for the initial evaluation, staging, and response assessment of Hodgkin and non-Hodgkin lymphoma: the Lugano classification. J Clin Oncol 32:3059–3067
2. Barrington SF, Mikhaeel GN, Kostakoglu L, Meignan M, Hutchings M, Müeller SP et al (2014) Role of imaging in the staging and response assessment of lymphoma: Consensus of the International Conference on Malignant Lymphomas Imaging Working Group. J Clin Oncol 32:3048–3058
3. Vassilakopoulos TP, Prassopoulos V, Rondogianni P, Chatziioannou S, Konstantopoulos K, Angelopoulou MK (2015) Role of FDG-PET/CT in staging and first-line treatment of Hodgkin and aggressive B-cell lymphomas. Memo 8:105–114
4. Sehn LH, Klasa R, Shenkier T, Villa D, Slack GW, Gascoyne RD et al (2013) Long-term experience with PET-guided consolidative radiation therapy (XRT) in patients with advanced stage diffuse large B-cell lymphoma (DLBCL) treated with R-CHOP. Hematol Oncol 31(S1):137 (abstr 123)
5. Pfreundschuh M, Trumper L, Osterborg A et al (2006) CHOP-like chemotherapy plus rituximab versus CHOP-like chemotherapy alone in young patients with good-prognosis diffuse large-B-cell lymphoma: a randomised controlled trial by the MabThera International Trial (MInT) Group. Lancet Oncol 7:379–391
6. Pfreundschuh M, Schubert J, Ziepert M et al (2008) Six versus eight cycles of bi-weekly CHOP-14 with or without rituximab in elderly patients with aggressive CD20+ B-cell lymphomas: a randomized controlled trial (RICOVER-60). Lancet Oncol 9:105–116
7. Vassilakopoulos TP, Pangalis GA, Katsigiannis A et al (2012) Rituximab, cyclophosphamide, doxorubicin, vincristine, and prednisone with or without radiotherapy in primary mediastinal large B-cell lymphoma: the emerging standard of care. Oncologist 17:239–249
8. Martelli M, Ceriani L, Zucca E, Zinzani PL, Ferreri AJ, Vitolo U et al (2014) [^{18}F] fluorodeoxyglucose positron emission tomography predicts survival after chemoimmunotherapy for primary mediastinal large B-cell lymphoma: results of the International Extranodal Lymphoma Study Group IELSG-26 study. J Clin Oncol 32:1769–1775
9. Sehn LH, Scott DW, Chhanabhai M et al (2011) Impact of concordant and discordant bone marrow involvement on outcome in diffuse large B-cell lymphoma treated with R-CHOP. J Clin Oncol 29:1452–1457
10. Paone G, Itti E, Haioun C et al (2009) Bone marrow involvement in diffuse large B-cell lymphoma: Correlation between FDG-PET uptake and type of cellular infiltrate. Eur J Nucl Med Mol Imaging 36:745–750
11. Adams HJA, Kwee TC, Finjnheer R, Dubois SV, Nievelstein AJR, de Klerk JMH (2014) Bone marrow ^{18}F-fluoro-2-deoxy-D-glucose positron emission tomography/computed tomography cannot replace bone marrow biopsy in diffuse large B-cell lymphoma. Am J Hematol 89:726–731
12. Hong J, Lee Y, Park Y et al (2012) Role of FDG-PET/CT in detecting lymphomatous bone marrow involvement in patients with newly diagnosed diffuse large B-cell lymphoma. Ann Hematol 91:687–695
13. Cerci JJ, Gyorke T, Fanti S, Paez D, Meneghetti JC, Redondo F et al (2014) Combined PET and biopsy evidence of marrow involvement improves prognostic prediction in diffuse large B-cell lymphoma. J Nucl Med 55:1591–1597
14. Berthet L, Cochet A, Kanoun S, Berriolo-Riedinger A, Humbert O, Toubeau M et al (2013) In newly diagnosed diffuse large B-cell lymphoma, determination of bone marrow involvement with ^{18}F-FDG PET/CT provides better diagnostic performance and prognostic stratification than does biopsy. J Nucl Med 54:1244–1250
15. Khan AB, Barrington SF, Mikhaeel NG, Hunt AA, Cameron L, Morris T et al (2013) PET-CT staging of DLBCL accurately identifies and provides new insight into the clinical significance of bone marrow involvement. Blood 122:61–67
16. Adams HJA, Kwee TC (2015) Do not abandon the bone marrow biopsy yet in diffuse large B-cell lymphoma. J Clin Oncol 33:1217
17. Meignan M, Itti E, Gallamini A, Younes A (2015) FDG PET/CT imaging as a biomarker in lymphoma. Eur J Nucl Med Mol Imaging 42(4):623–633
18. Sasanelli M, Meignan M, Haioun C, Berriolo-Riedinger A, Casasnovas RO, Biggi A et al (2014) Pretherapy metabolic tumor volume is an independent predictor of outcome in diffuse large B-cell lymphoma. Eur J Nucl Med Mol Imaging 41:2017–2022
19. Song MK, Chung JS, Shin HJ, Lee SM, Lee SE, Lee HS et al (2012) Clinical significance of metabolic tumor volume by PET/CT in stages II and III of diffuse large B cell lymphoma without extranodal site involvement. Ann Hematol 91:697–703
20. Kim TM, Paeng JC, Chun IK, Keam B, Jeon YK, Lee SH et al (2013) Total lesion glycolysis in positron emission tomography is a better predictor of outcome than the international prognostic index for patients with diffuse large B cell lymphoma. Cancer 119:1195–1202
21. Ceriani L, Martelli M, Zinzani PL et al (2015) Utility of baseline 18FDG PET/CT functional parameters in defining prognosis of primary mediastinal (thymic) large B-cell lymphoma. Blood 126(8):950–956
22. Dupuis J, Itti E, Rahmouni A, Hemery F et al (2009) Response assessment after an inductive CHOP or CHOP-like regimen with or without rituximab in 103 patients with diffuse large B-cell lymphoma: integrating 18fluorodeoxyglucose positron emission tomography to the International Workshop Criteria. Ann Oncol 20:503–507
23. Dabaja BS, Phan J, Mawlawi O, Medeiros LJ, Etzel C, Liang FW et al (2013) Clinical implications of positron emission tomography-negative residual

computed tomography masses after chemotherapy for diffuse large B-cell lymphoma. Leuk Lymphoma 54:2631–2638
24. Vassilakopoulos TP, Kanellopoulos A, Papageorgiou S, Pangalis GA, Anastasopoulou A, Moschogianni M et al (2014) Clinical implications and prognostic significance of positron emission tomography (PET/CT) in patients with diffuse large B-cell lymphoma (DLBCL) after R-CHOP chemoimmunotherapy. Hematol J 99(Suppl 1):702 (abstr. 1831)
25. Thomas A, Gingrich RD, Smith BJ et al (2010) 18-fluoro-deoxyglucose positron emission tomography report interpretation as predictor of outcome in diffuse large B-cell lymphoma including analysis of "indeterminate" reports. Leuk Lymphoma 51: 439–446
26. Pregno P, Chiappella A, Bello M, Botto B, Ferrero S, Franceschetti S et al (2012) Interim 18-FDG-PET/CT failed to predict the outcome in diffuse large B-cell lymphoma patients treated at the diagnosis with rituximab-CHOP. Blood 119:2066–2073
27. Mamot C, Klingbiel D, Hitz F et al (2015) Final results of a prospective evaluation of the predictive value of interim positron emission tomography in patients with diffuse large B-cell lymphoma treated with R-CHOP-14 (SAKK 38/07). J Clin Oncol 33:2523–2529
28. Vassilakopoulos TP, Pangalis GA, Chatziioannou S et al (2016) PET/CT in patients with primary mediastinal large B-cell lymphoma responding to Rituximab-CHOP: an analysis of 106 patients regarding prognostic significance and implications for subsequent radiotherapy. Leukemia 30:238–242
29. Dunleavy K, Pittaluga S, Maeda LS et al (2013) Dose-adjusted EPOCH-rituximab therapy in primary mediastinal B-cell lymphoma. N Engl J Med 368: 1408–1416
30. Filippi AR, Piva C, Giunta F et al (2013) Radiation therapy in primary mediastinal B-cell lymphoma with positron emission tomography positivity after rituximab chemotherapy. Int J Radiat Oncol Biol Phys 87:311–316
31. Ceriani L, Martelli M, Zinzani P et al (2015) Use of the Lugano classification criteria for PET/CT assessment of primary mediastinal B-cell lymphoma after immunochemotherapy and irradiation in the IELSG-26 study. Hematol Oncol 33(S1):143 (abstr. 081)
32. Vassilakopoulos TP, Pangalis GA, Polliack A (2015) A "PET" topic in primary mediastinal large B-cell lymphoma: positive or negative, and how to handle it in the end. Leuk Lymphoma 56:3–5
33. Martelli M, Zucca E, Gospodarowicz M, Johnson PWM, Ricardi U (2013) A randomized, multicentre, two-arm phase III comparative study assessing the role of mediastinal radiotherapy after rituximab-containing chemotherapy regimens to patients with newly diagnosed primary mediastinal large B-cell lymphoma (PMLBCL): the IELSG-37 study. Hematol Oncol 31(S1):140
34. Itti E, Juweid ME, Haioun C et al (2010) Improvement of early 18F-FDG-PET interpretation in diffuse large B-cell Lymphoma: importance of the reference background. J Nucl Med 51:1857–1862
35. Moskowitz CH, Schoder H, Teruya-Feldstein J et al (2010) Risk-adapted dose-dense immunochemotherapy determined by interim FDG-PET in advanced-stage diffuse large B-cell lymphoma. J Clin Oncol 28:1896–1903
36. Avigdor A, Sirotkin T, Kedmi M, Ribakovsy E, Berkowicz M, Davidovitz Y et al (2014) The impact of R-VACOP-B and interim FDG-PET/CT on outcome in primary mediastinal large B cell lymphoma. Ann Hematol 93:1297–1304
37. Moskowitz C, Hamlin PA, Maragulia J, Meikle J, Zelenetz AD (2010) Sequential dose-dense RCHOP followed by ICE consolidation (MSKCC protocol 01–142) without radiotherapy for patients with primary mediastinal large B-cell lymphoma. Blood 116:abstr 420
38. Horning SJ, Juweid ME, Schoeder H et al (2010) Interim positron emission tomography scans in diffuse large B-cell lymphoma: an independent expert nuclear medicine evaluation of the Eastern Cooperative Oncology Group E3404 study. Blood 115:775–777
39. Meignan M, Gallamini A, Itti E, Barrington S, Haioun C, Polliack A (2012) Report on the third international workshop on interim positron emission tomography in lymphoma held in Menton, France, 26–27 September 2011 and Menton 2011 consensus. Leuk Lymphoma 53:1876–1881
40. Carr R, Fanti S, Paez D, Cerci J, Gyorke T, Redondo F et al (2014) Prospective international cohort study demonstrates inability if interim PET to predict treatment failure in diffuse large B-cell lymphoma. J Nucl Med 55:1936–1944
41. Itti E, Meignan M, Berriolo-Riedinger A, Biggi A, Cashen AF, Verra P et al (2013) An international confirmatory study of the prognostic value of early PET/CT in diffuse large B-cell lymphoma: comparison between Deauville criteria and ΔSUVmax. Eur J Nucl Med Mol Imaging 40:1312–1320
42. Casasnovas RO, Meignan M, Berriolo-Riedinger A et al (2011) SUVmax reduction improves early prognosis value of interim positron emission tomography scans in diffuse large B-cell lymphoma. Blood 118:37–43
43. Duehrsen U, Hüttmann A, Müller S, Hertenstein B, Kotzerke J, Mesters R et al (2014) Positron emission tomography (PET) guided therapy of aggressive lymphomas – a randomized controlled trial comparing different treatment approaches based on interim PET results (PETAL Trial). Blood. (ASH Annual Meeting Abstracts) 124:Abstract 391
44. Swinnen LJ, Li H, Quon A, Gascoyne RD, Ranheim EA, Hong F et al (2013) Response-adapted therapy and predictive value of mid-treatment PET scanning for diffuse large B-cell lymphoma. ECOG study

E3404. Hematol Oncol 31(S1):138 (abstr. 126). Hematol Oncol. 2013; 31(S1): 101 (abstr. 016)
45. Sehn LH, Hardy ELG, Gill KK, Al-Tourah AJ, Shustik J, Macpherson MA et al (2014) Phase 2 trial of interim PET scan-tailored therapy in patients with advanced stage diffuse large B-cell lymphoma (DLBCL) in British Columbia (BC). Blood. (ASH Annual Meeting Abstracts) 124:Abstract 392
46. Recher C, Coiffier B, Haioun C et al (2011) Intensified chemotherapy with ACVBP plus rituximab versus standard CHOP plus rituximab for the treatment of diffuse large B-cell lymphoma (LNH03-2B): an open-label randomised phase 3 trial. Lancet 378:1858–1867
47. Cheson BD, Pfistner B, Juweid ME et al (2007) Revised response criteria for malignant lymphoma. J Clin Oncol 25:579–586
48. Juweid ME, Stroobants S, Hoekstra OS et al (2007) Use of positron emission tomography for response assessment of lymphoma: consensus of the Imaging Subcommittee of International Harmonization Project in Lymphoma. J Clin Oncol 25:571–578
49. Wirk B (2010) Sarcoid reactions after chemotherapy for Hodgkin's lymphoma. Clin Med Insights Case Rep 3:21–25
50. Papageorgiou SG, Sachanas S, Pangalis GA et al (2014) Gastric involvement in patients with primary mediastinal large B-cell lymphoma. Anticancer Res 34:6717–6723

8 Follicular Lymphomas (FL)

John P. Apostolidis, Roxani D. Efthymiadou, and Theodoros A. Pipikos

Case 1

A 62-year-old male visited his doctor because of swelling and discomfort at the left parotid area. After 1 week of anti-inflammatory medication without relief of symptoms, he underwent a skull MRI. MRI scan revealed abnormal signal in the left parotid gland and an enlarged parotid lymph node. The patient underwent surgery, with the left parotid removed. Histopathology revealed infiltration of the parotid gland of low-grade follicular lymphoma (FL) (grade I). The enlarged lymph node was also infiltrated.

Whole-body CT imaging did not reveal any other pathological findings, while a bone marrow biopsy was negative for disease infiltration. The initial staging of the disease suggested that the patient had localized stage I disease, a potentially curable disease when locoregional radiation therapy is applied [1]. The patient's physician requested an FDG PET/CT scan for more precise staging and treatment decision making.

FDG PET/CT revealed postsurgery findings of the left parotid area with no abnormal metabolic activity as seen in Fig. 8.2. The rest of whole-body imaging showed multiple hypermetabolic lymph nodes in the thorax, abdomen and pelvis (Figs. 8.1 and 8.3). Patient's staging was changed from stage I to stage III. Advanced stage III–IV disease is not curable with conventional treatment, and therapeutic options range from a "watch-and-wait" approach to systemic immunochemotherapy, depending on the presence of disease-related symptoms and tumor burden [2]. The patient's physician opted to treat the patient with six cycles of immunochemotherapy (rituximab-CVP).

Discussion

FL is the second most frequent subtype of lymphoma. Clinically, it is usually characterized by a relapsing and remitting pattern, with mainly nodal and bone marrow involvement. This results in a chronic illness, which is managed with close observation and immunochemotherapy when appropriate [2]. There is no consensus on the optimal management of FL, and it remains essentially an incurable disease. A notable exception are patients with limited stage I–II disease (15–20 % of cases), with a long-term disease-free survival rate of 40–50 % when treated with locoregional

J.P. Apostolidis
Department of Hematology, Bone Marrow Transplant Unit, Evangelismos Hospital, 10th Floor AHEPA Building, Room 1031, Ipsilandou, Athens 10676, Greece
e-mail: japostol@otenet.gr

R.D. Efthymiadou (✉)
Director of PET/CT Department, "HYGEIA" Hospital, Erythrou Stavrou 4 and Kifissias, Maroussi 15123, Greece
e-mail: r.efthimiadi@hygeia.gr

T.A. Pipikos
Department of Nuclear Medicine and PET/CT, "HYGEIA" Hospital, Erythrou Stavrou 4 and Kifissias, Maroussi 15123, Greece
e-mail: tpipikos@hygeia.gr

J.A. Andreou et al. (eds.), *PET/CT in Lymphomas: A Case-Based Atlas*,
DOI 10.1007/978-3-319-27380-8_8

radiation. FDG PET/CT can identify more nodal and extranodal lesions compared to CT imaging in FL patients [3]. It can lead to patient's stage alteration in up to 45–50 % of the cases of limited stage disease as determined by CT [4, 5]. In this particular case, the patient would be falsely staged as stage I. A critical question is the prognostic relevance of detecting small-volume disease on FDG-PET but not on CT in this setting. Although there is a rationale for using PET for imaging of patients with limited stage disease to either change the size of the radiation field or avoid due to upstaging fruitless involved field radiotherapy (IFRT), the outcome of IFRT for localized FL staged by PET has not yet been reported. Therefore, in FL it is unknown whether improved staging accuracy will result in improved outcome [6]. Prospective trials will need to address these issues.

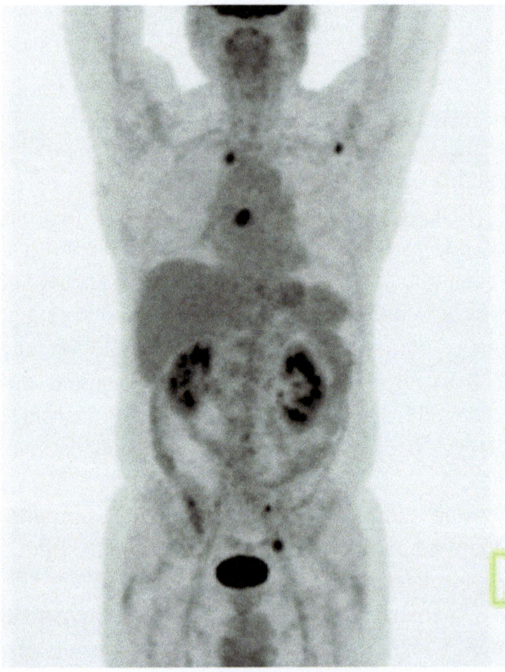

Fig. 8.1 In the MIP projection, multiple hypermetabolic lesions are found

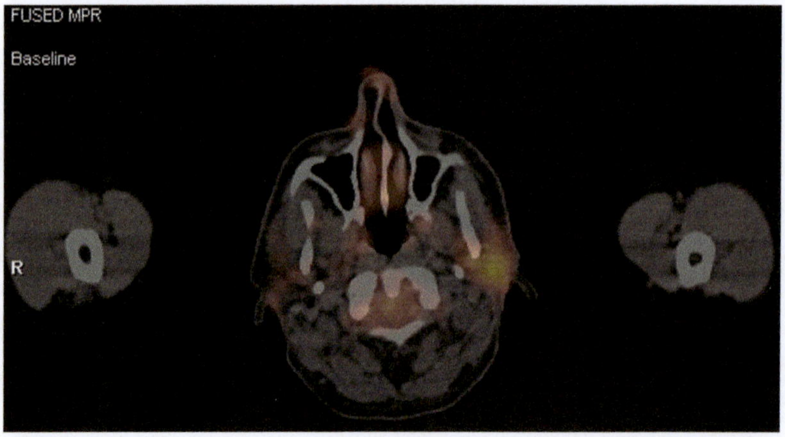

Fig. 8.2 Postsurgery findings in the left parotid

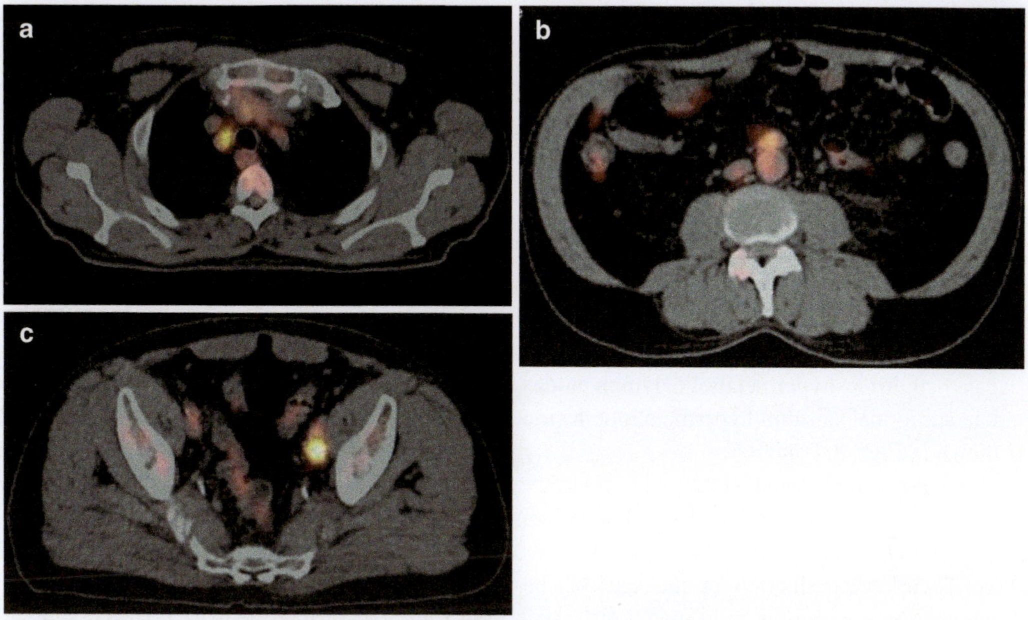

Fig. 8.3 Hypermetabolic lymph nodes in the thorax (**a**) abdomen (**b**) and pelvis (**c**)

Case 2

A 64-year-old with diffuse abdomen discomfort underwent sonography of the abdominal area which revealed a 17 cm mesenteric mass located in the left abdominal area. Initial suspicion was that of a GIST tumor. A biopsy was performed, and histopathology results were that of a follicular NHL grade 1/2. CT imaging demonstrated the mesenteric mass and enlarged para-aortic and retroperitoneal lymph nodes.

FDG PET/CT imaging for initial staging revealed multiple hypermetabolic lymph nodes and an additional sternum hypermetabolic lesion as shown in Figs. 8.4 and 8.5.

The patient underwent systematic immunochemotherapy with rituximab-CHOP and had an interim FDG PET/CT for therapy response evaluation. There was reduction in the size of the abdominal mass with only mild metabolic activity (SUV_{max} 2, 7). There were no other lesions of abnormal metabolic activity in the whole-body imaging (Fig. 8.6).

Two months following completion of therapy, the patient underwent a new PET/CT scan, with further reduction of abdominal mass size and no pathological metabolic activity. The patient had achieved a complete remission (Figs. 8.7 and 8.8).

Discussion

The role of FDG PET/CT in response assessment after immunochemotherapy in FL has been evaluated in a limited number of retrospective and prospective studies. One study retrospectively evaluated the role of postinduction PET/CT scans in patients enrolled onto the PRIMA study and treated with rituximab-CHOP or rituximab-CVP. Patients with PET-positive scans after induction had significantly worse progression-free survival (PFS) and overall survival (OS) than patients with PET-negative scans. [7] PET-based response assessment was more predictive than conventional response assessment using international working criteria (IWC). This study was limited by its retrospective nature and the PET methodology.

A prospective study by Depuis et al. evaluated the prognostic role of interim and end-of-treatment PET scans in patients with high-tumor burden FL (in need of treatment) and uniformly treated with rituximab-CHOP [8]. The Deauville criteria with a cutoff of ≥4 were used to determine positivity. Both interim and end-of-treatment PET scans were predictive of 2-year PFS, but only end-of-treatment PET scans were predictive of 2-year OS with rates of 88 % versus 100 % ($P = .0128$) for positive and negative scans, respectively. The authors concluded that a scan at the end of treatment was sufficient. PET was also superior to the Follicular Lymphoma International Prognostic Index (FLIPI) score, remaining predictive of survival across FLIPI risk groups.

Overall, although follow-up is limited in both studies, it seems that PET-assessed response is better in predicting PFS and possibly OS in patients with FL. Still, there is no evidence to suggest that response-guided treatment will improve the outcome of these patients, and any alteration of treatment based on PET results remains experimental. Prospective studies are currently addressing these issues.

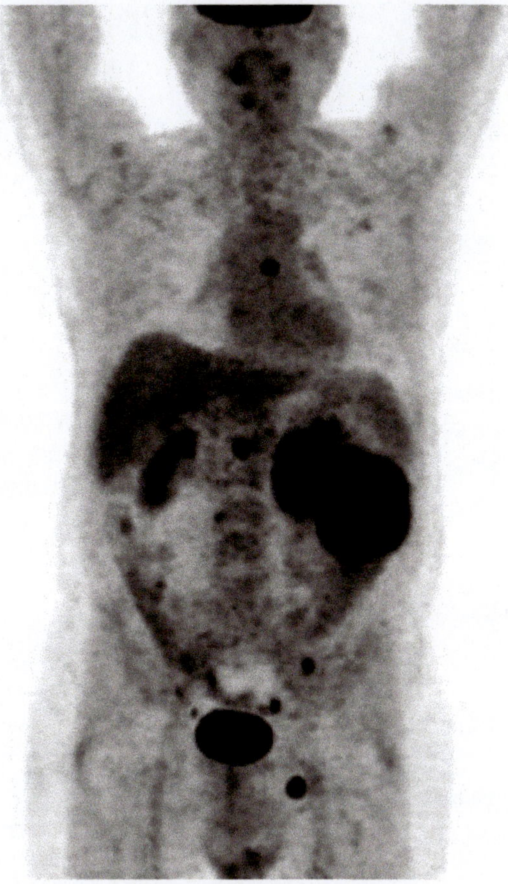

Fig. 8.4 Initial pretherapy scan showing multiple hypermetabolic lesions. Stage IV

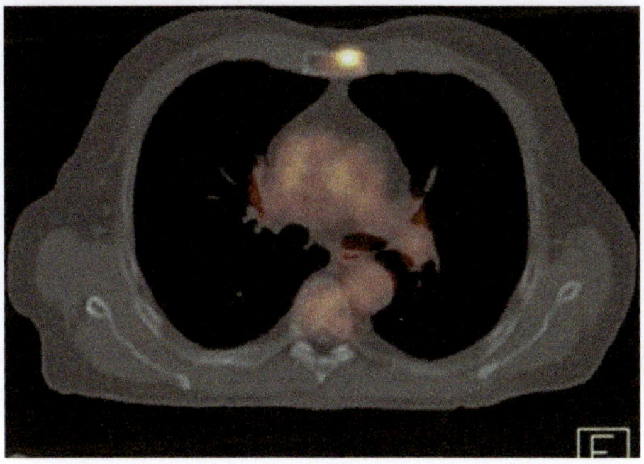

Fig. 8.5 Sternum lesion with no corresponding CT findings

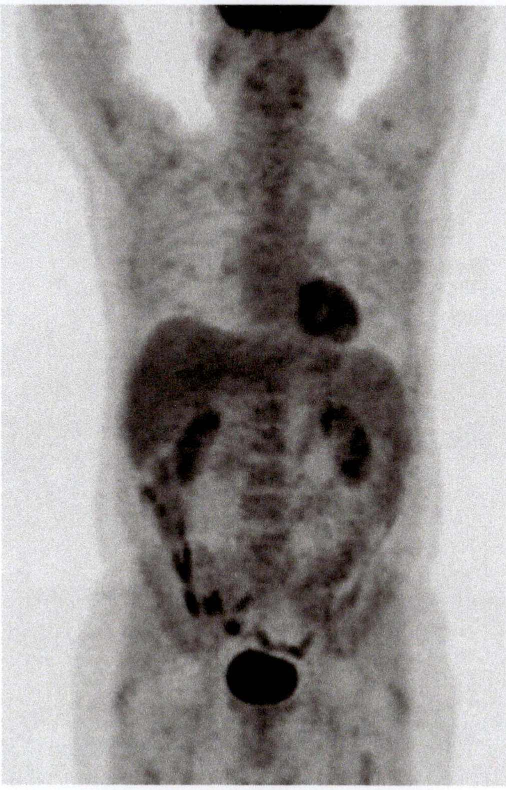

Fig. 8.6 Interim PET with findings of complete response

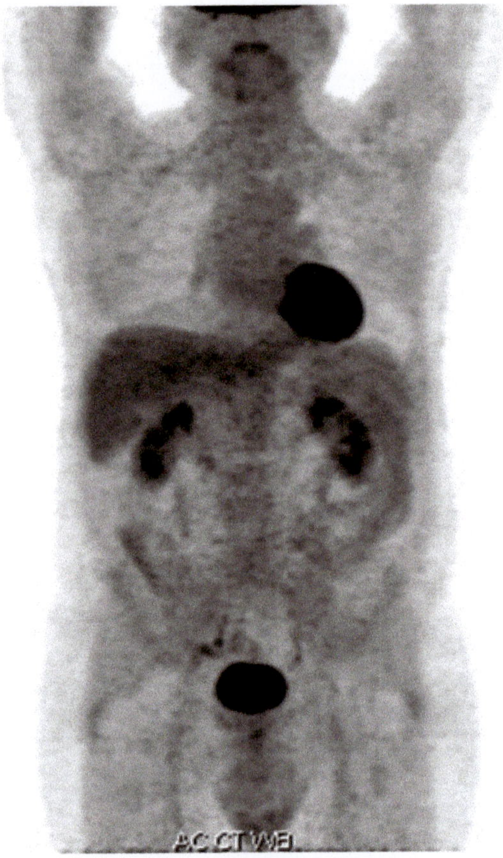

Fig. 8.7 End-therapy scan. No findings of pathological metabolic activity

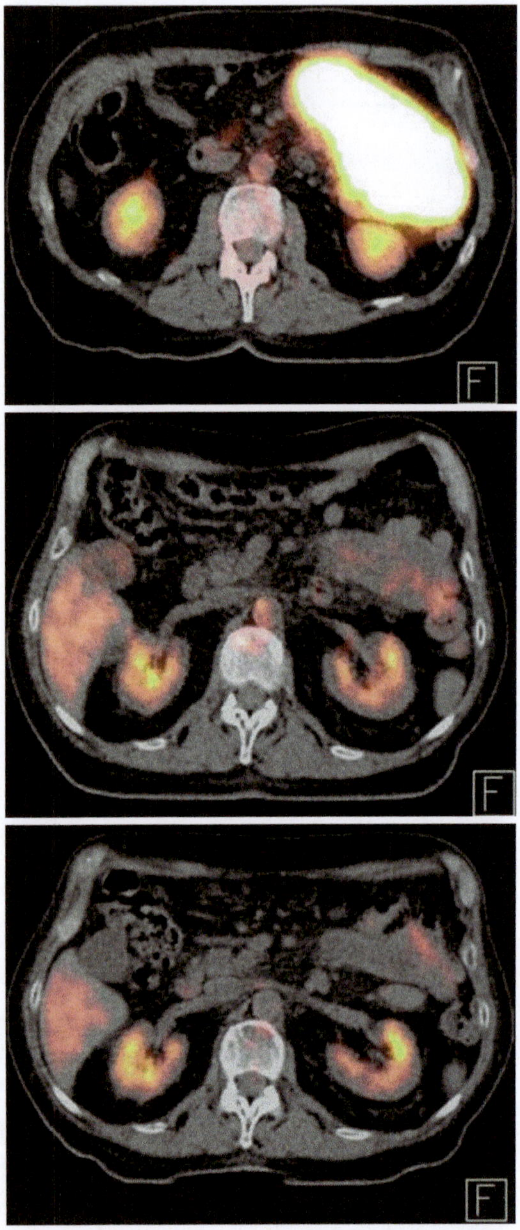

Fig. 8.8 Superiority of metabolic evaluation of treatment response compared to CT imaging. Gradual significant reduction of the size of the lesion in the CT images, with early absence of metabolic activity

Case 3

A 62-year-old female presented with left axillary lymph node enlargement and underwent a biopsy which revealed a grade 1/2 follicular lymphoma. Further staging with CTs demonstrated a few borderline cervical lymph nodes and enlarged para-aortic, iliac, and inguinal lymph nodes. A bone trephine biopsy was negative.

The patient underwent an FDG PET/CT study for initial staging in the spectrum of doubtful CT findings. As shown in Fig. 8.9, multiple hypermetabolic lymph nodes were found in the area of the neck, thorax, abdomen, and pelvis. Moreover, there were splenic hypermetabolic lesions and hypermetabolic lesions in the subcutaneous tissue of the right gluteal area.

The patient underwent systematic immunochemotherapy with rituximab-CHOP, and an interim PET/CT study demonstrated great reduction of metabolic activity, as seen in Fig. 8.10, indicating response to the systematic therapy.

Two months after the completion of therapy, a posttherapy PET scan was performed with no findings of abnormal metabolism and a complete remission was established (Fig. 8.11).

A new PET/CT scan was performed 4 months later because of equivocal findings on CT imaging suggestive of splenic lesions. The PET scan revealed splenic hypermetabolic lesions, with no other pathological findings in whole-body imaging as seen in Fig. 8.12.

The patient proceeded to a splenectomy that revealed infiltration of the initial disease. The patient has since been followed up expectantly with no indication for further treatment. A follow-up PET/CT was performed 3 months later that had no abnormal findings (Fig. 8.13).

Discussion

FDG PET/CT or CT imaging is not routinely recommended for the detection of relapse in patients with follicular lymphoma who have achieved a complete remission with induction therapy [9, 10]. Because of high sensitivity of FDG PET/CT, false-positive findings that can cause diagnostic problems can occur. Follow-up is usually based on physical examination, blood and biochemistry tests, or minimal imaging such as x-rays and ultrasonography.

However, PET/CT can be considered in selected cases based on clinical judgment and when therapeutic decisions are to be made. In this patient early identification of spleen lesions leads to the right therapeutic decision. Apart from diagnostic, splenectomy was also therapeutic, since no further treatment is indicated.

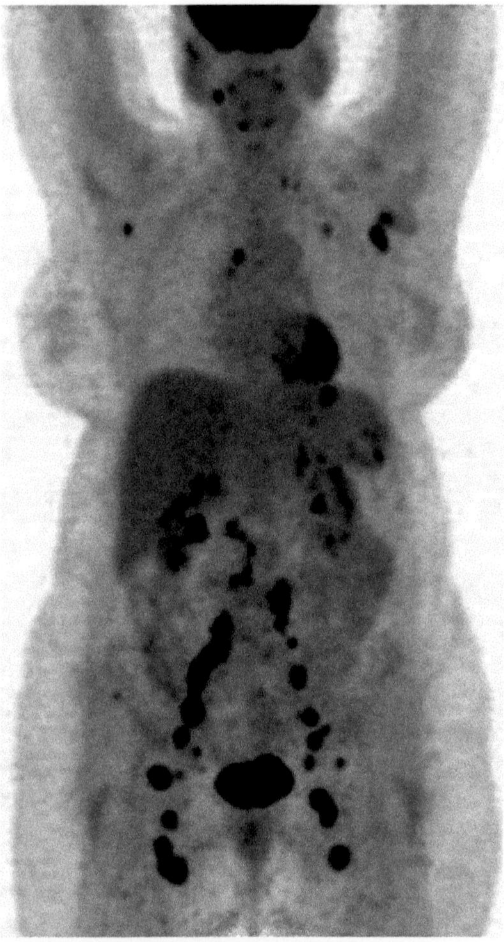

Fig. 8.9 MIP of the initial staging showing multiple hypermetabolic lymph node areas

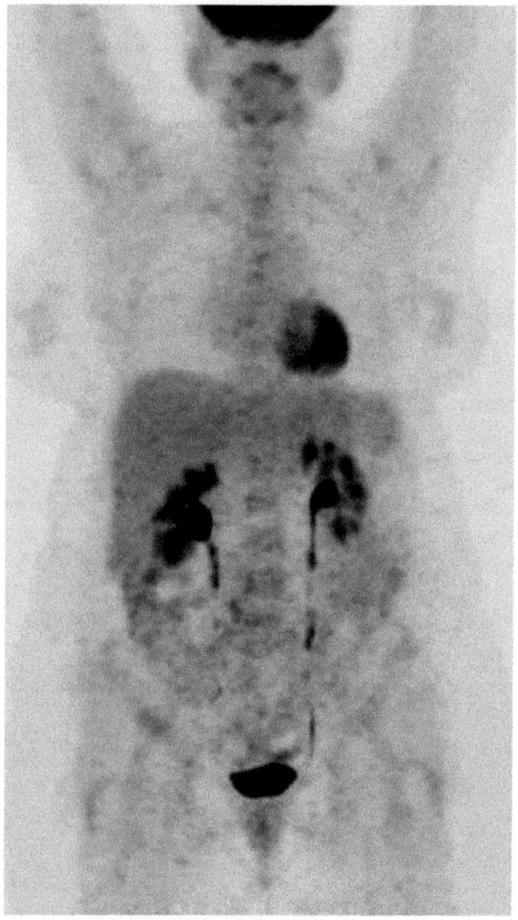

Fig. 8.10 MIP of interim PET/CT. There is almost disappearance of pathologically increased metabolic activity

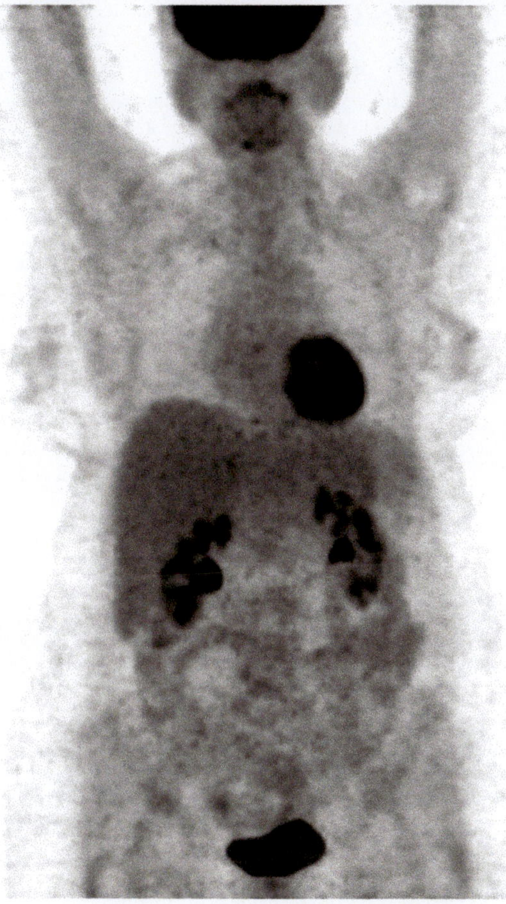

Fig. 8.11 Findings of CR in posttherapy PET/CT scan

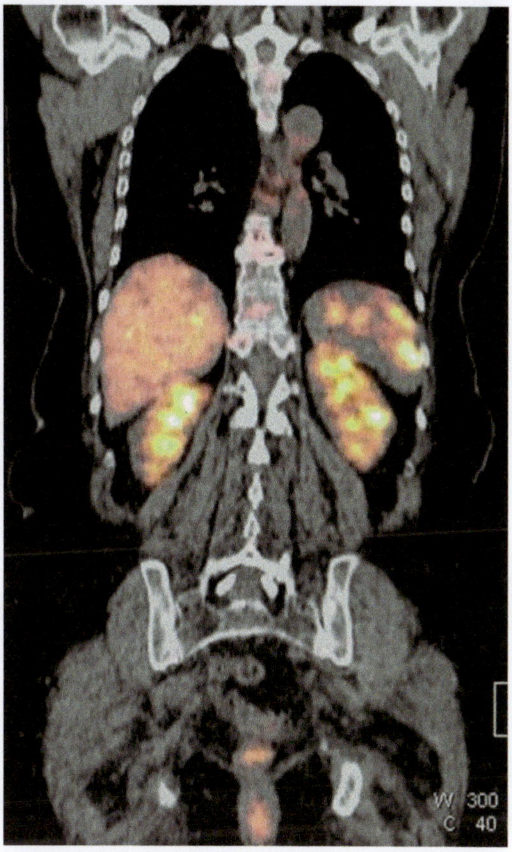

Fig. 8.12 Splenic hypermetabolic lesions. No other pathology in the rest of whole-body imaging was found

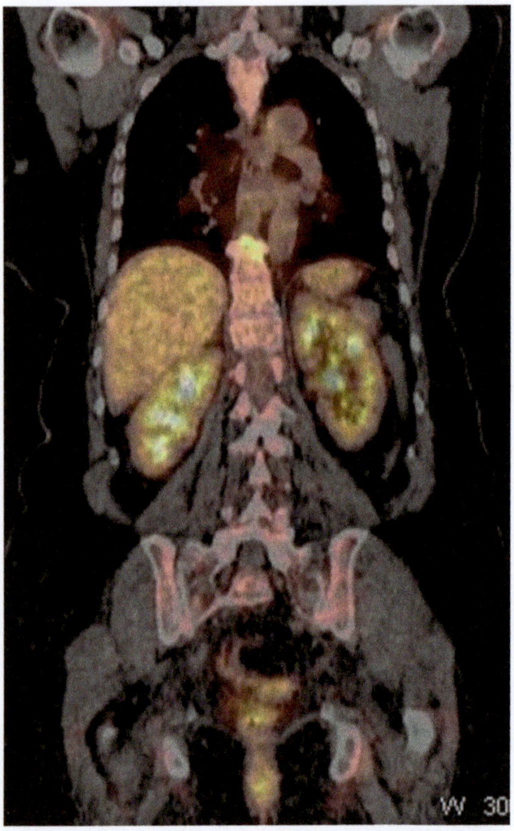

Fig. 8.13 No findings of active disease. Image after splenectomy

References

1. Pugh TJ, Ballonoff A, Newman F, Rabinovitch R (2010) Improved survival in patients with early stage low-grade follicular lymphoma treated with radiation: a Surveillance, Epidemiology, and End Results database analysis. Cancer 116:3843–3851
2. Hiddemann W, Cheson BD (2014) How we manage follicular lymphoma. Leukemia 28:1388–1395
3. Janikova A, Bolcak K, Pavlik T et al (2008) Value of [18F]fluorodeoxyglucose positron emission tomography in the management of follicular lymphoma: the end of a dilemma? Clin Lymphoma Myeloma 8:287–293
4. Wirth A, Foo M, Seymour JF et al (2008) Impact of [18f] fluorodeoxyglucose positron emission tomography on staging and management of early-stage follicular non-Hodgkin lymphoma. Int J Radiat Oncol Biol Phys 71:213–219
5. Le Dortz L, De Guibert S, Bayat S et al (2010) Diagnostic and prognostic impact of 18F-FDG PET/CT in follicular lymphoma. Eur J Nucl Med Mol Imaging 37:2307–2314
6. Barrington SF (2012) Imaging follicular lymphoma using positron emission tomography with [^{18}F]fluorodeoxyglucose: to what purpose? J Clin Oncol 35:4285–4287
7. Trotman J, Fournier M, Lamy T et al (2011) Positron emission tomography-computed tomography (PET-CT) after induction therapy is highly predictive of patient outcome in follicular lymphoma: analysis of PET-CT in a subset of PRIMA trial participants. J Clin Oncol 29:3194–3200
8. Dupuis J, Berriolo-Riedinger A, Julian A et al (2012) Impact of [18F]fluorodeoxyglucose positron emission tomography response evaluation in patients with high-tumor burden follicular lymphoma treated with immunochemotherapy: a prospective study from the groupe d'Etudes des lymphomas de l'Adulte and GOELAMS. J Clin Oncol 30:4317–4322
9. Ghielmini M, Vitolo U, Kimby E et al (2013) ESMO guidelines consensus conference on malignant lymphoma 2011 part 1: diffuse large B-cell lymphoma (DLBCL), follicular lymphoma (FL) and chronic lymphocytic leukemia (CLL). Ann Oncol 24:561–576
10. Cheson BD, Fisher RI, Barrington SF et al (2014) Recommendations for initial evaluation, staging, and response assessment of Hodgkin and non-Hodgkin lymphoma: the Lugano Classification. J Clin Oncol 32:3059–3068

Mantle Cell Lymphoma (MCL) 9

John P. Apostolidis, Maria G. Skilakaki, and Alexandra V. Nikaki

Case 1

A 52-year-old male presented with a diagnosis of mantle cell lymphoma (MCL) following a left inguinal lymph node biopsy. Initial staging with conventional imaging modalities revealed nodal disease both above and below the diaphragm. The largest nodal lesion was noted at the left para-aortic region, just below the renal vessels, measuring 7 cm in cephalocaudal diameter. Bone marrow biopsy was negative. The patient was treated with eight cycles of immunochemotherapy (rituximab-bendamustine).

An end-of-treatment FDG PET/CT performed revealed persistent disease: Anterior and lateral views of maximum intensity projection FDG PET image (Fig. 9.1a, b) show abnormal metabolic activity (SUVmax = 16) in the left para-aortic nodal enlargement.

The patient received additional chemotherapy with an anthracycline-containing regimen (R-CHOP × two cycles) and in March 2015 underwent a new PET/CT study to evaluate for response. Anterior and lateral views of maximum intensity projection FDG PET image (Fig. 9.2a, b) reveal increased FDG uptake (SUVmax = 9) in the known left para-aortic nodal enlargement, which remained stable in size. Although there is a 55 % decrease in the metabolic activity of the lesion, the finding is indicative of persistent disease.

Further treatment options for this patient would include salvage chemotherapy followed by high-dose therapy and autologous hematopoietic stem cell transplantation (auto-HSCT) or treatment with the novel oral BTK inhibitor ibrutinib as "bridging" to proceed with an allogeneic hematopoietic stem cell transplant (allo-HSCT), if a compatible donor is available.

Discussion

MCL is a relatively rare lymphoma entity accounting for an estimated 3–6 % of all NHL cases. Patients are predominantly male with a median age at diagnosis of 60–65 years. The disease combines the incurability of indolent lymphomas with the rapid growth of aggressive lymphomas and is characterized by an unfavorable clinical course with median overall survival of only 4–5 years [1, 2].

Standard therapy for MCL consists of immunochemotherapy such as R-CHOP or R-bendamustine or more aggressive regimens including high-dose

J.P. Apostolidis
Department of Hematology, Evangelismos General Hospital, Ypsilantou 45-47, Athens, 10676, Greece
e-mail: japostol@otenet.gr

M.G. Skilakaki (✉)
Department of Radiology, G.N.A. "Annunciation", Ypsilantou 45-47, Athens 10676, Greece
e-mail: skmaria@otenet.gr

A.V. Nikaki
Department of Nuclear Medicine, D.TH.K.A. "HEALTH", Kifissias Av. & Q. Cross 4, Maroussi 15123, Greece

J.A. Andreou et al. (eds.), *PET/CT in Lymphomas: A Case-Based Atlas*,
DOI 10.1007/978-3-319-27380-8_9

cytarabine (R-DHAP or R-HyperCVAD/MA) alongside high-dose chemotherapy auto-HSCT [3, 4].

Large prospective randomized studies are lacking in MCL due to the rarity of the disease, and the choice of appropriate treatment remains a complex problem that still requires evidence-based guidance. In general, therapeutic approaches include the treatment of patients who are eligible for autologous hematopoietic stem cell transplantation and those who are not. Unfortunately, despite the improved activity of first-line treatment, with time nearly all patients relapse with a clinically aggressive course, and salvage therapy is usually followed by only a short duration of response [1]. Allo-HSCT is a potential curative therapeutic strategy for selected patients [5]. Overall, MCL shows the worst long-term survival among all B-cell lymphoma subtypes. However, a number of active targeted therapies look promising and are currently being incorporated into the treatment algorithms of this disease [6].

MCL is a FDG-avid tumor, particularly for nodal disease. This is typically apparent in the above case, which has residual bulky nodal disease. However, in contrast to other high grade NHLs, studies have demonstrated that a positive PET scan did not predict for an inferior overall survival when used either as an interim assessment or at the end of therapy [7, 8]. Therefore response criteria based on PET scanning rather than conventional imaging in MCL, outside the context of a clinical trial, cannot be routinely recommended.

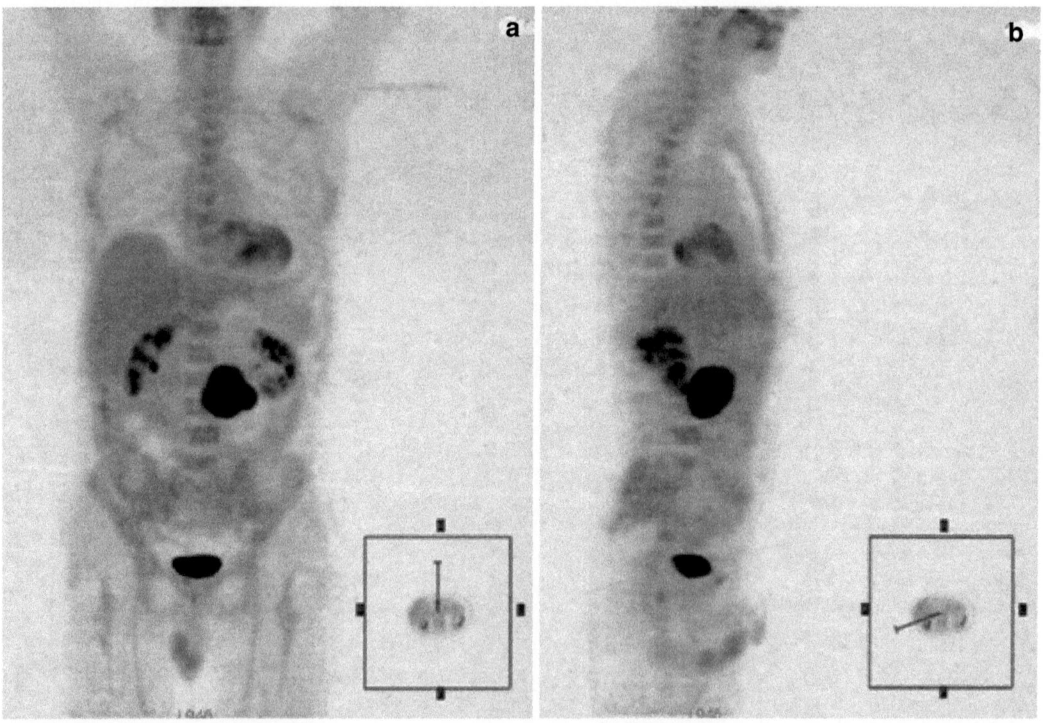

Fig. 9.1 (**a**, **b**) Anterior (**a**) and lateral (**b**) views of multiple intensity projection image show an area of increased metabolic activity in the left abdomen

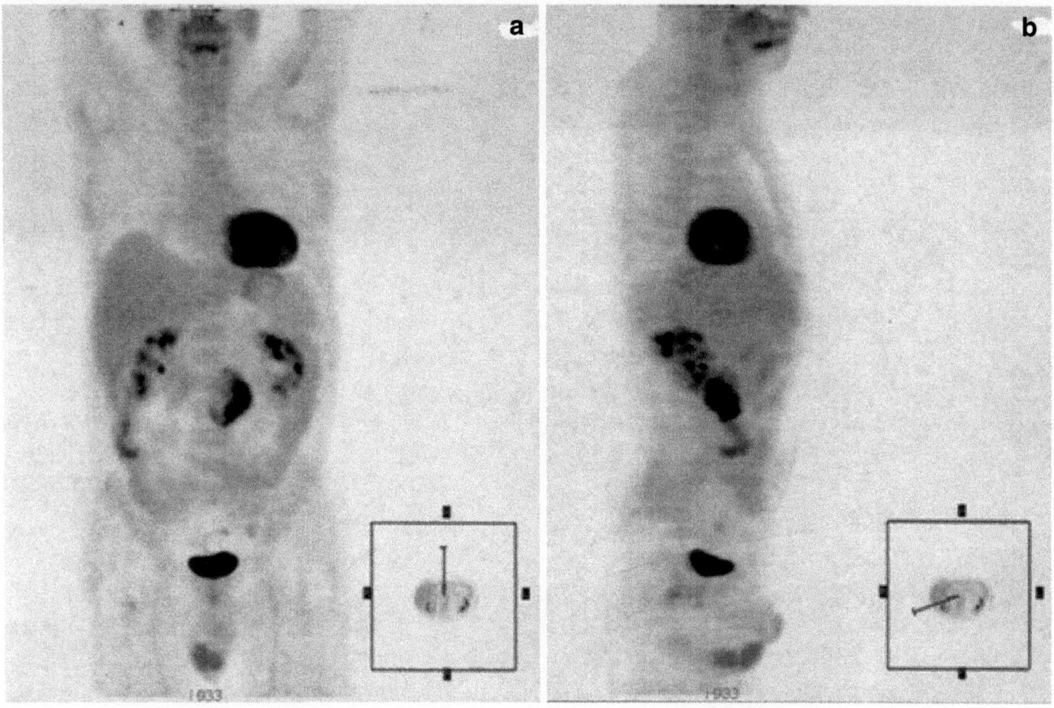

Fig. 9.2 (**a**, **b**) Anterior (**a**) and lateral (**b**) views of multiple intensity projection image reveal persistent focal metabolic activity in the left abdomen

Case 2

A 79-year-old male was diagnosed with MCL following a hepatogastric ligament lymph node biopsy. Imaging with CT of the abdomen and pelvis revealed lymphadenopathy at the area of hepatogastric ligament in contiguity with the lesser bow of the stomach. A FDG PET/CT was requested to by the treating physician.

Anterior and lateral views of maximum intensity projection FDG PET image (Fig. 9.3a, b) show focal abnormal metabolic activity in the left upper abdominal area representing the known nodal disease. They also reveal a focus of increased FDG uptake in the right lower chest and increased metabolism in the lower esophagus.

Figure 9.4: Axial CT and corresponding axial fused PET/CT image of the chest (Fig. 9.4a, b) show a FDG-avid nodular lesion in the lower lobe of the right lung

Figure 9.5: Axial fused PET/CT image at the level of the diaphragm (Fig. 9.5) revealed increased metabolic activity (SUV max = 3,2) in the gastroesophageal junction. The finding was considered as nonspecific and further evaluation with endoscopy was recommended

The lung lesion was resected and histology was "negative for malignancy." The increased metabolic activity in the lower esophagus was interpreted as clinically insignificant finding of functional origin. The patient was treated with first-line immunochemotherapy with six cycles of R-CHOP.

Twelve months following completion of treatment, the patient had a repeat PET/CT for evaluation of possible relapse. Anterior and lateral views of maximum intensity projection image (Fig. 9.6a, b) show several foci of increased metabolic activity in the chest and the upper abdomen.

Axial CT and corresponding axial fused PET/CT images of the chest (Fig. 9.7) reveal multiple nodular FDG-avid lesions in both lungs.

Axial CT, corresponding axial fused PET/CT images (Fig. 9.8a–d) at the level of the lower chest-upper abdomen and coronal fused PET/CT image (Fig. 9.9) show intense (SUVmax = 13) metabolic activity in the gastroesophageal junction and the gastric fundus. Remarkable concentric stenosis of the gastric lumen is also noted on CT images.

The findings were indicative of recurrence.

Discussion

MCL has been reported to have a FDG avidity of 85–100 % [9, 10]. Most patients initially present with stage III–IV generalized, nonbulky lymphadenopathy, often with extranodal involvement. The bone marrow, tonsils, spleen, liver, and gastrointestinal (GI) tract are among the most common extranodal sites.

Thirty percent of the patients present with obvious GI symptoms, but the actual incidence of GI involvement is much higher. 10 % of cases present with macroscopic disease (multiple lymphomatous polyposis), while prospective studies have identified microscopic disease of the GI tract in 92 % of cases [11]. However, it has been demonstrated that this finding only rarely (in less than 4 % of cases) changes clinical management [12]. Therefore, routine endoscopy and colonoscopy cannot be recommended for all patients at baseline staging. Thus, enteroscopy should be reserved for patients with clinical indications, such as significant enteric symptoms [13]. Although FDG PET/CT is generally highly sensitive in the initial staging of MCL, it does not reliably detect bowel disease (11–20 % of cases) or bone marrow infiltration [7, 14]. Thus, the involvement of the GI tract should be assessed with endoscopy and biopsy when clinically indicated.

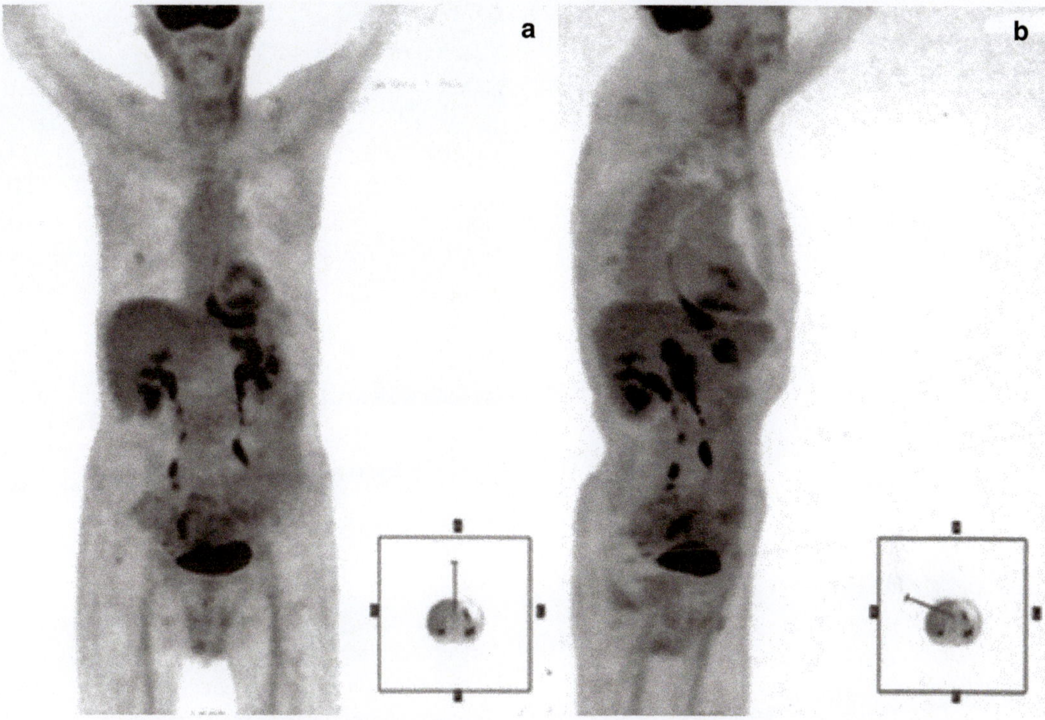

Fig. 9.3 (**a**, **b**) Anterior (**a**) and lateral (**b**) views of maximum intensity projection image show a hypermetabolic lesion in the upper left abdomen, a focus of increased FDG uptake in the right lower chest and increased metabolic activity in the lower esophagus

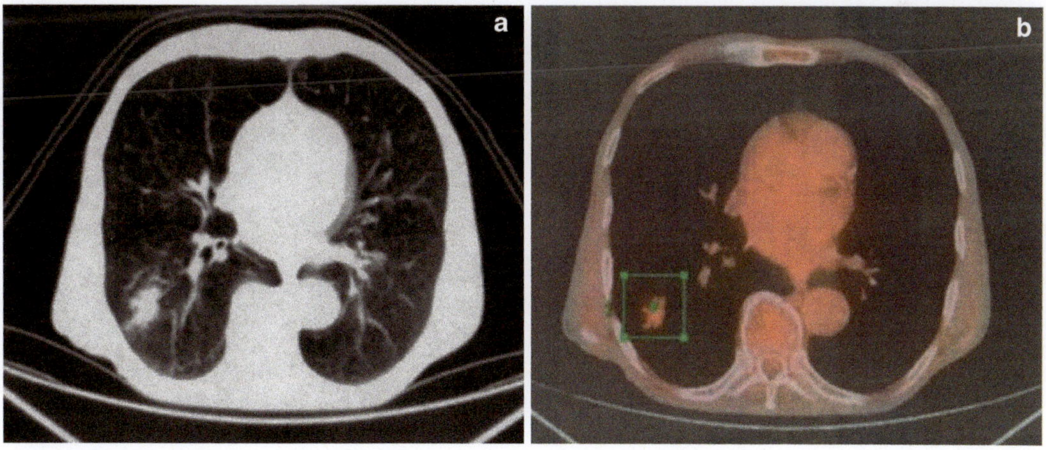

Fig. 9.4 (**a**, **b**) Axial CT (**a**) and corresponding axial fused PET/CT (**b**) image of the chest reveal a hypermetabolic lesion in the lower lobe of the right lung

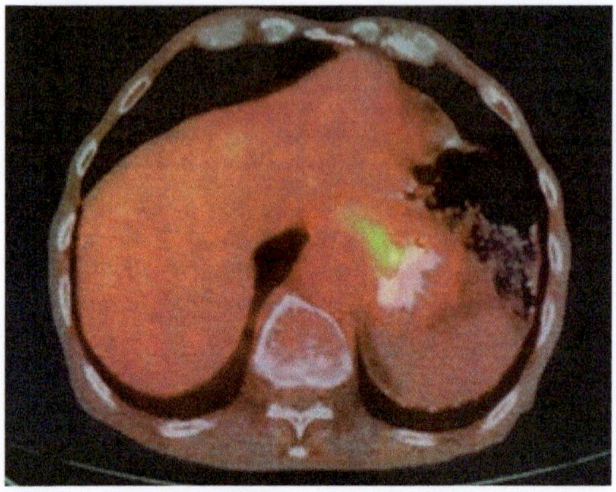

Fig. 9.5 Axial fused PET/CT image at the level of the diaphragm shows increased metabolism in the gastroesophageal junction

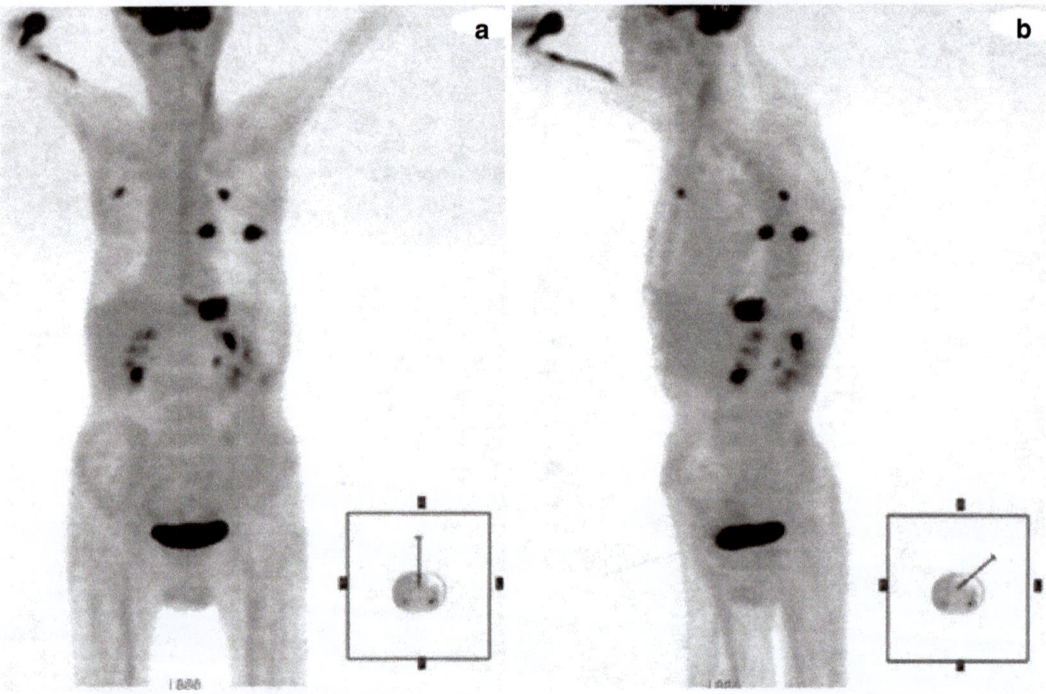

Fig. 9.6 (**a**, **b**) Anterior (**a**) and lateral (**b**) views of maximum intensity projection image show several hypermetabolic lesions in the chest and the upper abdomen

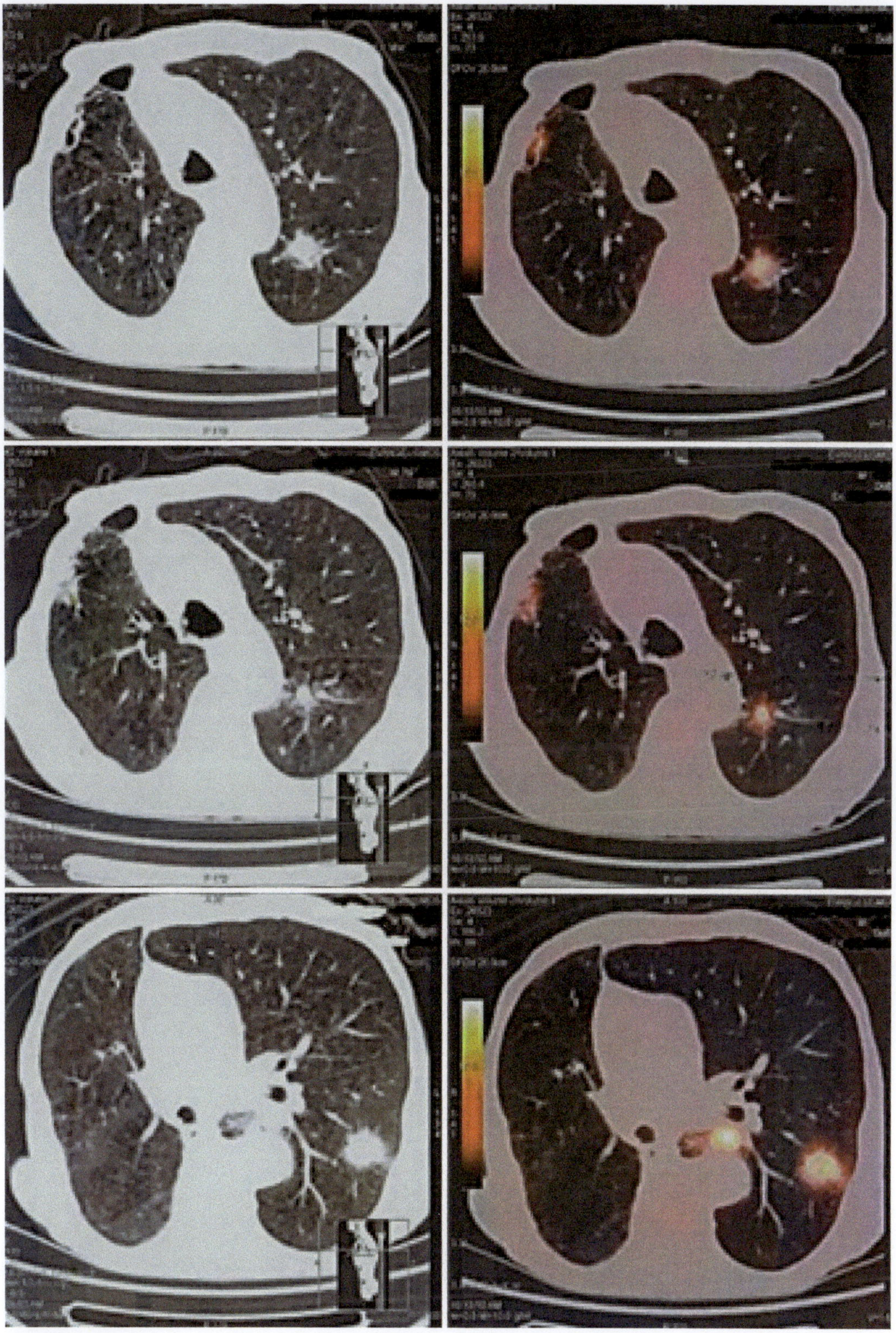

Fig. 9.7 Axial CT and corresponding axial fused PET/CT images of the chest reveal multiple nodular FDG-avid lesions in both lungs

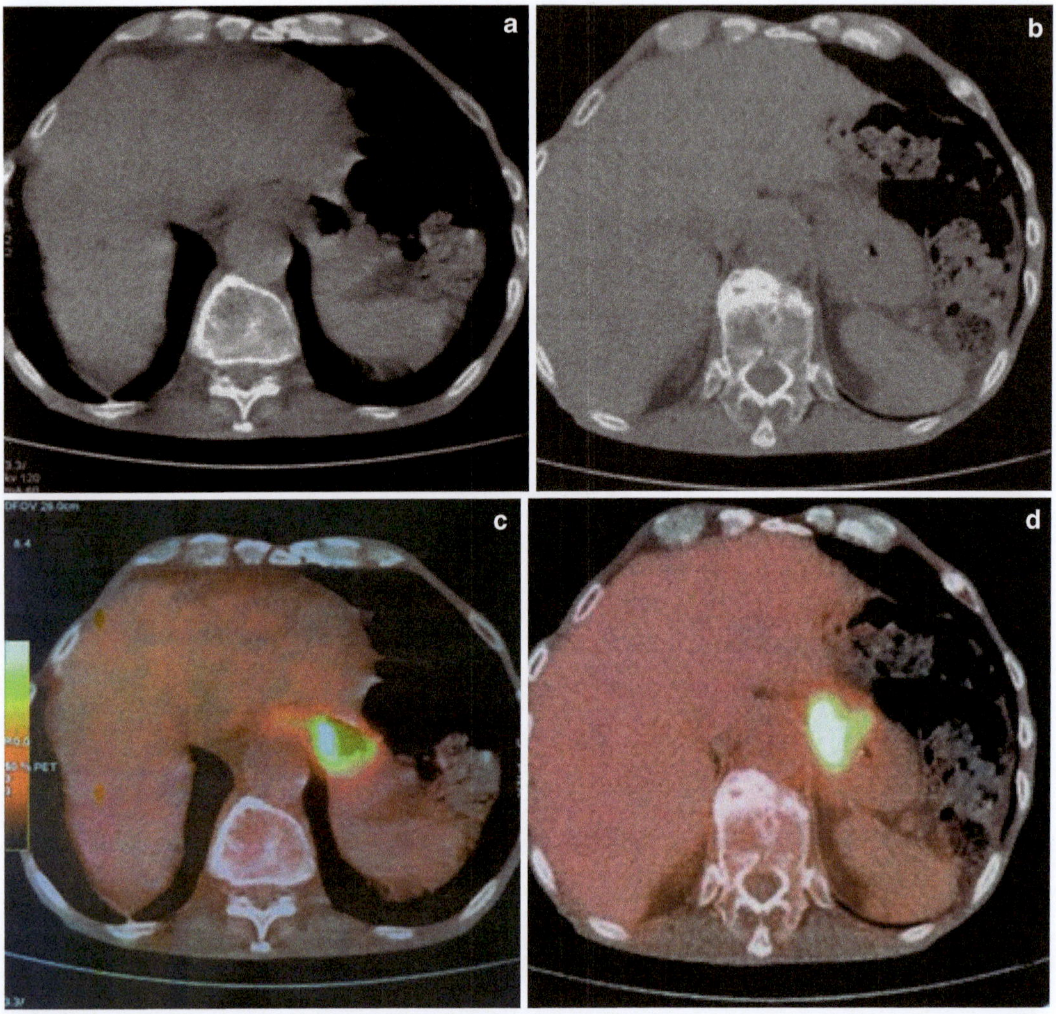

Fig. 9.8 (**a–d**) Axial CT (**a**, **b**) and corresponding axial fused PET/CT (**c**, **d**) images at the level of the lower chest-upper abdomen show concentric stenosis of the esophagogastric lumen and intense metabolic activity in the gastroesophageal junction

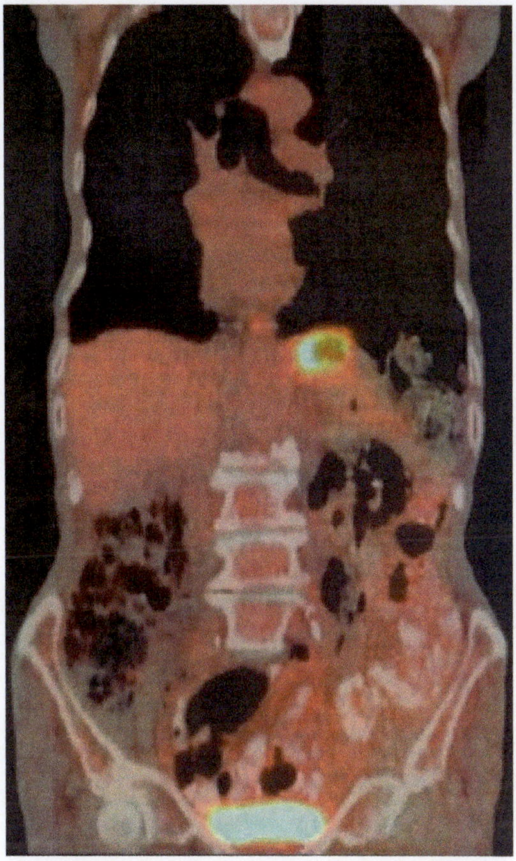

Fig. 9.9 Coronal fused PET/CT image reveals hypermetabolism in gastric fundus

Case 3

A 61-year-old male with a history of relapsed Hodgkin lymphoma involving the left inguinal lymph nodes and treated with high-dose chemotherapy and autologous hematopoietic stem cell transplantation presents with anorexia, loss of weight, and fever. Initial investigation with CT of the chest, abdomen, and pelvis showed several liver lesions and some lymph nodes behind the head of the pancreas. A liver lesion biopsy was indicative of MCL, and the patient was referred to our department for more accurate staging of his disease.

Anterior and lateral views of maximum intensity projection FDG PET image (Fig. 9.10a, b) show multiple foci of abnormal metabolic activity in the abdomen. There is also diffuse FDG uptake in the bone marrow, a finding suggestive of reactive hematopoietic changes within the marrow.

Axial fused PET/CT images of the upper abdomen (Fig. 9.11a–c) reveal several hypermetabolic lesions in the right liver lobe.

Axial fused PET/CT images of the abdomen (Fig. 9.12a, b) confirm abnormal metabolic activity in lymph nodes behind the pancreatic head.

Axial fused PET/CT images of the abdomen (Fig. 9.13a–d) reveal hypermetabolic lesions in the small and large bowel.

Discussion

For FDG-avid NHL subtypes, PET and PET/CT improve the accuracy of staging compared with CT scans for nodal and extranodal sites. However, because of its low sensitivity for the detection of GI involvement (11–20 %), FDG PET/CT is not currently recommended for initial staging of MCL [7, 15].

FDG PET/CT may be useful in patients with limited-stage disease in order to confirm that the extent of their disease has not been underestimated. There is also preliminary evidence that posttreatment PET/CT results may predict clinical outcome in MCL patients treated with high-dose chemotherapy [16]. The current National Comprehensive Cancer Network guidelines (NCCN) recommend baseline PET/CT imaging as a useful diagnostic tool in selected cases in MCL [17].

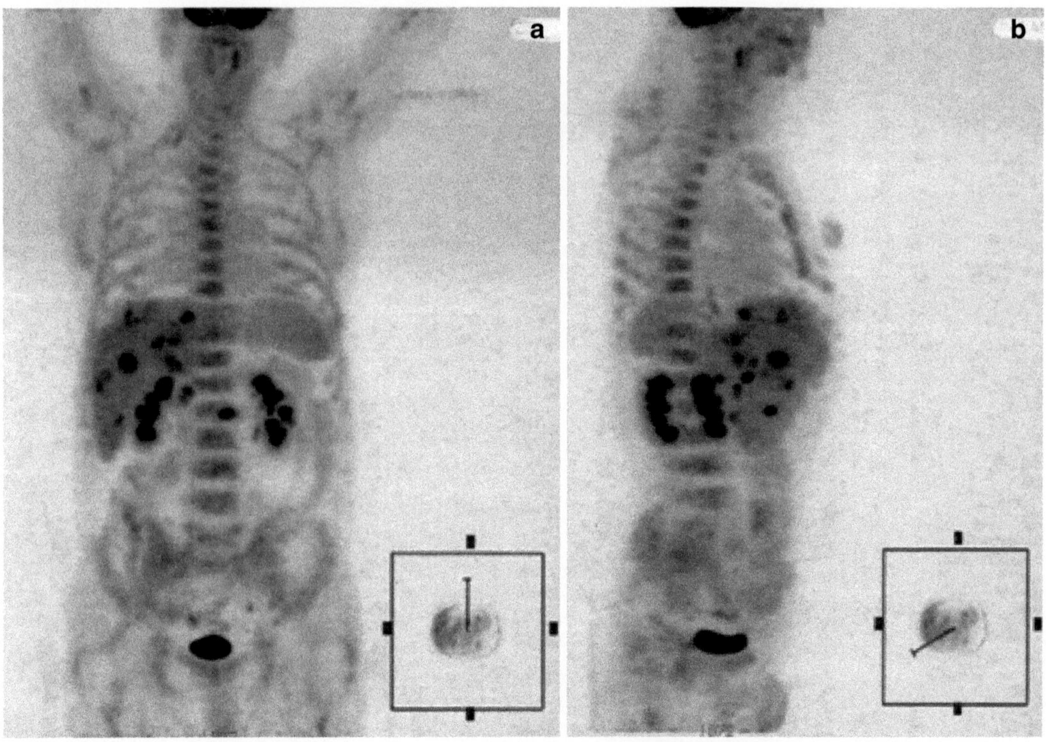

Fig. 9.10 (**a**, **b**) Anterior (**a**) and lateral (**b**) views of maximum intensity projection FDG PET image show multiple foci of abnormal metabolic activity in the abdomen and diffuse FDG uptake in the bone marrow

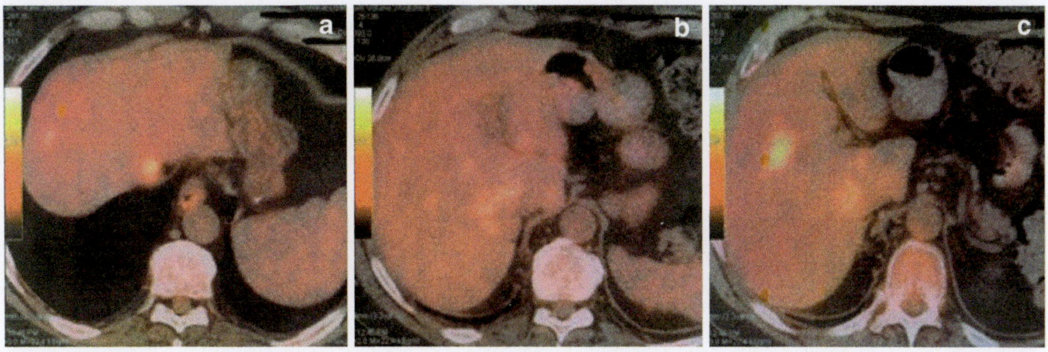

Fig. 9.11 (**a**–**c**) Axial fused PET/CT images of the upper abdomen reveal several hypermetabolic lesions in the right liver lobe

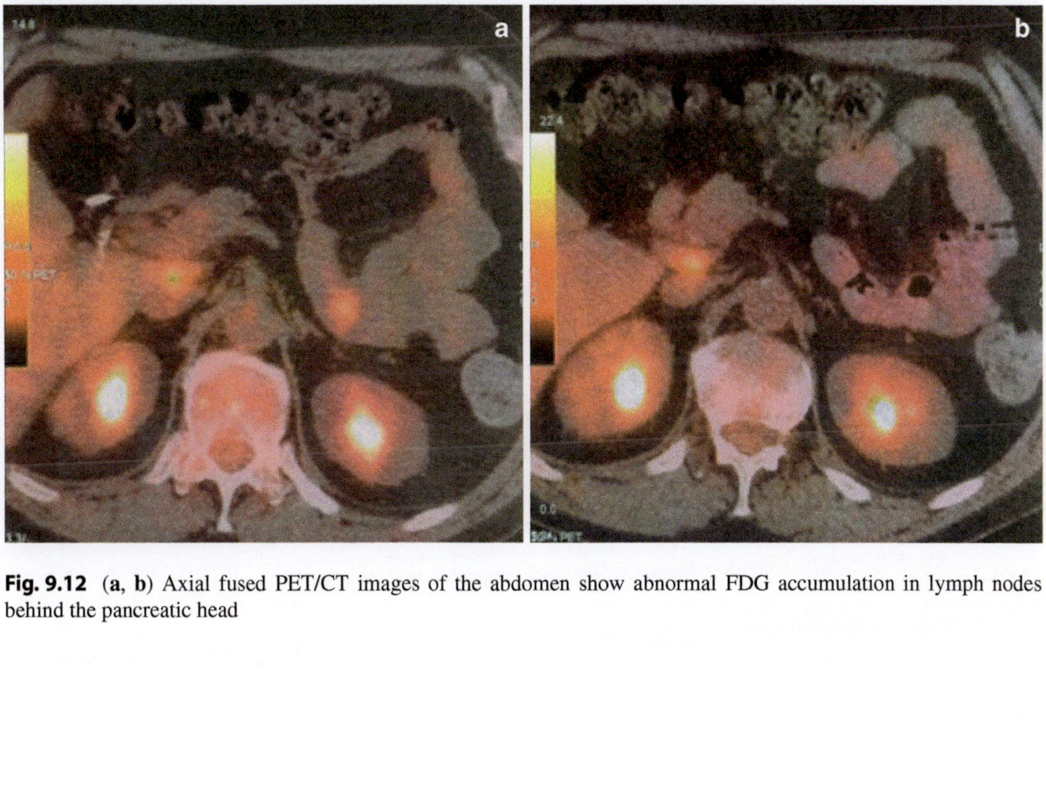

Fig. 9.12 (**a**, **b**) Axial fused PET/CT images of the abdomen show abnormal FDG accumulation in lymph nodes behind the pancreatic head

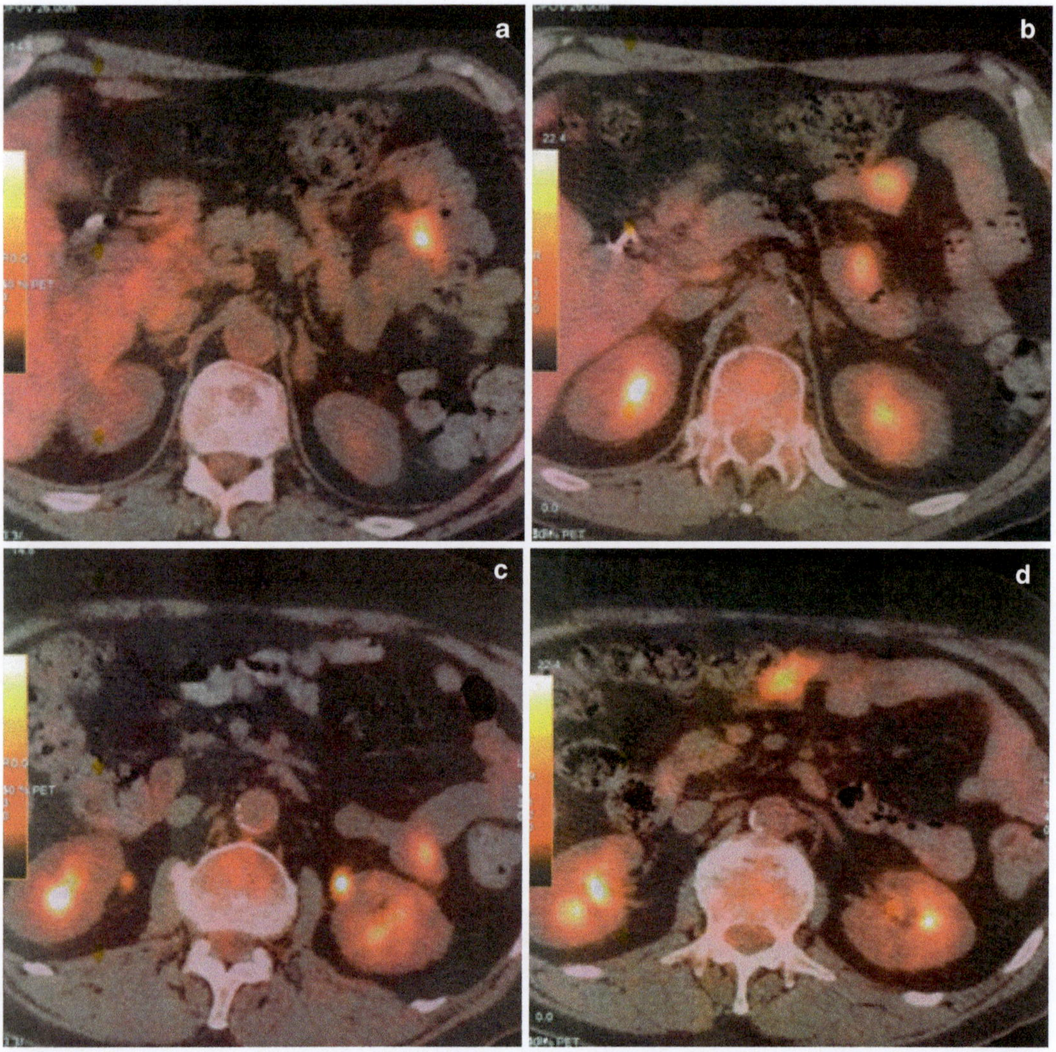

Fig. 9.13 (**a**–**d**) Axial fused PET/CT images of the abdomen show several hypermetabolic lesions in the small and large bowel

References

1. Herrmann A, Hoster E, Zwingers T et al (2009) Improvement of overall survival in advanced stage mantle cell lymphoma. J Clin Oncol 27:511–518
2. Vose JM (2012) Mantle cell lymphoma: 2012 update on diagnosis, risk-stratification and clinical management. Am J Hematol 87:604–609
3. Rummel MJ, Niederle N, Maschmeyer G et al (2013) Bendamustine plus rituximab versus CHOP plus rituximab as first-line treatment for patients with indolent and mantle cell lymphomas: an open-label, multicentre, randomized, phase 3 non-inferiority trial. Lancet 381:1203–1210
4. Hermine O, Hoster E, Walewski J et al (2012) Alternating courses of 3xCHOP and 3xDHAP plus rituximab followed by high dose ARA-C containing myeloablative regimen and autologous stem cell transplantation (ASCT) increases overall survival when compared to 6 courses of CHOP plus rituximab followed by myeloablative radiochemotherapy and ASCT in mantle cell lymphoma: final analysis of the MCL younger trial of the European Mantle Cell Lymphoma Network (abstract). Blood 120:151, ASH Annual Meeting Abstracts
5. Robinson S, Dreger P, Caballero D et al (2015) The EBMT/EMCL consensus project on the role of autologous and allogeneic stem cell transplantation in mantle cell lymphoma. Leukemia 29:464–473
6. Campo E, Rule S (2015) Mantle cell lymphoma: evolving management strategies. Blood 125:48–55
7. Hosein PJ, Pastorini VH, Paes FM et al (2011) Utility of positron emission tomography scans in mantle cell lymphoma. Am J Hematol 86:841–845
8. Kedmi M, Avivi I, Ribakovsky E et al (2014) Is there a role for therapy response assessment with FDG-PET/CT in Mantle Cell Lymphoma? Leuk Lymphoma 55:2484–2489
9. Weiler-Sagie M, Bushelev O, Epelbaum R et al (2010) 18F-FDG avidity in lymphoma readdressed: a study of 766 patients. J Nucl Med 51:25–30
10. Kostakoglu L, Cheson BD (2013) State-of-the-art research on lymphomas: role of molecular imaging for staging, prognostic evaluation and treatment response. Front Oncol. 3(212):1–9. 04/09/13. doi:10.3389/fonc.201300
11. Salar A, Juanpere N, Bellosillo B et al (2006) Gastrointestinal involvement in mantle cell lymphoma: a prospective clinical, endoscopic, and pathological study. Am J Surg Pathol 30:1274–1280
12. Romaguera JE, Medeiros LJ, Hagemeister FB et al (2003) Frequency of gastrointestinal involvement and its clinical significance in mantle cell lymphoma. Cancer 97:586–591
13. McKay P, Leach M, Jackson R et al (2012) Guidelines for the investigation and management of mantle cell lymphoma. Br J Haematol 159:405–426
14. Bodet-Milin C, Touzeau C, Leux C et al (2010) Prognostic impact of 18F-fluoro-deoxyglucose positron emission tomography in untreated mantle cell lymphoma: a retrospective study from the GOELAMS group. Eur J Nucl Med Mol Imaging 37:1633–1642
15. Saito M, Miyazaki M, Tanino M et al (2014) 18F-FDG PET/CT imaging for a gastrointestinal mantle cell lymphoma with multiple lymphomatous polyposis. World J Gastroenterol 20(17):5141–5146
16. Mato AR, Svoboda J, Feldman T et al (2012) Post treatment (not interim) positron emission tomography-computed tomography scan status is highly predictive of outcome in mantle cell lymphoma patients treated with R-HyperCVAD. Cancer 118:3565–3570
17. National Comprehensive Cancer Network Non-Hodgkin Lymphoma (2015) NCCN Version2; http://www.nccn.org/professionals/physician_gls/f_guidelines.asp#nhl

Peripheral T-Cell Lymphomas

10

Maria K. Angelopoulou, Fani J. Vlachou, and Dimitrios T. Kechagias

Peripheral T-cell lymphomas represent very rare entities comprising 8–15 % of all non-Hodgkin lymphomas. This broad category includes lymphomas arising of mature T lymphocytes. They are divided in leukemic, nodal, and extranodal ones. This section focuses on nodal T-cell lymphomas (TCL), which are the most frequently encountered in the Western World and include the entities of ALK+ and ALK− systemic anaplastic T-cell lymphoma (ALK+ ALCL and ALK− ALCL, respectively), angioimmunoblastic T-cell lymphoma (AITL), and peripheral T-cell lymphoma – not otherwise specified (PTCL-NOS) [1]. Due to the rarity of these diseases, there are no prospective randomized trials including specifically patients with these histologies. Thus, prognostic scores and treatment strategies have been adopted from aggressive B-cell lymphomas (DLBCL). CHOP combination chemotherapy with or without etoposide still remains the first-line treatment of choice for many decades. The prognosis of TCL is dismal. Even with the adaptation of more aggressive strategies incorporating high-dose therapy and autologous stem cell transplantation (ASCT) at first remission, the cure rate is approximately 30 %, with the exception of ALK+ ALCL (5-year progression-free survival: 60 %) [1]. At diagnosis, the majority of patients present with generalized lymphadenopathy, advanced-stage disease, frequent extranodal involvement, and poor performance status leading to a high-risk profile. Common extranodal sites are the skin, GI tract, subcutaneous tissue, bones, liver, and lung [1]. The prognostic significance of PET/CT in Hodgkin lymphoma and DLBCL has prompted the investigation of its role in TCL as well. However, its role is less well established in TCL, since data come from single-institution retrospective studies and are often contradictory. Herein, we review the existing data on PET/CT scan in nodal TCL.

M.K. Angelopoulou (✉)
Department of Hematology and Bone Marrow Transplantation, National and Kapodistrian University of Athens, Athens, Greece
e-mail: mkangelop@gmail.com

F.J. Vlachou
Department of Nuclear Medicine, D.TH.K.A. "HEALTH", Kifissias Av. & Q. Cross 4, Maroussi 15123, Greece
e-mail: fanivlachou@yahoo.com

D.T. Kechagias
Ultrasound, Curator Department of PET/CT, D.TH.K.A. "HEALTH", Kifissias Av. & Q. Cross 4, Maroussi 15123, Greece
e-mail: dikechagias@hotmail.com

10.1 Baseline PET/CT

Although initial reports suggested that TCL are less frequently FDG avid [2], subsequent studies revealed that nodal TCL display PET/CT positivity in the majority of cases in percentages ranging between 86 and 100 % of the

J.A. Andreou et al. (eds.), *PET/CT in Lymphomas: A Case-Based Atlas*,
DOI 10.1007/978-3-319-27380-8_10

patients. More specifically ALCL is almost 100 % FDG avid [2–9], whereas in AITL and PTCL-NOS, FDG avidity has been reported in 78–100 % [3–10] and 86–100 % of the cases, respectively [2–10].

At diagnosis, PET/CT scan may detect more disease sites than conventional staging with the exception of skin and bone marrow disease [11]. In a large retrospective study from Memorial Sloan Kettering with 75 patients with nodal TCL [5] who had undergone baseline PET/CT, PET detected new sites in 50 % of the patients, with the more frequent new site being bone. However, stage was modified in only 5.2 %, since TCL patients already present with advanced disease [5]. Thus, baseline PET findings have little impact on treatment strategy, but it may help in the interpretation of subsequent interim- or posttherapy PET/CT. In the retrospective study by GOELAMS [6], all 40 nodal TCL cases were FDG avid. Twenty percent were upstaged and especially ALK+ ALCL histology. Feeney et al. studied 135 patients, among whom 34 had PTCL-NOS, 16 ALCL, and 18 AITL, and reported FDG avidity in 97 %, 94 %, and 78 %, respectively [10]. They observed that in 29 % of the cases, new sites detected by PET/CT were outside the range of conventional CT imaging. Such sites were cutaneous, subcutaneous, or muscular masses of the scalp, upper/lower extremities, and epitrochlear and popliteal lymph nodes. ALCL is associated with the highest SUV_{max} values (median: 22.9–25.3) compared to AITL (median: 12.6–13.5) and PTCL-NOS (median: 11.4–12.3) [8, 10].

10.2 Interim and Posttreatment PET

Studies focusing on the prognostic significance of interim or end-of-treatment PET have many methodological disadvantages: they are retrospective with limited number of patients and heterogeneous histologies. Patients are not homogenously treated, and occasionally ASCT is incorporated in frontline strategy, a fact that introduces a selection bias. In addition, the decision to treat with salvage therapy is individually taken by the treating physicians and is based on PET/CT results randomly. Moreover, the method of PET/CT interpretation differs among studies: some researchers use the International Harmonization Project Criteria [12, 13], whereas others the 5-point Deauville scale [14] or other non-standardized methods [6, 15]. It has to be stressed that a high positive predictive value (PPV) is a requirement, especially for interim PET, in order to intensify treatment and offer ASCT based on PET results.

10.2.1 Posttreatment PET

The GOELAMS group describes TCL patients among whom 31 underwent posttreatment PET/CT [6]. They found no significant correlation between PET results and either progression-free survival (PFS) or overall survival (OS). The negative predictive value (NPV) and the PPV were reported as 61 % and 33 %, respectively, with a higher NPV for ALK+ ALCL (83 %). However, in this study, ASCT was part of first-line treatment in a significant number of patients. Moreover, patients who progressed during first-line treatment did not undergo posttreatment PET, a fact that can explain the very low PPV. On the contrary, two recent studies show a strong correlation of posttreatment PET with PFS and OS. In the study by Tomita et al., on 36 nodal TCL treated homogenously with anthracycline-containing chemotherapy, 69 % of the patients were PET negative at the end of first-line treatment and had a 62 % 3-year PFS compared to 18 % for PET-positive patients [16]. In the second study by Li et al., evaluating 47 patients, among whom 30 patients with nodal TCL, 2-year PFS was 55 % for PET− patients vs. 0 % for PET+ ones [8]. In this latter study posttherapy PET was an independent predictor for PFS and OS. From both these studies, it seems that posttreatment PET has a relatively high PPV (82 % and 88.9 %, respectively), but a low NPV (64 % and 58.6 %) for PFS [8, 16]. Horwitz et al. evaluated response according to PET/CT in 110 patients treated with romidepsin at the relapsed setting and showed that the duration of response was significantly longer in PET-negative compared to PET-positive cases [9]. In addition, it seems that PET can discriminate patients who are considered as partial or nonresponders by conventional criteria, but have a more favorable prognosis [9]. Thus, PET-negative complete responders had the best outcome, followed by PET-negative partial or no responders (median PFS: 18.2 months), whereas PET+ patients had a poor outcome irrespective of conventional response status (median PFS for PET+ CRs: 7.2 months and for PET+ PRs/SDs: 7.1 months) [9]. The prognostic significance of PET was also verified in the post-ASCT setting in a study evaluating 41 patients, among whom 23 had nodal TCL: PET-positive patients had a significantly inferior event-free survival and OS compared to negative ones [17]. From these studies, discordant results between conventional staging and PET/CT are reported in 13–27 % of the cases. In this setting, PET can identify truly negative residual masses.

In conclusion, PET/CT performed after first-line treatment seems to have strong prognostic significance for outcome and is associated with relatively high PPV. However, its NPV is rather low, indicating that a considerable fraction of patients without FDG avidity after the end of treatment still relapse.

10.2.2 Interim PET

Interim PET, after 2–4 cycles of chemotherapy, could be of great clinical utility, since TCLs are characterized by a particularly poor outcome. Patients tend to progress either during or close to the end of first-line treatment. Thus, early identification of patients who will progress would lead to early intensification of treatment, e.g., with ASCT. With the exception of the GOELAMS study [6], the remaining ones indicate that interim PET has a strong prognostic significance for outcome. Thus, in four studies, a negative interim PET/CT scan is associated with a significantly superior PFS (Table 10.1) [5, 8, 18, 19]. The PPV for interim PET has been reported between 77.8 and 92.8 % and the NPV between 76.5 and 96.5 % [8, 19]. The study by Jung et al. is the only prospective study evaluating interim PET in TCL. It includes 63 patients (30 with nodal PTCL), among whom 59 underwent interim PET [19]. They used 3 different methodologies for PET interpretation: the visual method by the 5-point Deauville scale (cutoff: grades 4 and 5), the ΔSUV method (cutoff: 67.6 %), and % change in metabolic tumor volume or ΔMTV2.5 (cutoff: 98.7 %). Interim PET was of prognostic significance for PFS and OS by all three methods. The authors applied a model combining the results of all three methods that could stratify patients better. Thus, patients who were negative by all 3 methods had a median PFS of 64 months vs. 7.9 months for those who were positive by 1–2 methods vs. 4.1 months for those who were positive by all 3 methods. The corresponding values for OS were not reached vs. 23.5 months vs. 9.6 months, respectively. The authors also observed that among 35 PET-negative patients according to the Deauville scale, PFS was significantly lower for the 9 patients with grade 3 positivity (median: 8.8 months) compared to 26 patients with grade 1–2 positivity (median: 64 months). This observation reveals that the criteria for positivity for interim PET, as adopted from other diseases, might not apply in TCL and need to be standardized for these histologies.

Table 10.1 Studies evaluating the prognostic role of interim PET/CT in T-cell lymphomas

Study	Cahu 2011	Casulo 2013	Li 2013	Pellegrini 2014	Jung 2015
Patient #	54 (44)[a]	95 (50)[a]	88 (62)[a]	34	63 (59)[a]
Histology	ALK+ALCL: 10 ALK–ALCL: 14 PTCL–NOS: 15 AITL:11 Others: 4	ALK+ALCL: 9 ALK–ALCL: 5 PTCL–NOS: 19 AITL:6 Others: 11	ALK+ALCL: 0 ALK–ALCL: 9 PTCL–NOS: 13 AITL:3 Others: 37	ALK+ALCL: 9 ALK–ALCL: 6 PTCL-NOS: 11 AITL:6 Others: 2	ALK+ALCL: 0 ALK–ALCL: 6 PTCL–NOS: 17 AITL:10 Others: 30
Anthracycline-based first-line treatment	96 %	86 %	51 %	100 %	84.1 %
SCT at first line	44 %	58 %	–	24 %	14.3 %
Timing of interim PET	After cycle 3 or 4	After a median of 4 cycles	After a median of 3 cycles	After cycle 3	After cycle 3 or 4
PET interpretation	3-point scale IHP criteria	Deauville 5-PS	IHP criteria	IHP criteria	Deauville 5-PS ΔSUV ΔMTV
Interim PET (+) patients (–) patients	 43 %/59 %[b] 57 %/41 %[b]	 30 % 68 %	 68 %[c] 32 %[c]	 20.5 % 79.5 %	 38.1 %[d] 61.9 %[d]
PFS PET+ PET–	*p*=NS 4 y: 49 % 4 y: 69 %	*p*=0.03 Median: 10 mo Median: 5.1 y	*p*=0.002[c] 2 y: 19 % 2 y: 70 %	*p*=0.02 3 y: 17 % 3 y: 73 %	*p*<0.0001[d] Median: 5 mo Median: 27 mo
OS PET+ PET–	*p*=NS 4 y: 47 % 4 y: 76 %	*p*=NS 3 y: 26 % 3 y: 63 %	*p*=0.026[c] 2 y: 30 % 2 y: 85 %	*p*=0.02 3 y: 21 % 3 y: 79 %	Not reported

[a]The number in brackets indicates the number of patients who actually underwent interim PET/CT scan
[b]The second number is according to the IHP criteria.
[c]Numbers and percentages refer to nodal T-cell lymphomas, only.
[d]Numbers and percentages refer to visual PET interpretation according to the Deauville 5-point scale.
ALK+ ALCL ALK+ anaplastic large cell lymphoma, *ALK- ALCL* ALK- anaplastic large cell lymphoma, *PTCl-NOS* peripheral T-cell lymphoma not otherwise specified, *AITL* angioimmunoblastic T-cell lymphoma, *SCT* stem cell transplant, *IHP* international harmonization project, *PS* point scale, *PFS* progression-free survival, *OS* overall survival, *y* years, *mo* months, *NS* not significant

Case 1

A 52-year-old male presented to the outpatient unit with a right inguinal mass. The history of present illness started 1 year before, when he first noticed the abovementioned enlargement. Otherwise, he was completely asymptomatic.

Performance status was zero. Clinical examination disclosed bilateral cervical and axillary lymphadenopathy (maximal diameter 1×1.5 cm), a right inguinal mass measuring 8×3 cm, with 2 more lymph nodes adjacent to the mass, measuring 3×1 and 2×1 cm, as well as left inguinal lymph nodes, approximately 1×1 cm. The liver and spleen were non-palpable. His blood counts were normal, and his chemistries revealed a slightly elevated LDH. Whole-body CT scans confirmed the generalized lymphadenopathy as described above. In addition, there were mediastinal, left hilar, multiple para-aortic, and bilateral iliac lymph nodes. The patient underwent biopsy of the right inguinal mass, and the pathology report was consistent with systemic CD30+ ALK negative anaplastic large T-cell lymphoma (ALCL). Bone marrow trephine biopsy was negative for involvement. Thus, the clinical stage was IIIA, whereas PIT and IPI score were both 1 (low-intermediate and low respectively).

The patient received CHOP combination chemotherapy×8 cycles. Clinical examination and mid-treatment CT scans showed complete resolution of lymphadenopathy, with the exception of a residual lymph node <2 cm at the right inguinal area. After the completion of treatment, reevaluation of his disease showed complete response by clinical examination and CT scans. PET/CT scan showed normal distribution of 18-FDG, except of increased focal uptake at the right 4th and 11th ribs bilaterally (Fig. 10.1).

After questioning the patient, he reported an accident after which he experienced rib fractures, few months before. Thus, the patient was considered as a complete responder, both by conventional methods and PET/CT scan. In our institution we consider consolidation of first remission with ASCT in patients with nodal TCL, if IPI is high-intermediate or high. Thus, the patient was placed on follow-up. Four and a half months later, he presented with a subcutaneous, erythematous nodule at the right inguinal area, the biopsy of which disclosed infiltration of the subcutaneous tissue by CD30+ALCL. Further staging showed bilateral inguinal lymphadenopathy; thus, clinical stage was IIA. The patient received salvage chemotherapy with 2 cycles of ESHAP chemotherapy (etoposide, methylprednisolone, cytarabine and cisplatin). He achieved a PET/CT-negative complete remission (Fig. 10.2) and proceeded to ASCT.

Three months later, he experienced a second relapse at the upper third of his right thigh, close to the area of first relapse (Fig. 10.3). He was treated initially with interferon-alfa for 7 months, without response. Disease remained localized. Accordingly, he was placed on brentuximab vedotin (BV), showing response after the first cycle (Fig. 10.4).

Recently he has just completed 16 cycles of BV, and restaging was consistent with clinical complete remission. PET/CT scan showed a weak focal uptake at a left upper cervical lymph node (SUV_{max}: 2), most likely due to inflammation (Fig. 10.5).

Points of interest:

- This case is representative of the low negative predictive value (NPV) of posttreatment PET in nodal T-cell lymphomas, as indicated in the chapter of this section. However, caution should be taken because conventional staging may miss sites of disease that are outside of the range of CT imaging. PET/CT may prove helpful in this setting.
- PET/CT scan has low sensitivity for cutaneous or subcutaneous lymphoma involvement.
- It is important to stress that PET/CT findings should be always interpreted in the clinical context of each case. False-positive findings should always be kept in mind, such us inflammation, infection, intramuscular injections, and vaccination. In particular, small upper cervical, nonpalpable lymph nodes with low uptake are a common finding, associated with viral infections. This should not be considered as probable relapse, and a follow-up PET is recommended. In case of persistent uptake, a biopsy is mandatory for confirmation of disease relapse/progression.

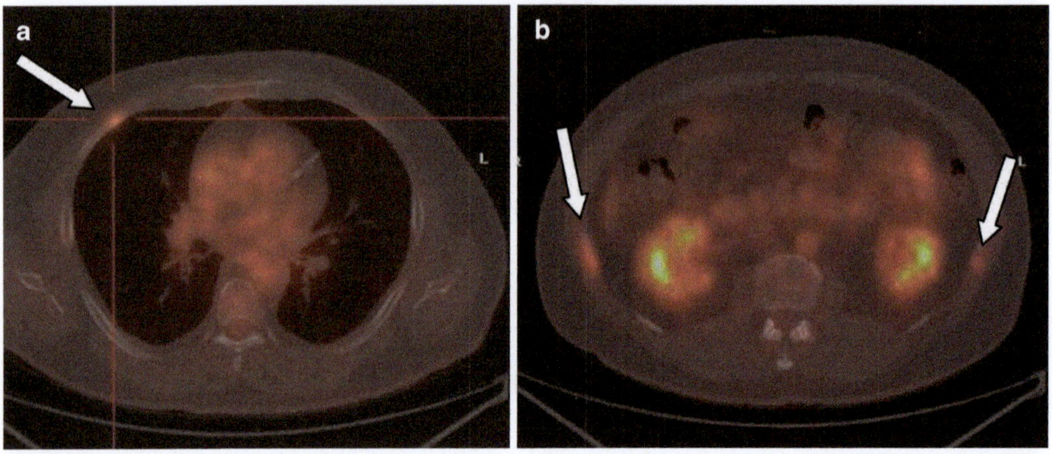

Fig. 10.1 Axial PET/CT after first-line therapy (**a**, **b**) shows increased metabolic activity in the right 4th rib and 11th rib bilaterally (*arrows*)

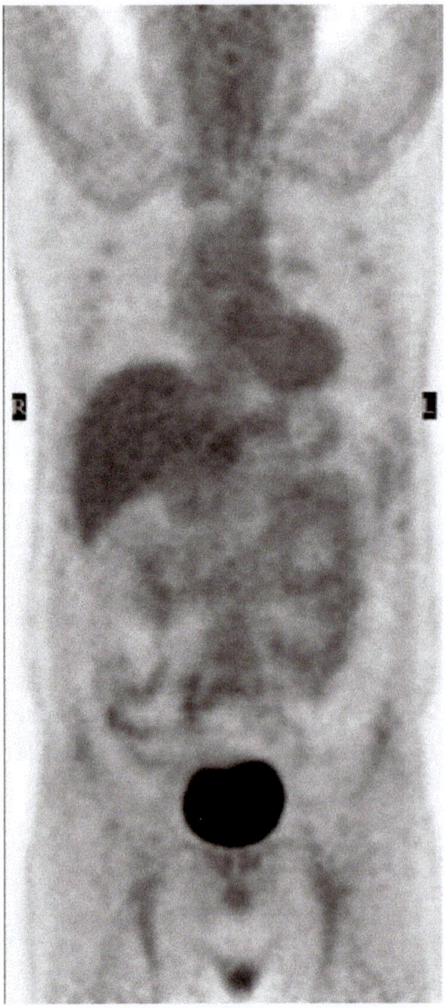

Fig. 10.2 PET/CT after second-line therapy is normal

Fig. 10.3 Picture of 2nd relapse, showing erythematous subcutaneous nodules, close to the previous disease site

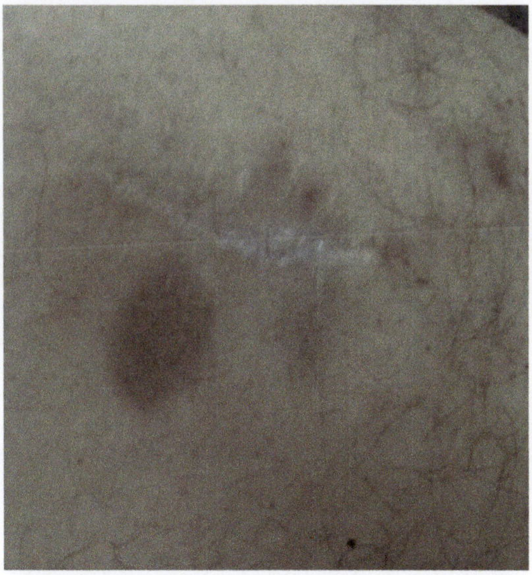

Fig. 10.4 Picture of the same area as in Fig. 10.3, showing the resolution of nodules after one cycle of treatment with brentuximab vedotin. Note the residual skin melanchrosis

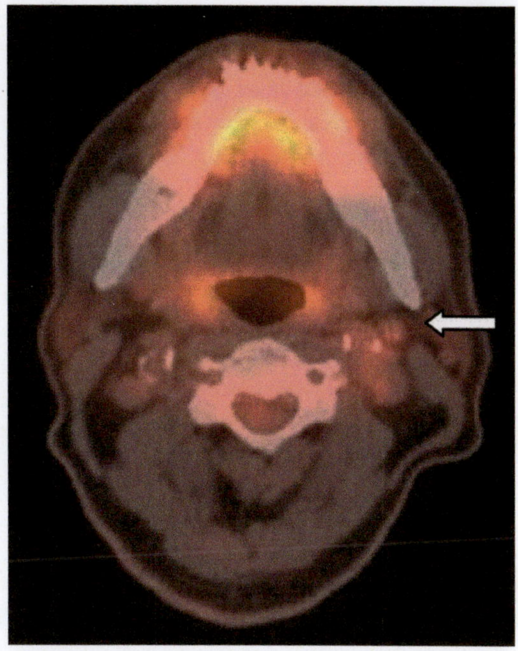

Fig. 10.5 Axial PET/CT after 4th line treatment shows a left cervical mild hypermetabolic lymph node (*arrow*)

Case 2

A 36-year-old female was admitted to the hospital due to prolonged fever of 1-month duration and painful bilateral cervical swelling. Her past medical history was significant for multiple sclerosis diagnosed 6 years before.

Clinical examination disclosed bilateral cervical (submandibular) lymphadenopathy (maximal diameter 1×2 cm). No enlarged lymph nodes were initially palpated at the axillary and inguinal areas. No organomegaly was present. Her blood counts showed borderline anemia that worsened during her hospitalization (Ht: 21.1 %%, Hb: 7.1 g/dL), leukopenia with a normal differential (WBC: 2.6×10^9/L), and thrombocytopenia (PLT: 30×10^9/L). Her chemistries revealed a slightly elevated LDH. Whole-body CT scans soon after her admission revealed bilateral submandibular lymph nodes (maximum diameter: 2×1 cm), a left axillary (2×1.5 cm) lymph node, a mesenteric lymph node mass measuring 4.5×4.5 cm, as well as multiple small para-aortic and left inguinal lymph nodes. The liver and spleen had normal dimensions and imaging. The patient underwent a biopsy of the left submandibular lymph node that was nondiagnostic. The patient deteriorated with high fevers and hepatomegaly, while alkaline phosphatase and gamma glutamyltransferase were 5× above normal values. Performance status was 2. A percutaneous liver biopsy was not diagnostic.

Subsequent MRI and CT scan of the abdomen confirmed hepatomegaly (sagittal diameter, 29 cm) with multiple hypodense lesions, with a low T2 signal and mild splenomegaly with small focal lesions and a low T2 signal.

At that juncture the patient underwent a PET/CT scan that showed the following findings: increased 18FDG uptake at submandibular lymph nodes bilaterally (SUV_{max}: right: 6.3 and left: 2.7), at a left axillary lymph node (SUV_{max}: 5.6), at the hilum bilaterally (SUV_{max}: 2.6) – most likely due to inflammation, at multiple lesions in the liver (SUV_{max}: 4.0–7.0), one splenic lesion (SUVmax: 3.3) at multiple mesenteric lymph nodes (SUVmax: 6.2), and para-aortic and left inguinal lymph nodes (SUVmax: 3.8 and 3.3, respectively). A mild diffuse uptake at the two upper thirds of the femurs bilaterally was also evident (Fig. 10.6).

The patient underwent exploratory laparotomy and biopsy from four mesenteric lymph nodes and the liver. A diagnosis of a peripheral T-cell lymphoma not otherwise specified (PTCL-NOS) was established. Bone marrow trephine biopsy and immunophenotype were both negative for involvement. Thus, the clinical stage was IVB, whereas PIT score was 2 and IPI score was 3 (risk groups high-intermediate for both systems).

The patient started high-dose CHOP alternating with ESHAP. The patient defervesced after the first cycle of chemotherapy and her PS improved. After 4 cycles, she underwent a mid-treatment (interim) PET/CT scan. The findings were the following: (1) no abnormal uptake above the diaphragm, (2) increased uptake by mesenteric lymph nodes (SUV_{max}: 3.4), and (3) no other hypermetabolic lymph nodes noted. The PET/CT was considered positive according to the Deauville criteria (Deauville 4) for the abdominal lymph nodes, since their FDG uptake was above the liver (Fig. 10.7).

The patient was scheduled for ASCT after completing 6 cycles of CHOP/ESHAP combination. However, while on treatment, she developed disease progression complicated with hemophagocytic syndrome and succumbed to her disease two months later.

Points of interest:

- This case is representative of FDG avidity in nodal TCL at diagnosis. Specifically the histologic category of PTCL-NOS is FDG avid in 86–100 % of the cases. SUV_{max} has been reported to be lower in PTCL-NOS compared to other histologies of nodal TCL.
- PET/CT detects new sites of disease in half of the patients, but only a minority is upstaged, since they already present with advanced disease. The most frequent new site is bone. In this case, all sites detected by conventional staging coincided with the ones by PET/

CT. The diffuse uptake by the femurs should not be considered as disease involvement and can be explained in the context of possible hypersplenism, leading to hyperfunctioning bone marrow. From studies in Hodgkin lymphoma, it has been shown that only focal uptake by the bones/bone marrow is highly suspicious for disease.

- The role of interim PET in nodal TCL has not been established yet. Recent data show that it has a strong positive predictive value for progression, as it was the case in this patient. If this is confirmed by further studies, interim PET would be a valuable tool for early treatment intensification. Important limitations include the lack of validation of the criteria that should be used for its interpretation. From the published retrospective series, it appears that many physicians change treatment according to interim PET. However, this should be done with caution and not on an individual patient basis.

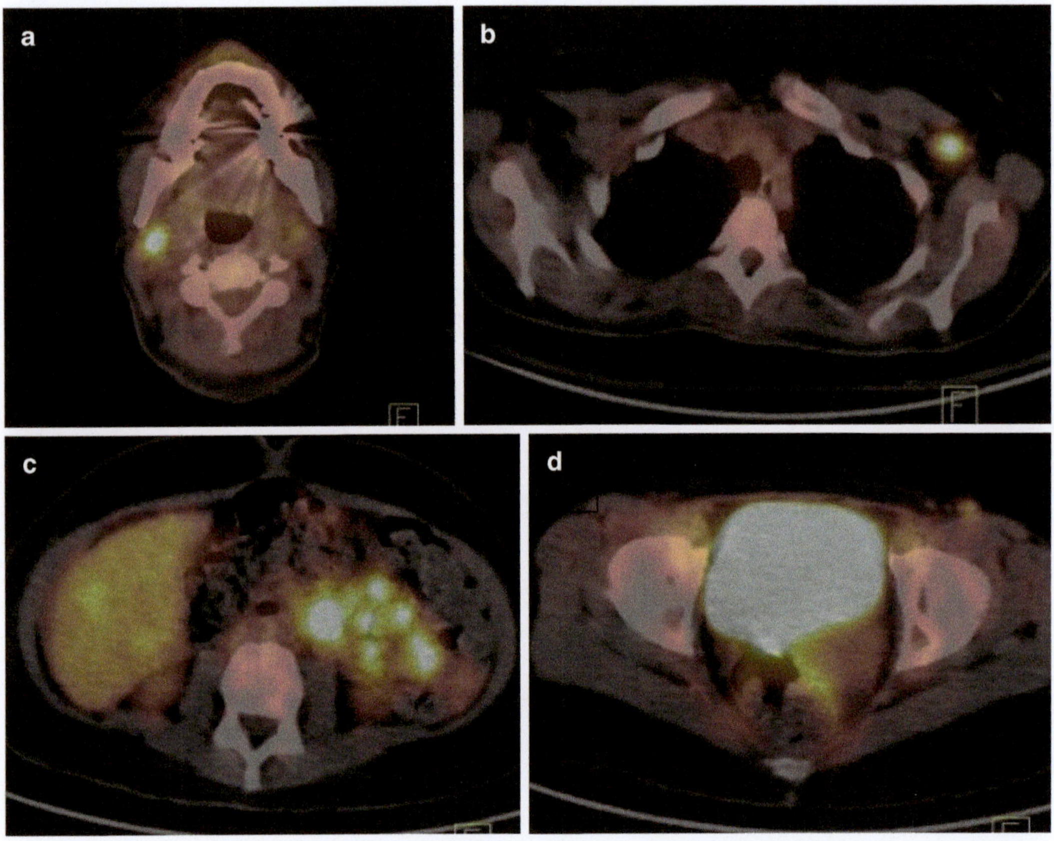

Fig. 10.6 PET/CT shows hypermetabolic submandibular (**a**), left axillary (**b**), mesenteric (**c**), and left inguinal (**d**) lymph nodes. Lesions with increased metabolic activity are seen in the liver and spleen (**e–h**)

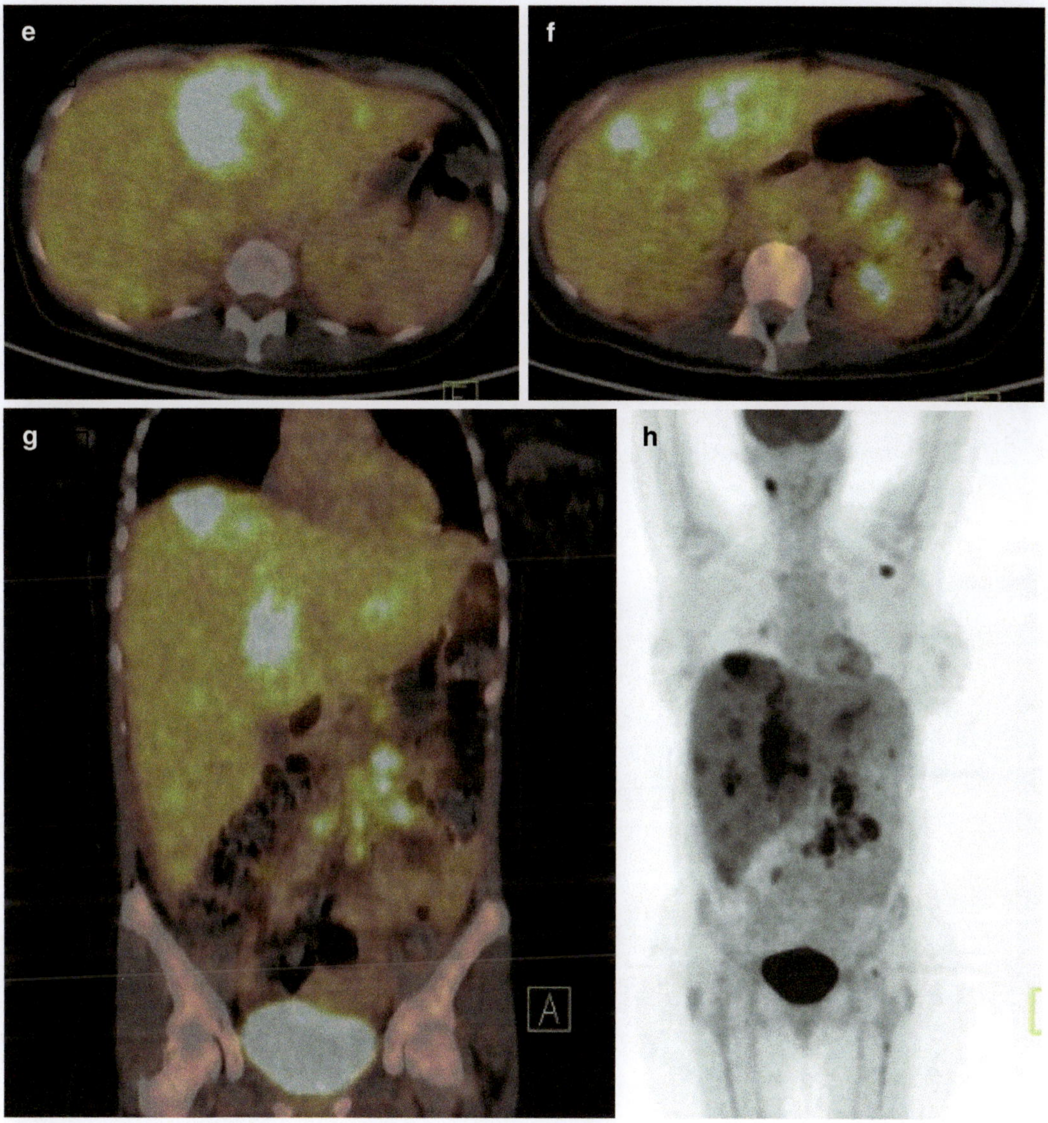

Fig. 10.6 (continued)

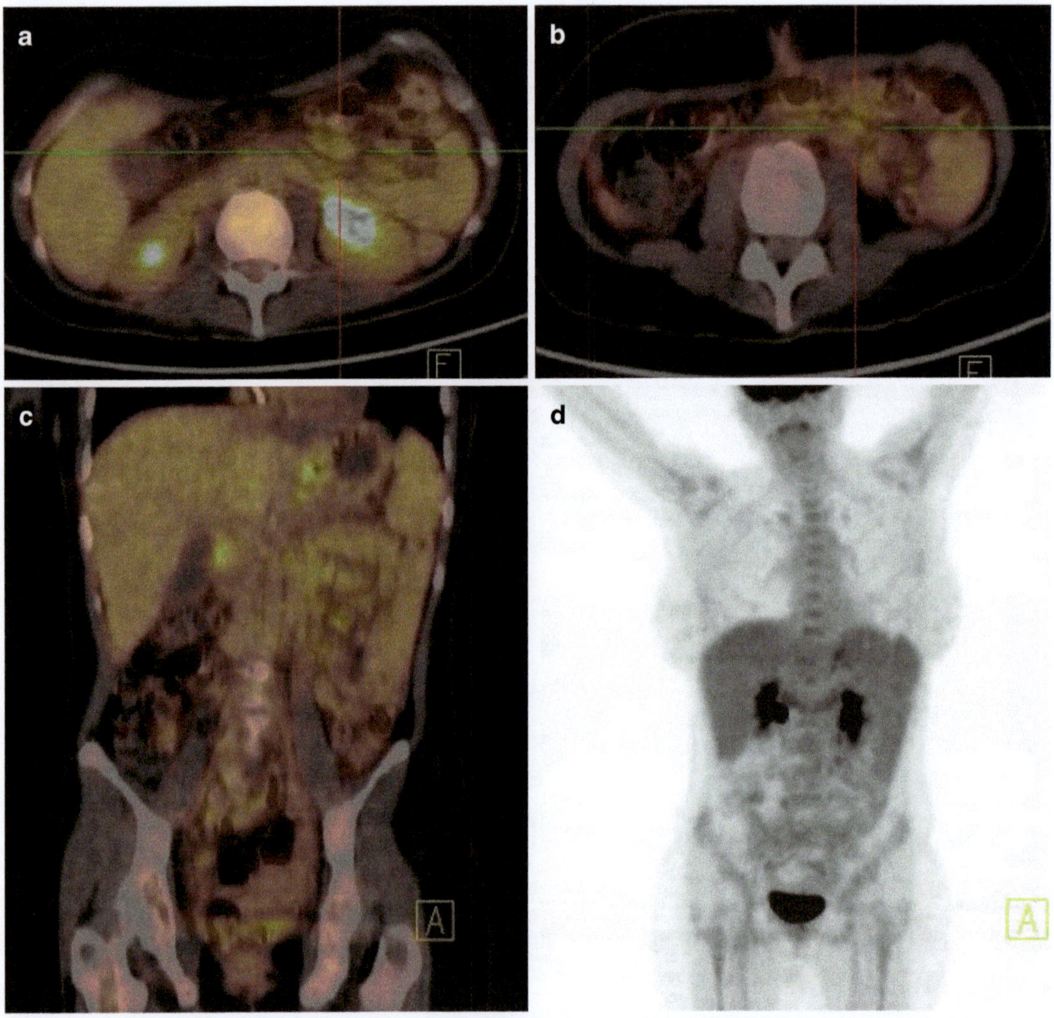

Fig. 10.7 Interim PET/CT shows mild hypermetabolic mesenteric lymph nodes, which were however interpreted as positive by the Deauville 5-point scale (score: 4) (**a**–**d**)

Case 3

A 60-year-old male presented to our outpatient unit due to right lower extremity swelling and a right inguinal mass of 2 weeks' duration. He was otherwise asymptomatic. His past medical history was significant for Hodgkin lymphoma, nodular sclerosis, clinical stage IIB in 1996, for which he was treated with the alternating MOPP/ABVD regimen.

Clinical examination disclosed a right inguinal lymph node mass measuring 5×4 cm and right lower extremity pitting edema. The patient underwent biopsy of the right inguinal mass that was consistent with ALK– CD30+ ALCL. Whole-body CT imaging showed right inguinal (maximal diameter 5×5 cm) and right iliac lymph nodes (maximal diameter 4×4 cm). Bone marrow trephine biopsy was negative for involvement. Performance status was 0. His blood counts and chemistries were normal. Thus, the clinical stage was IIA, whereas PIT and IPI score were both 1 (risk groups: low-intermediate and low, respectively). The patient underwent a baseline PET/CT scan that showed FDG avidity at the right iliac (SUV_{max}: 4.4) and the right inguinal lymph nodes (SUV_{max}: 12). In addition, it disclosed increased uptake at a small right upper cervical lymph node (SUV_{max}: 6.4), which was neither palpable nor evident by conventional imaging (Fig. 10.8).

The patient started CHOEP-14 combination chemotherapy for 6 cycles. Clinical examination and mid-treatment CT scans were consistent with a very good partial remission. Evaluation of his disease after the end of chemotherapy showed complete disappearance of the involved lymph nodes both by clinical examination and CT scans. End-of treatment PET/CT scan showed normal distribution of 18FDG. Multiple subpleural granulomatous lesions and interstitial disease were evident from the CT scan of the thorax that were considered nonspecific, inflammatory, chronic changes and were negative by PET/CT (Fig. 10.9).

The patient was considered a complete responder and was placed on follow-up every 3 months. Eight months later, he presented two new lymph nodes at the left inguinal area, measuring 2×2 cm and 1×1 cm, confirmed by CT scans. The biopsy of a left inguinal node was consistent with relapse of ALK– CD30+ ALCL. The patient had localized disease (clinical stage IA). He received salvage chemotherapy with 2 cycles of ESHAP combination chemotherapy. At restaging clinical examination was normal and CT scan showed that the previously noted left inguinal lymph nodes were smaller than 1 cm in their longest diameter. Two small (<1 cm) lymph nodes were described: the first in the right parotid and the second at the upper right cervical area. Both were considered as normal by CT scan criteria. PET/CT showed increased 18FDG uptake by a small (7.1 mm) lymph node within the right parotid with SUV_{max} of 3.8 and by another small right upper cervical lymph node, measuring 8.1 mm with SUV_{max} of 1.4 (Fig. 10.10).

PET/CT scan was considered positive according to the post-therapeutic PET criteria of that time. An effort was made to locate the cervical lymph node in order to perform a biopsy; however, this was not accomplished. Clinically, the patient was a complete responder, and as such he proceeded to ASCT.

Reevaluation of his disease 3 months post-ASCT disclosed the following: CT scans was unchanged, still showing the two small (<1 cm) lymph nodes within the right parotid and at the upper right cervical area. Otherwise, there was no evidence of disease. PET/CT showed that these two lymph nodes were still 18FDG avid: SUV_{max} was 4.7 for the former and 2.2 for the latter (Fig. 10.11).

Ten months after ASCT, the patient progressed with a palpable right upper cervical lymph node 1.5×1 cm. CT scan showed bilateral small lymph nodes at the cervical area as well as within both parotids. PET/CT scan confirmed abnormal uptake by intraparotid and cervical lymph nodes bilaterally and a left supraclavicular one. These findings were scored as Deauville 5 and confirmed progression (Fig. 10.12).

The patient was treated with therapeutic radiotherapy at a dose of 4000 cGy to the cervical area bilaterally. Unfortunately, he experienced generalized progression, both within the irradiated field and at the lung hilum, right axillary area, the liver, and the skin (Fig. 10.13). He is currently receiving systemic treatment with brentuximab vedotin and has responded (Fig. 10.14).

Points of interest:

- This case is representative of FDG avidity in nodal TCL at diagnosis. Specifically the histologic category of ALCL is FDG avid in almost 100 % of the cases. SUV_{max} has been reported as the highest, when compared with other histologic categories of nodal TCL. However, this case displayed lower SUV_{max} than the median values reported in the literature.
- As already stated, PET/CT detects new sites of disease in half of the patients, but only a minority is upstaged. In this case, the right upper cervical lymph node that was detected by PET/CT did actually change the stage of the patient from IIA to IIIA. However, treatment would still be the same.
- This case is also representative of the low negative predictive value (NPV) of posttreatment PET in nodal T-cell lymphomas, similarly to case 1. The PET scan performed after first-line treatment was completely negative, yet the patient relapsed in a short period of time at the left inguinal area.
- The criteria by which end-of-treatment PET should be interpreted are not established in nodal TCL. For Hodgkin lymphoma and DLBCL, the Cheson criteria were applied until recently. According to these, nodes measuring less than 2 cm were considered positive if their uptake was above the surrounding tissues, whereas masses larger than 2 cm were considered positive if their uptake was above the mediastinal blood pool. Recently the criteria have changed, and every node/mass with an uptake above the liver (Deauville 4 or 5) is considered positive regardless of its size. If these criteria are applicable in TCL remains to be verified. In this case, the interpretation of posttreatment PET after ESHAP chemotherapy might be different depending on the criteria used. However, the follow-up PET confirmed active disease.
- This case is representative of the high PPV of posttreatment PET in nodal TCL. Both the post-salvage (ESHAP) and post-ASCT PET were positive, although clinical staging was consistent with a complete remission. The patient experienced a frank relapse few months later.

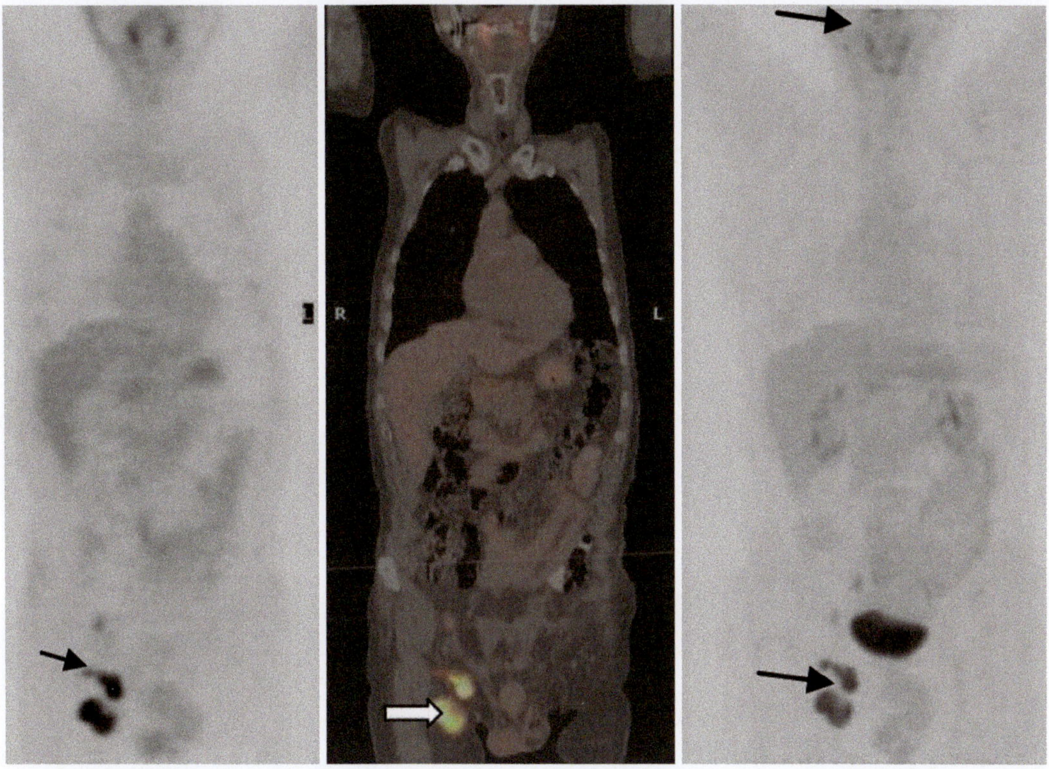

Fig. 10.8 Baseline FDG PET/CT shows hypermetabolic right inguinal, right iliac, and small right cervical lymph nodes (*arrows*)

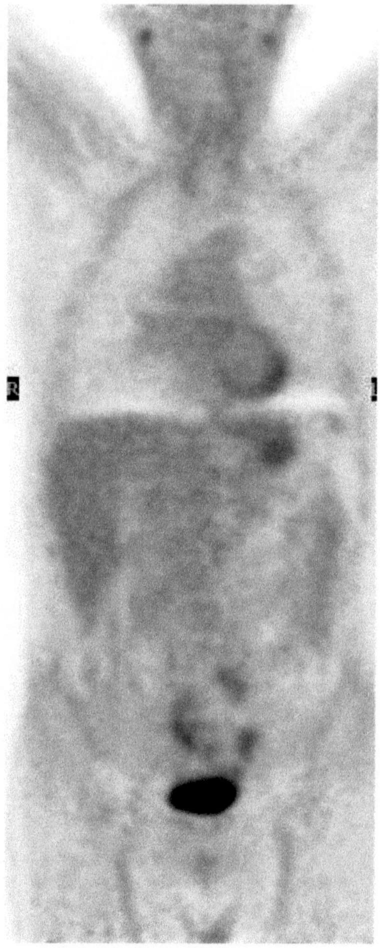

Fig. 10.9 One month after the end of first-line chemotherapy, PET/CT shows complete remission

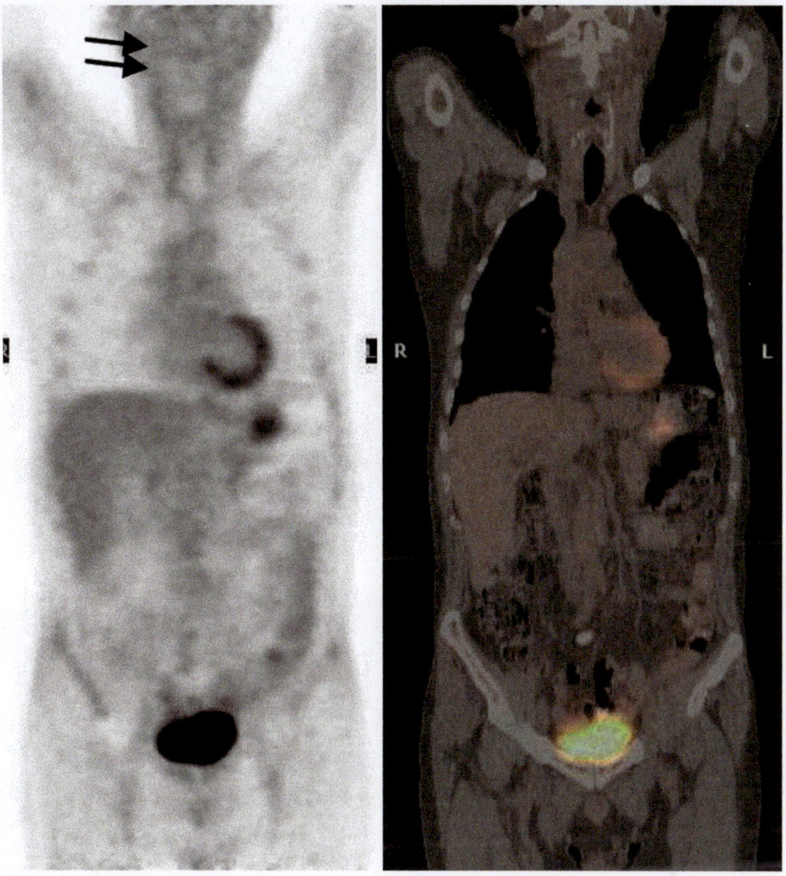

Fig. 10.10 Posttreatment PET/CT after ESHAP chemotherapy shows two small hypermetabolic lymph nodes in the right parotid and at the upper right cervical area (*arrows*)

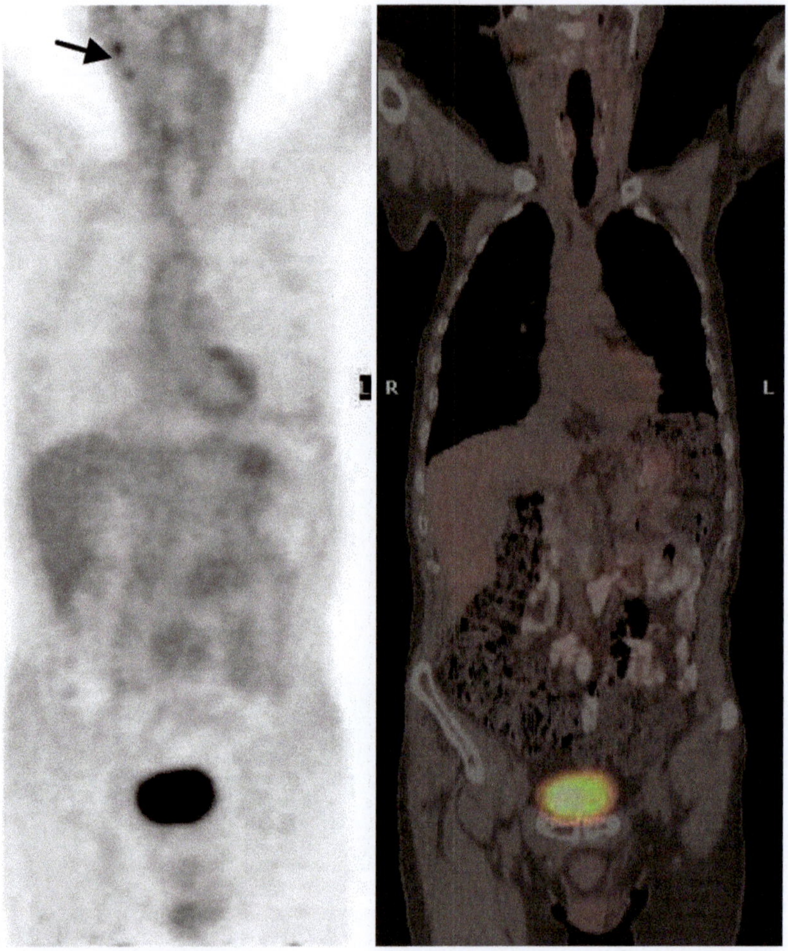

Fig. 10.11 Three months after ASCT, PET/CT shows hypermetabolic lymph nodes in the right parotid and at the upper right cervical area (*arrow*)

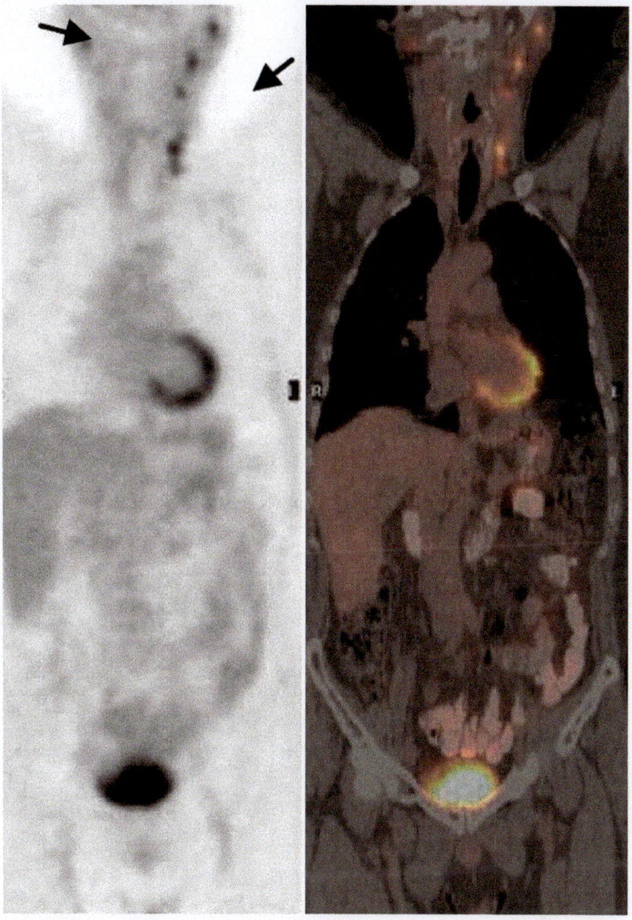

Fig. 10.12 Eight months later, PET/CT shows progression of the disease in the cervical area. Small hypermetabolic lymph nodes are observed in both parotids and in cervical region bilaterally as well as left supraclavicular (*arrows*)

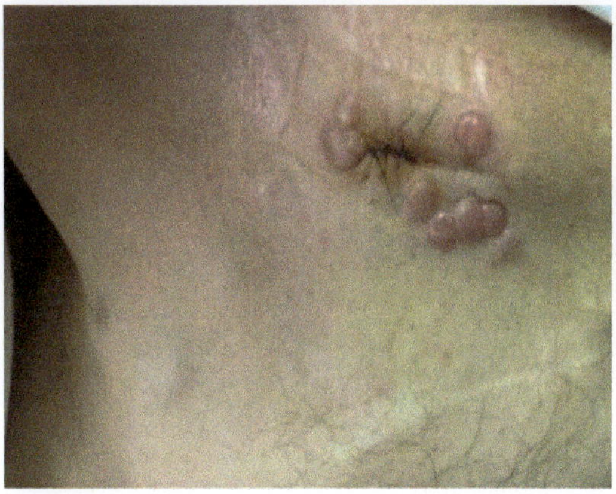

Fig. 10.13 Skin nodules due to disease relapse before treatment with brentuximab vedotin

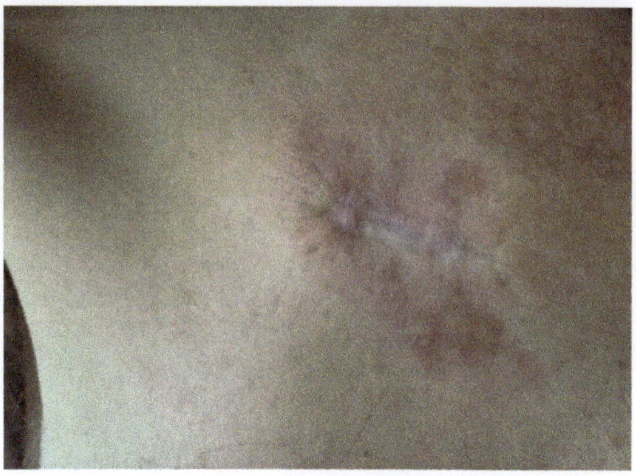

Fig. 10.14 Complete resolution of skin nodules after treatment with brentuximab vedotin

References

1. Vose J, Armitage J, Weisenburger D (2008) International peripheral T-cell and natural killer/T-cell lymphoma study: pathology findings and clinical outcomes. J Clin Oncol 26:4124–4130
2. Elstrom R, Guan L, Baker G et al (2003) Utility of FDG-PET scanning in lymphoma by WHO classification. Blood 101:3875–3876
3. Tsukamoto N, Kojima M, Hasegawa M et al (2007) The usefulness of 18F-fluorodeoxyglucose positron emission tomography (18FDGPET) and a comparison of 18FFDG- PET with 67gallium scintigraphy in the evaluation of lymphoma. Relation to histologic subtypes based on the World Health Organization classification. Cancer 110:652–659
4. Khong P-L, Pang CBY, Liang R et al (2008) Fluorine-18 fluorodeoxyglucose positron emission tomography in mature T-cell and natural killer cell malignancies. Ann Hematol 87:613–621
5. Casulo C, Schöder H, Feeney J et al (2013) 18F-fluorodeoxyglucose positron emission tomography in the staging and prognosis of T cell lymphoma. Leuk Lymphoma 54:2163–2167
6. Cahu X, Bodet-Milin C, Brissot E et al (2011) 18F-fluorodeoxyglucose-positron emission tomography before, during and after treatment in mature T/NK lymphomas: a study from the GOELAMS group. Ann Oncol 22:705–711
7. Weiler-Sagie M, Bushelev O, Epelbaum R, Dann EJ, Haim N, Avivi I, Ben-Barak A, Ben-Arie Y, Bar-Shalom R, Israel O (2010) (18)F-FDG avidity in lymphoma readdressed: a study of 766 patients. J Nucl Med 51:25–30
8. Li YJ, Li ZM, Xia XY et al (2013) Prognostic value of interim and posttherapy 18F-FDG PET/CT in patients with mature T-cell and natural killer cell lymphomas. J Nucl Med 54:507–515
9. Horwitz S, Coiffier B, Foss F et al (2015) Utility of 18fluoro-deoxyglucose positron emission tomography for prognosis and response assessments in a phase 2 study of romidepsin in patients with relapsed or refractory peripheral T-cell lymphoma. Ann Oncol 26:774–779
10. Feeney J, Horwitz S, Gonen M, Schoder H (2010) Characterization of T-cell lymphomas by FDG PET/CT. AJR 195:333–340
11. Kako S, Izutsu K, Ota Y et al (2007) FDG-PET in T-cell and NK-cell neoplasms. Ann Oncol 18: 1685–1690
12. Juweid ME, Stroobants S, Hoekstra OS et al (2007) Use of positron emission tomography for response assessment of lymphoma: consensus of the Imaging Subcommittee of International Harmonization Project in Lymphoma. J Clin Oncol 25:571–578
13. Cheson BD, Pfistner B, Juweid ME et al (2007) Revised response criteria for malignant lymphoma. J Clin Oncol 25:579–586
14. Meignan M, Barrington S, Itti E, Gallamini A, Haioun C, Polliack A (2014) Report on the 4th International Workshop on Positron Emission Tomography in Lymphoma held in Menton, France, 3–5 October 2012. Leuk Lymphoma 55:31–37
15. Haioun C, Itti E, Rahmouni A et al (2005) [18F] fluoro-2-deoxy-D-glucose positron emission tomography (FDG-PET) in aggressive lymphoma: an early prognostic tool for predicting patient outcome. Blood 106:1376–1381
16. Tomita N, Hattori Y, Fujisawa S et al (2015) Post-therapy ^{18}F-fluorodeoxyglucose positron emission tomography for predicting outcome in patients with peripheral T cell lymphoma. Ann Hematol 94(3): 431–436
17. Sohn BS, Yoon DH, Kim KP et al (2013) The role of 18F-fluorodeoxyglucose positron emission tomography at response assessment after autologous stem cell transplantation in T-cell non-Hodgkin's lymphoma patients. Ann Hematol 92:1369–1377
18. Pellegrini C, Argnani L, Broccoli A et al (2014) Prognostic value of interim positron emission tomography in patients with peripheral T-cell lymphoma. Oncologist 19:746–750
19. Jung S-H, Ahn J-S, Kim Y-K et al (2015) Prognostic significance of interim PET/CT based on visual, SUV-based, and MTV-based assessment in the treatment of peripheral T-cell lymphoma. BMC Cancer 15:198–206

Highly Aggressive Lymphomas 11

Panagiotis D. Tsirigotis,
Nikolaos D. Papathanasiou,
and Arkadios Ch. Rousakis

11.1 Diagnosis: Burkitt Lymphoma

A 43-year-old HIV seronegative male was admitted for evaluation of fatigue, low grade fever, and dyspnea on exertion. Past history was unremarkable and clinical examination revealed nothing except pallor. Complete blood count (CBC) revealed pancytopenia, and microscopy of the peripheral blood smear showed the presence of blast cells with characteristically deeply basophilic and vacuolated cytoplasm. Biochemistry was normal except for the presence of a highly elevated serum LDH. Bone marrow aspiration and biopsy showed almost complete replacement of normal myeloid elements by a diffuse blastoid infiltrate consisting of medium-sized blast cells, with round nuclei, dispersed chromatin, and multiple nucleoli. Cytoplasm was deeply basophilic with many vacuoles. Blast cells showed moderate expression of surface IgM and strong expression of the B-cell markers CD19, CD20, and CD22. Lymphoid cells were positive for CD10, BCL6, and CD38 and negative for TdT and BCL2. Ki67 proliferation marker was uniformly expressed in 100 % of lymphoid cells. Morphology and immunophenotype of neoplastic cells were compatible with the diagnosis of Burkitt lymphoma.

FDG-PET/CT was performed for initial staging and revealed diffuse bone marrow infiltration and multiple peritoneal deposits (Figs. 11.1, 11.2 and 11.3). Although the patient had no neurological symptoms, cerebrospinal fluid (CSF) examination, which is part of the initial staging workup in patients with highly aggressive lymphomas, revealed the presence of leptomeningeal involvement. Clinical stage was IVB.

Patient received treatment with the CODOX-M/IVAC regimen consisting of cyclophosphamide, vincristine, doxorubicin, high-dose methotrexate/ifosfamide, etoposide, and high-dose cytarabine, with the addition of rituximab. He had a favorable response to induction treatment and achieved complete resolution of all clinical and laboratory signs of disease. Follow-up FDG-PET/CT showed resolution of metabolic active disease (Fig. 11.4). Currently he is still on treatment, in excellent clinical condition, and disease-free.

P.D. Tsirigotis, MD
Division of Hematology, 2nd Dept of Internal Medicine, ATTIKON, General University Hospital, Rimini-1, Haidari PO: 12462, Athens, Greece
e-mail: panagtsirigotis@gmail.com

N.D. Papathanasiou, MSc
Nuclear Medicine and PET-CT Department, Metropolitan Hospital, Ethnarhou Makariou & El. Venizelou St, Neo Faliro 18547, Greece
e-mail: nikopapath@googlemail.com

A.C. Rousakis (✉)
CT & MRI department, "HYGEIA" & "MITERA" hospitals, Kifissias Av. & Erythrou Stavrou 4, Maroussi 15123, Greece
e-mail: a.rousakis@hygeia.gr

J.A. Andreou et al. (eds.), *PET/CT in Lymphomas: A Case-Based Atlas*,
DOI 10.1007/978-3-319-27380-8_11

Discussion

Burkitt lymphoma (BL) originates from germinal or postgerminal center B cells and is a highly aggressive non-Hodgkin lymphoma with very high proliferative activity and avid FDG uptake [1, 2]. Three different disease variants are recognized, with different clinical presentations. Endemic BL represents the most common malignancy of childhood in equatorial Africa and is characterized by a predilection for jaw involvement. Sporadic BL occurs through the developed world in children and young adults commonly presenting with abdominal masses and frequent ileocecal region involvement. Immunodeficiency-associated BL is primarily seen in the context of HIV infection. Bone marrow involvement and leptomeningeal dissemination are common through the course of disease. Moreover, presentation as acute leukemia is not rare, especially in the setting of immunodeficiency [3]. FDG-PET is very sensitive for the detection of bone marrow involvement, which is present in up to 40 % of highly aggressive non-Hodgkin lymphomas, even in cases with no concomitant bone abnormality on anatomic imaging. Bone marrow involvement may present with heterogenous focal/multifocal lesions or with diffuse disease, showing intense abnormal FDG activity throughout the whole bone marrow extent [4].

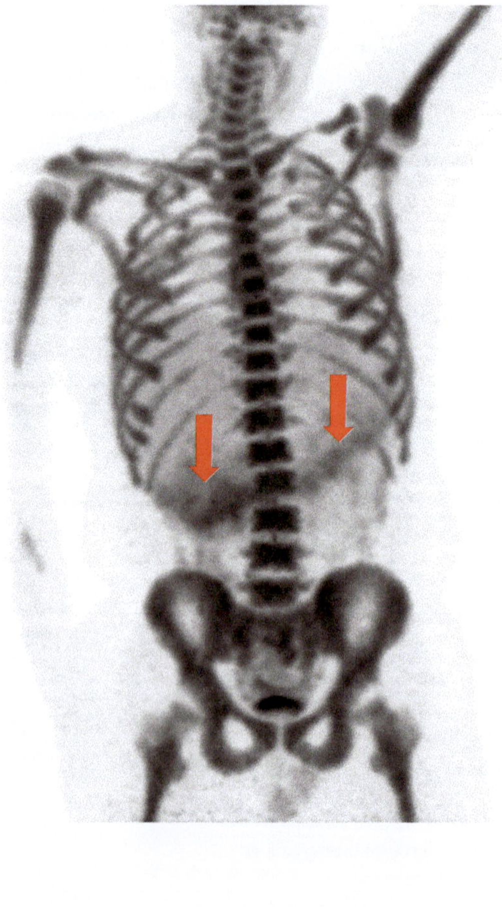

Fig. 11.1 Whole-body PET maximum intensity projection (MIP) image shows abnormal, diffuse increased FDG uptake in both axial and proximal appendicular skeleton, in keeping with bone/bone marrow infiltration. There is also FDG-avid peritoneal disease in the omentum (*red arrows*)

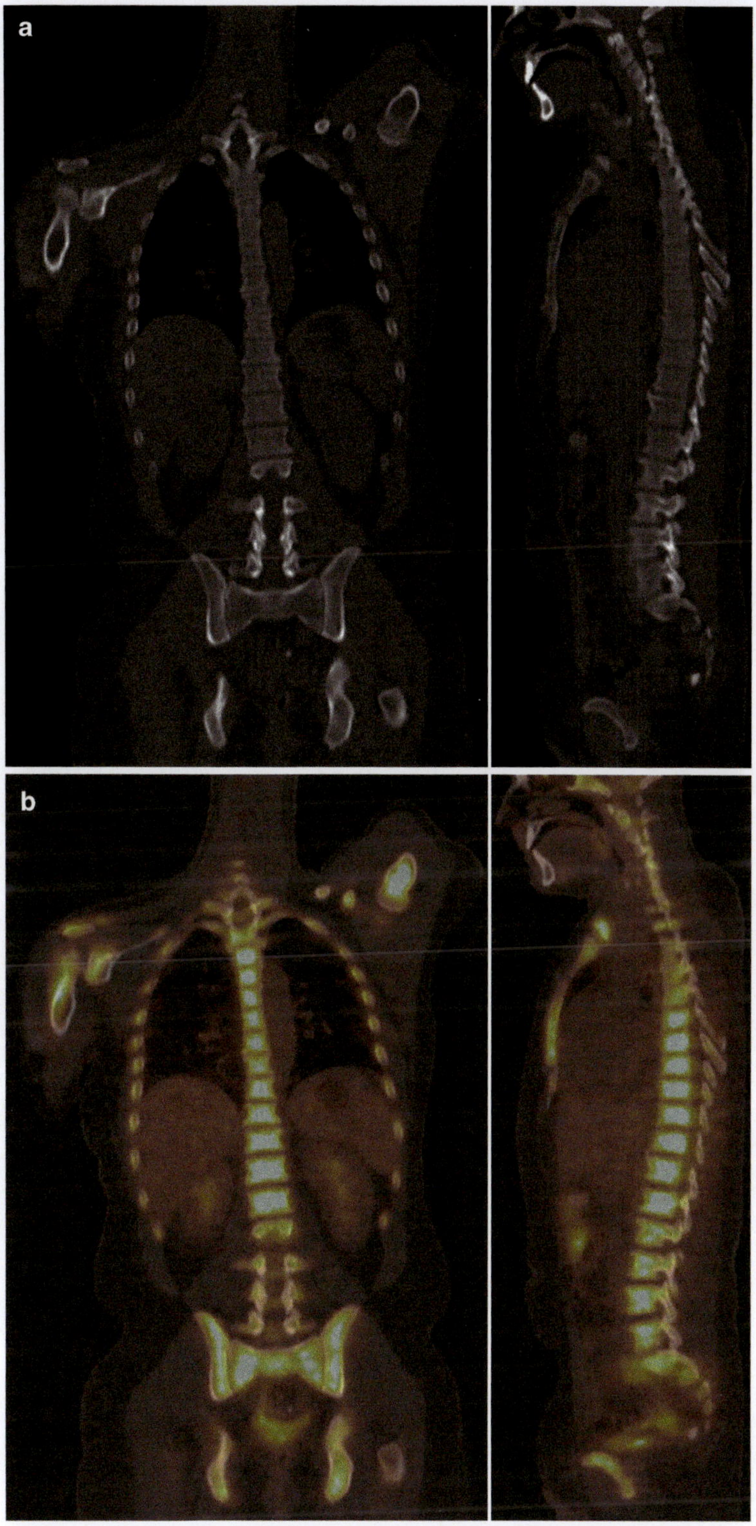

Fig. 11.2 Coronal and sagittal fused PET/CT images (**b**) show intense skeletal FDG activity (SUVmax: 16.4), in keeping with diffuse bone marrow involvement. There is no obvious bone abnormality on the CT component of the study (**a**)

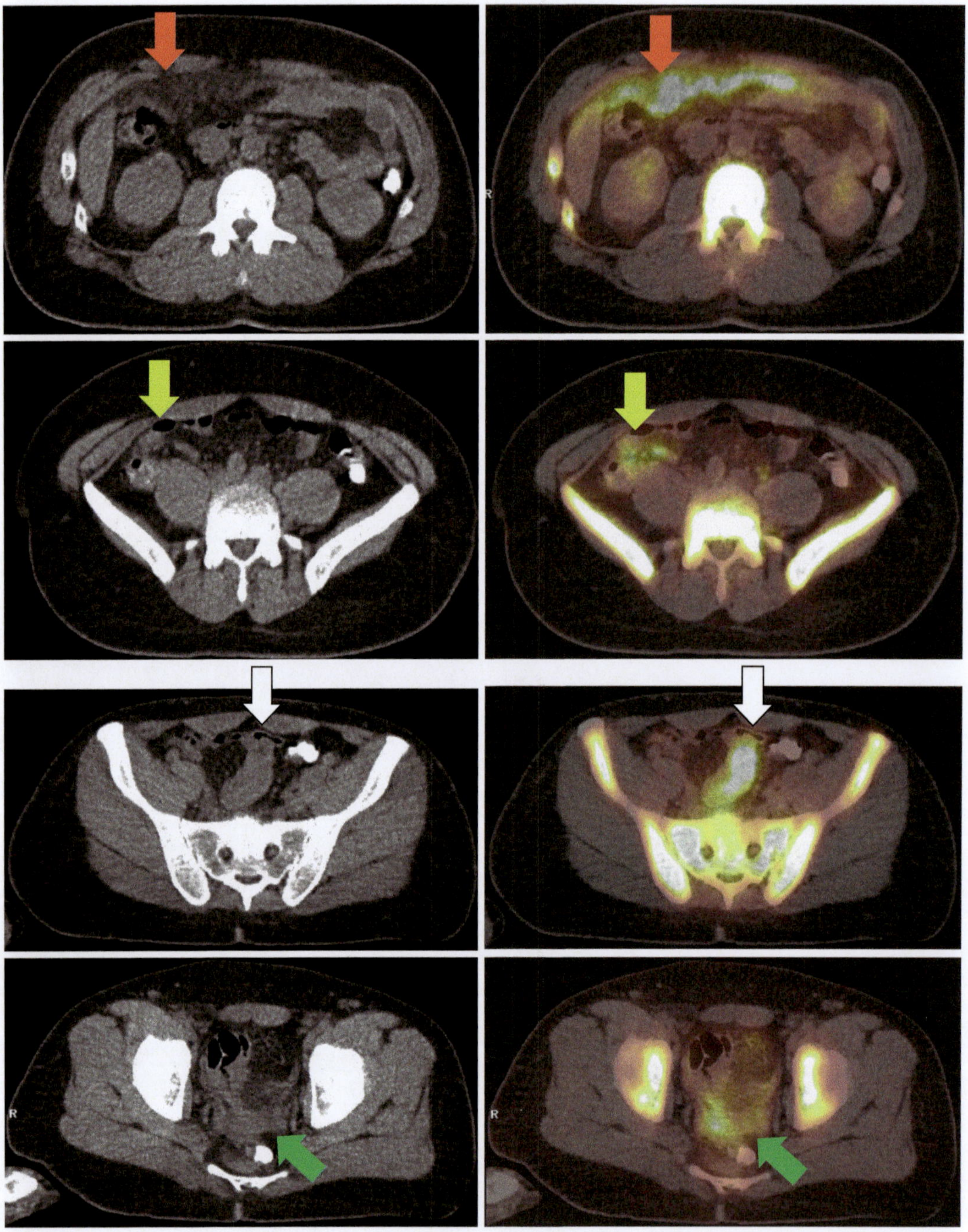

Fig. 11.3 Axial CT (*left column*) and corresponding fused PET/CT images (*right column*) show lymphomatous involvement of the peritoneum. There is omental soft-tissue stranding and multiple, ill-defined nodules with intense FDG uptake (SUVmax: 16.8, *red arrows*). There is FDG-avid peritoneal disease at the ileocecal region (*yellow arrow*), along bowel loops (*white arrow*) and in the pelvis, in the rectovesical pouch (*green arrow*)

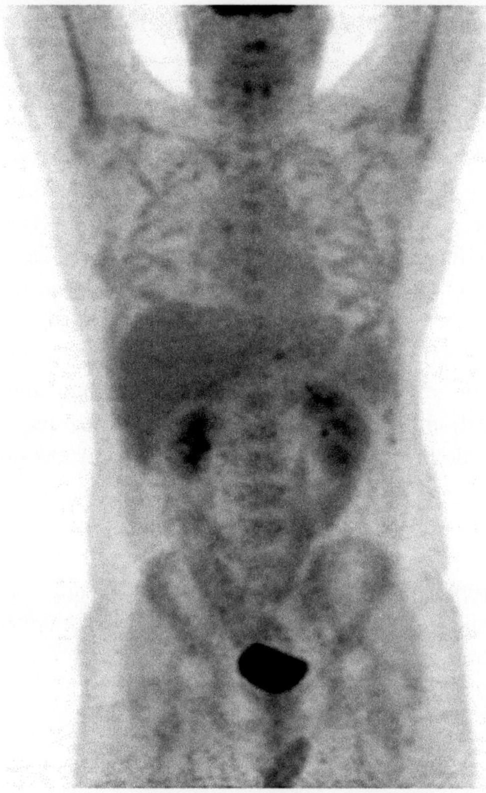

Fig. 11.4 Whole-body maximum intensity projection (MIP) image of follow-up PET/CT shows no hypermetabolic lesions in the bone marrow or elsewhere in the body, in keeping with metabolic treatment response

11.2 Lymphoblastic Lymphoma

Case 1: Diagnosis – B-Cell Lymphoblastic Lymphoma

A 62-year-old female was admitted for evaluation of severe pain in the left groin and thigh. Past history and clinical examination were unremarkable. Complete blood count (CBC) and biochemistry were all normal. CT scan of the left femur showed a lytic lesion in the corresponding intertrochanteric region. CT scans of the chest and abdomen did not reveal any additional abnormal finding. CT-guided fine-needle biopsy (FNB) of the left femoral lesion was performed, and histological examination showed the presence of a dense infiltrate consisted of medium-sized blast cells with scant cytoplasm, finely dispersed chromatin, and one to three small nucleoli. Immunohistochemistry showed expression of the B-cell markers CD19, CD79a, CD20, CD22, and cytoplasmic TdT positivity. Bone marrow aspiration and biopsy were normal. Clinical and laboratory workup was compatible with B-cell lymphoblastic lymphoma (B-LBL), stage IAE. Patient received treatment with an acute lymphoblastic leukemia (ALL) regimen consisting of repeated cycles of high-dose cyclophosphamide, vincristine, doxorubicin, and dexamethasone alternating with high-dose methotrexate and high-dose cytarabine (HyperCVAD-HiMTX-HiDAC). She had an excellent treatment response with complete resolution of all clinical signs after induction chemotherapy. However, 4 months after the completion of treatment, she was readmitted for pain in the same anatomical area (left groin and thigh). Restaging PET/CT showed abnormal increased FDG activity in the intertrochanteric region of the left proximal femur and no disease elsewhere (Figs. 11.5, 11.6 and 11.7). Repeated CT-guided FNB confirmed relapse of B-LBL.

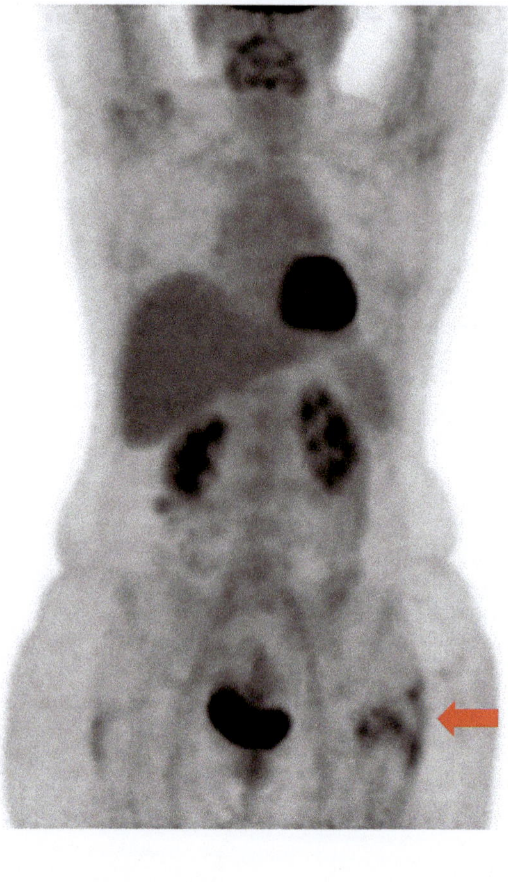

Fig. 11.5 Whole-body PET maximum intensity projection (MIP) image reveals abnormal increased FDG activity in the intertrochanteric region of the left proximal femur (*red arrow*). There is no FDG-avid disease elsewhere

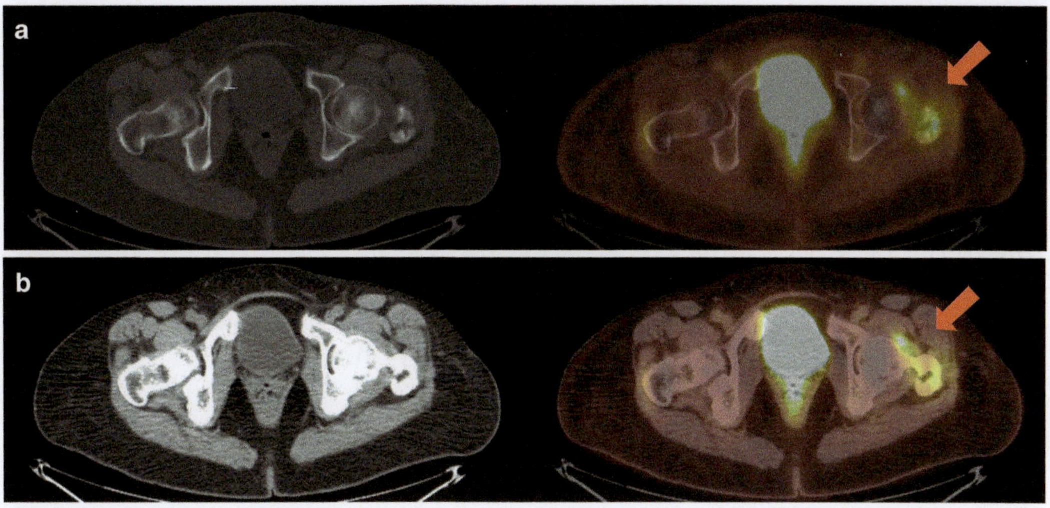

Fig. 11.6 Transaxial CT and fused PET/CT images in bone (**a**) and soft-tissue windows (**b**) show a heterogenous lytic-sclerotic lesion (*red arrow*) in the intertrochanteric region of the left femur with increased metabolic activity (SUVmax: 3.9). There is extension of the abnormal metabolic activity in the adjacent musculature of the ipsilateral hip

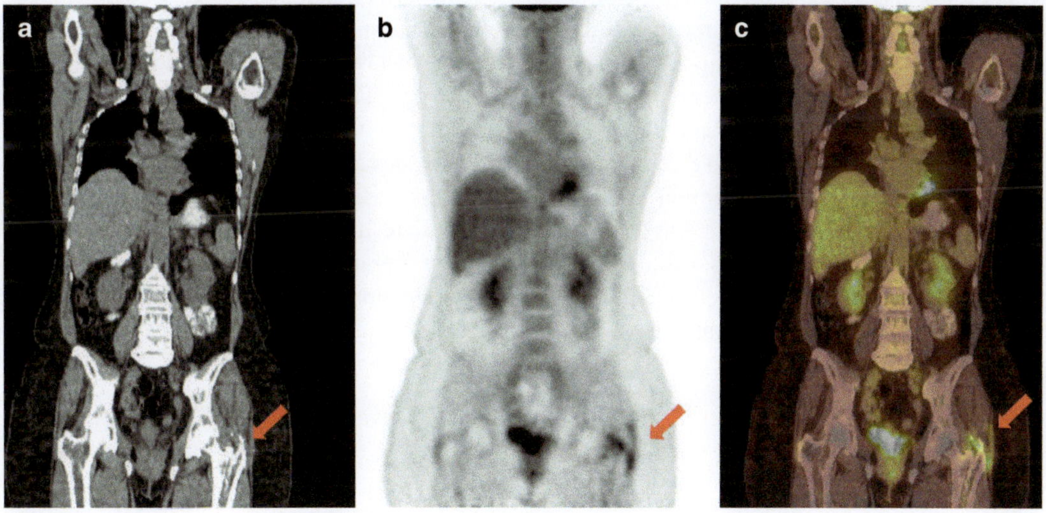

Fig. 11.7 Coronal CT (**a**), PET (**b**), and fused PET/CT (**c**) images show the hypermetabolic lesion of the intertrochanteric region of the left proximal femur with concomitant infiltration of the adjacent muscles/soft tissues of the hip (*red arrow*)

Case 2: Diagnosis – T-Cell Lymphoblastic Lymphoma

A 33-year-old female was admitted with a diagnosis of T-cell lymphoblastic lymphoma (T-LBL) following a large mediastinal mass biopsy representing thymus enlargement. She received treatment according to GMALL 07/2003 study protocol consisting of repeated cycles of intensive chemotherapy followed by maintenance treatment with low-dose chemotherapy administered in an outpatient basis. Initially, she achieved complete remission, but 2 months after the completion of intensive chemotherapy, during maintenance treatment, clinical examination revealed the presence of a right breast mass with regional lymphadenopathy. Surgical biopsy of a right axillary lymph node was consistent with T-LBL relapse.

Repeated staging with FDG-PET/CT revealed a hypermetabolic lesion in the right breast coupled with confluent, ipsilateral axillary and supraclavicular lymphadenopathy (Figs. 11.8 and 11.9). Bone marrow aspiration and biopsy were normal. She received salvage chemotherapy with a nelarabine-based regimen for tumor debulking. Subsequently she underwent allogeneic stem cell transplantation (allo-SCT) following myeloablative conditioning with 12 Gy total body irradiation (TBI) and cyclophosphamide. The donor was her HLA-matched sister. Three months later, restaging FDG-PET/CT showed complete resolution of disease in keeping with a complete metabolic response (Fig. 11.10).

Discussion

T-cell and B-cell lymphoblastic leukemia/lymphoma (T, B-ALL/LBL) is a neoplasm originating from lymphoid precursors committed to T- or B-cell lineage respectively [5]. Disease usually manifests itself as acute lymphoblastic leukemia (ALL) with peripheral blood (PB) and bone marrow (BM) involvement. However, in some cases, the disease presents with nodal or extranodal involvement with no or minimal bone marrow infiltration. By definition, the term lymphoma (LBL) is used when the main bulk of disease is confined to extramedullary sites, while the term leukemia (ALL) is used for cases with extensive PB and BM involvement [6]. T-LBL is more common than B-LBL, with 80–90 % of all LBL cases being of T-cell origin. T-LBL usually presents as a mediastinal mass due to thymic enlargement. On the contrary, the presence of a mediastinal mass is very rare in B-LBL, where the most frequent sites of involvement are lymph nodes, skin, soft-tissue, and bone.

LBL is a rare type of aggressive non-Hodgkin lymphoma and has been reported to be intensely FDG-avid [1]. Since it belongs to the group of very aggressive lymphomas, it shows higher FDG uptake than indolent lymphomas [7]. PET/CT provides accurate staging of nodal and extranodal disease, as in these cases, leading to appropriate management stratification. A baseline pre-therapy PET is strongly advised for initial evaluation and mapping of disease extent. Moreover, it enables interpretation of subsequent posttreatment scan.

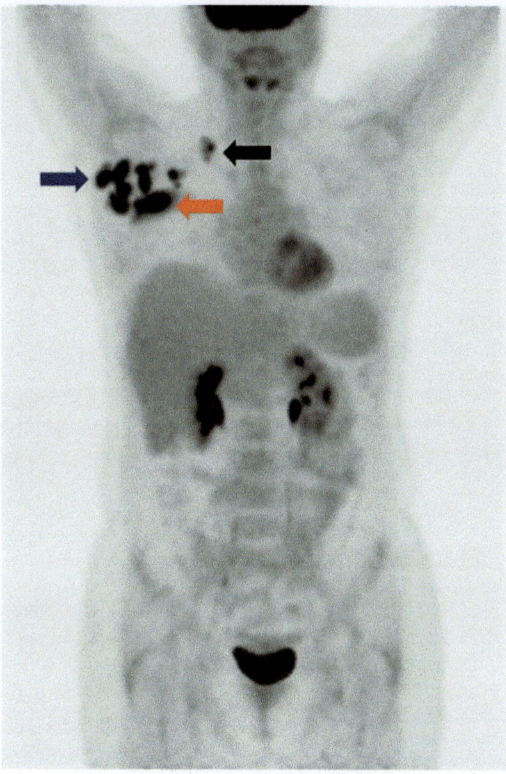

Fig. 11.8 Whole-body PET maximum intensity projection (MIP) image shows an intensely FDG-avid lesion in the right breast (*red arrow*) with concomitant, hypermetabolic, confluent right axillary (*blue arrow*) and ipsilateral supraclavicular (*black arrow*) lymphadenopathy. According to Deauville scale, this is a score 5 study (uptake markedly higher than liver). There are no bone/bone marrow FDG-avid lesions

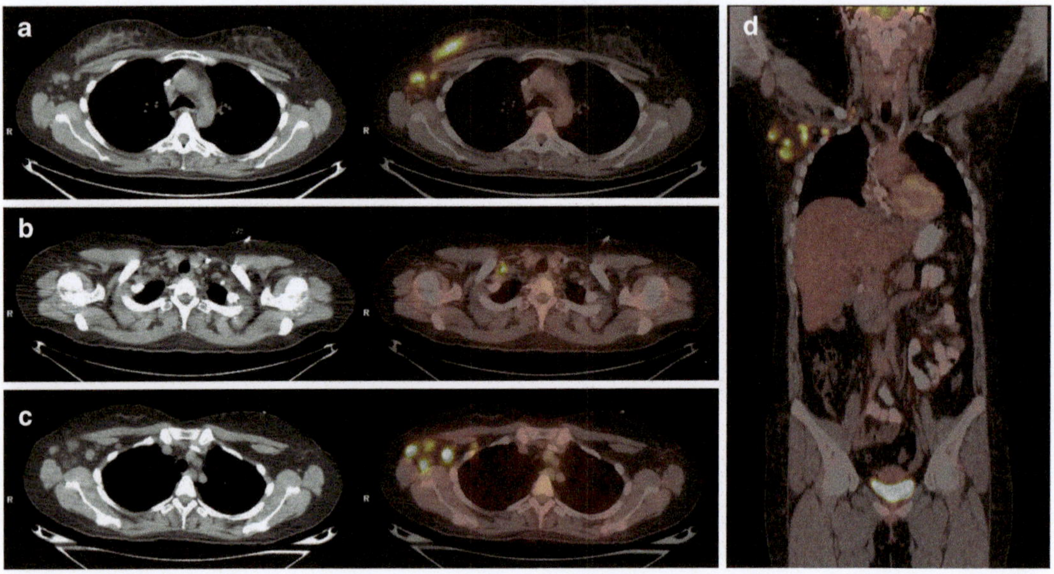

Fig. 11.9 Transaxial CT and fused PET/CT images show an FDG-avid lesion (SUVmax: 13.7) in the upper outer quadrant of the right breast and ipsilateral hypermetabolic axillary subpectoral and supraclavicular lymph nodes. (**a**, **b**, **c**) Coronal fused PET/CT (**d**) image shows multiple hypermetabolic right axillary, subpectoral/infraclavicular, and ipsilateral supraclavicular nodal disease

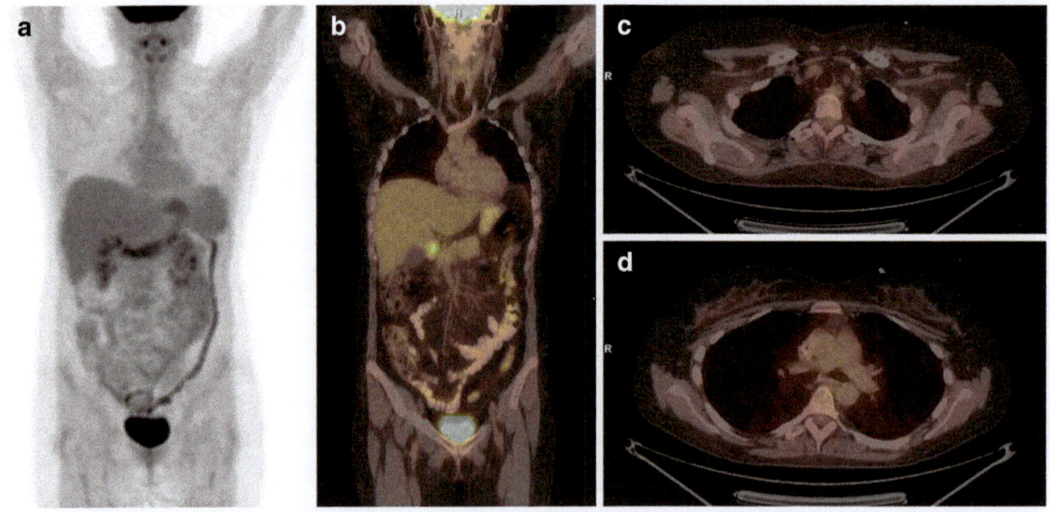

Fig. 11.10 Posttreatment whole-body PET MIP (**a**) and coronal fused PET/CT (**b**) images show no hypermetabolic foci in the right breast-axillary region or elsewhere in the body, in keeping with a compete metabolic response to treatment. This is essentially a Deauville score 1 study. There is only some diffuse FDG activity along the gastric wall, probably of inflammatory etiology (gastritis), and diffuse colonic uptake of functional or inflammatory etiology. Successful treatment result is further elucidated on transaxial-fused PET/CT images (**c** and **d**) showing no hypermetabolic breast lesion and no hypermetabolic or enlarged lymph nodes, in keeping with a complete metabolic and anatomic response

Acknowledgments

Case 1 Images courtesy of Vlachou F and Pipikos Th., Nuclear Medicine Physicians, PET/CT Unit, Hygeia Hospital.

Case 2 Patient was scanned in PET/CT Unit of Evangelismos General Hospital. We acknowledge the contribution of Boudali M and Gregorakou K, PET/CT technologists. Images courtesy of Rondogianni Ph, Nuclear Medicine Physician, PET/CT Unit, Evangelismos General Hospital.

References

1. Weiler-Sagie M, Bushelev O, Epelbaum R et al (2010) (18)F-FDG avidity in lymphoma readdressed: a study of 766 patients. J Nucl Med 51(1):25–30
2. Zeng W, Lechowicz MJ, Winton E et al (2009) Spectrum of FDG PET/CT findings in Burkitt lymphoma. Clin Nucl Med 34(6):355–358
3. Molyneux EM, Rochford R, Griffin B et al (2012) Burkitt's lymphoma. Lancet 379(9822):1234–1244
4. Pelosi E, Penna D, Deandreis D et al (2008) FDG PET in the detection of bone marrow disease in Hodgkin's disease and aggressive non-Hodgkin's lymphoma and its impact on clinical management. Q J Nucl Med Mol Imaging 52:9–16
5. Inaba H, Greaves M, Mullighan CG (2013) Acute lymphoblastic leukaemia. Lancet 381(9881): 1943–1955
6. Cortelazzo S, Ponzoni M, Ferreri AJ, Hoelzer D (2011) Lymphoblastic lymphoma. Crit Rev Oncol Hematol 79(3):330–343
7. Barrington SF, Mikhaeel NG (2014) When should FDG-PET be used in the modern management of lymphoma? Br J Haematol 164(3):315–28

Splenic Lymphomas

12

Christina Kalpadakis, Gerassimos A. Pangalis, Dimitrios T. Kechagias, Xanthi Yiakoumis, and Fani J. Vlachou

12.1 Splenic Lymphomas

Spleen is involved in approximately one third of patients with non-Hodgkin lymphoma (NHL), usually secondarily, either at presentation or at the time of disease progression. On the contrary, primary splenic lymphoma is rare, comprising only 1 % of all lymphomas, although its incidence is probably underestimated. The definition of primary splenic lymphoma is controversial. Herein, we adopt a less restrictive definition of splenic lymphomas, encompassing cases presenting with splenic involvement and in which the disease may also extend to the bone marrow, blood, and liver without prominent lymphadenopathy. Splenic lymphomas include mainly the following categories: splenic marginal zone lymphoma (SMZL), hairy cell leukemia (HCL), and the provisional entities: HCL variant (HCLv), splenic diffuse red pulp small B-cell lymphoma (SDRPL), primary splenic diffuse large B-cell lymphoma (DLBCL), and T-γδ hepatosplenic lymphoma [1].

Mantle cell lymphoma, follicular lymphoma, chronic lymphocytic leukemia (CLL), T-large granular leukemia, prolymphocytic leukemia, and lymphoplasmacytic lymphoma/Waldenstrom's macroglobulinemia may also present with splenomegaly without lymphadenopathy, along with bone marrow involvement in most cases.

The patterns of lymphomatous infiltration of the spleen are classified into the following four types based on the gross appearance: (1) homogeneous involvement without masses (diffuse pattern), (2) milliary masses (micronodular pattern), (3) 2–10 cm masses, and (4) large solitary mass (types 3 and 4 represent the macronodular pattern of involvement) [2].

In general, NHLs have an overall ^{18}F-FDG avidity of almost 90 %. However, the avidity is lower in indolent lymphomas than in aggressive ones with the exception of follicular lymphomas. ^{18}F-FDG avidity correlates better with the histopathologic subtype of NHL. Follicular lymphoma, regardless of grade, shows high ^{18}F-FDG avidity, whereas most of other low-grade lymphomas have low ^{18}F-FDG avidity. Its overall usefulness in indolent lymphomas (e.g., CLL/SLL, lymphoplasmacytic lymphoma, marginal zone lymphoma) remains unclear. In splenic lymphomas with low-grade histology, diffusely

C. Kalpadakis (✉)
Department of Haematology, University Hospital of Heraklion, Heraklion, Crete, Greece
e-mail: xkalpadaki@yahoo.gr

G.A. Pangalis • X. Yiakoumis
Department of Haematology, Athens Medical Center, Psychikon Branch, Athens, Greece

D.T. Kechagias • F.J. Vlachou
PET/CT Department, Hygeia Hospital, Athens, Greece

J.A. Andreou et al. (eds.), *PET/CT in Lymphomas: A Case-Based Atlas*,
DOI 10.1007/978-3-319-27380-8_12

increased uptake is usually observed, while in DLBCL cases with primary involvement of the spleen, there is more often focal uptake in the spleen on a whole-body PET/CT. On a pre-therapeutic scan for lymphoma, splenic uptake, greater than hepatic uptake, is a relative reliable indication of lymphomatous involvement of the spleen [3]. However, diffusely increased splenic uptake is not characteristic only for lymphoproliferative disorders, since it can also be seen in other clinical settings, such as administration of granulocyte colony-stimulating factor, sarcoidosis, malaria, and many inflammatory or hematopoietic diseases [4].

12.1.1 Splenic Marginal Zone Lymphoma

Splenic marginal zone lymphoma (SMZL) is considered as a distinct entity in the World Health Organization classification. It is a relatively rare low-grade B-cell lymphoma, comprising less than 2 % of non-Hodgkin's lymphomas. SMZL affects mainly elderly patients with a median age of 65 years without gender predilection. It is characterized by splenomegaly and bone marrow infiltration. Spleen histology typically shows a micronodular involvement of the white pulp with a biphasic pattern of infiltration and a variable degree of red pulp involvement. Diffuse, uniform infiltration is the most common pathological form of SMZL. Typically, lymph node involvement is absent, with the exception of splenic hilum. Lymphocytosis is present in almost half of the patients, while circulating lymphoma cells are present in the vast majority of cases. The immunophenotype is nonspecific, and SMZL B cells express pan-B-cell markers CD19, CD20, CD22, and CD79a and surface IgM ± IgD of moderate to strong intensity, while CD5 is found only in 15 % and CD23 in 30 % of cases. Bone marrow is invariably infiltrated by the disease (>95 %). Diagnosis is based on the integration of the clinical findings, lymphocyte morphology, immunophenotype, and bone marrow histology, while spleen histology is not mandatory for the establishment of diagnosis in most cases [5]. SMZL usually runs an indolent clinical course with a median survival of approximately 10 years. Rituximab monotherapy and splenectomy are among the most effective treatment modalities [6]. Currently, the role of PET scan in SMZL staging and response evaluation is limited. Based on the published data in very small series of patients, PET scan shows a moderate sensitivity in the range of 50–67 %. However, the emergence of foci of intense uptake in a patient with SMZL should raise suspicion of histologic transformation to a more aggressive NHL variant.

Case 1: Diagnosis – Splenic Marginal Zone Lymphoma

A 65-year-old male presented on June 2006 with lymphocytosis and splenomegaly, without any constitutional symptoms. Blood morphology showed villous lymphocytes admixed with small lymphocytes. Flow cytometry analysis of circulating lymphocytes disclosed a clonal B-cell population with strong CD20 expression and intermediate expression of sIgM/IgD with κ light chain restriction, along with expression of CD5, CD25, CD11c, and CD38 antigens. CD23 was weakly expressed. Conventional staging with CT scan revealed a homogeneously enlarged spleen (maximum diameter 17.5 cm), without any lymphadenopathy. A bone marrow biopsy showed 50 % infiltration by clonal B cells with a nodular and intrasinusoidal pattern of involvement. A diagnosis of splenic marginal zone lymphoma was established. Since the patient was asymptomatic without any cytopenias, he was placed in a watch-and-wait policy. On February 2009, he presented with anemia and further increase in spleen size (22.5 cm) along with abdominal pain. Due to the disease progression, treatment with rituximab monotherapy was initiated. He received six weekly cycles of rituximab at the standard dose of 375 mg/m^2. Evaluation of response 2 months after the completion of treatment disclosed stable disease. A few months later, a PET/CT was performed in order to exclude disease transformation. PET/CT at the time of rituximab failure confirmed the presence of splenomegaly without any mass lesions indicative of disease transformation (Fig. 12.1).

The patient underwent splenectomy which confirmed the diagnosis of SMZL, without evidence of histologic transformation. Splenectomy resulted in complete hematologic response, which lasted for 5 years. At that time, the patient experienced disease progression with bulky abdominal lymphadenopathy, very high lymphocyte counts, and anemia. He received combination therapy with rituximab and bendamustine and achieved a complete response. Patient remains in remission 1 year after the end of treatment.

Discussion

SMZL is typically characterized by infiltration of the splenic white pulp, with a micronodular pattern of involvement. Splenic hilar lymph nodes are usually infiltrated as well. Radiographic findings are not specific. Spleen is usually homogeneously enlarged, without any masses. The presence of solitary or multiple nodules should raise concerns for histologic transformation of the disease. SMZL diagnosis should be based on the integration of clinical findings, blood morphology, immunophenotype, bone marrow histology, and cytogenetics. Some atypical cases in order to be diagnosed may require splenectomy. Published data is limited regarding the utility of PET/CT in SMZL. Current data, in a very small number of cases, indicate that SMZL demonstrate relatively low FDG avidity. In a study contacted by our group, including ten SMZL cases, PET/CT was negative in three of them [7]. To date, there is no indication for PET/CT in the diagnostic approach and staging of SMZL.

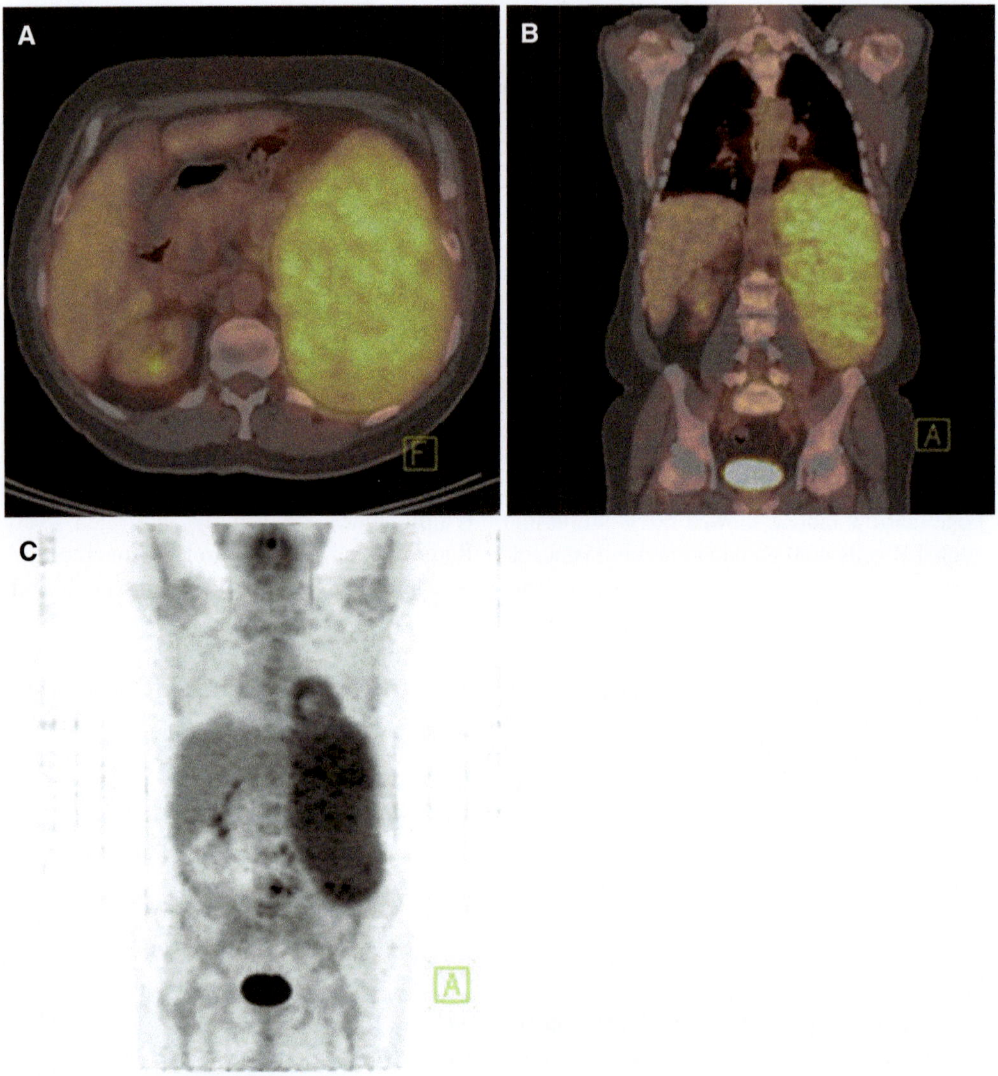

Fig. 12.1 Axial and coronal PET/CT images (**A**, **B**) and PET MIP image (**C**) show enlarged spleen and diffuse uptake of FDG from the splenic parenchyma (SUVmax 5.5)

12.1.2 Hairy Cell Leukemia

Hairy cell leukemia (HCL) is also an uncommon low-grade B-cell lymphocytic proliferation, representing approximately 1 % of lymphoid neoplasms. The median age at onset is 52 years. There is a strong male predominance of approximately four to one. Lymphoma cells are medium size mature B cells with abundant cytoplasm and "hairy" projections infiltrating the blood, the bone marrow, and the splenic red pulp. Usually, patients present with splenomegaly, while pancytopenia and monocytopenia are found in the majority of cases. The bone marrow is often inaspirable (dry tap) due to HCL-induced marrow fibrosis. "Hairy" cells display expression of pan-B-cell antigens (e.g., CD19, CD20, CD22) along with positivity for CD103, CD11c, and CD25. Expression of annexin A1 in B cells is specific, but not sensitive enough for the diagnosis of HCL. The diagnosis of HCL is usually made by blood morphology and immunophenotype along with bone marrow biopsy. BRAF mutations are a disease-defining event among patients with classical HCL who do not express IGHV4-34. Purine analogs, cladribine and pentostatin, are treatment of choice in HCL patients. Prognosis is excellent with long survival in most patients. There is no data regarding PET/CT findings in HCL. Very limited number of published cases reported on the role of PET/CT in identification of disease in extrasplenic areas mainly at relapse setting [8, 9].

Case 2: Diagnosis – Hairy Cell Leukemia

A 36-year-old female was admitted to our Department on October 2011 because of asymptomatic splenomegaly and leukopenia. At presentation, her physical examination disclosed splenomegaly (8 cm blcm) and slight hepatomegaly with the following blood counts: Hgb 12.2 gr/dl, WBCs 3.4×10^9/L, and PLT 190×10^9/L. Blood smear morphology revealed a few abnormal small-sized lymphoid cells with villi. CT scan disclosed only homogeneous enlargement of the spleen (max length 25 cm). Bone marrow aspiration was copious but not dry tap. Blood and bone marrow flow cytometry analysis revealed a monoclonal B-cell population consistent with the diagnosis of either variant HCL or SMZL or diffuse red pulp splenic B-cell lymphoma (expression of CD20, CD22, CD11c, CD103, FMC7, CD200, and TCL1, while CD25 was not expressed). Bone marrow biopsy showed a 60 % infiltration, mainly interstitial and partially intrasinusoidal, by a B-cell monoclonal population CD20+, DBA44+, CD23+, TRAP+, CD25+(weak), annexinA1(+/–), CD27–, and cyclinD1–, and expression of surface IgM, IgD+/–. PCR analysis for the presence of BRAF V600E mutation was negative. PET/CT disclosed an abnormal uptake by the spleen (max SUV 5.8) (Fig. 12.2a).

Based on the above data, a diagnosis of a splenic lymphoma/leukemia unclassifiable was made. She was treated with rituximab monotherapy for six weekly cycles, starting on November 2011, with no significant response (<PR). On June 2012, she received second-line therapy with pentostatin. After the completion of four cycles, splenomegaly was stable. A second PET scan was performed at that time, in order to exclude histologic transformation to a high-grade lymphoma. PET scan on March 2012 was similar to the previous one but with less metabolic activity (Fig. 12.2b).

On October 2012, she underwent splenectomy, which established the diagnosis of HCL. She received no further treatment and remains in complete remission 2.5 years after splenectomy.

Discussion

HCL represents a relatively rare chronic lymphoproliferative disorder with specific clinical, morphologic, histologic, immunophenotypic, and molecular characteristics. By integrating these clinical and laboratory data, diagnosis can be made relatively easily, without the need for splenectomy. Our case was interesting because there were overlapping characteristics between HCL and splenic lymphoma unclassifiable (HCL variant or SDRPL) and despite extensive evaluation a definitive diagnosis could not be made. Since splenectomy is a major surgical procedure, our approach is generally to avoid it in cases with a generic diagnosis of a chronic B-cell lymphoproliferative disorder. However, splenectomy is recommended in cases in which the possibility of a mantle cell lymphoma exists as well as cases in which an underlying high-grade lymphoma is suspected. In the case under discussion, splenectomy was performed due to suboptimal response to therapy. The present case is also interesting because it gives information on PET/CT findings in patients with HCL that is currently not available in the literature. PET/CT showed a diffusely increased uptake of FDG in the spleen, without focal lesions.

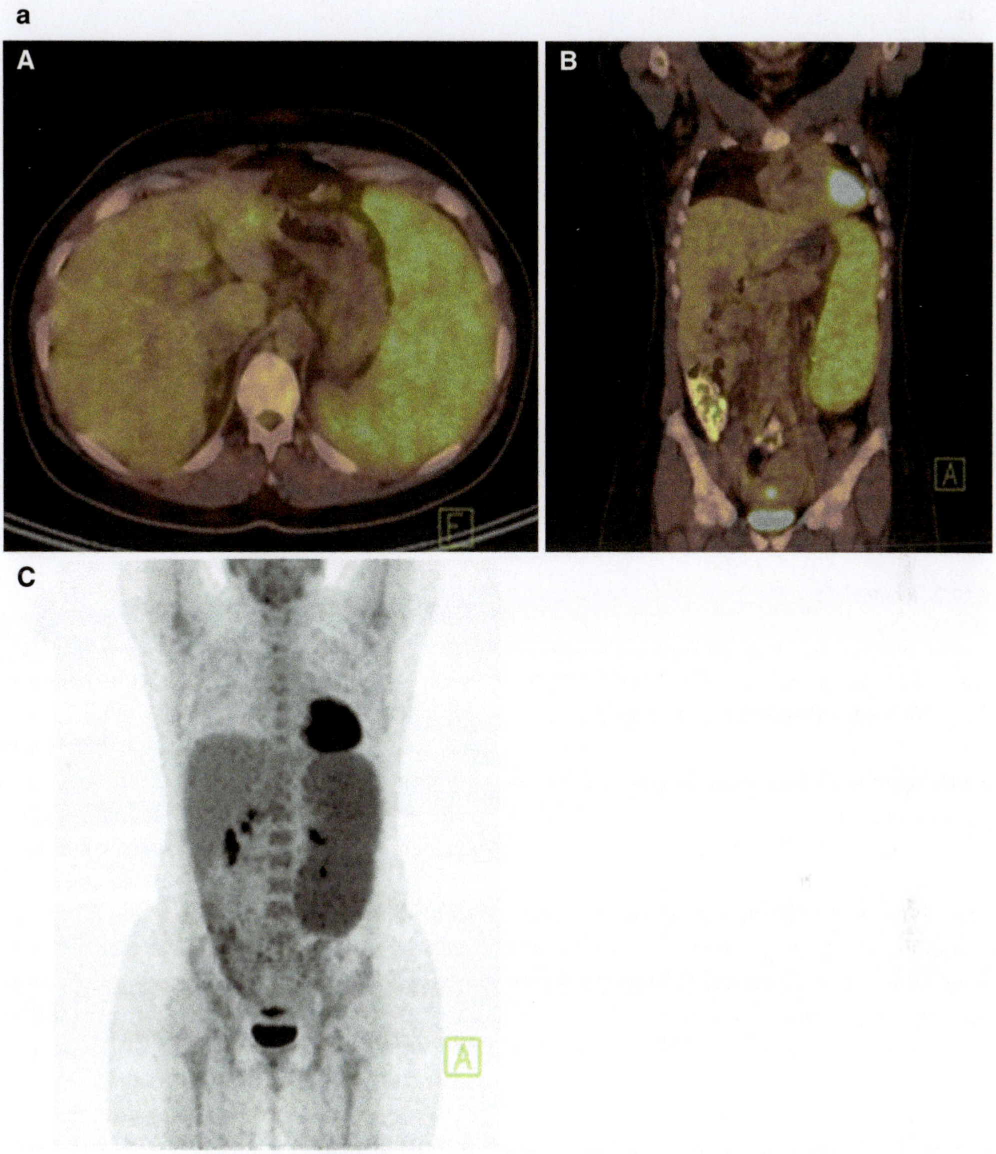

Fig. 12.2 (**a**) Axial and coronal PET/CT images (*A*, *B*) and PET MIP image (*C*) show the enlarged spleen with diffusely increased uptake of the radiopharmaceutical (SUVmax 5,8). (**b**) In axial and coronal PET/CT images (*A*, *B*) 5 months later, the size of the spleen and the metabolic activity are practically unchanged (slight metabolic reduction, SUVmax 5.6)

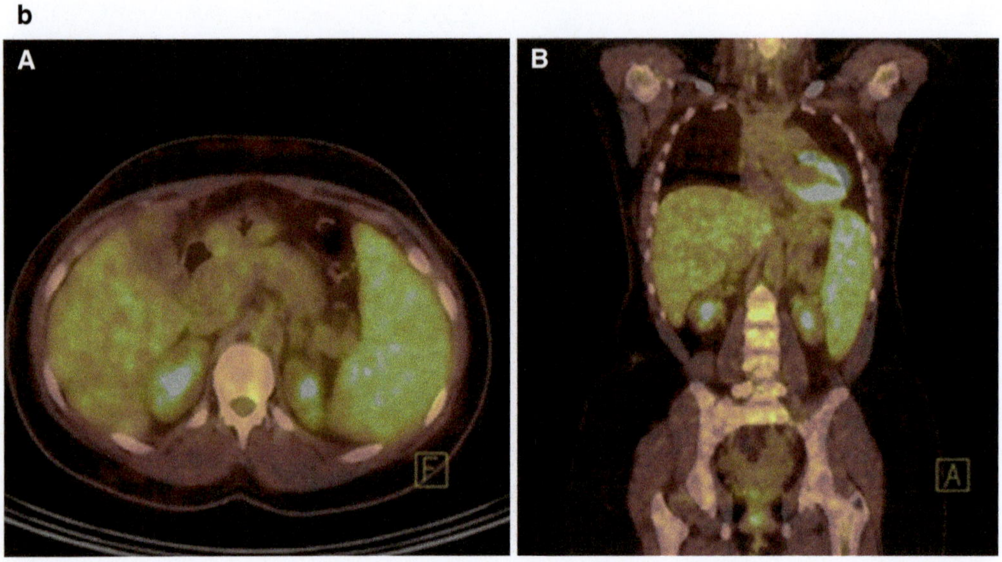

Fig. 12.2 (continued)

12.2 Primary Splenic Diffuse Large B-Cell Lymphoma (DLBCL)

Primary splenic diffuse large B-cell lymphoma is an uncommon entity, representing less than 1 % of NHLs [10]. However, it represents the most common histologic subtype of primary splenic lymphomas if the restrictive definition of lymphomatous involvement of spleen and splenic hilar lymph nodes only is applied. There is usually single tumor mass, which is large occupying more than 50 % of the spleen. The second most common type of splenic infiltration is multiple (confluent) nodules. Necrosis is very common. Local invasion of neighboring structures is commonly observed. Patients usually present with symptomatic splenomegaly, B symptoms, and localized disease. Therefore, DLBCL of the spleen should be considered in the differential diagnosis of patients presenting with B symptoms associated with radiographic evidence of single or multiple focal lesions in the spleen. Therapy is based on the R-CHOP combination, while splenectomy may play a role not only in the establishment of diagnosis but also in the improvement of long-term outcome. A rare type of primary splenic DLBCL with infiltration of the splenic red pulp has also been described. It is characterized by a more aggressive clinical picture with disseminated disease, cytopenias, bone marrow infiltration and worse outcome. As DLBCL in general is characterized by high FDG avidity, PET/CT is currently recommended for staging, as well as for response assessment [11]. In DLBCL, PET/CT positivity after R-CHOP is associated with long-term PFS of <40 %. A negative PET/CT after R-CHOP carries a rather low negative predictive value, with 5-year PFS of 70–80 %, [12, 13].

Case 3 – Diagnosis: Splenic Diffuse Large B-Cell Lymphoma

A 40-year-old woman presented on March 2012 with abdominal distention and left shoulder pain of acute onset. She also complained of drenching night sweats and weakness. Her spleen was palpable on physical exam, but no lymphadenopathy was present. Complete blood count and serum chemistry were normal. Abdominal ultrasonography showed splenomegaly (15.6 cm) along with a large mass in the spleen (10.3 cm). She underwent whole-body CT scan, which revealed an enlarged spleen with a large splenic mass and a marginally enlarged intraabdominal lymph node (1.5 cm). Abdominal MRI was also performed, which confirmed the presence of a large mass in the spleen (11 × 10 × 9 cm) along with multiple marginally enlarged peripancreatic and perigastric lymph nodes. Whole-body PET–CT scan showed a hyperactive mass involving the spleen with a maximum SUV of 27.8, clearly separated from normal spleen tissue. Multiple lymph nodes in the abdomen were also identified with a maximum SUV of 21.4 (Fig. 12.3a).

On May 2012 splenectomy was performed, which ameliorated the local symptoms and established the diagnosis of diffuse large B-cell lymphoma of activated type. The procedure was well tolerated without complications. Bone marrow aspiration and biopsy demonstrated no infiltration of lymphoma. Thus, the patient had stage IIB DLBCL. On June 2012 before treatment initiation, a CT scan was repeated, which showed enlarged para-aortic and retroperitoneal lymph nodes (max 5.5 cm). The patient received R-CHOP combination immunochemotherapy. An interim CT scan was performed after four cycles of treatment, which showed a decrease in the size of the previously enlarged lymph nodes (max 1.9 cm vs 5.5 cm). After the completion of two more cycles of therapy, evaluation of the disease was performed both by CT scan and PET/CT. CT scan findings were stable as in the interim analysis, whereas PET/CT showed no FDG uptake, as indicated in Fig. 12.3b (Nov-2012).

Our patient remains in complete remission 2.5 years after the end of therapy.

Discussion

DLBCL is characterized by high FDG avidity of approximately 97 %. For this reason, PET/CT is strongly recommended for initial staging. Primary splenic DLBCL is very rare. Splenic involvement may be characterized by homogeneous splenomegaly, diffuse infiltration with military lesions, focal nodular lesions, or a large solitary mass, as in this case. Assessment of response after treatment is more accurate with PET/CT, especially for patients with complete remission unconfirmed or partial remission by conventional staging (CT). The current recommendation is to use the 5-point scale for end-of-treatment assessment [11].

a

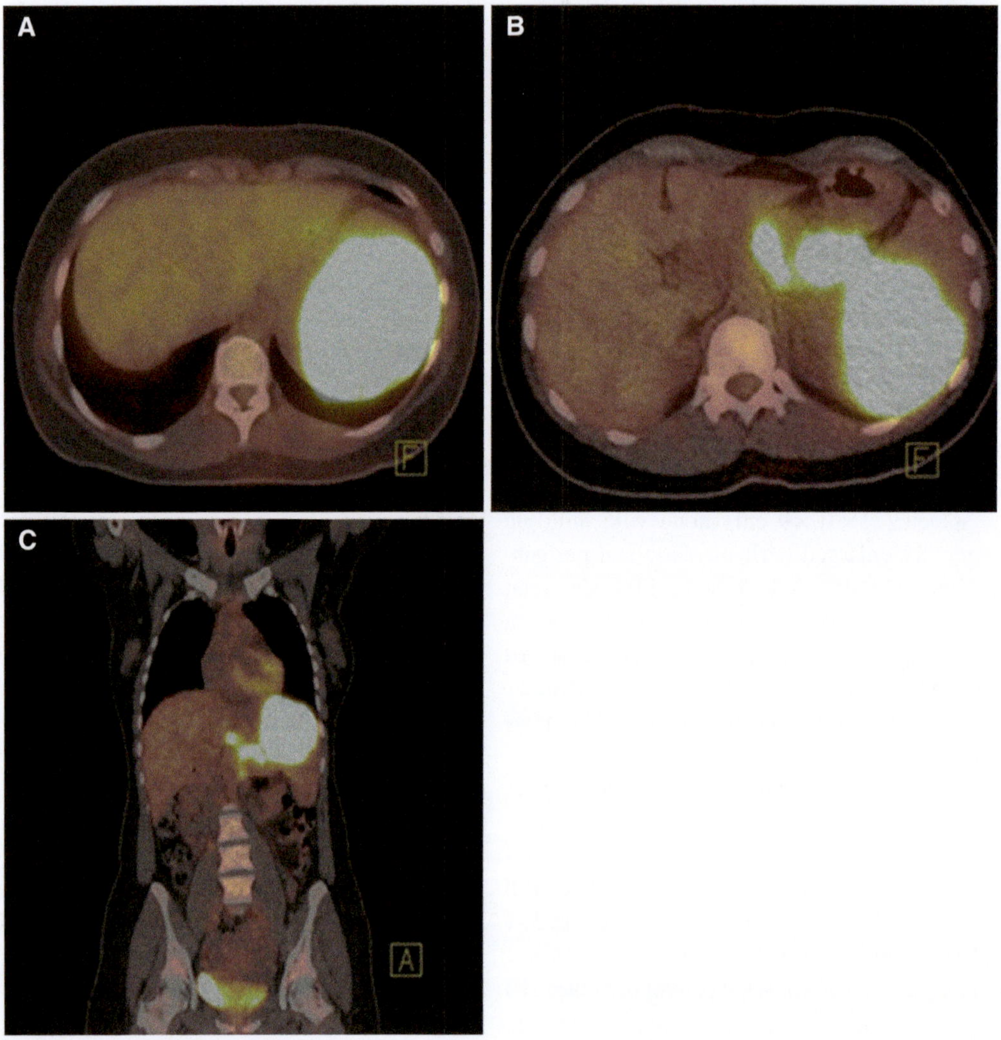

Fig. 12.3 (**a**) Axial PET/CT images (*A*, *B*) show hypermetabolic lesion of the spleen (SUVmax 27.8) and hypermetabolic lymph nodes (SUVmax 21,4) in the abdomen. Coronal PET/CT image (*C*) shows the extent of the disease in the abdomen. (**b**) PET/CT study 7 months later shows great improvement after splenectomy and chemotherapy. Axial PET/CT image (*A*) and PET MIP image (*B*) show postoperative findings without foci of increased metabolic activity

b

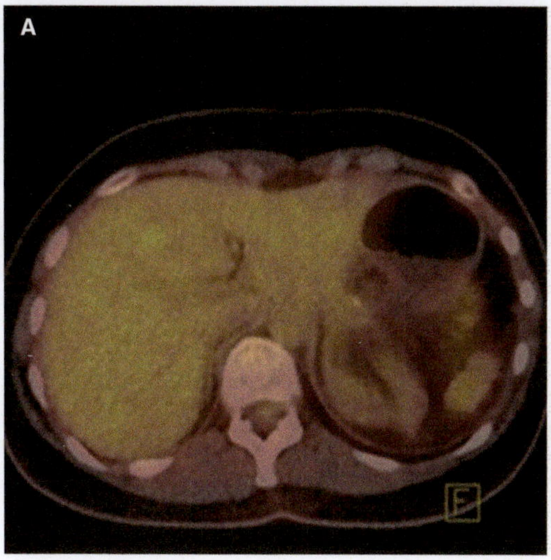

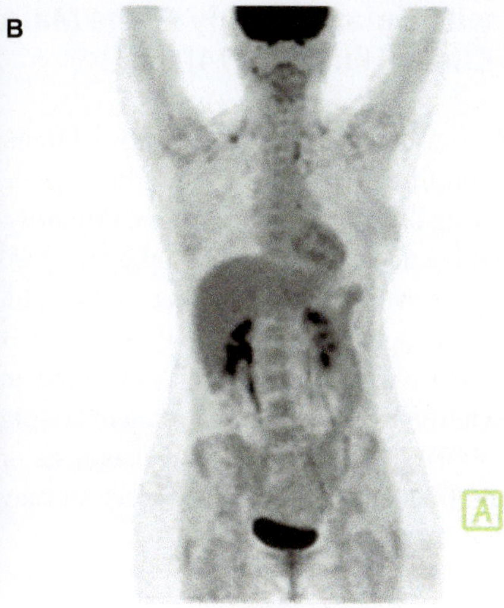

Fig. 12.3 (continued)

12.3 Chronic Lymphocytic Leukemia with Splenomegaly as the Main Clinical Finding [14]

CLL is the most common of the small B-cell lymphocytic proliferations to involve the spleen, mainly during the course of the disease. Primarily, white pulp is affected, while red pulp is involved during disease evolution. Lymphoma cells exhibit the typical immunophenotype of CLL. SUV is low in patients with CLL, but may increase in Richter syndrome (RS) [15]. According to current practice, PET/CT has no role in the diagnosis or follow-up of patients with CLL. However it may be important in CLL cases with evidence of histologic transformation. In such cases, PET/CT may guide the choice of the site for biopsy. Furthermore, recent data indicate that PET/CT may be of prognostic significance. In the largest series of patients reported so far, including 332 CLL cases at different phases, histologically aggressive CLL and RS cases presented higher maximum uptake value (SUV_{max}), than histologically indolent CLL cases. An $SUV_{max} \geq 10$ strongly correlated with mortality (overall survival 56.7 vs 6.9 months in patients with $SUV_{max} < 10$ vs ≥ 10 respectively). Patients with different CLL phases, but similar SUV_{max} had similar outcome [16].

Case 4: Diagnosis – Chronic Lymphocytic Leukemia

A 55-year-old woman diagnosed with typical CLL (Rai-0) in 2003, was admitted to our Department in 2010 for further evaluation of night sweats and anorexia for the last 2 months. At physical examination she presented splenomegaly (15 cm below left costal margin), without any lymphadenopathy. Complete blood count showed lymphocytosis (ALC = 10.610/μL), without any other abnormal findings. Biochemical profile was normal as well as serology for hepatitis B and C. Blood immunophenotype showed the presence of a B-cell clonal population with weak CD20 and sIg expression, along with expression of CD5, CD23, CD43. Whole-body CT scan revealed enlarged lymph nodes of marginal size (max 1.4 cm) in cervical, axillary and inguinal areas, along with splenomegaly (26 cm). Bone marrow biopsy was also consistent with CLL diagnosis. So, the patient progressed from Rai stage 0 in 2003 to Rai stage II after a 7-year history of indolent, untreated disease. In order to exclude the possibility of histologic transformation, since she was complained for B symptoms, a PET/CT was performed, which showed an area of increased FDG uptake in the upper pole of the enlarged spleen (SUV_{max} 9.5) (Fig. 12.4).

Splenectomy was planned in order to further evaluate the above-described splenic mass, but patient did not consent. Moreover, she presented a gradual resolution of B symptoms, and she was placed in a closed watch-and-wait policy. Five years later, she is alive without any symptoms, with further increase in spleen size and development of anemia. Splenectomy is once again planned, and this time patient has accepted it.

Discussion

The available studies do not justify using PET/CT routinely in the staging or response assessment in patients with CLL. FDG/PET is a useful diagnostic tool in patients with CLL and suspected transformation [15]. Histologic transformation is not infrequent in CLL, and Richter syndrome is estimated to occur in approximately 10 % of patients. Recent data suggests that PET/CT is important for detecting disease transformation [16, 17]. Disease transformation is usually associated with aggressive clinical course and short survival. For this reason, it requires early diagnosis and prompt therapy. A positive PET/CT supports the possibility of transformation, and moreover it indicates the site where a biopsy is more likely to be informative [16].

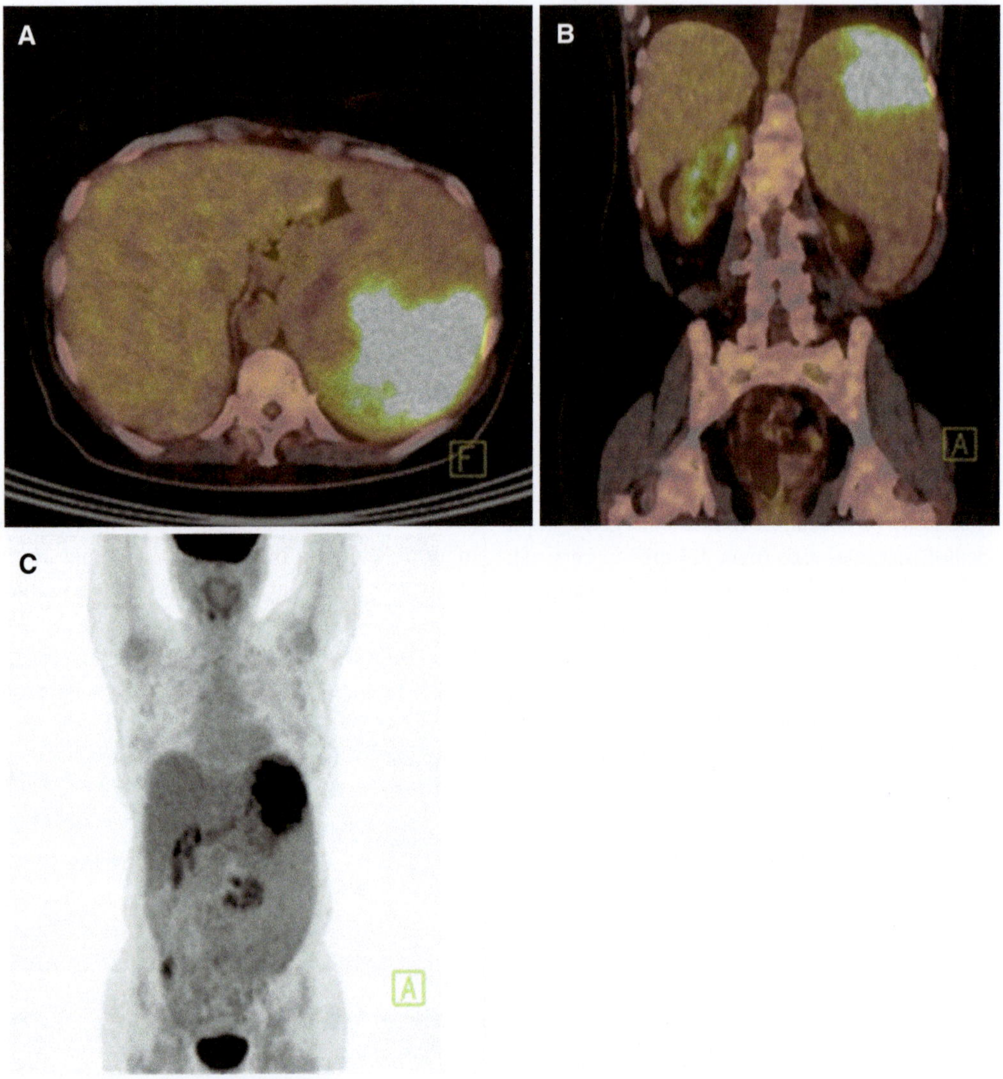

Fig. 12.4 In axial and coronal PET/CT images (**A**, **B**) and PET MIP image (**C**), an area of increased FDG uptake is seen in the upper pole of the enlarged spleen (SUVmax 9.5)

References

1. Isaacson PG, Piris MA, Berger F et al (2008) Splenic B-cell marginal zone lymphoma. In: World Health Organization Classification of Tumours: pathology and genetics of tumours of haematopoietic and lymphoid tissues. IARC, Lyon, pp 185–187
2. Ahmann DL, Kiely JM, Harrison EG Jr et al (1966) Malignant lymphoma of the spleen. A review of 49 cases in which the diagnosis was made at splenectomy. Cancer 19:461–469
3. Karunanithi S, Sharma AP, Shambo Guha R et al (2014) Use of 18F-FDG PET/CT imaging for evaluation of patients with primary splenic lymphoma. Clin N Med 39:772–778
4. Liu Y (2009) Clinical significance of diffusely increased splenic uptake on FDG-PET. Nucl Med Commun 30: 763–769
5. Matutes E, Oscier D, Montalban C et al (2008) Splenic marginal-zone lymphoma proposals for a revision of diagnosis, staging and therapeutic criteria. Leukemia 22:487–495
6. Kalpadakis C, Pangalis GA, Angelopoulou MK et al (2013) Treatment of splenic marginal zone lymphoma with rituximab: progress report and comparison with splenectomy. Oncologist 18:190–197
7. Yiakoumis X, Moschogiannis M, Vassilakopoulos T et al (2011) FDG PET CT scan role on diagnosis and initial staging of lymphoproliferative diseases. Haematologica 96:574 (Abstract)
8. Subhawong AP, Subhawong TK, Ali SZ (2012) Hairy cell leukemia presenting as a peripancreatic mass: cytomorphology and radiographic correlates. Acta Cytol 56:463–466
9. Rutherford SC, Andemariam B, Philips SM et al (2008) FDG-PET in prediction of splenectomy findings in patients with known or suspected lymphoma. Leuk Lymphoma 49:719–726
10. Mollejo M, Algara P, Mateo MS et al (2003) Large B-cell lymphoma presenting in the spleen: identification of different clinicopathologic conditions. Am J Surg Pathol 27:895–902
11. Cheson BD, Fisher RI, Barrington SF et al (2014) Recommendations for initial evaluation, staging, and response assessment of Hodgkin and non-Hodgkin lymphoma: the Lugano classification. J Clin Oncol 32:3059–3067
12. Dupuis J, Itti E, Rahmouni A, Hemery F et al (2009) Response assessment after an inductive CHOP or CHOP-like regimen with or without rituximab in 103 patients with diffuse large B-cell lymphoma: integrating 18 fluorodeoxyglucose positron emission tomography to the International Workshop Criteria. Ann Oncol 20:503–507
13. Thomas A, Gingrich RD, Smith BJ et al (2010) 18-fluoro-deoxyglucose positron emission tomography report interpretation as predictor of outcome in diffuse large B-cell lymphoma including analysis of "indeterminate" reports. Leuk Lymphoma 51: 439–446
14. Pangalis GA, Vassilakopoulos TP, Dimopoulou MN et al (2002) Chronic lymphocytic leukemia: practical aspects. Hematol Oncol 20:103–146
15. Bruzzi JF, Macapinlac H, Tsimberidou AM et al (2006) Detection of Richter's transformation of chronic lymphocytic leukemia by PET/CT. J Nucl Med 47:1267–1273
16. Falchi L, Keating MJ, Marom EM et al (2014) Correlation between FDG/PET, histology, characteristics, and survival in 332 patients with chronic lymphoid leukemia. Blood 123:2783–2790
17. Papajík T, Myslivećek M, Urbanová R et al (2014) 2-[18F] fluoro-2-deoxy-D-glucose positron emission tomography/computed tomography examination in patients with chronic lymphocytic leukemia may reveal Richter transformation. Leuk Lymphoma 55:314–319

Primary Non-Hodgkin's Lymphoma of the Central Nervous System (PCNSL)

13

Marina P. Siakantaris, Vasiliki P. Filippi, and Julia V. Malamitsi

13.1 Introduction

PCNSL is a rare aggressive lymphoma, which occurs mainly in the immunocompromised hosts (HIV), but is reported in immunocompetent patients as well, with a progressive incidence. It affects the brain in the majority of cases, whereas the spinal cord or the eye is more rarely involved. At presentation, there should be no evidence of lymphoma outside the CNS or systemic symptoms. The main histologic type of PCNSL is of the diffuse large B cell (DLBCL) (90 %). Other subtypes such as Burkitt, MALT, and T-cell lymphomas have been occasionally reported. The prognosis of PCNSL remains poor, with a median survival of 1.5–3 months in untreated patients. Debulking surgery is not recommended for this type of lymphoma. Radiotherapy produces high response rates (60–90 %) but nearly all patients relapse (median survival of 14 months). Until today, it remains the treatment of choice, for older patients with comorbidities who cannot tolerate toxic chemotherapy. The chosen chemotherapeutic agents must penetrate the blood-brain barrier in order to reach and kill the lymphoma cells [1]. High-dose methotrexate (MTX)-based regimens have been successfully employed with median failure-free survival (FFS) of 4 months. In a large randomized phase 2 study, the combination of high-dose methotrexate with high-dose cytarabine with or without brain radiation produced superior FFS to MTX alone, of 8 months [2]. Several studies have tried to improve survival with the employment of dose-intensive chemotherapeutic consolidation, including autologous stem cell rescue. Agents that penetrate the CNS such as carmustine, thiotepa, cyclophosphamide, busulfan, high-dose cytarabine, and etoposide have been used with promising results. In a similar context, the most recent and effective two-step program (CALGB 50202) has yielded a median time to progression of 4 years for all patients, where the responding patients to high-dose MTX-rituximab initial treatment received combination of high-dose infusional etoposide plus cytarabine [3]. An important issue is drug-related renal toxicity and another that remains to be seen is neurotoxicity. In nearly all studies the main adverse risk factor is age with a cutoff of 60 years. In contrast

M.P. Siakantaris, MD (✉)
Department of Internal Medicine, National and Kapodistrian University, Laiko General Hospital, Agiou Thoma 17,11527 Athens, Greece
e-mail: msiaka@med.uoa.gr; siakantaris@gmail.com

V.P. Filippi
Department of CT-MRI and PET/CT, Hygeia Hospital, Athens, Greece
e-mail: vicky.filippi@gmail.com

J.V. Malamitsi, MD, MSc
Department of Medical Physics, Medical School, National and Kapodistrian University of Athens, Mikras Asias 75, 11527 Athens, Greece
e-mail: imalamits@med.uoa.gr

J.A. Andreou et al. (eds.), *PET/CT in Lymphomas: A Case-Based Atlas*,
DOI 10.1007/978-3-319-27380-8_13

to the rest of DLBCL, a panel of different risk factors has been proposed by the International Extranodal Lymphoma Study Group for PCNSL, which include age >60 years, ECOG performance status >1, elevated LDH, elevated CSF protein concentration, and presence of deep brain lesions. Patients with 0–1, 2–3, or 4–5 of the above factors have a 2-year overall survival of 80 %, 48 %, or 15 %, respectively [4] A very important prognostic parameter identified in recent studies is the timing of treatment initiation which means that delayed diagnosis correlates with a worse outcome. Initial tools for diagnosis have traditionally been CT and MR imaging. According to the report of an international workshop to standardize baseline evaluation and response criteria for primary CNS lymphoma, the recommended imaging method is gadolinium-enhanced MRI scan and, if this is contraindicated, contrast-enhanced CT [5]. Solitary or multiple masses in the central or periventricular areas of the white matter with uniform enhancement are the most frequent findings, while the accompanying edema is sometimes impressive [6]. The lymphoma can involve the frontal lobe in up to 40 % of cases, the basal ganglia and the cerebellum in a smaller percentage. Even if the radiologic findings are highly suggestive of a malignant disease, the gold standard of diagnosis is the stereotactic biopsy with immunohistochemistry. In technically difficult cases, modern imaging modalities are valuable alternatives. The role of 18-FDG PET in the diagnosis and treatment outcome of lymphoma patients is well established although in PCNSL is not fully elucidated. From previous studies it is demonstrated that the PCNSL lesion uptake is usually homogeneous and much greater than that of other malignant tumors, with a mean SUV maximum value of 22.6 [7]. The SUV measurement is influenced by corticosteroids, high blood sugar, age, body weight, and tumor size. Patients with brain lymphoma often receive steroids on presentation due to neurological deficits and cerebral edema. The responsiveness of lymphoma cells to steroids is a known fact which may give falsely negative PET/CT results. According to published data, the accuracy of SUVmax by itself for distinguishing PCNSL from high-grade gliomas or glioblastomas was 86 %, the sensitivity was 100 %, and the specificity was 71.4 %, when the cutoff value of SUVmax was set at 12 [7]. In a recent analysis by Yamaguchi et al., a superiority of the ratio, tumor to the contralateral cortex (T/N ratio), for the characterization of brain tumors was stated [8]. This ratio was independent of the factors that influence SUVmax and is therefore suggested to be incorporated in further evaluations. Lastly, 18-FDG PET/CT can be a valuable tool for the response to treatment, although data are missing as to the perfect time of reevaluation, in order to change the modality treatment and to predict disease outcome [9].

13.2 Diagnosis: Primary Non-Hodgkin's Lymphoma of the Central Nervous System (PCNSL)

A male patient, 65 years old, was admitted to our department with the diagnosis of PCNSL. During the last 5 months, he complained of weakness of the lower extremities with nausea and occasional vomiting. As his past history included diabetes type II, hypertension, and total thyroidectomy due to papillary carcinoma, he underwent blood analysis which was inconclusive. One month before his admission, he developed left-sided hemiparesis with mild aphasia. Brain MRI findings were consistent with brain tumor in the right temporoparietal area with regional edema (abnormal signal intensity in the right periventricular white matter involving the right optical thalamus and the ipsilateral cerebral peduncle). Dexamethasone was introduced with improvement of the symptoms. Subsequent MRI spectroscopy was in favor of anaplastic astrocytoma grade III. Therefore a stereotactic biopsy was performed which demonstrated infiltration of the brain parenchyma by a diffuse large B-cell lymphoma (CD20+, Ki-67:85 %). The patient was negative for HIV, HCV, HBV, and HTLVI + II and negative for *Toxoplasma*, CMV, and EBV. CT scans of the thorax and abdomen, as well as blood immunophenotype and bone marrow aspiration plus biopsy, were free of disease. LDH and β2-microglobulin were within normal range. The cerebrospinal fluid had no cells and low protein. The patient received three cycles of high-dose cytarabine and methotrexate with improvement of the left upper and lower extremity mobility and strength. The previously described lesion of the right hemisphere had resolved in the new brain MRI (Fig. 13.1), and the patient was discharged for a few days, to recuperate from drug toxicity.

In order to answer the question whether he could omit further treatment, we performed a total body 18-FDG PET/CT, which surprisingly demonstrated a very avid lesion in the periventricular area of the right white matter (SUVmax 10) and three more foci in the left island of Reil and left external capsule (Fig. 13.2).

Since there was no PET/CT study at diagnosis for comparison, the patient received one more cycle of the same therapeutic agents and was reevaluated with MRI and PET/CT scans (Figs. 13.3 and 13.4). The disease had recurred to the periventricular area, right basal ganglia, and thalamus on MRI, while PET/CT detected extensive uptake in the right brain hemisphere and the liver with SUVmax 28 and 10, respectively.

The patient became gradually aphasic with paresis of the IX and X cranial nerves and left hemiplegia. Total brain irradiation of 30 Gy was offered afterward with minimal response. The patient died 1 month after the completion of radiotherapy while sleeping.

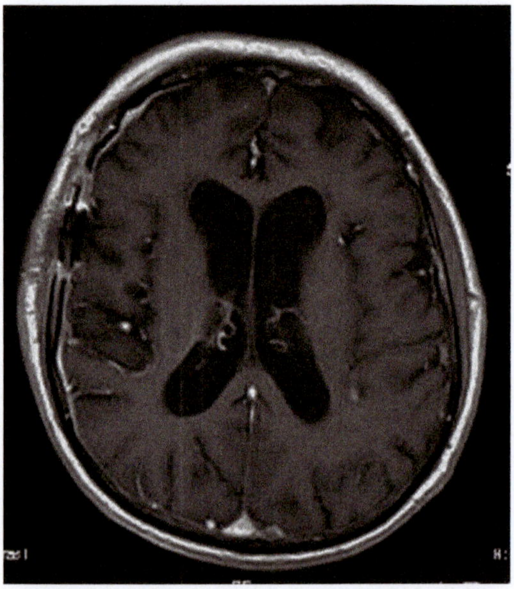

Fig. 13.1 Axial T1-weighted image, post contrast medium administration, shows no foci of abnormal contrast enhancement in the periventricular area of the right brain hemisphere. No evidence of residual disease is identified

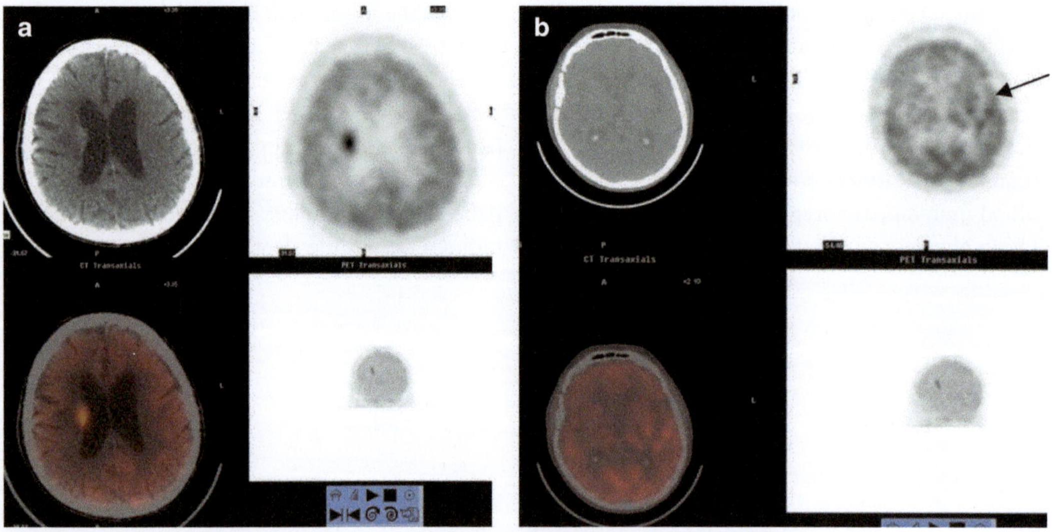

Fig. 13.2 (**a**) Abnormal FDG uptake is identified in the right periventricular white matter (SUV max 10). (**b**) Three more foci of abnormal uptake are seen in the left island of Reil and left external capsule (*arrow*)

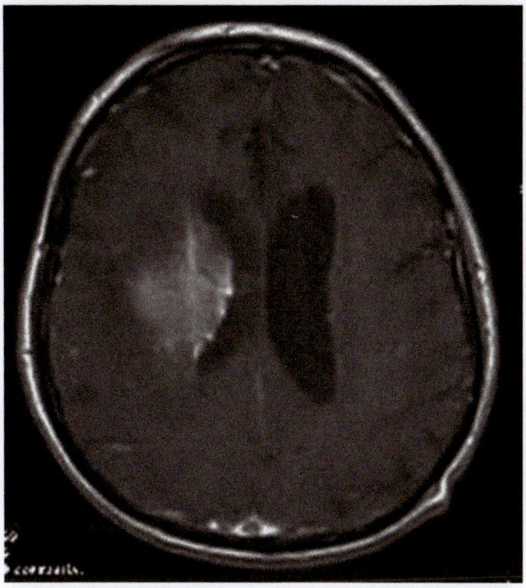

Fig. 13.3 T1-weighted image post contrast medium administration, showing an area with intense enhancement in the right periventricular area, a finding more compatible with recurrence

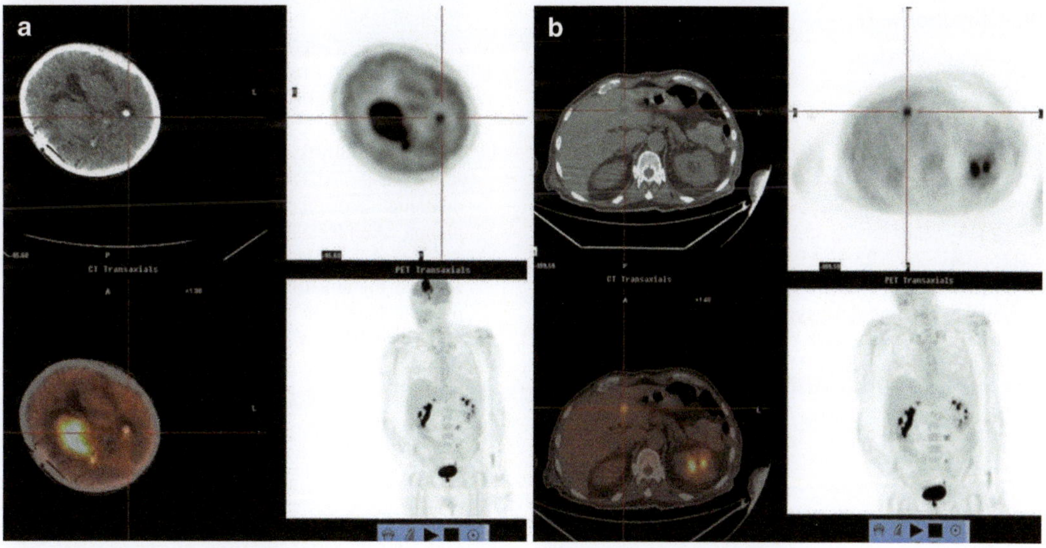

Fig. 13.4 (**a**) Abnormal FDG uptake in the periventricular area of the right brain hemisphere (SUVmax 28) and in the calcified choroid plexus of the occipital horns of the lateral ventricles. (**b**) Abnormal uptake is seen in segment III of the liver (SUVmax 10)

13.3 Discussion

The standard imaging method for initial diagnosis of PCNSL and response assessment to therapy is gadolinium-enhanced MRI scan and, when this is contraindicated, contrast-enhanced CT scan [5]. In the last decade, there is an increasing number of publications emphasizing on the added value of FDG PET/CT scan in initial diagnosis, and on follow-up of PCNSL, due to its high and homogeneous uptake of FDG [9]. In our case the result of MRI scan after three cycles of chemotherapy was negative, in contrast to PET/CT scan, which revealed foci of lymphoma, characterizing the status of the patient as partial remission. Within 2 months the patient developed a full-blown recurrence confirmed on both MRI and PET/CT. Interim PET/CT is not an established method for response assessment to therapy of DLBCL, which comprises the main histologic subtype of PCNSL. Studies examining the predictive value of interim PET, especially in the rituximab era, show conflicting results [10–12]. More studies are needed in that direction.

References

1. Rubenstein JL, Gupta NK, Mannis GN et al (2013) How I treat CNS lymphomas. Blood 122(14): 2318–2330
2. Ferreri AJ, Reni M, Foppoli M et al (2009) International Extranodal Lymphoma Study Group (IELSG). High-dose cytarabine plus high-dose methotrexate versus high-dose methotrexate alone in patients with primary CNS lymphoma: a randomised phase 2 trial. Lancet 31:1512–1520
3. Rubenstein JL, His ED, Johnson JL et al (2013) Intensive chemotherapy and immunotherapy in patients with newly diagnosed primary CNS lymphoma: CALGB 50202 (Alliance 50202). J Clin Oncol 31(25):3061–3068
4. Ferreri AJ, Blay JY, Reni M et al (2003) Prognostic scoring system for primary CNS lymphomas: the International Extranodal Lymphoma Study Group experience. J Clin Oncol 21(2):266–272
5. Abrey LE, Batchelor TT, Ferreri AJ et al (2005) Report of an International Workshop to standardize baseline evaluation and response criteria for Primary CNS Lymphoma. J Clin Oncol 23:5034–5043
6. Haldorsen IS, Espeland A, Larsson EM (2011) Central nervous system lymphoma: characteristic findings on traditional and advanced imaging. AJNR Am J Neuroradiol 32(6):984–992
7. Makino K, Hirai T, Nakamura H et al (2011) Does adding FDG-PET to MRI improve the differentiation between primary cerebral lymphoma and glioblastoma? Observer performance study. Ann Nucl Med 25:432–438
8. Yamaguchi S, Hirata K, Kobayashi H et al (2014) The diagnostic role of (18) F -FDG PET for primary central nervous system lymphoma. Ann Nucl Med 28(7):603–609
9. Kawai N, Miyake K, Yamamoto Y et al (2013) 18F-FDG PET in the diagnosis and treatment of Primary Central Nervous System Lymphoma. BioMed Res Int 2013:247152
10. Zinzani PL, Gandolfi L, Broccoli A et al (2011) Midtreatment 18F-fluorodeoxyglucose positron emission tomography in aggressive non-Hodgkin lymphoma. Cancer 117(5):1010–1018
11. Avigdor A, Sirotkin T, Kedmi M et al (2014) The impact of R-VACOP-B and interim FDG-PET/CT on outcome in primary mediastinal large B cell lymphoma. Ann Hematol 93(8):1297–1304
12. Swinnen LJ, Li H, Quon A et al (2015) Response-adapted therapy for aggressive non-Hodgkin's lymphomas based on early [18F] FDG-PET scanning: ECOG-ACRIN Cancer Research Group study (E3404). Br J Haematol 170(1):56–65

The Role of PET/CT Scan in Primary Gastric Lymphomas

14

Sotirios G. Papageorgiou, Vasiliki P. Filippi, and Sofia N. Chatziioannou

14.1 Introduction

Primary gastric non-Hodgkin lymphomas (PG-NHL) are localized in the stomach, with or without perigastric and/or abdominal lymph node involvement, and represent 20–30 % of all primary extranodal NHL. PG-NHL show an incidence of 1 per 100,000 of the population in Western countries, but the incidence is progressively increasing [1]. Any histological subtype can arise in the stomach, but the main two histological subtypes of PG-NHL are diffuse large B-cell lymphoma (DLBCL) and MALT NHL which represent 60 % and 35 % of the cases, respectively [2, 3]. *Helicobacter pylori* infection has been implicated in the pathogenesis of PG MALT NHL[4, 5], but its role in gastric DLBCL is controversial [6] (Fig. 14.1).

S.G. Papageorgiou, MD, PhD (✉)
2nd Department of Internal Medicine, Propaedeutic, Hematology Unit, "Attikon" University General Hospital, Athens, Greece
e-mail: sotirispapageorgiou@hotmail.com

V.P. Filippi
Department of CT-MRI and PET/CT, Hygeia Hospital, Athens, Greece

S.N. Chatziioannou
Department of Nuclear Medicine, National and Kapodistrian University of Athens, Sotiria Hospital, Athens, Greece

Clinical presentation of PG-NHL is nonspecific and variable, with abdominal pain being the most common symptom followed by dyspepsia, vomiting, nausea, and anorexia. Gastric bleeding, as presenting symptom, occurs in 20–30 % of patients, while gastric occlusion and perforation are less common [2]. Weight loss is common, probably because of the localization of the disease rather than a constitutional symptom. Bone marrow involvement, elevated LDH, and B symptoms are less common in gastric compared to nodal lymphomas.

The diagnosis is usually set by endoscopy which mainly reveals nonspecific gastritis or peptic ulcer with mass lesions being unusual [7]. Occasionally, PG-NHL can present as a multifocal stomach disease with numerous clonally identical foci in macroscopically unaffected tissue [8]. Therefore, gastric mapping of unaffected mucosa is crucially recommended in order to establish diagnosis. PG MALT NHL is characterized by the presence of lymphoepithelial lesions that are formed by invasion of single glands by aggregates of neoplastic cells with centrocyte morphology [9], in contrast to DLBCL where lymphoma infiltrating cells show a centroblastic morphology [10].

Staging work-up for PG-NHL includes complete hematological biochemical examinations (including LDH and beta-2-microglobulin); computed tomography (CT) of the chest,

J.A. Andreou et al. (eds.), *PET/CT in Lymphomas: A Case-Based Atlas*,
DOI 10.1007/978-3-319-27380-8_14

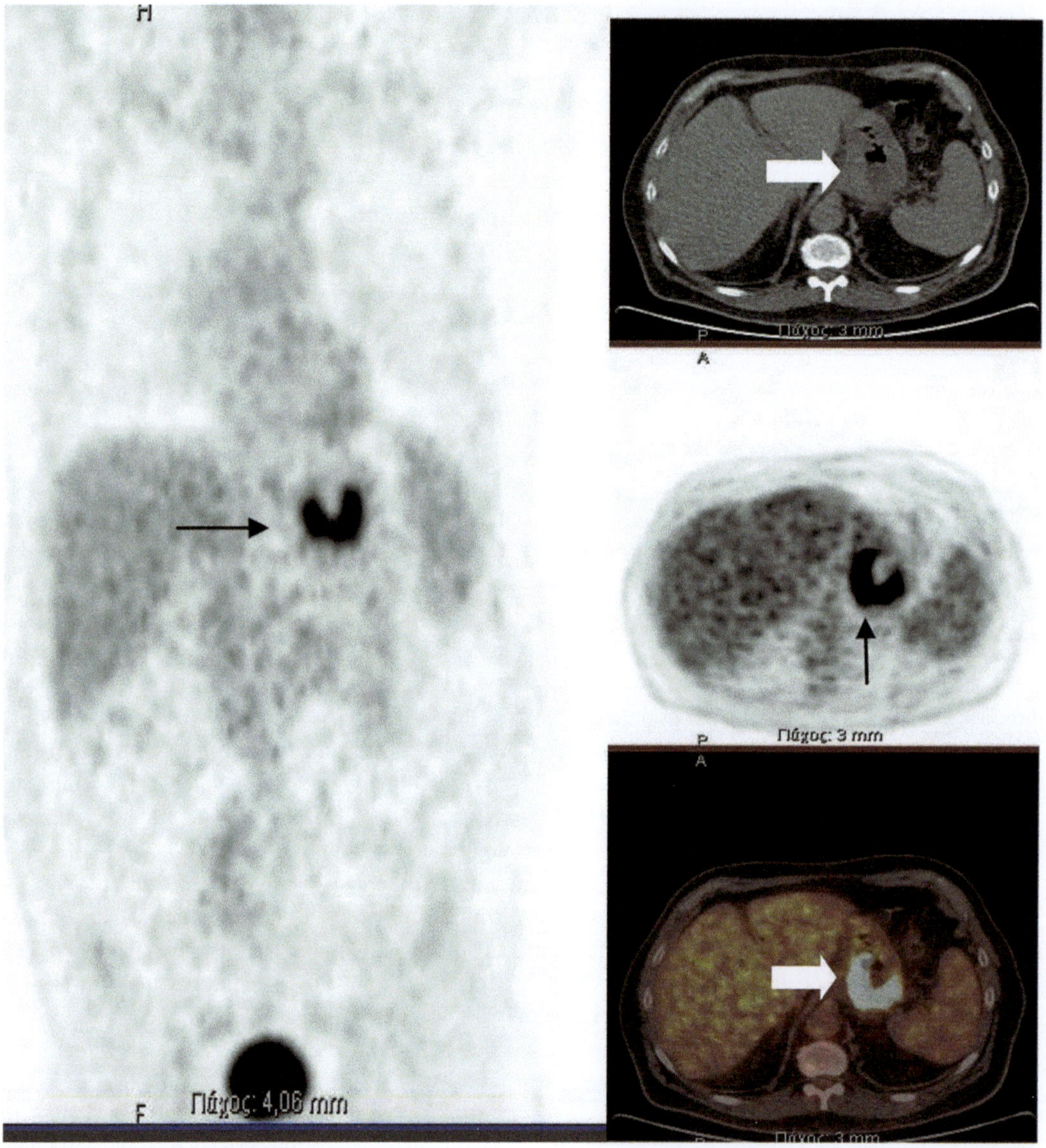

Fig. 14.1 A 67-year-old male with DLBCL. Initial staging evaluation with PET/CT (coronal PET images (*left*) and transverse CT, PET, and fused images (*right*)) demonstrates thickening of the fundus of the stomach on the CT (*thick arrow*) with markedly increased tracer activity on the PET images (*thin arrows*) (SUVmax=22.9) (*thin arrows*)

abdomen, and pelvis; and bone marrow aspiration and biopsy. Upper GI endoscopy and multiple biopsies of the stomach, duodenum, gastroesophageal junction and of abnormal-appearing lesions are required. An endoscopic ultrasound should be performed to determine the depth of invasion and the presence of perigastric nodes. Examination of the pharynx by an otorhinolaryngologist should be performed to exclude infiltration of Waldeyer ring that is occasionally associated with PG-NHL. Histochemistry (Genta stain or Warthin-Starry stain) and breath test should be carried out to determine the presence of active *H. pylori* infection. If histology is negative, serology should be undertaken to identify truly negative *H. pylori* gastric MALT NHL which is present in approximately 10 % of the cases [1] (Fig. 14.2).

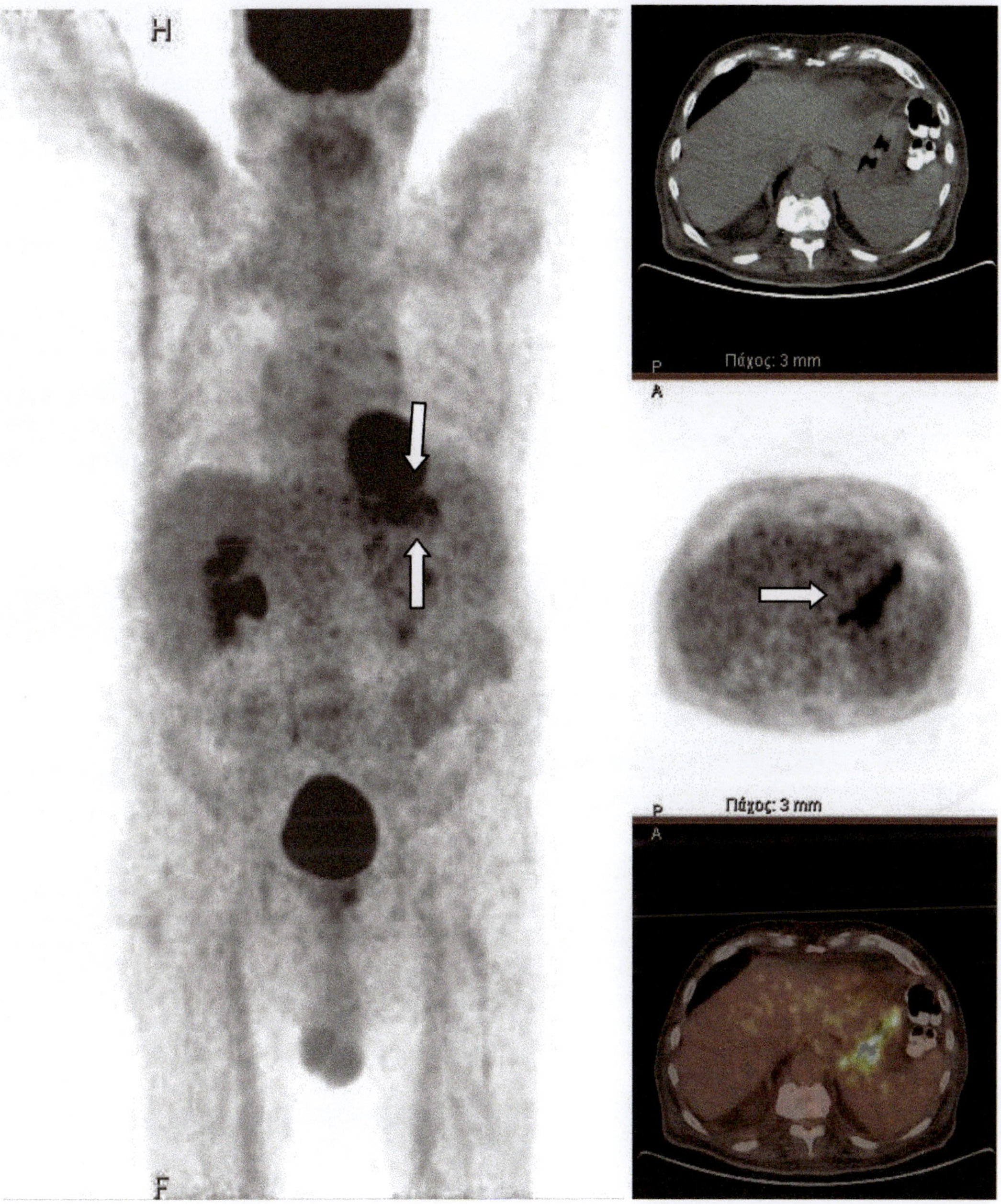

Fig. 14.2 An 85-year-old male with MALT lymphoma. Initial staging evaluation with PET/CT (coronal PET images (*left*) and transverse CT, PET, and fused images (*right*)) demonstrates markedly increased tracer activity in the stomach on the PET images (SUVmax = 6.8) (*arrows*)

The diagnostic value of fluorine-18-2-fluoro-2-deoxy-D-glucose positron emission tomography (^{18}F-FDG-PET) scan has been well established only in PG DLBCL while its use is controversial for PG MALT NHL. Although initial studies reported that ^{18}F-FDG-PET scan was not useful in the staging of PG MALT NHL [11], subsequent studies suggested otherwise. However, the sensitivity of ^{18}F-FDG-PET in detecting PG MALT NHL remains lower than the sensitivity for detecting PG DLBCL [12]. One study showed a detection rate of 80 % for PG MALT NHL [13]. More recently, Radan et al., using the combined technology of ^{18}F-FDG-PET with CT (^{18}F-FDG-PET/CT) scan, found its sensitivity to be 100 % for PG DLBCL and 71 % for PG MALT NHL [14]. The main limitation on the use of PET/CT in gastric MALT lymphoma is the low uptake of the ^{18}F-FDG. It has been hypothesized that the lower ^{18}F-FDG uptake in gastric MALT lymphoma may be due to a more heterogeneous cellular population with lower metabolic activity shown by small or large B cells or plasma cells [14]. In addition, diffuse physiologic background ^{18}F-FDG uptake in the stomach is another obstacle of PET/CT imaging for the evaluation of these tumors. The ^{18}F-FDG

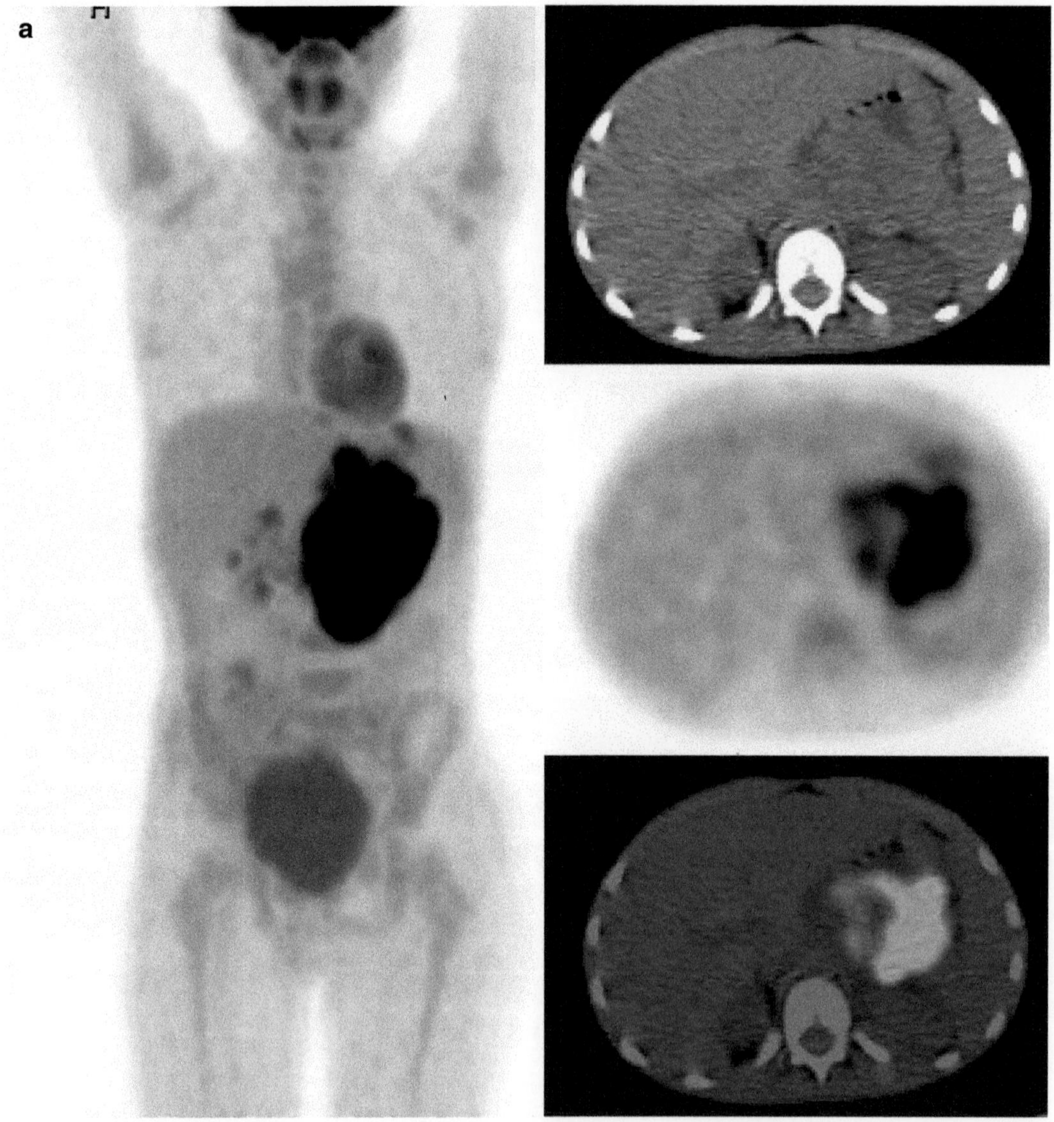

Fig. 14.3 A 9-year-old boy with Burkitt lymphoma. Initial staging evaluation with PET/CT (coronal PET images (**a** *left*) and transverse CT, PET, and fused images (**a** *right*)) demonstrates markedly increased tracer activity in the entire stomach on the PET images (SUVmax = 11.9). Following PET/CT (**b**) after four chemotherapy cycles demonstrates complete resolution of findings

b

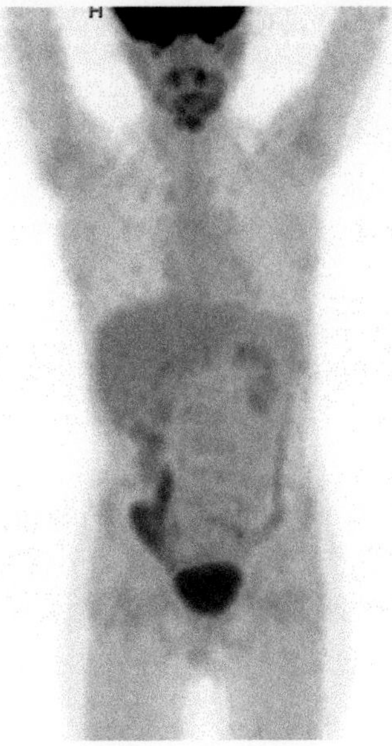

Fig. 14.3 (continued)

uptake pattern in PG-NHL is usually diffuse, less commonly focal, and can involve any portion of the stomach [15].

On the other hand, the majority of PG DLBCL shows increased ^{18}F-FDG uptake, with abnormal gastric wall thickening in CT [16]. The ^{18}F-FDG uptake is usually higher than normal liver uptake, with a maximum standardized uptake value (SUVmax) as high as 15 (±11). Differential diagnosis of gastric ^{18}F-FDG uptake includes physiologic background activity, inflammatory disease, and gastric adenocarcinoma. A major benefit of PET/CT imaging in the PG lymphomas is more accurate detection of the extent of disease. Regional lymph nodes (perigastric, mesenteric, and retroperitoneal lymph nodes) are revealed in 47 % of cases, whereas distant lymph nodes (supraclavicular, infraclavicular, mediastinal, pelvic) are less commonly affected. Extragastric disease is identified in 61 % of cases of PG lymphoma, usually in DLBCL cases [14]. Finally, ^{18}F-FDG-PET/CT has also been shown to be useful in evaluating the response to therapy of PG-NHL, and a positive ^{18}F-FDG-PET/CT scan after therapy is a strong predictor of relapse [17] (Fig. 14.3).

References

1. Psyrri A, Papageorgiou S, Economopoulos T (2008) Primary extranodal lymphomas of stomach: clinical presentation, diagnostic pitfalls and management. Ann Oncol 19:1992–1999
2. Koch P, del Valle F, Berdel WE et al (2001) Primary gastrointestinal non-Hodgkin's lymphoma: I. Anatomic and histologic distribution, clinical features, and survival data of 371 patients registered in the German Multicenter Study GIT NHL 01/92. J Clin Oncol 19:3861–3873
3. Papaxoinis G, Papageorgiou S, Rontogianni D et al (2006) Primary gastrointestinal non- Hodgkin's lymphoma: a clinicopathologic study of 128 cases in Greece. A Hellenic Cooperative Oncology Group study (HeCOG). Leuk Lymphoma 47:2140–2146
4. Nakamura S, Yao T, Aoyagi K et al (1997) Helicobacter pylori and primary gastric lymphoma. A histopathologic and immunohistochemical analysis of 237 patients. Cancer 79:3–11
5. Hussell T, Isaacson PG, Crabtree JE, Spencer J (1993) The response of cells from lowgrade B-cell gastric lymphomas of mucosa-associated lymphoid tissue to Helicobacter pylori. Lancet 342:571–574
6. Chen LT, Lin JT, Tai JJ et al (2005) Long-term results of anti-Helicobacter pylori therapy in early stage gastric high-grade transformed MALT lymphoma. J Natl Cancer Inst 97:1345–1353
7. Andriani A, Zullo A, Di Raimondo F et al (2006) Clinical and endoscopic presentation of primary gastric lymphoma: a multicentre study. Aliment Pharmacol Ther 23:721–726
8. Wotherspoon A, Doglioni C, Isaacson PG (1992) Low-grade gastric B-cell lymphoma of mucosa-associated lymphoid tissue (MALT): a multifocal disease. Histopathology 20:29–34
9. Papadaki L, Wotherspoon AC, Isaacson PG (1992) The lymphoepithelial lesion of gastric low-grade B-cell lymphoma of mucosa-associated lymphoid tissue (MALT): an ultrastructural study. Histopathology 21:415–421
10. Isaacson PG, Du MQ (2005) Gastrointestinal lymphoma: where morphology meets molecular biology. J Pathol 205:255–274
11. Hoffmann M, Kletter K, Diemling M et al (1999) Positron emission tomography with fluorine-18-2-fluoro-2-deoxy-D-glucose (F18-FDG) does not visualize extranodal B-cell lymphoma of the mucosa-associated lymphoid tissue (MALT)-type. Ann Oncol 10:1185–1189
12. Ambrosini V, Rubello D, Castellucci P et al (2006) Diagnostic role of 18F-FDG PET in gastric MALT lymphoma. Nucl Med Rev Cent East Eur 9:37–40
13. Beal KP, Yeung HW, Yahalom J (2005) FDG-PET scanning for detection and staging of extranodal marginal zone lymphomas of the MALT type: a report of 42 cases. Ann Oncol 16:473–480

14. Radan L, Fischer D, Bar-Shalom R et al (2008) FDG avidity and PET/CT patterns in primary gastric lymphoma. Eur J Nucl Med Mol Imaging 35: 1424–1430
15. Paes FM, Kalkanis DG, Sideras PA, Serafini AN (2010) FDG PET/CT of extranodal involvement in non-Hodgkin lymphoma and Hodgkin disease. Radiographics 30:269–291
16. Yun M, Yang W, Lee Y, Kim T-S, Cho A, Lee J (2006) Patterns of FDG uptake in primary gastric lymphoma including MALT lymphoma. J Nucl Med 47 (Suppl 1):452
17. Kumar R, Xiu Y, Potenta S et al (2004) 18F-FDG PET for evaluation of the treatment response in patients with gastrointestinal tract lymphomas. J Nucl Med 45:1796–1803

Primary Cutaneous Lymphomas

15

Marina P. Siakantaris, Alexandra V. Nikaki, and Despina J. Savvidou

15.1 Introduction

Primary cutaneous lymphomas (PCL) are defined as non-Hodgkin lymphomas affecting primarily the skin. They are the second most frequent extranodal lymphomas after the gastrointestinal ones. The vast majority of PCL are of the T-cell lineage (≈75 %), whereas the B-cell types account for 20–25 % [1, 2]. The PCL are unique diseases, different from their nodal counterparts in terms of pathogenesis, prognosis, and treatment. According to the most recent WHO-EORTC classification, where PCL are described as separate entities, an important effort has been made in order to accurately diagnose these uncommon diseases and treat them in a more uniform manner [3]. Concerning the primary cutaneous B-cell lymphomas (PCBCL), three main subgroups have been well recognized: the primary cutaneous marginal zone lymphoma (PCMZL), the primary cutaneous follicle center lymphoma (PCFCL), and the primary cutaneous diffuse large B-cell lymphoma, leg type (PCLBCL, LT). The first two exhibit an excellent prognosis (5-year survival >90 %), while the latter is more aggressive with a worse survival (5-year survival: 20–50 %). The etiology of the indolent forms (PCMZL, PCFCL) is not clear, and although there were some previous data connecting the tumors with *Borrelia burgdorferi* infection, such a correlation was not confirmed in a large case-controlled study [4]. An antigenic selection has been proposed in the pathogenesis of PCBCL through the evidence of somatic hypermutations of the cases studied by Dijkman et al. [5]. The abnormal expression of activation-induced cytidine deaminase (AID) in PCLBCL, LT patients could add information in our understanding as to the origin of the disease [6]. Both PCMZL and PCFCL can be treated with local therapy, either excision ± radiotherapy or intralesional immunotherapy with anti-CD20 monoclonal antibodies [7]. There is rarely need for systemic treatment, especially in multifocal disease. The PCMZL tends to recur more often than PCFCL, but the overall survival is not significantly altered. On the other hand, PCLBCL, LT should be treated upfront as the nodal diffuse large B-cell lymphomas with systemic chemoimmunotherapy. Primary cutaneous T-cell lymphomas (PCTCL) constitute a heterogenous group of diseases affecting all layers

M.P. Siakantaris, MD
Department of Internal Medicine, National and Kapodistrian University, Laiko general Hospital, Agiou Thoma 17, Athens, Maroussi 15123, Greece
e-mail: msiaka@med.uoa.gr; siakantaris@gmail.com

A.V. Nikaki
Department of Nuclear Medicine and PET/CT, Hygeia Hospital, Kifissias Av and Erythrou Stavrou 4, Athens, Maroussi 15123, Greece
e-mail: anikaki@gmail.com

D.J. Savvidou (✉)
CT and MRI Department, Hygeia Hospital, Kifissias Av and Erythrou Stavrou 4, Athens, Maroussi 15123, Greece
e-mail: despinasavvidou@yahoo.com

J.A. Andreou et al. (eds.), *PET/CT in Lymphomas: A Case-Based Atlas*,
DOI 10.1007/978-3-319-27380-8_15

of the skin. Mycosis fungoides (MF) is the most common subtype and has an indolent prognosis in the early stages (patch-plaque). The MF cell of origin is a mature (CD3+, CD5+, CD45RO+, TCRβ+), helper (CD4+, CD8−) T lymphocyte, which expresses the cutaneous lymphocyte antigen (CLA), lacks surface antigen CD7, exhibits epidermotropism, and has a characteristic appearance with cerebriform nucleus. It also expresses chemokine receptors as the CXCR4, which facilitates the migration to the dermis through endothelial adherence [8]. Advanced-stage patients present with one or more of the following: tumors (IIB), erythroderma (III), infiltration of lymph nodes (IVA), and visceral spread of the disease (IVB). Advanced-stage cutaneous lymphoma has a poor prognosis [9]. Patients with erythroderma or tumors have a median 5-year OS of 4 years, patients with lymph node disease have a median 5-year OS of 2–3 years, and patients with extracutaneous disease have the worst outcome with a median 5-year OS of 1.5 years. Prognosis is also influenced by age, abnormal LDH, β2-microglobulin, and large cell transformation which occurs in 8–39 % of cases [10].

A thorough staging investigation is important in order to exclude systemic lymphoma that infiltrates the skin secondarily, for the extent of disease and in order to plan the appropriate treatment. CT scan is employed for the detection of lymph node enlargement and organomegaly. It cannot detect the infiltration of the normal-sized lymph nodes or the small extracutaneous sites. Although 18-FDG-PET/CT has been extensively used in various types of lymphoma, its value in PCL is not clearly stated. Small retrospective studies have demonstrated that the limitations of CT can be overcome by the newer methodology of PET, combined with CT [11]. On initial staging, 18-FDG-PET was able to detect cutaneous disease and extracutaneous sites of involvement with a sensitivity of 82 % and 80 %, respectively, while the CT sensitivity was 55 % for local disease and 100 % for extracutaneous lesions [12]. There are concerns about the false negative results of 18-FDG-PET scans especially in early stages where the lesions are small and of low metabolic state. In this setting, the clinical examination is essential in leading biopsy and diagnosis of an abnormal lesion. On restaging after treatment, 18-FDG-PET detected recurrence or residual cutaneous disease with a sensitivity of 86 % and specificity of 92 %, better than CT. The majority of PET studies in PCL have been conducted in cutaneous T-cell lymphoma patients where the FDG uptake was found moderate and was furthermore able to detect areas of high-grade transformation, which reflects poor prognosis [13]. The prompt timing for reevaluation is a matter of discussion. Usually, PET is advised 4–6 weeks after chemotherapy and 8–12 weeks after radiation therapy due to accumulation of nonspecific inflammatory cells and false positive results [14].

Case #1

A 54-year-old male patient presented to our department with the histological diagnosis of primary cutaneous T-cell non-Hodgkin lymphoma of the NOS type. The patient had multiple cutaneous nodules of various sizes ($d \sim 1–3$ cm), on the trunk and extremities. The immunohistochemical study demonstrated the infiltration of the dermis by a medium-sized lymphocytic population which was CD4(±), CD8(−), CD5(±), CD30(−), ALK1(−), TIA-1(+), PD-1(−), and CD56(−), exhibiting a nonactivated cytotoxic phenotype. His past history was unremarkable. The clinical staging according to the TNM staging system was IIB. Due to the adverse prognosis of the tumor-stage disease and the histological subtype, the patient received CHOP combination chemotherapy (cyclophosphamide, adriamycin, vincristine, prednisolone). After two cycles, he was almost free of lesions, but during the fourth cycle of chemotherapy, he recurred with various similar pruritic lesions. A second skin biopsy was performed which was consistent with the same histologic subtype but with an activated cytotoxic phenotype this time. Treatment was changed to CHOEP (CHOP plus Etoposide) every 14 days with quick clearance of the lesions. The patient was immediately harvested after the third cycle and was programmed for progenitor stem cell rescue with salvage treatment, but 2 weeks after the harvest, he again experienced a relapse with a cutaneous tumor at the left thoracic wall. At that time point, he was evaluated with 18-FDG-PET/CT for a detailed assessment of the disease burden which revealed an abnormal cutaneous nodular area at the left frontal chest wall with an SUV uptake of 3.8 and no extra cutaneous lesions (Fig. 15.1). Subsequently, the patient received gemcitabine and pegylated doxorubicin with no response and died with extensive disease including generalized lymphadenopathy and infiltration of Waldeyer's ring.

Discussion

Primary cutaneous T-cell NHL (PCTCL) constitutes 2 % of all lymphomas, with manifestations in all layers of the skin as well as the subcutaneous areas and extra cutaneous involvement of lymph nodes and visceral organs [15]. Diagnosis and staging include biopsy of the affected sites, clinical evaluation, and imaging procedures. FDG-PET/CT is not considered until now the method of choice for the evaluation of skin involvement especially for low-staged disease; however, better than CT alone, it could be used as an assistant tool in assessing the non-cutaneous disease [15–17]. For initial staging in a study including 31 pairs of PET and CT scans in peripheral T-cell lymphomas (19 patients, 15 with cutaneous T-cell lymphoma), the sensitivity of 18-FDG-PET for assessment of cutaneous and extra cutaneous lesions is referred as 82 and 80 %, respectively. Sensitivity and specificity of 18-FDG-PET for restaging is reported 86 and 92 %, respectively for cutaneous and 100 % for extra cutaneous involvement. All the above values were better than CT [12]. Of course, studies investigating the role of FDG-PET/CT in cutaneous lymphomas both in initial staging and for treatment response are scarce; however, the common sense is that 18-FDG-PET may be utilized mainly in evaluating aggressive and extra cutaneous disease, yet physical guided biopsy cannot be omitted.

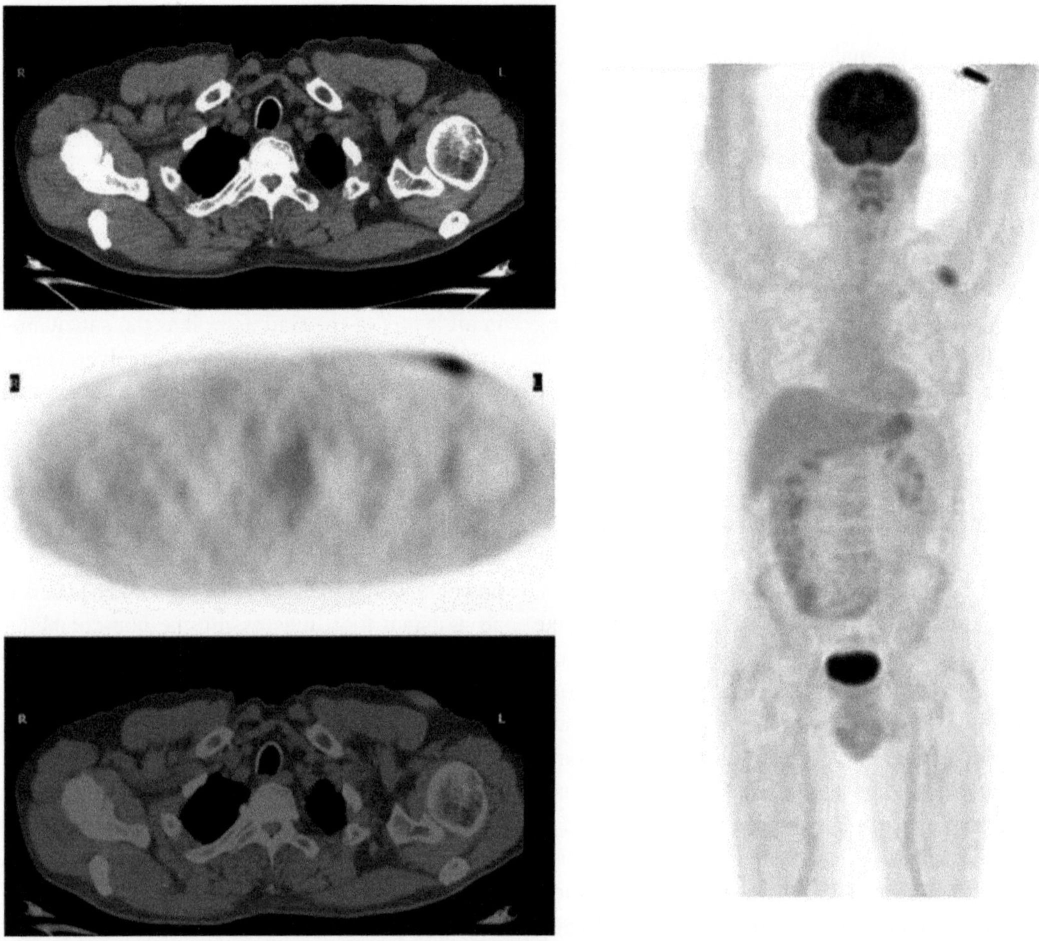

Fig. 15.1 CT, 18-FDG-PET, fused PET/CT, and MIP-PET images reveal the presence of hypermetabolic cutaneous nodule of the left thoracic wall. No other lesions of abnormal increased uptake of the radiopharmaceutical are observed

Case #2

A 65-year-old female patient presented to our department with primary cutaneous T-cell lymphoma of the mycosis fungoides type (MF), diagnosed 3 years before at the plaque stage. At the time of presentation, she had several infiltrated plaques and tumors with severe pruritus and palpable lymph nodes in both axillary and inguinal regions. She had not received any prior treatment and her past history was unremarkable. The skin biopsy showed extensive infiltration of the whole dermis and epidermis by medium to large lymphocytes that expressed CD2, CD3, and CD4>>CD8, while only a few of them were CD30+. The CT scans of the thorax and abdomen detected enlarged lymph nodes in both axillae of 2.4 cm maximum diameter and a left inguinal lymph node of 2.3 cm. The staging investigation was supplemented with a whole-body 18-FDG-PET/CT which demonstrated an SUVmax: 6.2 of the axillary lymph nodes and 6.3 of the left inguinal node (Fig. 15.2). Moreover, there was extensive cutaneous uptake (SUVmax: 12.8) especially on the rear surface of the trunk (Fig. 15.3). The biopsy of the left inguinal lymph node was consistent with T-cell lymphoma of the same type as the skin without a large cell transformation. Therefore, the patient was diagnosed with clinical stage IV, with a high risk of infections due to damaged skin barrier. She received interferon-α at a dose of 3 MIU/d sec combined with local radiation at the largest lesions, with a 50 % reduction of the cutaneous disease and relief of pruritus for a 6 months period. Soon after that, she developed new tumors with ulcers and experienced weakness and B symptoms. The treatment was switched to bexarotene 150 mg/kg po for 4 months without further response and eventually was put on CHOP combination chemotherapy. After two cycles, the patient felt better but refused to continue chemotherapy and discontinued her visits.

Discussion

Mycosis fungoides represents more than 50 % of all cutaneous T-cell lymphomas. 18-FDG-PET, although with better sensitivity than CT in identifying cutaneous involvement, cannot be utilized as the modality of choice in assessing skin lymphoma sites, especially in the patch, plaque, and erythroderma stage [15, 16]. However, 18-FDG-PET is an accurate imaging method in identifying nodal involvement in MF and Sezary syndrome (SS) high-risk patients and can detect lymph node involvement even in normal-sized lymph nodes, with better sensitivity than CT [18]. Moreover and importantly, 18-FDG-PET can be a marker of aggressive large cell transformation in MF and SS cases, as these cases exhibit higher metabolic activity measured as SUV [18, 19].

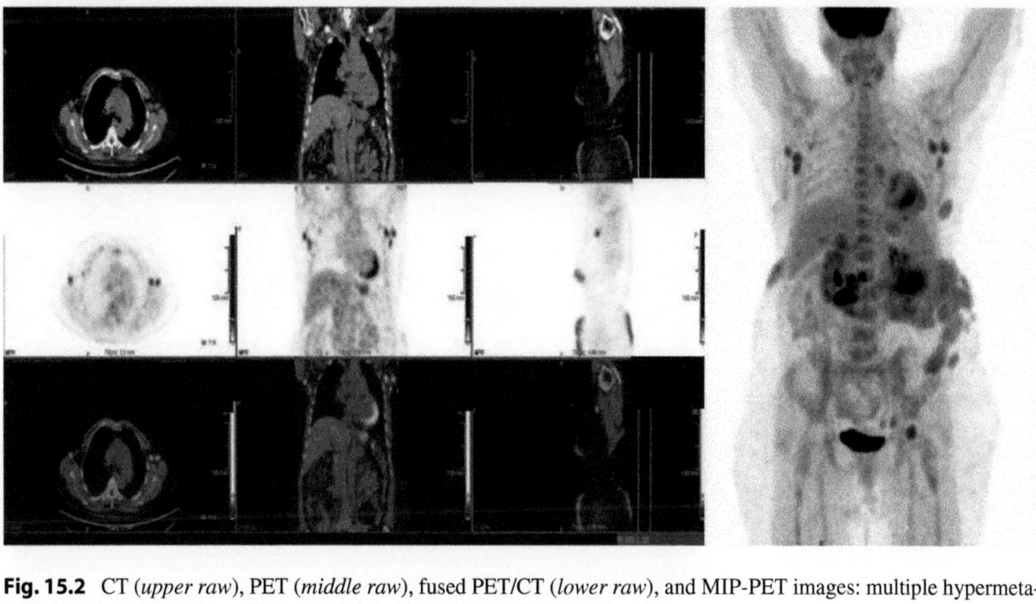

Fig. 15.2 CT (*upper raw*), PET (*middle raw*), fused PET/CT (*lower raw*), and MIP-PET images: multiple hypermetabolic lymph nodes at the axillary area bilaterally and the left inguinal region

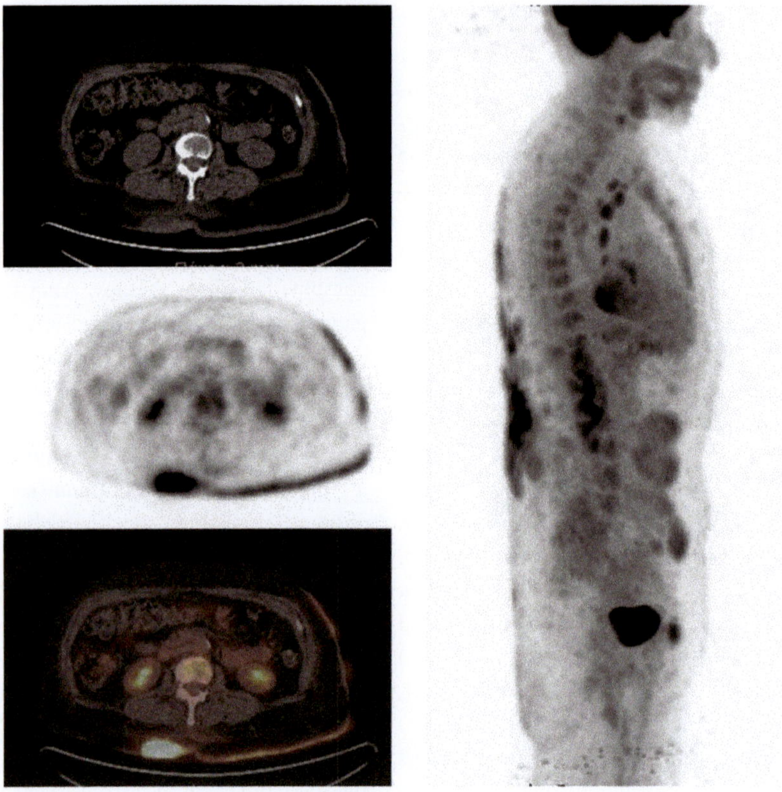

Fig. 15.3 CT (*upper raw*), PET (*middle raw*), fused PET/CT, and MIP-PET images: multiple cutaneous hypermetabolic lesions at the trunk

References

1. Pandolfino TL, Siegel RS, Kuzel TM et al (2000) Primary cutaneous B-cell lymphoma: review and current concepts. J Clin Oncol 18:2152–2168
2. Siegel RS, Pandolfino T, Guitart J et al (2000) Primary cutaneous T-cell lymphoma: review and current concepts. J Clin Oncol 18:2908–2925
3. Willemze R, Jaffe ES, Burg G et al (2005) WHO-EORTC classification for cutaneous lymphomas. Blood 105(10):3768–3785
4. Schöllkopf C, Melbye M, Munksgaard L et al (2008) Borrelia infection and risk of non-Hodgkin lymphoma. Blood 111(12):5524–5529
5. Dijkman R, Tensen CP, Buettner M et al (2006) Primary cutaneous follicle center lymphoma and primary cutaneous large B-cell lymphoma, leg type, are both targeted by aberrant somatic hypermutation but demonstrate differential expression of AID. Blood 107:4926–4929
6. Pasqualucci L, Bhagat G, Jankovic M et al (2008) AID is required for germinal center-derived lymphomagenesis. Nat Genet 40(1):108–112
7. Akhtari M, Reddy JP, Pinnix CC et al (2015) Primary cutaneous B-cell lymphoma (non-leg type) has excellent outcomes even after very low dose radiation as single-modality therapy. Leuk Lymphoma 12:1–5. [Epub ahead of print]
8. Ralfkiaer E, Cerroni L, Sander CA et al (2008) Mycosis fungoides. In: Swerdlow SH, Campo E, Harris NL, Jaffe ES, Pileri SA, Stein H, Thiele J, Vardiman JW (eds) WHO classification of tumours of haematopoietic and lymphoid tissues, 4th edn. International Agency for Research on Cancer, Lyon
9. Kim YH, Liu HL, Mraz-Gernhard S et al (2003) Long-term outcome of 525 patients with mycosis fungoides and Sezary syndrome: clinical prognostic factors and risk for disease progression. Arch Dermatol 139:857–866
10. Vergier B, de Muret A, Beylot-Barry M et al (2000) Transformation of mycosis fungoides: clinicopathological and prognostic features of 45 cases. Blood 95:2212–2218
11. Shapiro M, Yun M, Junkins-Hopkins JM et al (2002) Assessment of tumor burden and treatment response by 18F-fluorodeoxyglucose injection and positron emission tomography in patients with cutaneous T- and B-cell lymphomas. J Am Acad Dermatol 47: 623–628
12. Kumar R, Xiu Y, Zhuang HM, Alavi A (2006) 18F-fluorodeoxyglucose-positron emission tomography in evaluation of primary cutaneous lymphoma. Br J Dermatol 155:357–363
13. Kuo PH, McClennan BL, Carlson K et al (2008) FDG-PET/CT in the evaluation of cutaneous T-cell lymphoma. Mol Imaging Biol 10:74–81
14. Paes FM, Kalkanis DG, Sideras PA, Serafini AN (2010) FDG PET/CT of extranodal involvement in non-Hodgkin lymphoma and Hodgkin disease. Radiographics 30(1):269–291
15. Spaccarelli N, Gharavi M, Saboury B et al (2014) Role of (18)F-fluorodeoxyglucose positron emission tomography imaging in the management of primary cutaneous lymphomas. Hell J Nucl Med 17(2):78–84
16. Kako S, Izutsu K, Ota Y et al (2007) FDG-PET in T-cell and NK-cell neoplasms. Ann Oncol 18(10): 1685–1690
17. Bishu S, Quigley JM, Schmitz J et al (2007) F-18-fluoro-deoxy-glucose positron emission tomography in the assessment of peripheral T-cell lymphomas. Leuk Lymphoma 48(8):1531–1538
18. Tsai EY, Taur A, Espinosa L et al (2006) Staging accuracy in mycosis fungoides and sezary syndrome using integrated positron emission tomography and computed tomography. Arch Dermatol 142(5):577–584
19. Feeney J, Horwitz S, Gönen M, Schöder H (2010) Characterization of T-cell lymphomas by FDG PET/CT. AJR Am J Roentgenol 195(2):333–340

16 Other Rare Extranodal Lymphomas

Catherine G. Stefanoudaki-Sofianatou,
Chariklia D. Giannopoulou,
and Dimitrios T. Kechagias

16.1 Multifocal Primary Bone Lymphoma

Primary bone lymphoma (PBL) is a rare disease exclusively involving the skeleton, accounting for <5 % of extra-nodal lymphomas and 1–2 % of all lymphomas in adults.

Most common is the limited I and II stages of disease, affecting one bone, with or without involvement of regional lymph nodes. A rarer form of PBL is the "multifocal bone lymphoma" (MBL) or "polyostotic" with exclusive multifocal involvement of the skeleton, but not of the lymph nodes or other visceral organs. This constitutes around 3–16 % of cases of the largest reported series of bone lymphomas [1–3]. The most common histological subtype of MBL is diffuse large B-cell lymphoma (DLBCL), also known as MB-DLBCL, occurring in 90 % of cases in western series [2, 4], as opposed to 68 % in Japanese. The immunophenotype of the cells in DLCL is consistent with a germinal center origin [5]. Other histological subtypes of MBL include follicular, marginal zone, NK/T cell, anaplastic large cell, and Burkitt's lymphoma and, more rarely, Hodgkin's lymphoma [4].

MB-DLCL presents particular clinical and prognostic characteristics.

There is a slight male predominance, with the median age 53 years, but cases involving children have also been reported [2, 4, 6].

Bone pain is the main symptom, 92 %, which may be accompanied by palpable mass of soft tissue attached to the affected bones, in 20–50 % of cases [2–5]. Any bone can be affected, but most often they are the weight-bearing long bones, the spine, the skull, and the pelvis. However, complications which do not seem to be irreversible occur when the location is on the vertebrae and the ribs, resulting in compression and/or dislocation of the spinal cord [4, 6]. Spine was the most frequently presented site of MBL in another recent study [5]. The diaphysis is the most common site of the lesions of the long bones, with a later progression to the metaphysis and epiphysis [5, 6]. Bone lesions can result in pathological fractures in 15–20 % of cases, but skeletal complications do not seem to confer a worse prognosis [7].

General symptoms of weight loss and fever can occur in 30 %. With progressive disease and

C.G. Stefanoudaki-Sofianatou, MD, PhD (✉)
Haematologist, Department of Haematology,
Agioi Anargiroi General & Oncological Hospital,
N. Kifissia, Raidestou 2, Athens 16122, Greece
e-mail: katy.stefanoudaki@gmail.com

C.D. Giannopoulou
Nuclear Medicine Department, Evangelismos
Hospital, G.N.A. "ANNUNCIATION",
Ypsilantou 45-47, Athens 10676, Greece
e-mail: harisg@otenet.gr

D.T. Kechagias
Ultrasound, Curator Department of PET/CT,
D.TH.K.A. "HEALTH",
Kifissias Av. & Q. Cross 4, Maroussi 15123, Greece

J.A. Andreou et al. (eds.), *PET/CT in Lymphomas: A Case-Based Atlas*,
DOI 10.1007/978-3-319-27380-8_16

the presence of osteolysis, hypercalcemia, rarely accompanied by symptoms, is observed in 5–15 % [6].

Though the above symptoms can affect general fitness, patients usually have good ECOG performance status, 0–1.

Radiological image findings are positive in more than 90 % and reveal the location and extent of the disease. Both lytic and osteoblastic patterns can be shown by plain films; nevertheless, CT and MRI scans give a more detailed picture concerning not only the presence of extraosseous extension but also the infiltration of the bones by the tumor. But again, the CT and MRI findings are nonspecific indicating usually an aggressive pattern of bone destruction [8]. Bone scan with technetium-99 m-MDP radionuclide imaging contributes to the discovery of additional sites of bone involvement. Functional imaging with ^{18}FDG-positron emission tomography/computed tomography, ^{18}FDG-PET/CT (^{18}FDG-PET), more thoroughly discloses sites of the disease by exploiting ^{18}FDG avid cells, usually suggesting an aggressive histology [9]. The ^{18}FDG-PET scan surpasses CT in that it provides greater sensitivity, specificity, and accuracy, 97 %, 100 %, and 98 %, respectively, compared to 87 %, 85 %, and 84 % of CT [8].

^{18}FDG-PET has been shown to be more sensitive and specific than 99 m Tc scan for the detection of osseous and extraosseous lesions by lymphoma, as well as for the early lymphomatous infiltration, before it has caused extensive bone destruction [10–12]. With the combined use of CT, MRI, and PET, MBL stage IV disease is more accurately and in a higher proportion of patients diagnosed, which is essential for the decision of the therapeutic strategy [9]. Furthermore, ^{18}FDG-PET is able to distinguish between posttreatment fibrosis and residual viable tumor, as it is suggested from a number of studies, thus contributing to a more precise post treatment restaging [13].

Adequate tissue sample for histological examination and immunophenotyping is the gold standard for diagnosis [4]. Excision biopsy of the bone is not usually recommended due to the risk of pathological fracture, inaccessibility, or false-negative results.

A staging system different from the Ann Arbor has been proposed for the staging of MB-DLBCL in a recent analysis of the International Extra Nodal Lymphoma Study Group (IELSG), based on the different outcome and prognosis between the patients of MB-DLBCL and disseminated DLBCL with secondary skeleton involvement, who share similar clinical features and treatment modalities [6]. According to this proposal, bone lymphomas are classified into four different stages: stage IE = single bony lesion, IIE = single bony lesion plus regional lymphadenopathy, IVE = polyostotic lymphoma, and IV = conventional stage IV lymphoma with skeletal involvement [6].

Radiotherapy, chemotherapy, or their combination has been used with varying results on this rare condition. Until recently, most information was available from anecdotal cases and unselected bone lymphoma series that were not consistent throughout. Already from the initial studies, it has been suggested that MBL can be acknowledged as a specific clinicopathologic entity of PBL due to the surprisingly high (61 %) overall survival (OS) at 5 years, even with stage IV disease patients [3].

In the IELSG-14 retrospective study mentioned above, the comparison of 37 MB-DLBCL patients to 63 controls of advanced stage DLCL with skeletal involvement and similar clinical and treatment characteristics (anthracycline containing regimens ± radiotherapy) demonstrated a significantly better response rate (RR) 92 % vs. 65 %, 5-year progression-free survival (PFS) 57 % vs. 35 %, and 5-year OS 75 % vs. 37 %, of the group with MB-DLBCL [6]. The improved outcomes were independent of the international prognostic index (IPI) and other prognostic variables, further indicating that MB-DLBCL should be considered a different condition [2, 3]. A positive effect of radiotherapy in MB-DLBCL, noticed in the above study with 5-year OS 83 % in the combined modality treatment (CMT) arm vs. 55 % in the chemotherapy (CT) arm, was attributed by the authors to probable patient selection bias [6]. In spite of this, they conclude that radiation could be recommended on special occasions and if the expected toxicity from radiotherapy is acceptable [6]. However, regarding the usefulness of consolidative radiotherapy, in a large series of 131 patients of the British Columbia Cancer Agency, it was not confirmed that advanced stage patients of PBL receiving CMT on an individualized basis experienced a better 10-year OS than those on chemotherapy alone (25 % vs. 56 %) [7].

With the advent of rituximab, there seems to have been significant improvement in results. Consequently, the comparison between CHOP or CHOP-like chemotherapy and CHOP combined with rituximab showed that the latter brought about an improvement in progression-free survival, from 52 to 88 % at 3 years and overall response rates of 92 % [6, 7]. Using similar chemotherapy plus rituximab and consolidative radiotherapy on half the patients of a recent smaller series, which however also included limited stage PBL cases, the reported 8-year OS was 95.2 % and the disease free survival (DFS) 100 % with no relapses reported after a median follow-up of 43.9 months [14]. In the post-rituximab and post-positron emission tomography era, "it is not entirely clear if CMT could be the standard of care for all cases of PBL or CT alone should be adequate in some cases" [4].

The general prognosis of the disease is not consistent throughout. The small number of patients per study and unselected bone lymphoma cases has contributed to this inconsistency. The IPI cannot, on the other hand, be used comprehensively, as stage and number of extra-nodal sites have no variability in polyostotic bone lymphoma and PBL [6]. However, age, performance status, and serum LDH were all prognostic variables associated with survival [3, 6, 7].

Additionally, as the bones of the skull are a frequent site of disease, it has been suggested that there is an increased risk of central nervous system (CNS) dissemination [4]. CNS involvement in the ENLSG-14 study was 5 % in patients with polyostotic DLBCL [6]. However, the above rates would be even lower in the rituximab era since reduced CNS dissemination has been reported in DLBCL patients treated with the anti-CD20 monoclonal antibody [15]. Theoretically, skull and spine lesions could disseminate to the CNS by direct invasion and this possibility cannot be ignored [6, 7].

There are some issues concerning the evaluation of patient response both during and after the treatment. The alleviation of symptoms and the decrease of the soft tissue element in image examinations, mainly CT or MRI scans, are the first signs of remission of the disease. Posttreatment examination will most probably reveal persistent bone abnormalities due to the time needed for bone remodeling. As far as ^{18}FDG-PET is concerned, no increased uptake would be a sign of complete response even in the persistence of radiological or MRI abnormalities [4]. Similarly, residual increased uptake of the tracer may still result in the case of bone healing and remodeling, since increased metabolism and malignancy are indistinguishable [4].

16.2 Case Study: Multifocal Primary Bone Lymphoma

An 82-year-old woman patient was admitted to hospital because of intense bone pain in the chest, the back and extremities, swelling of the left elbow, and low-grade fever which gradually had deteriorated during the last year.

On clinical examination she appeared suffering and disabled due to bone pain. Another soft tissue mass, 3.3 cm, was palpable on the left frontal. No other abnormalities were detected.

Laborative investigation revealed Hb 10.2 g/dl, Hct 30.3 %, ESR 47 mm, LDH 362 U/L (230–450), alkaline phosphatase 155 U/L (80–270 U/L), C-reactive protein 24.2 mg/L (<5 mg/L), beta-2 microglobulin 5.93 mg/L (1.2–2.0 mg/L), and protein electrophoresis borderline hypoglobulinemia. The viral serologies for HIV, hepatitis B, and hepatitis C were negative.

Plain x-ray films and CT and MRI scans disclosed osteolytic and sclerotic lesions in multiple bones including the vertebrae, ribs, skull, femur, and humerus. Bone lesions presented increased uptake on Tc-99 m-MDP bone scan.

In addition to the abnormal bone findings, soft tissue masses were disclosed, one extrapleural originating from the posterior aspects of the 9th right rib and entering the spinal canal causing pressure and dislocation of the spinal cord; another subcutaneous under the left frontal, adjacent to bone damage; and a third one surrounding the distal part of the left humerus. Biopsy of the chest wall mass revealed the diagnosis of an extranodal diffuse non-Hodgkin's lymphoma (NHL) infiltrating the muscles and the connective tissue of the thoracic wall, consisting mostly of large lymphoid B cells (DLBCL) CD20+, CD79a+, BCL-6+ (Fig. 16.1).

Lymph nodes or other visceral involvements were not detected in the chest, abdomen, and pelvis contrast CT scans. Bone marrow biopsy did not show any evidence of lymphoma infiltration.

Further staging with ^{18}FDG-PET/CT (^{18}FDG-PET) scan showed multiple foci of increased FDG uptake in the left elbow, left shoulder, middle and lower part of the right hemithorax, multiple vertebrae, the pelvis, the right hip, and the right and left femur, involving on some sites the adjacent soft tissues (Fig. 16.2).

Based on the above findings, the diagnosis of polyostotic or multifocal primary bone lymphoma (M-PBL), stage IVE, was established. The patient proceeded to immunochemotherapy with eight cycles of the CHOP-R regimen, with significant alleviation of symptoms soon after the start of therapy. During treatment and upon the completion of therapy, new CT and MRI scans of the affected areas showed the disappearance, before the third cycle of chemotherapy, of the paravertebral and left elbow masses, with no more epidural pressure. Persistence of all, almost unchanged bone damage was demonstrated on the subsequent MRI's and CT's, as well as residual poorly defined lesion in the thoracic wall, which was no longer visible after 1 year, without the continuation of any treatment.

No communication with the patient was possible for a 7 year period, but when contact was recently restored, it was confirmed that she is alive, apparently in complete remission.

Discussion

Polyostotic or M-PBL is an extremely rare and distinct subtype of PBL affecting multiple osseous sites without lymph node or visceral involvement [16]. It is a peculiar clinicopathological entity from the aspect of prognosis and treatment outcome [5, 7, 14]. The axial skeleton is more commonly involved with potential spinal cord complications. The interval between the onset of symptoms and diagnosis is about 8 months [7].

In approximately 50 % of cases, soft tissue extension of the osseous disease can occur, producing palpable masses which can be accessible for biopsy. In the rest of the cases, a surgical procedure would be necessary for performing a diagnostic biopsy [17]. Bone image findings are not always characteristic or uniform at PBL, not only in diagnosis but also throughout treatment and follow-up, and abnormalities can persist for a long period of time. In addition, tumor necrosis or inflammation changes create difficulties in differentiation from residual bone disease [17]. ^{18}FDG-PET scan is a well-established technique, not only for initial staging but also for evaluating the response to treatment. A negative ^{18}FDG-PET scan indicates complete response; however, a positive scan is not always indicative of disease [18]. Clinical improvement and the accompanied disappearance of soft tissue mass are the first indicators of positive response. The most common histological subtype is DLBCL, for which contemporary immunochemotherapy plus radiotherapy when needed gives high response rates and prolonged survival [7, 14, 18].

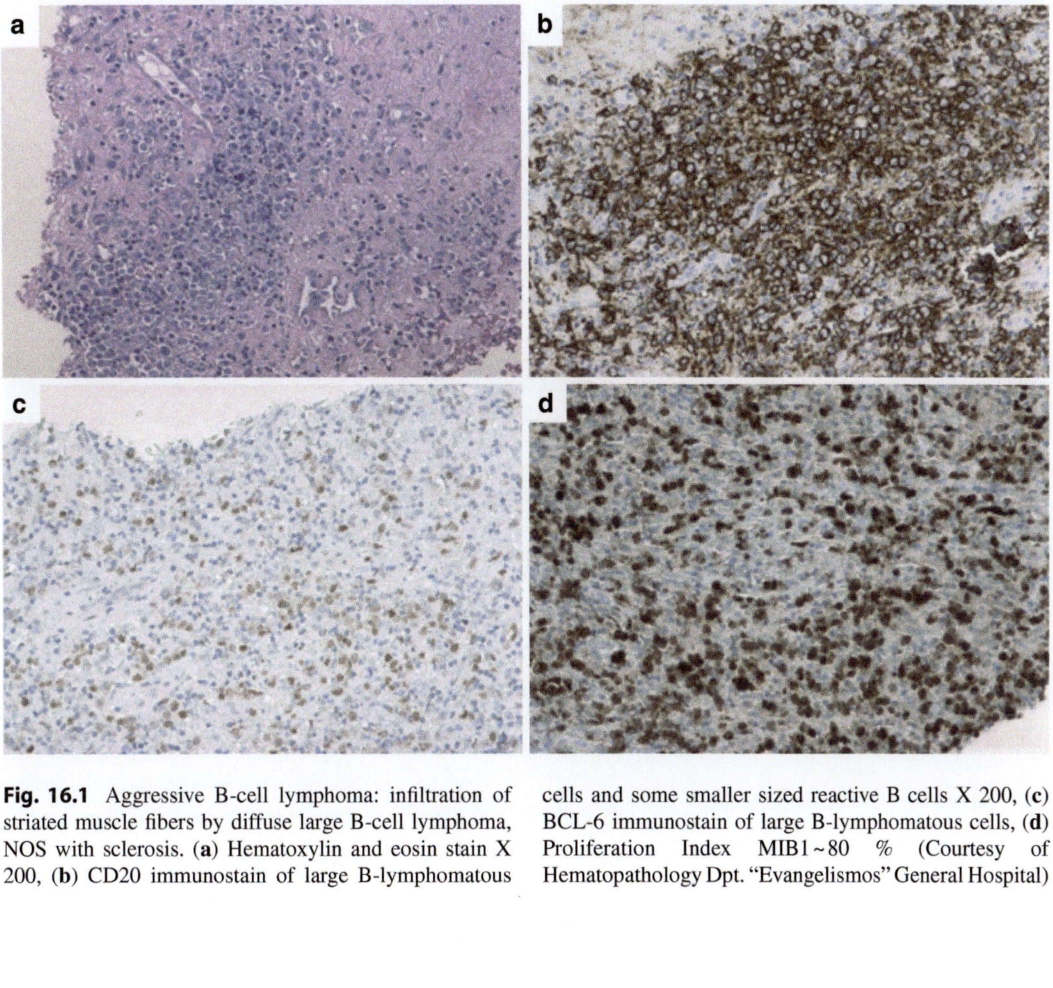

Fig. 16.1 Aggressive B-cell lymphoma: infiltration of striated muscle fibers by diffuse large B-cell lymphoma, NOS with sclerosis. (**a**) Hematoxylin and eosin stain X 200, (**b**) CD20 immunostain of large B-lymphomatous cells and some smaller sized reactive B cells X 200, (**c**) BCL-6 immunostain of large B-lymphomatous cells, (**d**) Proliferation Index MIB1 ~ 80 % (Courtesy of Hematopathology Dpt. "Evangelismos" General Hospital)

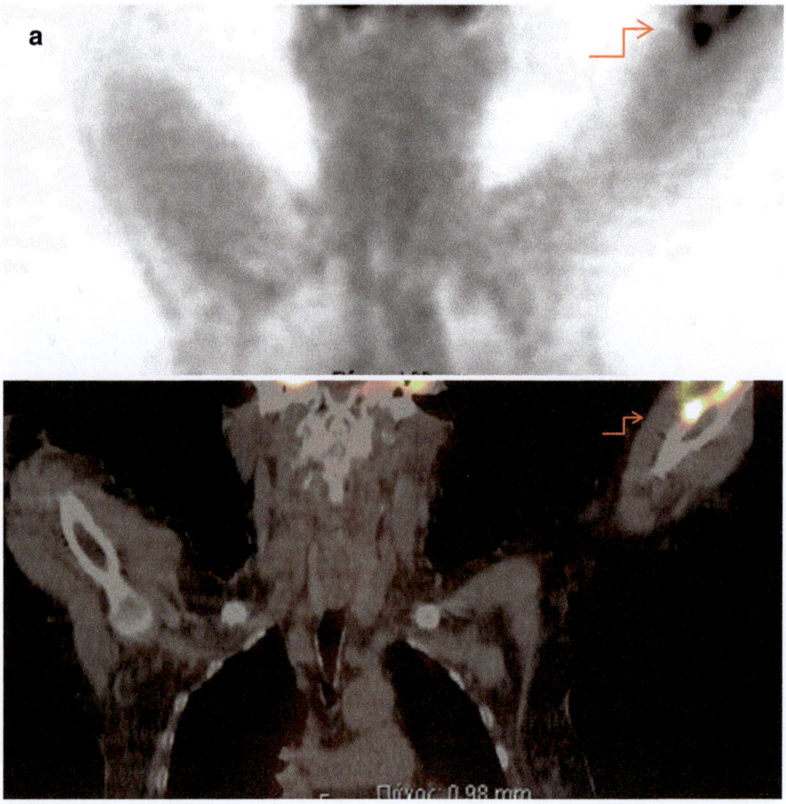

Fig. 16.2 Hypermetabolism in the bones and adjacent soft tissues: in the region of the left elbow (**a**) (*red arrows*, corona l PET and fused PET/CT images), in the region of the left shoulder, in the middle and the lower part of the right hemithorax and in the left rib (**b**) (*red arrows*, coronal PET and fused PET/CT images), in multiple vertebrae (**c**) (*red arrows*, sagittal PET and fused PET/CT images), in the right hip, in the middle of the right femur and in the left upper femur (**d**) (*red arrows*, coronal PET and fused PET/CT images), as well as in the pelvis (**e**) (*red arrows*, transverse PET and fused PET/CT images)

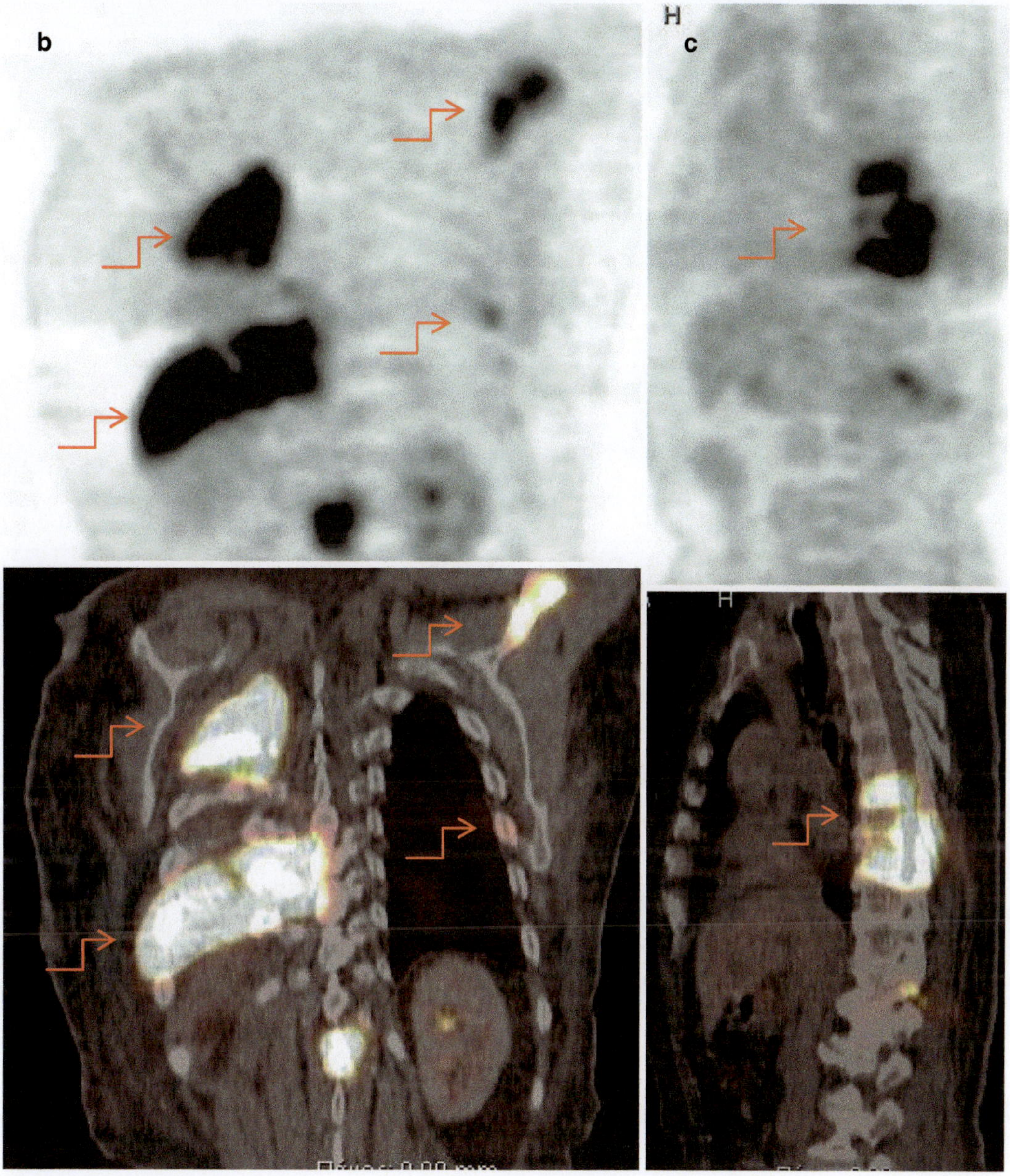

Fig. 16.2 (continued)

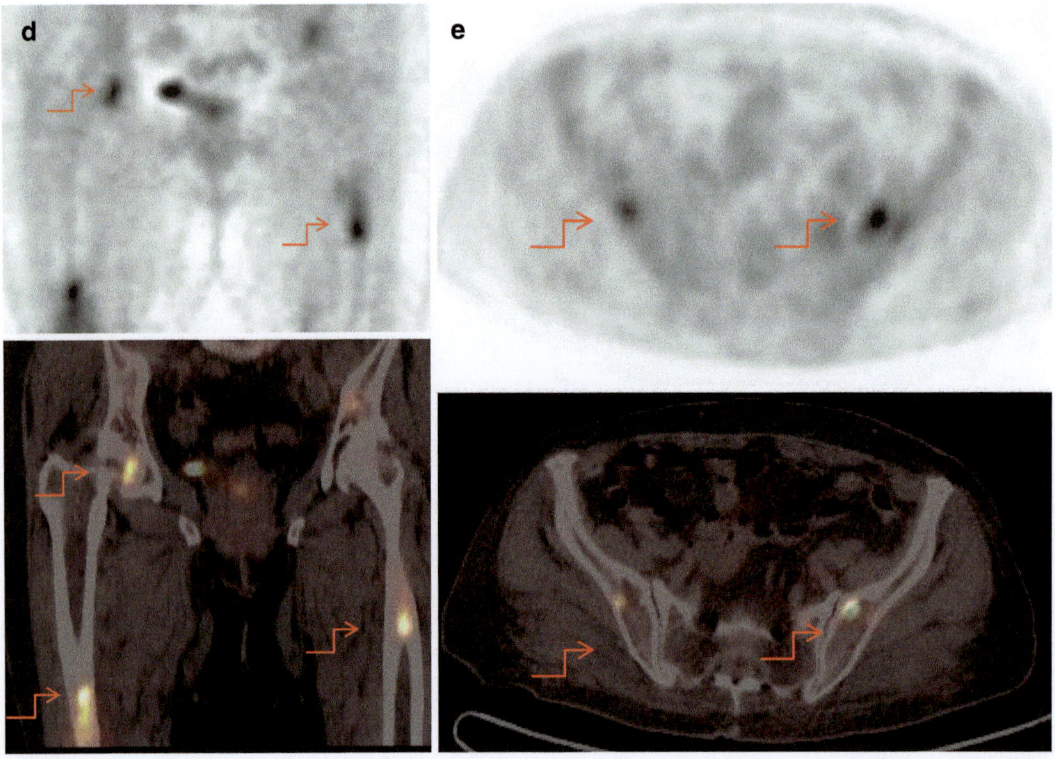

Fig. 16.2 (continued)

16.3 Primary Extranodal Hodgkin's Lymphoma of the Liver: Imaging Findings with Focus on Post-therapy Residual Disease in Spleen in Spite of a Negative ^{18}FDG-PET/CT Scan

Hodgkin's lymphoma (HL) lesions can arise primarily in 10 % of cases in nonlymphoid areas, under unknown circumstances. Evidence of primary extra-nodal HL (E-HL) comes from case reports or small groups of patients; therefore results of clinical characteristics and outcome of organ-specific involvement are difficult to access [19]. It is significant to clarify whether extranodal HL indicates primary disease or secondary, from invasion of adjacent tissue or dissemination, since the latter has a poorer prognosis [12]. Clinical features of E-HL are mainly manifestations of the affected visceral organs without any evidence of lymphadenopathy on physical examination. The affected organ usually exhibits enlargement and dysfunction which is not always accompanied by alterations in routine hematological and biochemistry investigation [12, 19].

The outcome of patients with the standard care approaches seems favorable with OS 89.6 %, DFS 87.7 %, and relapse rate 16.7 % at 5 years in the limited number of reports [20]. The usual risk factors, according to the International Prognostic Index (IPI) for HL, do not necessarily have the same prognostic value as in nodal disease patients [19].

Primary HL of the liver is extremely rare, accounting for <1 % of all extranodal lymphomas. Almost invariably it is accompanied by involvement of the spleen, which is regarded as a nodal organ in HL and as an extra-nodal organ in non-Hodgkin's lymphoma [21, 22].

In particular, diseased spleen can appear enlarged as a result of infiltration by HL, but the size is not always indicative of disease presence. Mild or moderate splenomegaly can occur without evidence of disease in about 30 % of cases, especially in the post-therapy setting, due to reactive changes. On the other hand, disease may be demonstrated in apparently clinically and radiologically normal spleen in another 30 % of lymphoma cases [12, 13]. However massive splenomegaly always suggests infiltration by lymphoma.

Infiltration by HL in the liver and spleen appears in a diffuse or nodular pattern or their combination and infrequently as a mass [9, 11, 12]. Image findings of HL of the liver and spleen are of great importance in the initial diagnosis, treatment response, and follow-up of the patients, because they may change tumor staging, treatment protocols, and overall prognosis.

The diffuse pattern appears on U/S and CT as inconsistent infiltrates particularly in the portal areas but is nonspecific and not always detectable. The nodular pattern in both liver and spleen may be seen either as small nodules of few centimeters or as miliary lesions <1 cm in diameter. U/S, CT, and MR imaging can similarly characterize nodular liver and spleen disease as low attenuation areas compared with normal tissue, but the accuracy of ultrasound and CT is comparatively low, ranging from 37 to 91 % in CT, as a consequence of the inability to detect occult HL in the spleen [23, 24]. Careful interpretation of CT findings is imperative because extranodal lesions may be subtle or even invisible in conventional enhanced CT [12, 25].

Although MR imaging can be more revealing in detecting disease in the liver and spleen, it may not provide conclusive results for the spleen, owing to the similarity in signal intensity between the normal spleen and lymphomatous tissue.

The superiority of ^{18}FDG-PET/CT (^{18}FDG-PET) in the detection of spleen and liver lymphoma cannot be challenged. Even in the absence of lesions demonstrated by CT, imaging of tumor metabolism with FDG, 2-[fluorine-18] fluoro-2-deoxy-D-glucose, and positron emission tomography (^{18}FDG-PET) may identify the extra-nodal sites. ^{18}FDG PET/CT has the highest sensitivity and specificity rates in detecting extra-nodal disease in the spleen, liver, cortical bone, bone marrow, and the normal-sized lymph nodes, compared to CT (88 % and 100 % vs. 50 % and 90 %) whether homogenous splenomegaly, diffuse infiltration with miliary lesions, focal nodular lesions, or a large mass is present [26–29].

In particular, in primary spleen involvement the diagnostic sensitivity and specificity of ^{18}FDG-PET can reach 100 %, which may not apply to the posttreatment setting due to reactive splenic uptake giving false-positive results [8, 29].

Involvement of the liver is manifested as patchy foci of FDP uptake with higher SUV than those of the surrounding parenchyma, present in the portal areas.

In the post-therapy setting, residual masses can be demonstrated in up to 80 % of HL patients who have completed successful treatment, although less than half of these will harbor residual disease [27].

The assessment of residual masses with ^{18}FDG-PET reaches 84 % in sensitivity and 90 % in specificity for HL and, most importantly, a clear distinction between residual metabolic active tumor and sites of necrosis or fibrosis can be done [8, 30]. The posttreatment response and restaging of HL patients with PET, in early and advanced disease stage, report results of positive predictive value (PPV) >90 % and of negative predictive value (NPV) 95–100 % following an aggressive chemotherapy vs. 75–80 % after low-intensity regimens [27, 28, 30].

The accuracy of end of treatment assessment with ^{18}FDG-PET in HL is much greater for patients with radiological (in CT), complete (unconfirmed), or partial remission. Regarding the complete metabolic response in ^{18}FDG-PET scan, it is considered as complete remission of lymphoma, even at the presence of a persistent mass of any size [30]. On the contrary metabolically active residual disease is an indication for further biopsies, scans, and treatment.

Therefore, ^{18}FDG-PET is the noninvasive modality of choice for staging and follow-up in patients with HL [28].

However, false-negative (FN) findings can result from a relatively small number of viable cancer cells in the splenic parenchyma, i.e., lesion's size – foci smaller than 5–8 mm, which is at the limits of systems' resolution [31]. Partial volume effect in such small lesions may cause lower ^{18}FDG uptake and thereby result in an FN study [32]. Another reason for FN results is the histological subtype. Although HL has 100 % ^{18}FDG avidity in at least one site at the initial staging [33], the avidity of subtypes may vary; nodular sclerosis shows the optimal ^{18}FDG avidity with mixed cellularity, lymphocyte depletion, and lymphocyte predominant type showing lower ^{18}FDG avidity, resulting in lower uptake and FN results.

Therefore, in spite of the existence of highly updated and innovative imaging procedures, noninvasive diagnosis of HL in the spleen remains uncertain and becomes obvious only after histological examination and splenectomy, which would be advised, as long as the discovery of residual disease in it would change the patient's treatment.

Since some individual cases may be inconclusive, a thorough interpretation of the radiological findings with the close collaboration between the specialists involved (hematologist, oncologist, radiologist, and nuclear medicine physician) can help. Additionally, throughout the lengthy treatment and follow-up period of the patient, good clinical judgment, careful history and physical examination, and meticulous interpretation of all the investigational results are all of crucial importance for the patient's life.

16.4 Case Study: Primary Hodgkin's Lymphoma of the Liver: Occult Disease in Spleen After Successful Initial Treatment Albeit a Negative ^{18}FDG-PET/CT Scan

A 49-year-old man, a smoker since the age of 15, was admitted to the clinic experiencing a 6-month period of fever, chills, night sweats, stomach pain, vomiting, and cough, all deteriorating gradually. His past history was significant for Crohn's disease treated with azathioprine and mesalazine.

On clinical examination he presented malaise and fever; the spleen and liver were palpable 2.5 cm and 2 cm, respectively, without lymphadenopathy.

Relevant laboratory findings included HGB 13.4 g/dL, HCT 39 %, ESR 69 mm, RTC 0.9 %, SAP 948 U/L, (8O-270 U/L), γ GT 175 U/L (10–50 U/L), SGOT 53 U/L (5–40 U/L), SGPT 46 U/L (5–40 U/L), LDH 626 U/L (230–450 U/L), HBAg (−), anti-HCV (−), and anti-HIV (−).

Imaging studies, and in particular MRI, disclosed enlargement of the liver and spleen with multiple lesions up to 4 cm diameter present in the liver as well as four foci up to 5 cm in the spleen and a block of lymph nodes at the portal of the liver, up to 3 cm.

Enlarged lymph nodes were not detected elsewhere.

Liver-directed biopsy disclosed infiltration by Hodgkin's lymphoma cells, CD30+, CD15+, PAX5+, and no infiltration in bone marrow.

A diagnosis of extra-nodal primary Hodgkin's lymphoma (HL) of the liver and spleen stage IV B was established, after which the patient started on ABVD chemotherapy.

Following the start of treatment, there was immediate relief of his symptoms, which coincided with improved imaging findings and serological results which had normalized before the third cycle.

Vinblastine was discontinued after the 4th cycle of chemotherapy because of peripheral neuropathy grade 3.

In spite of his clinical and radiological improvement, splenomegaly with two splenic lesions of 5 cm and 2 cm still remained in CT at the end of therapy, albeit liver CT-directed needle biopsy revealed no infiltration (Fig. 16.3a).

^{18}FDG-PET scan performed at the end of treatment (EoT) assessment showed no uptake of the tracer demonstrating a complete metabolic response (CMR) (Fig. 16.3b).

Because of the possibility of occult chemorefractory disease in the spleen, which if found would alter the therapeutic strategy as well as the patient's good clinical condition, the histological confirmation of splenic involvement was advised.

The surgically excised spleen had increased size (18 cm × 10 cm × 7 cm) with multiple dilatated light brownish foci of 0.6–1.8 cm in the parenchyma. Histology showed numerous non-necrotizing granulomas inside which infiltration by Hodgkin's Reed-Sternberg cells, CD30+, CD15+, PAX-5+, and EBV+ve was revealed (Fig. 16.4).

No infiltration by HL was demonstrated in a liver sample.

The patient afterward proceeded to high-dose therapy (HDT), with the TECAM conditioning regimen, followed by autologous stem-cell transplantation (ASCT), and remains, 6 years later, in complete remission.

Discussion

The existence of HL in patients with Crohn's disease is an extremely rare occurrence, with very few cases reported [34].

Non-necrotizing granulomas in spleen infiltrated by Hodgkin's cells have been reported quite commonly in the literature, either at the onset of HL or after chemotherapy, occasionally obscuring the malignant cells [35, 36]. Even more rarely granulomas of the spleen can be encountered in association with Crohn's disease [37].

^{18}FDG-PET scan is a very accurate imaging modality for the staging and restaging of HL patients with a high sensitivity and specificity value and thus PET response-adapted treatment programs have been developed.

Accurate EoT response assessment is critical to avoid over- or undertreatment, and post-therapy ^{18}FDG-PET/CT scan is the standard of care for the advanced disease treated with ABVD [28, 38]. A negative ^{18}FDG-PET scan is considered as CMR of the tumor, for which no more treatment is required.

The significance of residual radiological mass when CMR is achieved is still unclear, while some reports suggest improved outcomes when CMR is associated with a radiological CR [38]. If further treatment can be omitted in ABVD-treated patients who have PET-negative residual tissue >1.5 cm on CT remains unclear [39]. But because of the strong negative predictive value of ^{18}FDG-PET, residual CT nodules that are negative in ^{18}FDG-PET scan are quite unlikely to harbor persistent lymphoma, so treatment can be stopped, since such patients can be judged to have reached complete response [28, 40].

It has been indicated, however, that patients with a residual mass larger than 4 cm at CT and a negative ^{18}FDG-PET scan have a significant lower disease-free survival (DFS) comparing to those with smaller residual mass [41].

Particularly in the evaluation of the spleen, although the accuracy of ^{18}FDG-PET during initial staging has been reported to be 100 % compared to 57 % of CT alone [8], in very rare cases (2.7 %), a "false-negative" (FN) ^{18}FDG-PET has been reported which results to downstaging [42].

Concerning the FN ^{18}FDG-PET scan study results in the present case, the most possible explanation can be the infiltration extent or the relatively small number of viable cancer cells in the splenic parenchyma. In this context FN findings may be due to lesion's size (foci smaller than 5–8 mm) which is at the limits of systems' resolution [31].

On the other hand, the presence of granulomas in the spleen of the above patient should in theory be a source of "false-positive" findings, as granulomas usually take up ^{18}FDG [43]. A possible explanation for the negative ^{18}FDG-PET scan in this case, in spite of splenic non-necrotizing granulomas revealed, can be the metabolic status of the granulomatous cells. As in sarcoid disease – the most frequent granulomatous disease – ^{18}FDG-PET uptake is a marker of disease metabolic activity [44]. Published data show a sensitivity of 90 % for the detection of active inflammation [45], so one can assume a lower sensitivity for a low-grade (inactive) inflammatory condition; hence, in the present case there may exist metabolically inactive granulomata, not taking up ^{18}FDG.

Relating to failure of initial treatment, it has become very uncommon in the last decades; approximately 10 % of patients with advanced HL and more than two adverse prognostic factors will not reach complete remission and have over 50 % risk of refractory or relapsed disease, eliminating the probability of cure with the standard strategies. Occult chemorefractory disease in the spleen has been associated with high rates of relapses. A readiness must be maintained for those patients with histologically proven persistent disease for a definite chance of cure [40].

HDT and ASCT appear to be the best available options, offering cure in 50–60 % of the failed patients with high overall survival (OS) up to 84 % at 7 years after ABVD initial chemotherapy, which appears to be the best choice for primary chemotherapy [46, 47].

Concerning the significance of negative functional imaging preceding the ASCT, a high OS of 90 % is provided to such patients, which is similar for those in complete remission with conventional imaging [48].

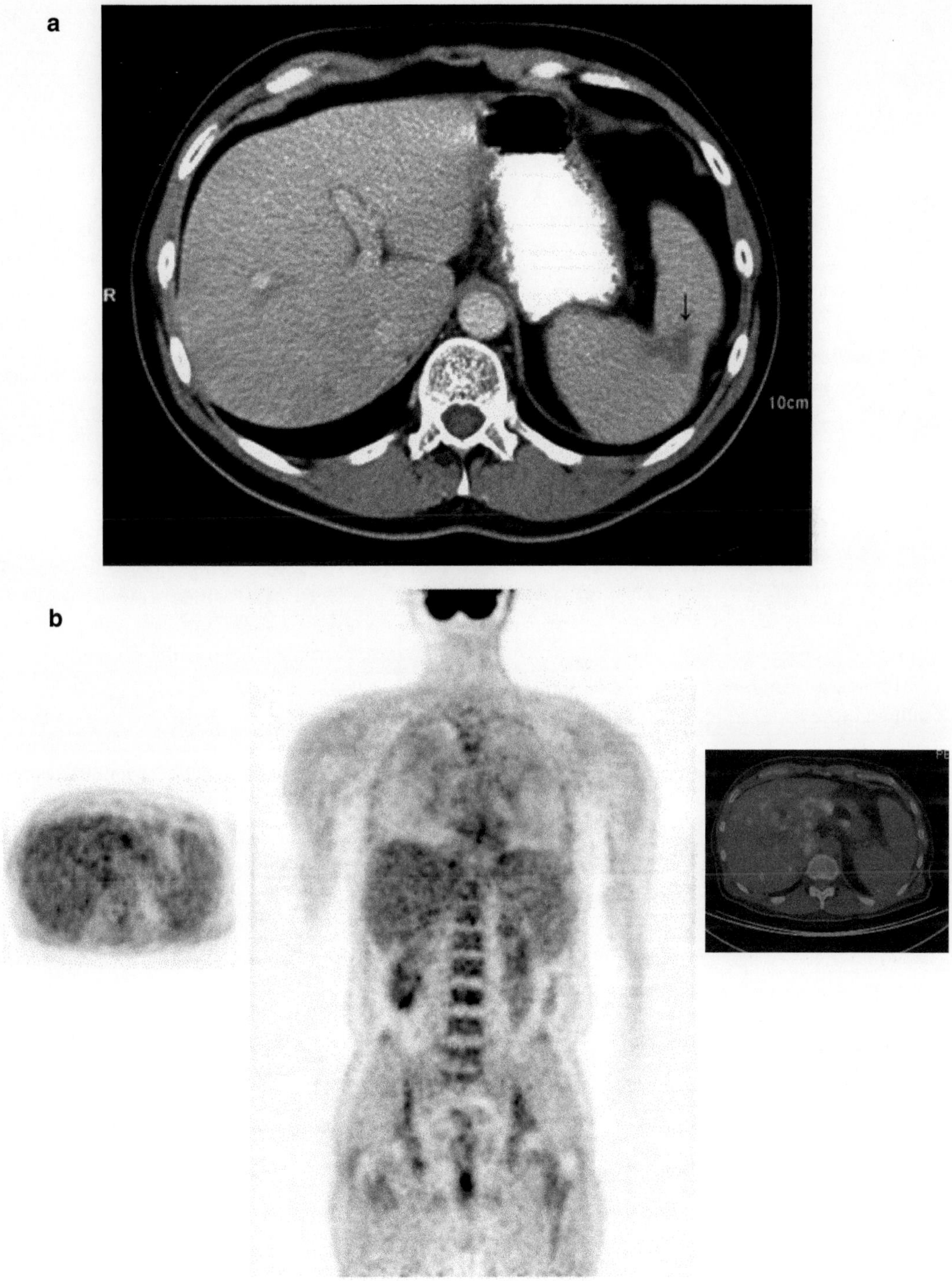

Fig. 16.3 (**a**) Post-therapy CT image shows residual lesion in spleen (*arrow*). (**b**) Coronal and transverse PET and fused PET/CT images show no focal increased radio-tracer uptake in the liver and spleen especially in the splenic lesion shown in CT image

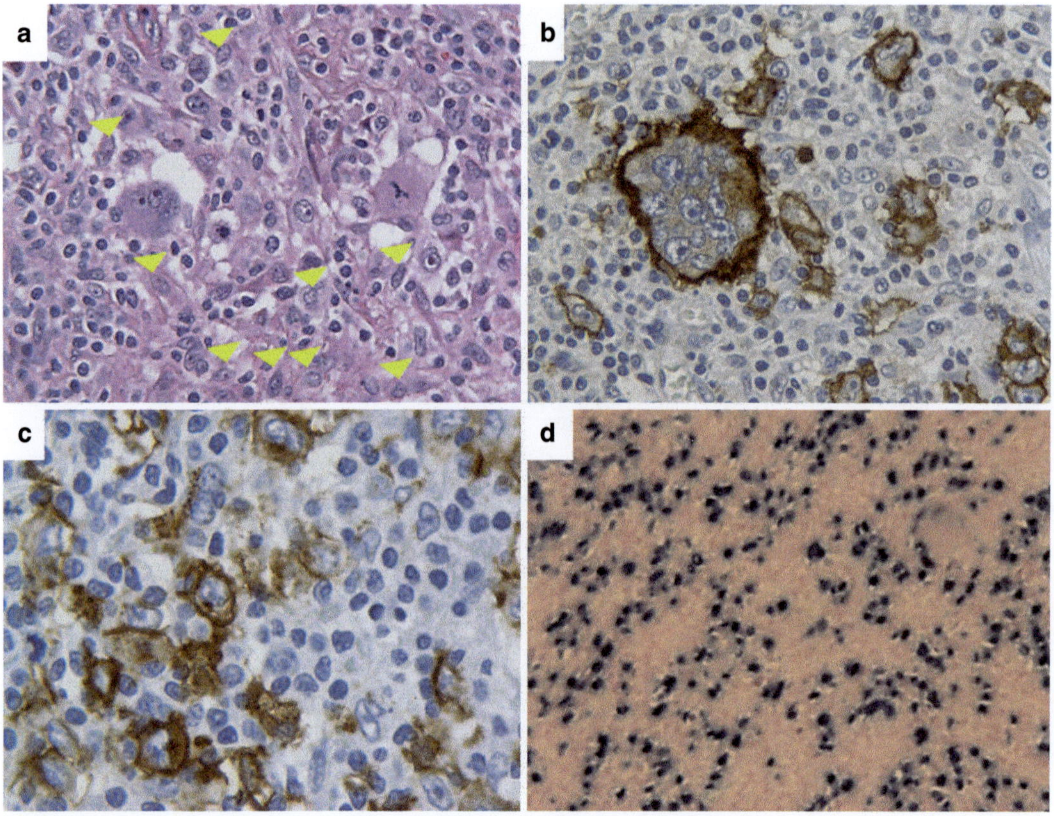

Fig. 16.4 Post-therapy spleen biopsy. Classical Hodgkin's lymphoma: (**a**) isolated Reed-Sternberg cells and lacunar cells and variants, intermixed with small lymphocytes and increased numbers of histiocytes (*arrowheads*) (H&E ×400). (**b**) CD30-positive Hodgkin's cells and variants (bizarre cells) ×400. (**c**) CD15-positive mainly Hodgkin's cells (×400) and (**d**) in situ hybridization for EBV-encoded early RNA (EBER) revealed detection of EBV in almost 100 % of neoplastic cells (×400) (Courtesy of Hematopathology Dpt. "Evangelismos" General Hospital, Athens, Greece)

16.5 Primary Vitreoretinal Lymphoma

Primary vitreoretinal lymphoma (PVRL), previously known as primary intraocular lymphoma (PIOL), is a very rare type of extranodal lymphoma which involves primarily the vitreous, the retinal pigment epithelium (RPE), and the optic nerve of the eye and is considered a rare subset of primary central nervous system lymphoma (PCNSL) with intraocular involvement. Ninety-eight percent of cases of PCNSL are aggressive diffuse large B-cell lymphomas (DLBCL), but more rare T-cell variants have also been reported [49–51].

PIOL is a heterogeneous group of malignant lymphomas including primary lymphomas of the choroid, the iris, and the ciliary body (uveal lymphomas), in addition to PVRL [49, 52].

There are differences between the two in terms of histology and association with central nervous system (CNS) lymphomas. In contrast to PVRL, uveal lymphomas are usually extranodal indolent B-cell lymphomas of the marginal zone, not associated with PCNSL, although other organs may be involved [50].

Approximately one-third of PVRL patients have concurrent PCNSL at presentation, which is accompanied by a lower 5-year overall survival of 35 %, compared to those without CNS involvement, whose 5-year overall survival is 68 % [53]. Another 15 % of cases have meningeal dissemination at initial staging [54]. PVRL patients develop subsequent intracranial disease in 42–92 % of cases, with a mean interval period of 8–29 months [51, 52, 55]. This ultimate association with CNS is the reason for a high fatal outcome, thus making PVRL a challenging malignant condition [49]. The results above and the anatomical relation between the eyes and the brain have led some researches to recommend therapies similar to PCNSL [54].

There is increasing incidence of PVRL in the past 15 years in both immunocompromised populations, usually infected by the Epstein-Barr virus and immunocompetent individuals [49, 52].

The disease seems to affect women more frequently and patients aged between 50 and 70 [51, 53]. Due to the rarity of PVRL, no established standards have been developed, causing difficulties in the diagnosis, follow-up, and therapy of patients [53, 55].

PVRL is most often bilateral (64–83 %), whose clinical feature frequently masquerades as an infectious or noninfectious inflammatory condition of the eye [53, 55]. Blurred vision and vitreous floaters are the most frequent symptoms of the disease, which has an insidious onset and a delayed diagnosis [49]. Lymphomatous infiltrates, together with inflammation cells, produce sheets and clusters of cells which cause hazy appearance of the vitreous, detected by standard ocular examinations [55]. When CNS is involved, neurological symptoms may appear accompanied by personality changes and cognitive deficits.

Diagnosis is challenging and requires definite tissue diagnosis, the gold standard being the demonstration of monoclonal lymphoid cells in an adequate vitreous specimen; clinical examination and ocular imaging are also beneficial [53]. Increase of IL-10 and a ratio of IL-10 to IL-6 > 1 in the vitreous liquid are supportive to diagnosis, but IL-10 values alone cannot be used as a biomarker [49]. IL-10 $_{1082}$ A allele has been found to be correlated with higher IL-10 levels and more aggressive course in PVRL and PCNSL [50].

Apart from the skillful surgical technique and the process required to obtain the vitreous humor, equally important to increasing the likelihood of diagnosis is the handling of the specimen, as the cells outside the eye rapidly die.

^{18}FDG-PET/CT is an established investigational method with great accuracy in detection, treatment monitoring, and follow-up of extranodal lymphomas [56]. CNS dissemination in extranodal lymphomas may occur in the brain with intraparenchymal lesions and leptomeningeal infiltration, either at initial diagnosis or in the course of relapse, recurrence, or progressive disease [54]. ^{18}FDG-PET/CT (^{18}FDG-PET) is very useful in the diagnosis of PCNSL, with typical radiological findings, usually showing remarkably increased ^{18}FDG uptake in the tumor [57]. However those patients with atypical radiological findings may have lower ^{18}FDG uptake making it difficult to differentiate the lesion from the normal high background uptake of ^{18}FDG [58]. A few papers with a relatively small number of patients and great heterogeneity among them have been published using ^{18}FDG-PET in the management of PCNSL [57, 59], implying that ^{18}FDG-PET coregistered to CT may be a useful examination in the detection and monitoring for systemic spread of the disease in PCNSL patients [60] and adds valuable information to MRI studies especially in treatment response assessment [61].

Therapy of PVRL could be local, with radiation or direct intravitreal methotrexate (IV MTX) and more recently rituximab injection (IV R) and systemic chemotherapy in an appropriate combination with radiotherapy [62–65]. The impact of local treatment on patient survival has not yet been proved [62]. In spite of this, the International PCNSL group recommends the following therapeutic principles: for disease limited to one eye, local therapy; for PVRL with CNS involvement, systemic chemotherapy and radiotherapy; and for bilateral disease without CNS involvement, either local or systemic treatment [49, 53, 64].

Nevertheless, others advocate that initial treatment of isolated PIOL should be similar to PCNSL including high-dose MTX-based and aracytin chemotherapy, accompanied or not by whole-brain radiation, to eradicate possible microscopic disease contamination in the brain and the cerebrospinal fluid responsible for relapse [52, 54].

Local therapies, remarkably less toxic, have not conclusively demonstrated an impact on the overall patient survival and do not suppress the development of the CNS tumor which ultimately develops in 69 % of the patients without CNS disease at presentation, with a mean follow-up time of 46.6 months (range 23–109 months) [55, 63, 65].

Since the optimal therapy for PVRL has not yet been established, and there are contrasting views even between experts, the close collaboration of the specialists involved is required for a team approach to the patient [49, 53, 62, 65].

The role of the hematologist or oncologist in that team is to direct the investigation, to evaluate all the results, and to decide on the treatment together with the ophthalmologist, taking into consideration the patient's desire as well. Up-to-date information and awareness of the diagnostic difficulties and treatment options are of vital importance.

16.6 Case Study: Primary Vitroretinal Lymphoma

The patient, a 64-year-old man, visited his ophthalmologist because of blurred vision and multiple floaters experienced for a year. Diffuse vitreous opacities were present in both eyes without clinical and imaging signs of intraocular (optic nerve, choroid, retina, uveal) inflammation, nevertheless with a clinical suspicion of malignancy. Pars plana diagnostic/therapeutic vitrectomy revealed monoclonal B-cell population and IgM κ light-chain restriction in the flow cytometry study. Neuroimaging of central nervous system with MRI and immunological cerebrospinal fluid specimen analysis failed to reveal evidence of lymphoma. The ^{18}FDG-PET/CT (^{18}FDG-PET) scan did not show any uptake (Fig. 16.5).

Clinical findings and a full oncologic workup were normal. The diagnosis of bilateral primary vitreoretinal lymphoma without CNS dissemination was established after which the patient received intravitreal monotherapy with rituximab 1 mg weekly for 4 weeks, without apparent side effects. He is in good clinical condition, without local recurrence of the disease for the last 25 months, and regular MRI investigation has not revealed evolution of primary central nervous system lymphoma (PCNSL).

Discussion

Primary vitreoretinal lymphoma (PVRL) is a rare subtype of PCNSL, manifestations of which may not be present at the time of diagnosis.

PVRL exhibits peculiar characteristics of clinical course and behavior. First, an aggressive highly fatal condition ensues because ultimately central nervous system (CNS) disease evolves in most cases. This contrasts with other extra-nodal lymphomas which usually have more favorable prognosis, for instance, bone lymphoma. Second, recurrence of the disease outside the eye and brain is extremely rare, indicating a unique tropism of the lymphoid cell for the retina and CNS. The ectopic expression of cytokines within the intraocular environment may assist lymphoma cell homing to the retinal pigment epithelium. Third, response to doxorubicin-based chemotherapy is less effective although large lymphoid cells are predominant, for reasons not yet evaluated; however, response to methotrexate in particular is high [49].

The gold standard of diagnosis is the identification of monoclonal B-cell population in a cellular vitreous sample. Cytopathology, immunohistochemistry, flow cytometry, and molecular analysis for the detection of IgH gene rearrangement are all supportive to diagnosis [51]. Gentle manipulation of the diagnostic sample is of vital importance regarding the temperature, the timely delivery to the laboratory, and the appropriate media of transportation, since the cells easily die outside the eye [50, 66]. The main cytologic features of malignant lymphoid infiltration include increased cellularity and necrosis. The abnormal large lymphoid cells form a poorly cohesive population and present large nuclei and prominent nucleoli. The positivity to CD20 immunocytochemistry confirms the morphologic diagnosis [66].

The value of ^{18}FDG-PET in the diagnosis of CNS dissemination in patients in rare extranodal lymphomas has not yet been widely studied. Patients with diffusely disseminated lesions may have lower 18 F-FDG uptake and patients with small lesions, below the system's resolution of 5–7 mm, may have "false-negative" ^{18}FDG-PET studies. In a paper by Matsuo et al., the authors conclude that ^{18}FDG-PET could be considered to be a method to confirm brain lymphoma in patients with intraocular lymphoma or a reference for initiating additional therapy in the case of eye recurrence or residual lesions after vitrectomy [67]. In a more recent retrospective study of 41 patients with ocular adnexal lymphoma, it has been shown that ^{18}FDG-PET has a lower sensitivity than MRI to detect ophthalmic lymphoma, particularly in non-conjunctival sites [68]. The degree to which an initial negative ^{18}FDG-PET scan, as in the present case, can assist to stage local disease more precisely and to intervene to the therapeutic decision is still questionable.

The optimal therapy for PVRL has not been defined yet and requires the combined efforts of hematologists and ophthalmologists. Although the malignant cells are highly radiosensitive and chemosensitive, the survival rate is low [49]. It is a matter of debate if isolated PVRL should be treated by local treatments or combined chemoradiotherapy, with protocol that presumes the involvement of CNS.

In particular, for disease located in one eye, local ocular therapies using either intravitreal chemotherapy with methotrexate (MTX) or external beam ocular radiation have been tried. Nevertheless, complications from radiation treatment are far from negligible and local methotrexate administration is commonly accompanied by disease resistance and recurrence or severe corneal epitheliopathy, which obliges the cessation of treatment. Since the malignant cell in 98 % of PVRL cases originates from diffuse large B cells that express CD19 and CD20 molecules, targeting malignant cells with the monoclonal anti-CD20 antibody leads to inhibition of B-cell proliferation and differentiation. Consequently, the most novel therapy is intravitreal rituximab (IV R) which has been similarly effective as MTX but less toxic. IV R monotherapy, in biopsy-proven CD20-positive PVRL, has succeeded in controlling the local growth of the tumor and alleviating the ocular symptoms [63].

Improvement of the ocular lesions has been observed in almost all the cases; however complete remission does not necessarily follow since the local recurrence of PVRL has been recorded to range between 22.5 % and 55 %, after a median of 17.5 and 3 months, respectively [63, 69]. The most common topical complications from the use of IV R have been cataract and increased intraocular pressure, easily manageable with local measures. The combination of IV R with MTX has also been used with sufficient optimization of results of complete and partial response reaching almost 90 % [63, 69, 70].

When the disease is bilateral, however, there is controversy as to whether local treatment is adequate or whether additional systematic chemotherapy with or without CNS radiation is preferable [49, 55, 64, 71]. However, poor intraocular penetration of the chemotherapeutic agents has to be taken into consideration.

Furthermore, the use of systematic chemotherapy in PVRL has not been reported as creating any difference to PCNSL progression (50–90 % during

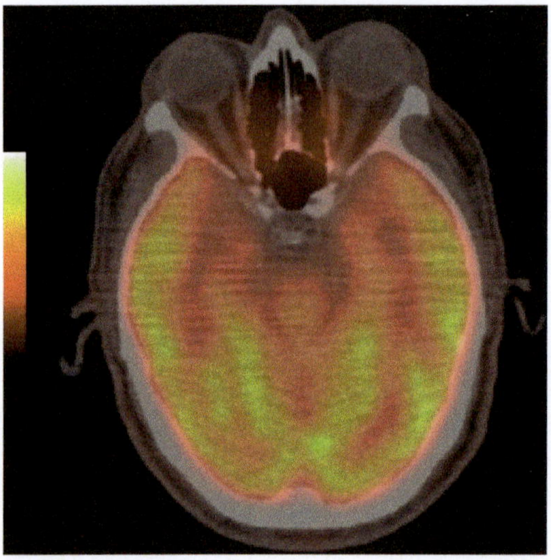

Fig. 16.5 Post-therapy PET/CT scan of the head shows no intraocular or brain uptake of ^{18}FDG

follow-up) and overall survival vs. local therapies [62]. Besides, in a recent European collaborative study, the impact of treatment on the incidence of CNS manifestations during the follow-up period was analyzed. These accounted for 36 % in a median time of 49 months. Results proved that no difference was observed between patients undergoing extensive treatment (systemic and intrathecal chemotherapy plus whole-brain radiation and peripheral stem-cell transplantation), those receiving local therapy (ocular radiotherapy and/or ocular chemotherapy), and those receiving a combination of the two. The survival rate was similar for the three groups and their conclusion summarized that the use of systematic chemotherapy was not proven to prevent evolution to PCNSL. On the contrary, chemotherapy related adverse effects such as acute renal failure followed in a substantial number of patients [65]. Currently, bilateral disease can still be treated with intraocular agents alone.

In view of the above results, it is suggested by some experts at the present that when CNS is involved at presentation, analogous therapeutic strategy should be followed, but when the disease is confined to the eyes, local therapy alone would be adequate*.

*A short time before the publication of this book, the patient in question presented with CNS relapse.

Acknowledgments The authors would like to thank to Dr Alexandros Charonis, ophthalmologist, Athens Vision Center Eye Institute, Athens Greece, and Dr Nicol Panou, ophthalmologist, Agii Anargiri General Cancer Hospital, Kifissia Athens, Greece, for the ophthalmologic history.

The author C.S. would like to express her gratitude to the staff of the Stanford Hospital Health Library Palo Alto CA, for their kindness and encouragement as well as their support in the search of the literature.

References

1. Fletcher CDM (2006) The evolving classification of soft tissue tumours: an update based on the new WHO classification. Histopathology 48:3–12
2. Messina C, Ferreri AJ, Govi S et al (2014) Clinical features, management and prognosis of multifocal primary bone lymphoma:a retrospective study of the international Extranodal Lymphoma Study Group (the IELSG 14 study). Br J Haematol 164(6):834–840
3. Heyning FH, Hogendoorn PCW, Kramer MHH et al (1999) Primary non-Hodgkin's lymphoma of bone: a clinicopathological investigation of 60 cases. Leukemia 13:2094–2098
4. Mikhaeell NG (2012) Primary bone lymphoma, overview. Clin Oncol 24:366e–370e
5. Wu H, Zhang L, Shao H et al (2014) Prognostic significance of soft tissue extension, International Prognostic Index, and multifocality in primary bone lymphoma: a single institutional experience. Br J Haematol 166:60–68
6. Messina C, Christie D, Zucca E et al (2015) Primary and secondary bone lymphomas. Tumor review. Cancer Treat Rev 41:235–246
7. Ramadan KM, Shenkier T, Sehn LH et al (2007) A clinicopathological retrospective study of 131 patients with primary bone lymphoma: a population-based study of successively treated cohorts from the British Columbia Cancer Agency. Ann Oncol 18(1): 129–135
8. Paes FM, Kalkanis DG, Sideras PA et al (2010) FDG PET/CT of extranodal involvement in non-Hodgkin lymphoma and Hodgkin disease. RSNA Radiographics 30:269–291
9. Das J, Ray S, Sen S et al (2014) Extranodal involvement in lymphoma-a pictorial essay and retrospective analysis of 281 PET/CT studies. Asia Oceania J Nucl Med Biol 2(1):42–56
10. Moog F, Kotzerke JK, Reske SN (1999) FDG PET can replace bone scintigraphy in primary staging of malignant lymphoma. J Nucl Med 40:1407–1413
11. Ilica AT, Kocacelebi K, Savas R (2011) Imaging of extranodal lymphoma with PET/CT. Clin Nucl Med 36:e127–e138
12. Guermazi A, Brice P, de Kerviler EE et al (2001) Extra-nodal Hodgkin disease: spectrum of disease. Radiographics 21:161–179

13. Chua SC, Rozalli FI, O'Connor S (2009) Imaging features of primary extranodal lymphomas. Clin Radiol 64:574–588
14. Pellegrini C, Gandolfi L, Quirini F et al (2011) Primary bone lymphoma: evaluation of chemoimmunotherapy as front-line treatment in 21 patients. Clin Lymphoma Myeloma Leuk 11:321–325
15. Guirguis HR, Cheung MC, Mahrous M et al (2012) Impact of central nervous system (CNS) prophylaxis on the incidence and risk factors for CNS relapse in patients with diffuse large B-cell lymphoma treated in the rituximab era: a single center experience and review of the literature. Br J Haematol 159:39–49
16. Fletcher CD, Bridge JA, Hogendoorn PC et al (2013) WHO classification of tumors of soft tissue and bone. World Health Organization, IARC, Lyon
17. Mengiardi B, Honegger H, Hodler J et al (2005) Primary lymphoma of bone: MRI and CT characteristics during and after successful treatment. AJR Am J Roentgenol 184(1):185–192
18. Mohamed M, Brain T, Sharma S (2013) Multifocal primary bone lymphoma: durable complete remission after R-CHOP chemotherapy. BMJ Case Rep. doi:10.1136/bcr-2013-009809
19. Ma J, Wang Y, Zhao H et al (2014) Clinical characteristics of 26 patients with primary extranodal Hodgkin lymphoma. Int J Clin Exp Pathol 7(8):5045–5050
20. Iyengar P, Mazloom A, Shihadeh F et al (2010) Hodgkin lymphoma involving extranodal and nodal head and neck sites characteristics and outcomes. Cancer 116(16):3825–3829
21. Gota VS, Gujral S, Nair R et al (2009) Positron emission tomography/computerized tomography evaluation of primary Hodgkins disease of liver. Ind J Cancer 46(3):237–239
22. Chim CS, Choy C, Ooi CG et al (2000) Hodgkin's disease with primary manifestation in the liver. Leuk Lymphoma 37:629–632
23. Saboo SS, Krajewski KM, O'Regan KN et al (2012) Spleen in haematological malignancies: spectrum of imaging findings. Br J Radiol 85(1009):81–92
24. Karlo CA, Stoolzmann P, Do RK et al (2013) Computed tomography of the spleen: how to interpret the hypodense lesion. Insights Imaging 4:65–76
25. Daskalogiannaki M, Prassopoulos P, Katrinakis G et al (2001) Splenic involvement in lymphomas: evaluation on serial CT examinations. Acta Radiol 42:326–332
26. Rini JN, Leonidas JC, Tomas MB et al (2003) 18 F-FDG PET versus CT for evaluating the spleen during initial staging of lymphoma. J Nucl Med 44:1072–1074
27. Gallamini A, Borra A (2014) Role of PET in lymphoma. Curr Treat Options Oncol 15:248–261
28. Cheson BD, Fisher RI, Barrington SF et al (2014) Recommendations for initial evaluation, staging, and response assessment of Hodgkin and non-Hodgkin lymphoma: the Lugano classification. J Clin Oncol 20:3050–3067
29. de Jong PA, van Ufford HM, Baarslag HJ et al (2009) CT and 18F-FDG PET for noninvasive detection of splenic involvement in patients with malignant lymphoma. Am J Roentgenol 192:745–753
30. Juweid ME (2011) FDG-PET/CT in lymphoma. Positron emission tomography. Methods Mol Biol 727:1–19
31. Kostakoglu L, Agress H, Goldsmith SJ (2003) Clinical role of FDG PET in evaluation of cancer patients. Radiographics 23:315–340
32. Purohit BS, Ailianou A, Dulguerov N et al (2014) FDG-PET/CT pitfalls in oncological head and neck imaging. Insights Imaging 5:585–602
33. Weiler-Sagie M, Bushelev O, Epelbaum R et al (2010) (18)F-FDG avidity in lymphoma readdressed: a study of 766 patients. J Nucl Med 51(1):25–30
34. Kappelman MD, Farkas DK, Long MD et al (2014) Risk of cancer in patients with inflammatory bowel diseases: a nationwide population-based cohort study with 30 years of follow up. Clin Gastroenterol Hepatol 12(2):265–273
35. Sacks EL, Donaldson SS, Gordon J et al (1978) Epithelioid granulomas associated with Hodgkin's disease: clinical correlations with 55 previously un-treated patients. Cancer 41:562–567
36. Paydas S, Yavuz S, Disel U et al (2002) Granulomatous reaction after chemotherapy for Hodgkin's disease. Leuk Res 26:967–970
37. Coyne JD (2006) Crohn's disease with inflammatory splenic granuloma. J Clin Pathol 59(8):889
38. Barrington SF, Mikhaeel NG, Kostekoglou L et al (2014) Role of imaging in the staging and response assessment of lymphoma: consensus of the International Conference on Malignant Lymphomas Imaging Working Group. J Clin Oncol 32: 3048–3058
39. Follows GA, Ardeshna KM, Barrington SF et al (2014) Guidelines for the first line management of classical Hodgkin lymphoma. British Committee for Standards in Haematology. Br J Haematol 166(1):34–49. doi: 10.1111/bjh.12878. Epub 2014 Apr 9.
40. Connors JM (2011) Hodgkin's lymphoma-the great teacher. N Engl J Med 365(3):264–265
41. Magagnoli M, Marzo K, Balzarotti M et al (2011) Dimension of residual CT scan mass in Hodgkin's Lymphoma (HL) is a negative prognostic factor in patients with PET negative after chemo+/–radiotherapy. Blood 118:93
42. Munker R, Glass J, Griffen LK et al (2004) Contribution of PET imaging to the initial staging and prognosis of patients with Hodgkin's disease. Ann Oncol 15:1699–1704
43. Ryu JS, Um JW, Min BW (2010) Inflammatory pseudotumour of the spleen: the findings on F-18 fluorodeoxyglucose positron emission tomography/computed tomography (FDG-PET/CT). ANZ J Surg 80(9): 650–652
44. Adams H, Keijsers RG, Korenromp IH, Grutters JC (2014) FDG PET for gauging of sarcoid disease activity. Semin Respir Crit Care Med 35(3):352–361

45. Balink H, Bennink RJ, Veeger NJ et al (2014) Diagnostic utility of (18) F-FDG PET/CT in inflammation of unknown origin. Clin Nucl Med 39(5): 419–425
46. Stathis A, Younes A (2015) The new therapeutical scenario of Hodgkin lymphoma. Ann Oncol 26(10):2026–2033. doi:10.1093/annonc/mdv256
47. Kuruvilla J, Keating A, Crump M (2011) How I treat relapsed and refractory Hodgkin lymphoma. Blood 117(16):4208–4217
48. Moskowitz CH, Matasar MJ, Zelenetz AD et al (2012) Normalization of pre-ASCT, FDG-PET imaging with second-line, non-cross-resistant, chemotherapy programs improves event-free survival in patients with Hodgkin lymphoma. Blood 119(7):1665–1670
49. Chan CC, Rubenstein JL, Coupland SE et al (2011) Primary vitreoretinal lymphoma: a report from an International Primary Central Nervous System Lymphoma Collaborative Group Symposium. Oncologist 16:1589–1599
50. Hwang CS, Yeh S, Bergstrom CS (2014) Diagnostic vitrectomy for primary intraocular lymphoma: when, why, how? Int Ophthalmol Clin 54(2):155–171
51. Levasseur SD, Wittenberg LA, White VA (2013) Vitreoretinal lymphoma: a 20-year review of incidence, clinical and cytologic features, treatment, and outcomes. JAMA Ophthalmol 131:50–55
52. Saggo MS, Mehta H, Swampillai AJ et al (2014) Primary intraocular lymphoma. Surv Ophthalmol 59(5):503–516
53. Davis JL (2013) Intraocular lymphoma: a clinical perspective. Eye (Lond) 27:153–162
54. Ferreri AJM (2014) Risk of CNS dissemination in extranodal lymphomas. Lancet Oncol 15:159–169
55. Mulay K, Narula R, Santosh HG (2015) Primary vitreoretinal lymphoma. Indian J Ophthalmol 63(3):180–186
56. Martelli M, Ceriani L, Zucca E (2014) [18F]fluorodeoxyglucose positron emission tomograph predicts survival after chemoimmunotherapy for primary mediastinal large B-cell lymphoma: results of the International Extranodal Lymphoma Study Group IELSG-26 Study. J Clin Oncol 32:1769–1775
57. Kawai N, Miyake K, Yamamoto Y (2013) 18F-FDG PET in the diagnosis and treatment of primary central nervous system lymphoma. Biomed Res Int. doi:10.1155/2013/247152, Epub 2013 Jun 17. Review
58. Kawai N, Okubo S, Miyake K et al (2010) Use of PET in the diagnosis of primary CNS lymphoma in patients with atypical MR findings. Ann Nucl Med 24:335–343
59. Yamaguchi S, Hirata K, Kobayashi H (2014) The diagnostic role of (18)F-FDG PET for primary central nervous system lymphoma. Ann Nucl Med 28: 603–609
60. Karantanis D, O'Neill BP, Subramaniam RM et al (2007) Contribution of F-18 FDG PET-CT in the detection of systemic spread of primary central nervous system lymphoma. Clin Nucl Med 32:271–274
61. Maza S, Buchert R, Brenner W et al (2013) Brain and whole-body FDG-PET in diagnosis, treatment monitoring and long-term follow-up of primary CNS lymphomas. Radiol Oncol 47:103–110
62. Grimm SA, Pulido JS, Jahnke K et al (2007) Primary intraocular lymphoma: an International Primary Central Nervous System Lymphoma Collaborative Group Report. Ann Oncol 18:1851–1855
63. Hashida N, Ohguro N, Nishida K (2012) Efficacy and complications of Intravitreal Rituximab Injection for treating Primary Vitreoretinal Lymphoma. Trans Vis Sci Technol 1:1
64. Chan CC, Sen HN (2013) Current concepts in diagnosing and managing primary vitroretinal (intraocular) lymphoma. Discov Med 15(81):93–100
65. Riemens A, Bromberg J, Touitou V (2015) Treatment strategies in primary vitreoretinal lymphoma a 17-Center European Collaborative Study. JAMA Ophthalmol 133(2):191–197
66. Rodriguez EF, Sepah YJ, Jang HS et al (2014) Cytologic features in vitreous preparations of patients with suspicion of intraocular lymphoma. Diagn Cytopathol 42(1):37–44
67. Matsuo T, Ishimura K, Ichigawa T et al (2009) Positron emission tomography/computed tomography after immunohistochemical and clonal diagnosis of intraocular lymphoma with vitrectomy cell blocks. J Clin Exp Hematopathol 49:77–87
68. Zanni M, Moulin-Romsee G, Servois V et al (2012) Value of ^{18}FDG PET scan in staging of ocular adnexal lymphomas: a large single-center experience. Hematology 17:768
69. Larkin KL, Saboo US, Comer GM et al (2014) Use of intravitreal rituximab for treatment of vitreoretinal lymphoma. Br J Ophthalmol 98:99–103
70. Hanson JA, Alexandru D, Bota DA (2013) The evaluation and treatment of primary intraocular lymphoma. J Cancer Ther Res 2:15
71. Hoang-Xuan K, Bessell E, Bromberg J, et al, for the European Association for Neuro-Oncology Task Force on Primary CNS Lymphoma (2015) Diagnosis and treatment of primary CNS lymphoma in immunocompetent patients: guidelines from the European Association for Neuro-Oncology. Lancet Oncol 16:e322–e333

Part IV

Lymphomas in Children and Adolescents

Lymphomas in Children and Adolescents: Introduction

17

Helen V. Kosmidis, Helen Dana, Catherine Michail-Strantzia, Georgia Ch. Papaioannou, and Vassilios K. Prassopoulos

17.1 General Information

Helen V. Kosmidis, MD and Helen Dana, MD

Hodgkin and non-Hodgkin lymphomas account for approximately 13 % of cancers in children and adolescents younger than 20 years of age and are the third most common childhood malignancies following leukemia and CNS tumors.

H.V. Kosmidis, MD (✉) • H. Dana, MD
Department of Pediatric Oncology, 'MITERA' Hospital, 4, Erythrou Stavrou and Kifissias Av, Maroussi-Athens, 15123, Greece
e-mail: helkosm@yahoo.com; danaeleni@hotmail.gr

G.Ch. Papaioannou, MD
Department of Pediatric Radiology, 'MITERA' Hospital, 4, Erythrou Stavrou and Kifissias Av, Maroussi-Athens, 15123, Greece
e-mail: gpapaio@hotmail.com

C. Michail-Strantzia, MD
Pathology Laboratory, P. and A. Kyriakou Children's Hospital, Thivon and Livadias Str., Athens, 11527, Greece
e-mail: cstrantzia@gmail.com

V.K. Prassopoulos, MD
Department of Nuclear Medicine and PET/CT, 'HYGEIA' Hospital, 4, Erythrou Stavrou and Kifissias Av, Maroussi-Athens 15123, Greece
e-mail: vprasso@otenet.gr

17.1.1 Non-Hodgkin Lymphoma

The incidence of non-Hodgkin lymphoma (NHL) is increasing mainly in ages 15–19 years and is not common in very young children (infants and toddlers). With the exception of mediastinal diffuse large B-cell lymphoma, males are affected more frequently [1–3]. Most of NHL are high-grade diseases and are classified according to immunophenotype (B-cell lineage, T-cell lineage, NK-cell lineage) and differentiation (precursor cell or mature cell) in the following subgroups (WHO and updated REAL classification) [1]:

1. *Mature B-cell NHL (Burkitt, Burkitt-like lymphoma or mature B-cell leukemia, and diffuse large B-cell lymphoma)*

   Main sites of involvement in Burkitt and Burkitt-like NHL are intra-abdominal, head and neck, bone marrow, and CNS (sporadic form) or jaw (endemic form). Tumor cells bear translocations, the most common being t(8;14)(q24;q32) and less frequently t(2;8)(p11;q24) and t(8;22)(q24;q11). In diffuse large B-cell lymphomas, the disease involves lymph nodes, bones, abdomen, mediastinum, and CNS (as primary lymphoma, if it is associated with immunodeficiency) [1, 2, 4–6].
2. *Lymphoblastic NHL (T-cell precursor NHL and rarely B-cell precursor NHL)*

J.A. Andreou et al. (eds.), *PET/CT in Lymphomas: A Case-Based Atlas*,
DOI 10.1007/978-3-319-27380-8_17

Main sites of involvement in the T-cell precursor NHL is mediastinum and bone marrow and, in the rare B-cell precursor, skin, bone, and mediastinum. In lymphoblastic lymphomas, t(1;14)(p34;q11) or t(11;14)(p13;q11) translocations are seen. Individuals with ataxia-telengiectasia syndrome (autosomal recessive heredity) have 10 % risk of developing T-cell lymphoid malignancies.

3. *Large-cell anaplastic lymphoma (mature T-cell NHL or non-T-non-B-cell NHL)*

   This type of lymphoma may exhibit systemic manifestations as is fever and may involve the lungs, lymph nodes, and skin, bearing the t(2;5)(p23;q35) translocation [8].

The precise role of FDG-PET/CT in NHL both at the time of initial presentation (staging) and as a key imaging study for evaluating response to treatment and therefore intensifying chemotherapy has been extensively studied. It has been demonstrated that during therapy and for the assessment of response, FDG-PET/CT has a very good negative predictive value [9, 10].

Children with immunodeficiency may develop less common lymphomas, such as HIV-associated NHL or primary CNS lymphoma. Immunodeficiency may be inherited or due to organ or bone marrow transplantation (posttransplant lymphoproliferative disorder – PTLD) [11, 12].

According to WHO, 4 major categories of PTLD are distinguished: *early lesions*, *polymorphic PTLD*, *monomorphic PTLD* (which are B- or T-cell neoplasms), and *classical Hodgkin lymphoma* [11–13]. In children, most PTLDs are seen 1 year after organ transplantation or later at 2–3 years. Factors influencing the development of PTLD are seronegativity to EBV and less to CMV, age <18 years and transplantation of intestine (15–25 % risk), lung (15 %), heart (6 %), liver (5–10 %), and kidney (2–3 %) [11–13]. CNS PTLD is mainly seen after renal transplantation (12 % risk) [15]. FDG-PET and FDG-PET/CT has a higher positive predictive value than CT alone, although still in PTLD, its use has some limitations [13].

Other less common NHL are *pediatric follicular lymphomas,* which occur mainly in males and are usually localized diseases; *MALT lymphomas,* presenting as low-stage disease and associated with helicobacter pylori; *primary CNS lymphomas,* being diffuse large B cell or anaplastic-ype lymphomas; and *peripheral T-cell lymphomas* [1, 3].

Children and adolescents with NHL at diagnosis usually have advanced disease (stages III and IV). Radiographic imaging is essential in the staging and evaluation of tumor response to chemotherapy and thereafter modification (as upgrading) of treatment [3].

With current treatment protocols which are specially designed for each subtype of lymphoma and are incorporating CNS prophylaxis schemes, the majority of patients are cured of their disease. In lymphoblastic lymphomas, protocols designed for acute lymphoblastic leukemia are used, whereas in B mature NHL, very intensive therapy of short duration is the gold standard [6, 7, 14].

17.1.2 Hodgkin Lymphoma

Hodgkin lymphoma (HL) comprises 6 % of pediatric cancers affecting mainly adolescents (15–19 years) and less frequently younger ages, with the age group of 0–4 years being very rarely affected. Children younger than 5 years are mainly boys, whereas in the adolescent age group, there is a slight female predominance. Children <14 years belong to larger families with lower socioeconomic status, in contrast to adolescents (and young adults), in whom higher socioeconomic status is appreciated. It was shown that positive family history for HL is associated with increased risk. Epstein Barr virus (EBV) has been implicated in the development of HL, with EBV positive titers in children with HL and age <14 years and in those with mixed cellularity subtype tumors [15–18].

The majority of children and adolescents have nodal disease (cervical, mediastinal, or abdominal lymphadenopathy) and/or spleen involvement (stages I–III), whereas only 20 % have extra nodal disease, namely lungs, liver, bones, and bone marrow (stage IV). Classical HL is categorized into four subtypes: lymphocyte rich, lymphocyte depleted, mixed cellularity, and nodular sclerosis HL. Pretreatment factors associated with poorer prognosis are advanced stage, bulky disease, presence of B symptoms (as are fever, weight loss, night sweats, and less importantly pruritus and alcohol-induced pain), anemia and leukocytosis, and slow response to therapy [18, 19].

Effective treatment for HL has been reported even with the early protocols. However, due to the fact that survivors of HL are of great risk of late effects and in particular of secondary cancers and subfertility [20, 21], more recent protocols advocate the avoidance of radiotherapy if functional imaging with FDG–PET/CT shows early response [22–25] and the substitution of fertility interfering agents with others [20].

17.2 Pathology of Pediatric Lymphoma

Catherine N. Michail-Strantzia, MD

17.2.1 Non-Hodgkin Lymphoma

Lymphomas account for 15 % of childhood malignancies, with nearly equal distribution of Hodgkin (HL) and non-Hodgkin lymphomas (NHL). Pediatric non-Hodgkin lymphomas include a group of neoplasms that derive from both mature and immature cells of B- and T-cell origin. The use of clinical presentation; morphology; and immunophenotypic, molecular, and cytogenetic features is integral in order to make a definite diagnosis and classify NHL in subgroups [26].

NHL in children are typically intermediate and high-grade tumors, usually aggressive, fast-growing neoplasms, requiring efficient and appropriate handling of pathologic materials in order to ensure that a precise diagnosis can be established [26, 27].

NHL in current pathology practice is usually following the World Health Organization (WHO) classification. The WHO classification, according to the 2008 modification, recognizes a large spectrum of mature and blastic B-cell NHLs, including primarily nodal lymphoma, lymphomas with primarily extra nodal disease ,and those with leukemic presentation [28].

Lymphoblastic neoplasms represent leukemias or lymphomas of B- or T-precursor lymphoid cells. Clinically, they are divided into two categories: lymphoblastic lymphomas (LBL) and acute lymphoblastic leukemias (ALL), both sharing similar clinical and pathologic features and biologic processes. Typically LBL represents neoplastic processes involving extramedullary lymphoid tissues with less than 25 % bone marrow involvement, whereas in ALL, more than 25 % of bone marrow is involved with or without extramedullary disease [27–29].

Mature B-cell NHLs in children are follicular center-derived neoplasms, whereas post follicular neoplasms are mainly seen in adults. Pediatric mature B-cell NHL has a high proliferation rate and over expression of pro-proliferative proteins, suggesting that the lymphomagenesis is due to abnormal proliferation rather than defective apoptosis. This may explain the relatively uniform fast response to therapy in children [27, 30]. B-cell NHLs in children are most typically Burkitt's lymphoma (BL) and diffuse large B-cell lymphoma (DLBCL) of mature B-cell origin. The immature B-cell NHLs are blastic and precursor B-cell neoplasms seen infrequently in children [1].

Other subtypes of mature B-cell neoplasms, such as small lymphocytic lymphomas, mantle cell lymphomas, plasma cell neoplasms, and lymphomatoid granulomatosis, are extremely rare and appear to represent unusual presentation of typical adult disease in children and adolescents [26–28].

Low-grade lymphomas follicular and marginal zone, which are seen in adults, are seen infrequently in children and have been recently recognized as distinct disease entities in children by the current WHO classification [28].

Mature T-cell neoplasms in children and adolescents comprise about 10–15 % of the NHLs. Specific subtypes of mature T-cell and NK-cell NHL have been recognized and defined by the WHO classification on the basis of clinical features, immunophenotype, cytogenetic, and molecular features. In this group, the anaplastic large-cell lymphoma (LCAL) is classified, which less commonly is null cell disease (non-T, non-B) [27, 28, 30]. In addition, there are some other mature T-NHL's that, although rare, occur predominantly in adolescents and young adults. These are [28, 30]:

- Extranodal NK/T-cell lymphoma nasal type: an angiocentric and angiodestructive neoplasm.
- Aggressive NK-cell leukemia: a genotypically and phenotypically similar tumor to extra nodal NK/T-cell neoplasm
- Hepatosplenic gamma-delta T-cell lymphoma
- Lymphoproliferative disorders associated with primary immune disorders as the posttransplant lymphoproliferative disease (PTLD)

Conclusion: Four subtypes comprise nearly 90 % of the NHL in children. These are Burkitt lymphoma, diffuse large B-cell lymphoma, lymphoblastic lymphoma (T- or B-cell precursor), and anaplastic large-cell lymphoma. The remaining 10 % include follicular lymphoma, marginal-zone lymphoma, cutaneous lymphoma, and peripheral T-cell lymphoma, which are common in adult population.

17.2.2 Hodgkin's Lymphoma

Hodgkin lymphoma (HL) is a clonal B-cell malignant neoplasm with unique clinical and pathologic features. It accounts for approximately 7 % of all childhood malignancies and 50 % of all lymphomas in children and is extremely uncommon in infancy, with a pick incidence in the 15–20 years age group [31].

Hodgkin lymphoma comprises a minority of neoplastic cells, the Reed–Sternberg cells and their variants, and a majority of reactive inflammatory cells in varying proportions. These include lymphocytes of various kinds, plasma cells, polymorphonuclear neutrophils and eosinophils, histiocytes, and fibroblasts, which form the bulk of the tumor. Based on its clinical behavior, as well as morphologic, immunophenotypic, and genetic profiles, Hodgkin lymphoma is divided into two entities, the nodular lymphocyte predominant Hodgkin lymphoma and the classical Hodgkin lymphoma, with the following subtypes according to the current WHO classification [31, 32]:

- Nodular lymphocyte predominant Hodgkin lymphoma (NLPHL)
- Classic Hodgkin lymphoma (CHL)
  - Nodular sclerosis (NSHL)
  - Mixed cellularity (MCHL)
  - Lymphocyte rich (LRCHL)
  - Lymphocyte depleted (LDHL)

These subtypes share the same immunophenotype of tumor cells but differ in their sites of involvement, clinical features, growth pattern, presence of fibrosis, composition of cellular background, degree of tumor cell's atypia, and the frequency of Epstein–Barr virus (EBV) infection [32].

17.3 Imaging Investigation in Children and Adolescents with Hodgkin and Non-Hodgkin Lymphoma

Georgia Papaioannou, MD
and Vassilios Prassopoulos, MD

17.3.1 Conventional Imaging

Diagnostic imaging in the initial diagnosis and staging of children with lymphoma using multimodality approach plays a substantial role in the evaluation of the extent of involvement. Imaging evaluation is unable to replace histologic analysis; however, it plays a crucial role in the staging which subsequently determines prognosis and treatment plan.

In children, the initial imaging exploration is usually performed with ultrasound (US). US is the ideal modality to evaluate superficial lymph nodes, in order to accurately detect abnormal texture and vascularity, and the modality of choice to detect testicular infiltration. US may also appear useful in identifying abnormally infiltrated bowel loops, parenchymal infiltrates in solid abdominal organs, and intra-abdominal lymph node enlargement.

However, since US has limitations with respect to the patient's body habitus and cooperation, cross-sectional imaging is irreplaceable during the staging phase. For reasons of radioprotection and according to availability, MRI is indicated for the investigation of the neck (additional evaluation of Waldeyer ring), the abdomen, and the CNS in clinical signs of CNS involvement. Evaluation of the chest could be initially performed with chest radiography, to assess mediastinal expansion and parenchymal disease and rarely chest wall invasion. However, there are reports suggesting that up to 50 % of chest disease may go undetected on plain chest radiographs in untreated patients [33] which raise the question whether chest CT should be performed routinely. Evaluation of bone disease (^{99m}Tc bone scan, MRI, FDG-PET) is recommended only in children with bone pain and elevated alkaline phosphatase concentration [33].

17.3.2 FDG-PET/CT

The role of FDG-PET/CT in evaluating adult Hodgkin and non-Hodgkin lymphoma is well documented. However, manifestations of lymphomas in childhood and adolescence are quite different, thus requiring different therapeutic and imaging approaches. Conventional imaging, although mandatory and helpful to accurate staging, restaging, and treatment response evaluation of lymphomas, may bear size, bone marrow, and visceral involvement limitations and further cross-sectional assessment is required.

FDG-PET has been employed recently for the evaluation of pediatric lymphomas; it has been advocated for the accurate staging, treatment planning, and response evaluation, exploiting its inherent ability to investigate and reveal areas of increased metabolic activity [34]. FDG-PET plays a documented role in determining the indication of radiotherapy and is routinely applied in the follow-up of children with HL. Thus, it has dramatically reduced the number of children that undergo additional radiotherapy as it allows differentiation between inactive residual lesions and active disease [22].

HL is routinely FDG avid (in 97–100 % of cases), while some caution should be paid in cases of lymphocyte-predominant HD, as this subtype may exhibit lower focal uptake [35]. The sensitivity and specificity of the method are reported high (96.5–98 % and >99 % specificity), higher than conventional imaging, with an accuracy of 96.7 % [36, 37]. Special attention has been attributed to bone marrow involvement imaging, where studies agree that uni- or multifocal pattern is evident of bone marrow dissemination, as well as that FDG-PET/CT bears a higher accuracy in detecting bone marrow infiltration than the biopsy of the ileum [38]. According to the EuroNet-PHL-Study Group, FDG-PET/CT is recommended in all children and adolescents with classic Hodgkin lymphoma before the initialization of therapy [39]. Moreover, bone marrow involvement is assumed if MRI and FDG-PET are both positive in the same area [39]. Radiotherapy plans are based on the initial affected areas. In this setting, FDG-PET may play an important role for planning determination, changing the involved fields in 1/3 of cases [35].

Interim PET for HL is recommended after two cycles of chemotherapy (strictly on day 14–17 after the last chemotherapy), and lesions initially affected should be assessed, as well as new sites only if progression is suspected. Bone marrow infiltration is only assessed by FDG-PET when findings are recognized at conventional imaging. FDG-PET is not recommended after the end of treatment. The same occurs for surveillance, with the exception that relapse is confirmed. In cases of adequate response with the utilization of FDG-PET after two cycles of chemotherapy, radiotherapy is omitted [39].

Non-Hodgkin lymphoma mainly consists of tumor cells, rather than inflammatory as in HL, which in fact indicates a different approach both to the interpretation criteria of FDG-PET and the therapeutic strategy followed. Furthermore, bone marrow involvement is reported more frequently, and emergency in initializing chemotherapy is not rare. However, most NHLs in childhood and adolescence are aggressive, therefore FDG avid [35]. FDG-PET is sensitive in detecting nodal (referred detecting 88.3 % of total lesions) and extranodal disease [40] in NHL children; outperforms contrast CT, leading to upstaging in 7/21 cases [40]; and thus may be used complementary to conventional imaging in this group of patients.

Studies investigating the role of FDG-PET/CT for treatment response evaluation in NHL pediatric patients are scarce and occupy small groups of patients. PET imaging is suggested to take place as close as possible to the next chemotherapeutic cycle, while standardized PET response criteria urge to be defined. However, the negative prognostic value and sensitivity of chemosensitivity assessment FDG-PET are reported, and PET may serve as a reliable imaging procedure for favorable response [10, 35]. Biopsy is recommended in PET-positive cases [10, 35]. Further studies are required to validate the usefulness of FDG-PET/CT in NHL patients.

References

1. Jaffe ES, Harris NL, Stein H et al (2008) Introduction and overview of the classification of the lymphoid neoplasms. In: Swerdlow SH, Campo E, Harris NL ét al (eds) WHO classification of tumors of haematopoietic and lymphoid tissues, 4th edn. IARC, Lyon, pp 157–166
2. Mbulaiteye SM, Biggar RJ, Bhatia K et al (2009) Sporadic childhood Burkitt lymphoma incidence in the United States during 1992–2005. Pediatr Blood Cancer 53(3):366–370
3. Sandlung JT, Downing JR, Crist WM (1996) Non-Hodgkin's lymphoma in childhood. N Engl J Med 334(19):1238–1248
4. Klapper W, Szczepanowski M, Burkhardt B et al (2008) Molecular profiling of pediatric mature B-cell lymphoma treated in population-based prospective clinical trials. Blood 112(4):1374–1381
5. Lones MA, Perkins SL, Sposto R et al (2002) Non-Hodgkin's lymphoma arising in bone in children and adolescents is associated with excellent outcome: a Children's Cancer Group report. J Clin Oncol 20(9):2293–2301
6. Reiter A, Klapper W (2008) Recent advances in the understanding and the management of diffuse large B cell lymphoma in childhood and adolescence. Br J Haematol 142(3):329–347
7. Reiter A, Schrappe M, Ludwig WD et al (2000) Intensive ALL-type therapy without local radiotherapy provides a 90% event-free survival for children with T-cell lymphoblastic lymphoma: a BFM group report. Blood 95(2):416–421
8. Lamant L, McCarthy K, d'Amore E et al (2011) Prognostic impact of morphologic and phenotypic features of childhood ALK positive anaplastic large cell lymphoma: results of the ALCL99 study. J Clin Oncol 29(35):4669–4676
9. Bailly C, Eugene T, Couec ML et al (2014) Prognostic value and clinical impact of FDG=PET in the management of children with Burkitt lymphoma after induction chemotherapy. Vol 1, article 54. www.frontiersin.org
10. Bhojwani D, McCarville MB, Choi JK et al (2015) The role of FDG-PET/CT in the evaluation of residual disease in paediatric non-Hodgkin lymphoma. Br J Haematol 168(6):845–853
11. Loren AW, Porter DL, Stadtmauer EA et al (2003) Post-transplant lymphoproliferative disorder: a review. Bone Marrow Transplant 31(3):145–155
12. Mynarek M, Schober T, Behrends U et al (2013) Post transplant lymphoproliferative disease after pediatric Solid organ transplantation. Clin Developmental Immunol: Article ID 814973
13. Parker A, Bowles K, Bradley A et al (2010) Diagnosis of post transplant lymphoproliferative disorder in solid organ transplant recipients – BCSH and BTS Guidelines. Br J Haematol 149:675–692
14. Patte C, Auperin A, Gerrard M et al (2007) Results of the randomized international FAB/LMB96 trial for intermediate risk B-cell non-Hodgkin lymphoma in children and adolescents: it is possible to reduce treatment for the early responding patients. Blood 109(7): 2773–2780
15. Armstrong AA, Alexander FF, Cartwright R et al (1998) Epstein Barr virus and Hodgkin's disease: further evidence for the three disease hypothesis. Leukemia 12(8):1272–1276
16. Chang ET, Montgomery SA, Richiardi L et al (2004) Number of siblings and risk of Hodgkin's lymphoma. Cancer Epidemiol Biomarkers Prev 13(7):1236–1244
17. Jarrett RF, Stark GL, White J et al (2005) Impact of tumor Epstein Barr virus status on presenting features and outcome in age-defined subgroups of patients with classic Hodgkin lymphoma: a population-based study. Blood 106(7):2444–2451
18. Macfarlane GJ, Evstifeeva T, Boyle P et al (1995) International patterns in the occurrence of Hodgkin's disease in children and young adult males. Int J Cancer 61(2):165–169
19. Mathas S (2007) The pathogenesis of classical Hodgkin's lymphoma: a model for B cell plasticity. Hematol Oncol Clin North Am 21(5):787–804
20. Mauz-Korholz C, Hasenclever D, Dorffel W et al (2010) Procarbazine free OEPA/COPDAC chemotherapy in boys and standard OPPA-COPP in girls have comparable effectiveness in pediatric Hodgkin's lymphoma: the GPOH-HD-2002 study. J Clin Oncol 28(23):3680–3686
21. O'Brien MM, Donaldson SS, Balise RR et al (2010) Second malignant neoplasms in survivors of pediatric Hodgkin's lymphoma treated with low dose radiation and chemotherapy. J Clin Oncol 28(7):1232–1239
22. Hudson MM, Krasin MJ, Kaste SC et al (2004) PET imaging in pediatric Hodgkin's lymphoma. Pediatr Radiol 34(3):190–198

23. Ilivitzki A, Radan L, Ben-Arush M et al (2013) Early interim FDG PET/CT prediction of treatment response and prognosis in pediatric Hodgkin disease-added value of low dose CT. Pediatr Radiol 43(1):86–92
24. Rathore N, Eissa HM, Margolin JF et al (2012) Pediatric Hodgkin lymphoma: are we over-scanning our patients? Pediatr Hematol Oncol 29(5):415–423
25. Ruhl U, Albrecht M, Dieckmann K et al (2001) Response adapted radiotherapy in the treatment of pediatric Hodgkin's disease: an interim response at 5 years of the German GPOH-HD 95 trial. Int J Radiat Oncol Biol Phys 51(5):1209–1218
26. Sm J, Linden E, Termuhlen AM, Flynn JM (2009) Lymphoma in adolescents and young adults. Semin Oncol 36(5):381–418
27. Cairo MS, Raetz E, Lim MS, Davenport V, Perkins LS (2005) Childhood and adolescent non-Hodgkin's lymphoma; new insights in biology and critical challenges for the future. Pediatr Blood Cancer 45(6):753–769
28. Swerdlow SH, Campo E, Harris NL et al (2008) WHO classification of tumors of haemotopaetic and lymphoid tissues, 4th edn. IARC Press, Lyon
29. Freedman AS, Aster JC (2014) Clinical manifestations, pathologic features, and diagnosis of precursor T cell acute lymphoblastic leukemia/lymphoma. www.uptodate.com
30. Jaffe ES, Harris NL, Stein H, Vardiman JW (2001) Pathology and genetics. Tumors of haematopoietic and lymphoid tissues. IARC Press, Lyon
31. Bai M, Panoulas V, Papoudou-Bai A, Horianopoulos N, Kitsoulis P, Stefanaki K, Rontagianni D, Agnantis NJ, Kanavaros P (2006) B-cell differentiation immunophenotypes in classical Hodgkin lymphomas. Leuk Lymphoma 47:495–501
32. Marafioti T, Hummel M, Foss HD, Laumen H, Korbjuhn P, Anagnostopoulos I et al (2000) Hodgkin and Reed – Sternberg cells represent an expansion of a single clone originating from a germinal center B-cell with functional immunoglobulin gene rearrangements but defective immunoglobulin transcription. Blood 95(4):1443–1450
33. Toma P, Granata C, Rossi A, Garaventa A (2007) Multimodality imaging of Hodgkin disease and non-Hodgkin lymphomas in children. Radiographics 27:1335–1354
34. Sioka C (2013) The utility of FDG PET in diagnosis and follow-up of lymphoma in childhood. Eur J Pediatr 172:733–738
35. Kluge R, Kurch L, Montravers F, Mauz-Körholz C (2013) FDG PET/CT in children and adolescents with lymphoma. Pediatr Radiol 43(4):406–417
36. Hutchings M, Loft A, Hansen M, Pedersen LM, Berthelsen AK, Keiding S, D'Amore F, Boesen AM, Roemer L, Specht L (2006) Position emission tomography with or without computed tomography in the primary staging of Hodgkin's lymphoma. Haematologica 91(4):482–489
37. London K, Cross S, Onikul E, Dalla-Pozza L, Howman-Giles R (2011) 18F-FDG PET/CT in paediatric lymphoma: comparison with conventional imaging. Eur J Nucl Med Mol Imaging 38(2):274–284
38. Purz S, Mauz-Körholz C, Körholz D, Hasenclever D, Krausse A, Sorge I, Ruschke K, Stiefel M, Amthauer H, Schober O, Kranert WT, Weber WA, Haberkorn U, Hundsdörfer P, Ehlert K, Becker M, Rössler J, Kulozik AE, Sabri O, Kluge R (2011) [18F]Fluorodeoxyglucose positron emission tomography for detection of bone marrow involvement in children and adolescents with Hodgkin's lymphoma. J Clin Oncol 29(26):3523–3528
39. EuroNet-Paediatric Hodgkin's Lymphoma Group Recommendations for the Diagnostics and Treatment of children and adolescents with a classical Hodgkin's Lymphoma during the Interim phase between the end of the EuroNet-PHL-C1 Study and the start of the EuroNet-PHLC2 Study 2013
40. Cheng G, Servaes S, Zhuang H (2013) Value of (18) F-fluoro-2-deoxy-D-glucose positron emission tomography/computed tomography scan versus diagnostic contrast computed tomography in initial staging of pediatric patients with lymphoma. Leuk Lymphoma 54(4):737–742

Hodgkin Lymphoma in Children

18

Dimitrios Doganis, Georgia Ch. Papaioannou, and Vassilios K. Prassopoulos

18.1 Introduction

Dimitrios Doganis, MD

Hodgkin lymphoma (HL) is the sixth most common type of cancer during childhood, accounting for approximately 5 % of all malignancies and half of all childhood lymphomas. HL is very rare in children under 5 years of age, whereas the incidence among patients younger than 15 years is 5.5 cases per million and for those aged 15–20 years reaches 12.1 cases per million [1–3]. A characteristic bimodal curve with an early peak during adolescence and a second peak in patients aged above 50 years old is well recognized.

HL is a lymphoreticular malignancy. Painless cervical or supraclavicular lymphadenopathy and mediastinal involvement are the most common sites of disease involvement in childhood HL. A definite diagnosis of HL needs a biopsy. HL is characterized by specific histopathological features which include a replacement of nodal architecture by an inflammatory cellular background containing Reed-Sternberg cells or their variants [4] and is classified into two disease entities: the classical HL (CHL, 95 % of cases, with four histology subtypes – nodular sclerosis, mixed cellularity, lymphocyte depleted, and lymphocyte-rich) and the nodular lymphocyte-predominant Hodgkin lymphoma (NLPHL, 5 % of cases) [5].

Accurate staging, including bone marrow and imaging evaluation, plays the major role in the management of patients with HL. Ultrasound, bone scanning, MRI, and computed tomography have been the gold standard for the initial staging, for assessing response to therapy, and for detecting tumor persistence or relapse. With the introduction of functional imaging modalities like gallium and positron emission tomography (PET) with 18F-fluorodeoxyglucose (18F-FDG), tumor activity could be correlated with anatomic features detected by conventional imaging [6, 7].

Factors such as the disease stage, patient's age, presence or absence of "B" symptoms (unexplained fever with temperature above 38 °C, drenching night sweats, weight loss of 10 %), presence of bulky nodal disease, and the response to treatment define the patient's management [2, 3, 8].

The introduction of combined/hybrid chemotherapy protocols, which have the advantage of lower cumulative doses of each agent, with or

D. Doganis, MD (✉)
Department of Oncology, P and A Kyriakou Children's Hospital, Levadias 6, Athens, 11527, Greece
e-mail: doganisd@gmail.com

G.Ch. Papaioannou, MD
Department of Pediatric Radiology, HOSPITAL 'MOTHER', Kifissias Av. and Q. Cross 4, Maroussi 15123, Greece
e-mail: gpapaio@hotmail.com

V.K. Prassopoulos, MD
Department of Nuclear Medicine and PET/CT, D.TH.K.A. "HEALTH", Kifissias Av. and Q. Cross 4, Maroussi 15123, Greece
e-mail: vprasso@otenet.gr

J.A. Andreou et al. (eds.), *PET/CT in Lymphomas: A Case-Based Atlas*,
DOI 10.1007/978-3-319-27380-8_18

without radiotherapy (RT), improved significantly the outcome of children with HL. The vast majority of these children nowadays have an excellent chance of definite cure. The 5-year event-free survival in childhood and adolescence exceeds 90 % for patients in the early stage of the disease and 70–80 % for those with advanced stage [9–11]. Even after relapse, the survival rate ranges between 50 and 80 %. For this group of patients, aggressive chemotherapy followed by bone marrow transplantation has proven to be beneficial [12].

The high curative rates that have been achieved modified treatment strategies, and currently, protocols aim at minimizing such late effects as cardiopulmonary toxicity, endocrine sequelae (hypothyroidism, gonad toxicity, and infertility), bone growth alterations, pulmonary sequelae, and secondary malignancies attributed to both radiotherapy and chemotherapy [7, 13].

To conclude, current management policy for childhood HL should focus on the patients who could be treated with the minimal required therapy and especially on those who can be cured without RT. Early response to chemotherapy is useful for the identification of patients with a lower risk for relapse, and consequently PET/CT scan could be used in selecting good-prognosis HL patients, who with less intensive and less morbid chemotherapy and without RT can be cured [3].

18.2 Cases Presentation

Dimitrios Doganis, MD,
Georgia Ch. Papaioannou, MD,
and Vassilios K. Prassopoulos, MD

Case 1

A 14-year-old adolescent girl was referred to our department with a history of right cervical and supraclavicular painless swelling. No symptoms were reported. At the time of her admission, ESR was 60 mm/h and LDH 245 U/L. Ultrasound (US) and computed tomography (CT) scan showed multiple enlarged lymph nodes in the right cervical, supraclavicular, and subclavian area, of 4 cm maximum diameter with parenchymal inhomogeneity and increased disorganized vascularity. Chest CT scan revealed multiple enlarged (maximum diameter of 5 cm) mediastinal lymph nodes, some of them in close proximity to the superior vena cava. Abdominal US and CT scan showed a hypoechoic, well-defined lesion (of 12 mm diameter) in the spleen.

Baseline PET/CT confirmed the presence of disseminated nodal disease in the cervical, supraclavicular, and subclavian regions (SUVmax of 6.2) and the mediastinum (SUVmax of 10.7). Severe compression to the trachea was noted on PET/CT, but it went undetected on conventional imaging. There was no evidence of active disease in the abdominal cavity on PET/CT, despite the splenic finding on US and CT scan (Fig. 18.1a, b).

Cervical lymph node biopsy revealed Hodgkin disease of nodular sclerosis according to the Rye classification [14]. She was staged as TG1, but because of bulky disease and elevated ESR, the patient was treated as TG2 according to the EuroNet-PHL-C1 protocol [15]. Our patient received two cycles of OPPA regimen (vincristine, prednisone, procarbazine, and doxorubicin) – procarbazine was used instead of etoposide because of allergic reaction to etoposide. US and CT scan demonstrated residual lymph node enlargement at the corresponding initially involved sites with remarkable interval reduction in size. Chest CT scan additionally revealed as a new finding lung nodules.

Interim PET/CT scan (Fig. 18.2) did not present any uptake at the previously affected areas, whereas the lung lesions, which were not evident on the baseline PET/CT scan, were attributed to infection (SUVmax of 1.7). Evaluation with QuantiFERON test and serum galactomannan assay was negative for *Mycobacterium* and *Aspergillus* infiltration, respectively.

Patient received two cycles of cyclophosphamide, vincristine, prednisone, and dacarbazine (COPDAC), and after the end of the chemotherapy, imaging studies including US and CT scan did not reveal any disease-related findings. PET/CT was also normal even for the lesions previously considered infectious. Because of imaging findings, the patient was classified as AR2 and no radiotherapy was provided. Eighteen months since the end of treatment, Hodgkin lymphoma is in complete remission.

Discussion

Therapeutic strategies have improved the survival of children with HL over the past decades, and, therefore, current treatment policy has prompted efforts to modify protocols to reduce the long-term toxicity and the risk for second malignancies caused especially by radiotherapy without jeopardizing the final outcome [3].

PET/CT scan has been introduced in children with HL for the initial staging but also for response assessment. Early response evaluation by PET/CT scan in pediatric HL patients might help physicians to identify those patients for whom radiotherapy is not necessary. In the protocol we administered to our patient (EuroNet-PHL-C1 study), radiotherapy is omitted, if interim – early PET becomes negative [7, 15]. Our patient did not receive radiotherapy since PET/CT scan did not present uptake in the initially involved fields after the first two cycles of chemotherapy. Moreover, PET/CT scan was also useful because our patient was staged as TG1 since no active disease of the spleen was detected in the PET/SCAN in contrast to conventional imaging.

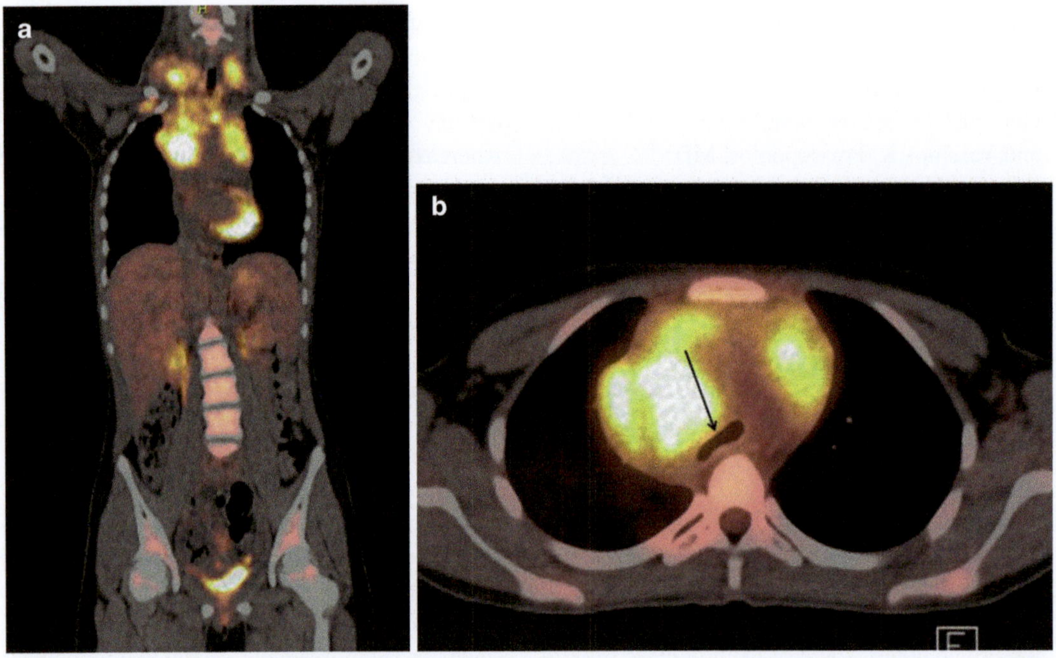

Fig. 18.1 (**a**, **b**) PET/CT scan (**a** coronal reformat, **b** axial) detected the presence of disseminated nodal disease in cervical, supraclavicular, subclavian (SUVmax of 6.2), and mediastinal area (SUVmax of 10.7). Severe compression to the trachea was also noted (*arrow* in **b**)

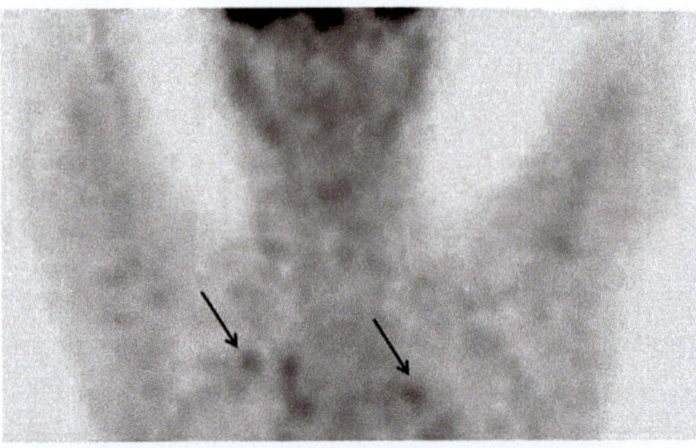

Fig. 18.2 Interim PET/CT scan did not present any uptake in the originally detected lymphoma sites. Lung lesions identified (*arrows*) were considered infectious (SUVmax of 1.7)

Case 2

We present the case of an 8-year-old girl with a history of fever up to 39 °C, sore throat, and abdominal pain during the last 3 days before her admission to our department. She looked sick, whereas pallor was obvious at clinical examination. At the time of her admission, WBC count was 29,500/mm^3 (neutrophils ratio 75 %), Hb 10.6 g/dl, CRP 282 mg/dl, ESR 88 mm/h, and LDH 245 U/L. After the administration of IV antibiotics, her temperature dropped and the infection markers (WBC and CRP) normalized. Imaging investigations including chest X-ray, ultrasound (US), and computed tomography (CT) scan showed multiple supraclavicular enlarged lymph nodes as well as a remarkably large lymphadenic block in the anterior and middle mediastinum. Additionally, CT scan detected two nodular lesions in the superior lobe of the right lung. Bone marrow aspiration and biopsy were negative for any type of infiltration, whereas abdominal imaging showed no enlarged abdominal lymph nodes or other organ involvement. Supraclavicular lymph node biopsy revealed Hodgkin disease of nodular sclerosis according to the Rye classification [14].

Regarding staging, our patient should have been staged as stage IV according to the Ann Arbor staging system with Cotswolds modifications [16, 17] due to the lesions that had been detected in the lung parenchyma. Nevertheless, PET/CT scan (Fig. 18.3) did not confirm hypermetabolic activity in the lung parenchyma allowing us to ignore CT scan pulmonary lesions. On the other hand, supraclavicular and mediastinal lymph node enlargement was affirmed by PET/CT scan (SUVmax of 5.4 and 6.5, respectively). No evidence of active disease was detected in the abdominal cavity in the PET/CT in concordance with the conventional imaging evaluation. Moreover, since fever was attributed to coexistent infection, no B symptoms were considered during staging workup. Consequently, our patient was staged as IIA with thoracic ratio of maximum transverse mass diameter of 0.45 and ESR >50/h.

Our patient received four cycles of COPP/ABV hybrid regimen (cyclophosphamide, vincristine, procarbazine, prednisone, doxorubicin, bleomycin, vinblastine). After two cycles of chemotherapy, a supraclavicular and mediastinal mass size reduction of more than 75 % was detected in conventional imaging evaluation. At the end of chemotherapy, the reduction ratio in comparison with the initial mass size was found to be more than 90 %. Radiotherapy (20Gy) was administered in the initially involved fields, and at the end of treatment, no residual mass was found. She is now 17 months off treatment and her Hodgkin lymphoma is in complete remission.

Discussion

Our patient underwent an initial PET/CT investigation which was part of the staging process. PET/CT scan clarified that conventional abnormal imaging findings were not Hodgkin lymphoma related, and consequently she was treated as of lower stage than that if PET/CT scan had not been performed.

Conventional imaging evaluation (CI), including X-ray, US, and CT scan, has been the recommended approach in the staging and assessment of response at the interim and the end of therapy in children with HL. The drawbacks of CI include its failure to differentiate lymphoma lesions from other benign ones creating a therapeutic dilemma whether the patient requires further treatment or not since, in case of no malignant lesions, CI overestimates the stage. On the other hand, CI fails to identify tumor deposits in normal-size lymph nodes, thus, underestimating the stage of the disease before starting therapy [18, 19]. After the introduction of PET/CT scan in the evaluation of Hodgkin lymphoma, it is being routinely used for staging, response monitoring, and prognosis of the disease [18]. PET-CT is a promising modality in determining the patient's management when there are ambiguous findings in the CI, therefore, helping physicians to avoid further unnecessary chemotherapy cycles and/or radiotherapy, as was the case with our patient. Additional and well-designed prospective studies of PET scan in pediatric Hodgkin lymphoma patients will increase the understanding about the optimal use of this imaging modality and will distinguish the nonmalignant findings that may be confusing for the interpretation of imaging evaluation.

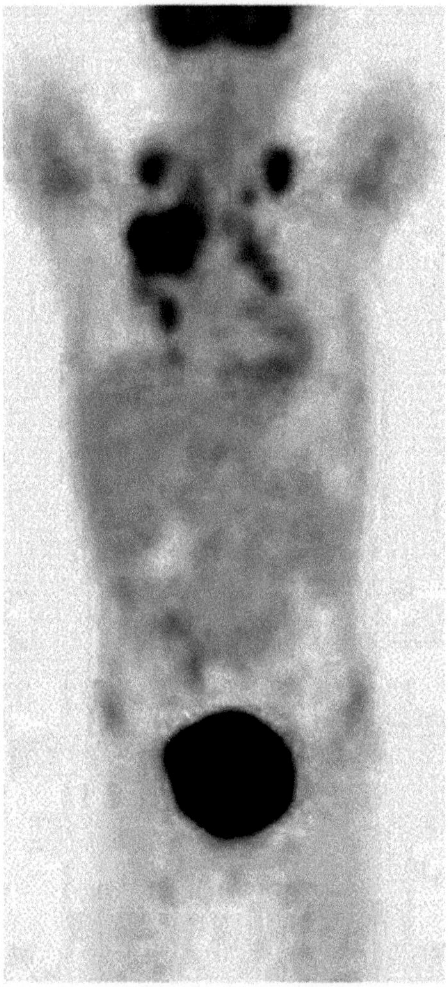

Fig. 18.3 PET/CT scan detected the presence of nodal disease in cervical and supraclavicular area (SUVmax of 5,4) as well as extensive nodal disease in the mediastinum (SUVmax of 10.7)

Case 3

A previously healthy 13-year-old girl was admitted to our department with a history of fever and sciatic neuralgia in the 2 months prior to her admission. Her evaluation with chest X-ray and computed tomography (CT) scan showed mediastinal enlargement and supraclavicular enlarged lymph nodes. Further imaging evaluation with magnetic resonance imaging (MRI), CT scan, and bone scan with Tc-99m revealed lesions in the sacrum, ilium, right femur, and the first sacral vertebra.

At the same time, PET/SCAN showed hypermetabolic activity in the left tonsil (SUVmax of 6.8), the supraclavicular lymph nodes bilaterally (SUVmax of 5.6), the mediastinum (SUVmax of 6.7), the ninth right rib (SUVmax of 2.6), the abdominal cavity (SUVmax of 5.7) and the sacrum (SUVmax of 7.2) (Fig. 18.4).

Bone marrow aspiration and biopsy were negative for any abnormal findings. At the time of her admission, WBC count was 13,700/mm^3 (neutrophils ratio 72 %), Hb 11.7 mg/dl, and ESR 61 mm/h. Supraclavicular lymph node biopsy revealed Hodgkin disease of nodular sclerosis according to the Rye classification [14], and our patient was staged as IV according to the Ann Arbor staging system with Cotswolds modifications [16, 17].

Our patient received two cycles of OPPA regimen (vincristine, prednisone, procarbazine, and doxorubicin) and four cycles of COPP (cyclophosphamide, vincristine, prednisone, and procarbazine). After two cycles of chemotherapy, interim PET/CT detected residual hypermetabolic activity restricted in the left tonsil (SUVmax of 4.2) and the sacrum (SUVmax of 2.8) (Fig. 18.5), whereas it became negative at the completion of chemotherapy. Radiotherapy (20 Gy) was administered after the end of chemotherapy in the initially involved fields and the sacrum. At the end of treatment, no hypermetabolic activity was found on the PET/CT.

Two months after the end of the treatment, she presented with pruritus, low-grade fever, and ESR 45 mm/h. At that time, the PET/CT presented avid uptake in abdominal lymph nodes (SUVmax of 7.5), liver (SUVmax of 4.5), and the right lung (SUVmax of 1.1) (Fig. 18.6). Conventional imaging confirmed PET/CT findings of relapse. She received two cycles of MINE regimen (mitoxantrone, ifosfamide, vinorelbine, and etoposide) as relapse treatment, and PET/CT turned negative for all the previously detected lesions. Following this, our patient underwent peripheral blood stem cell transplantation; she is now 9 months off treatment and her lymphoma in complete remission.

Discussion

Current protocols for pediatric Hodgkin lymphoma retain an excellent chance of definite cure. Even after relapse, survival rates are satisfactory, ranging between 50 and 80 %. In the case of relapse in HL patients, aggressive chemotherapy followed by bone marrow transplantation has proven to be beneficial [12].

PET/CT was not only helpful in the initial staging of our patient but also in establishing relapse. Furthermore, a high level of concordance with conventional imaging was detected. For patients in the first remission after the completion of treatment, current protocols mandate follow-up surveillance imaging depending upon the patient's risk stratification. On the other hand, many controversies have arisen concerning the type of imaging modalities that should be used for the follow-up as well as the frequency of surveillance. The need for frequent follow-up seems to be rational since the aim of physicians is to promptly detect relapse at a time of minimal disease burden. According to some studies, the majority of these relapses were detected by scans at a time when the patients were not symptomatic, but this is not universally accepted [20, 21].

Our patient was diagnosed with a relapse within only 2 months after the completion of her treatment – not during surveillance evaluation but because of symptoms and laboratory findings which necessitated an extensive imaging evaluation. PET/CT and conventional imaging were mandatory for both initial and relapse evaluation.

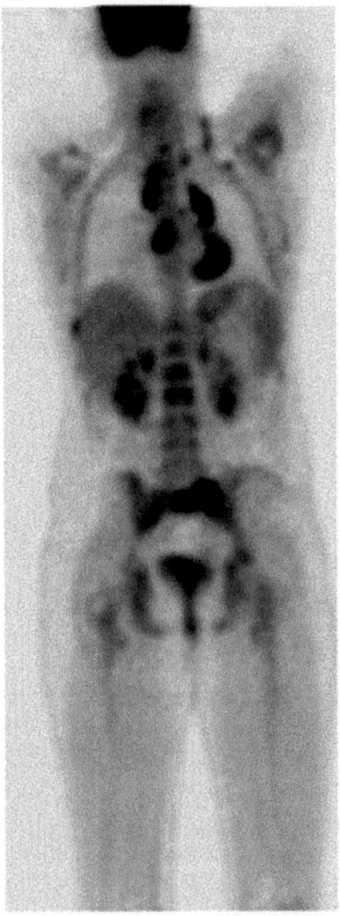

Fig. 18.4 The initial PET/CT showed hypermetabolic activity in the left tonsil (not evident on this figure), the supraclavicular lymph nodes bilaterally, the mediastinum, the ninth right rib, the abdominal cavity, and the sacrum

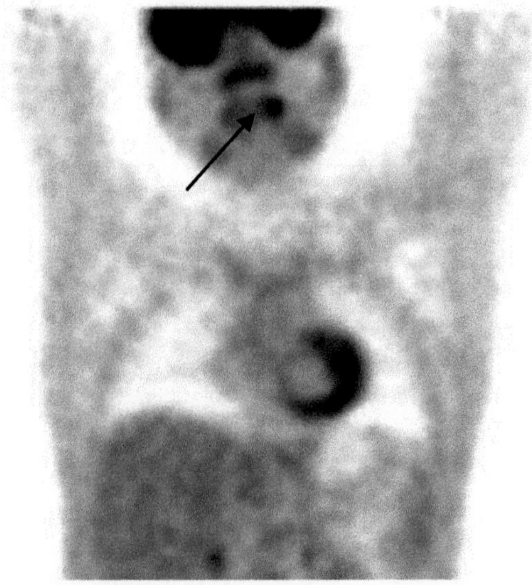

Fig. 18.5 The interim PET/SCAN detected hypermetabolic activity only in the left tonsil (*black arrow*) and the sacrum (not included in this figure)

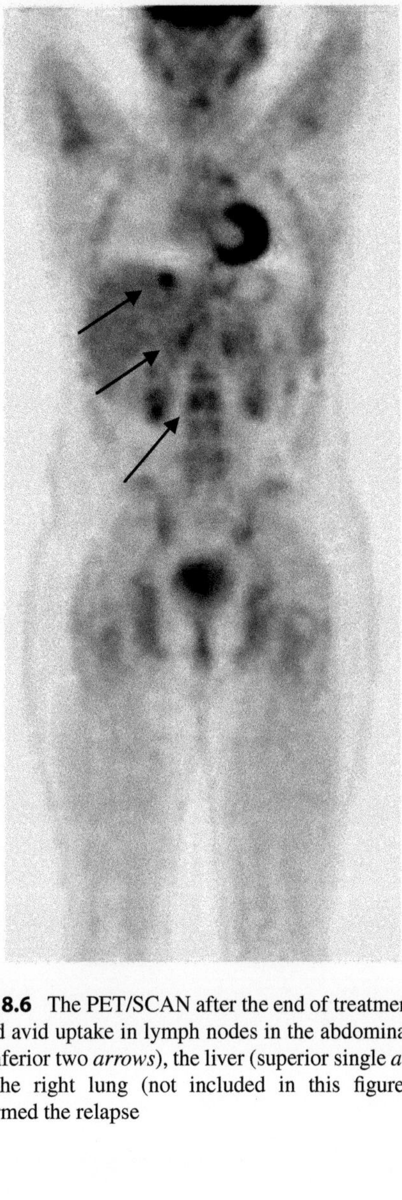

Fig. 18.6 The PET/SCAN after the end of treatment presented avid uptake in lymph nodes in the abdominal cavity (inferior two *arrows*), the liver (superior single *arrow*), and the right lung (not included in this figure) and confirmed the relapse

References

1. Gurney J, Bondy M (2006) Chapter 1. Epidemiology of childhood cancer. In: Pizzo AP, Poplack DG (eds) Principles and practice of pediatric oncology, 5th edn. Lippincott-Raven, Philadelphia, pp 1–13
2. Pourtsidis A, Doganis D, Baka M et al (2013) Differences between younger and older patients with childhood Hodgkin lymphoma. Pediatr Hematol Oncol 30:532–536
3. Pourtsidis A, Doganis D, Baka M et al (2012) Successful treatment in children with Hodgkin lymphoma in Greece; a 20-year experience in a single institution. Lymphoma 2012:Article ID 215868. doi:10.1155/2012/215868
4. Dinand V, Arya LS (2006) Epidemiology of childhood Hodgkin's disease: is it different in developing countries? Indian Pediatr 43:141–147
5. Feldman A, Pittaluga S, Jaffe E (2006) Classification and histopathology of the lymphomas. In: Canellos G, Lister T, Young B (eds) The lymphomas, 2nd edn. Saunders Elsevier, Philadelphia, pp 2–25
6. Nievelstein R, Quarles van Ufford H, Kwee T et al (2012) Radiation exposure and mortality risk from CT and PET imaging of patients with malignant lymphoma. Eur Radiol 22:1946–1954
7. Furth C, Steffen IG, Amthauer H, Ruf J, Misch D, Schönberger S et al (2009) Early and late therapy response assessment with [18F]fluorodeoxyglucose positron emission tomography in pediatric Hodgkin's lymphoma: analysis of a prospective multicenter trial. J Clin Oncol 27:4385–4391
8. Hudson M, Onciu M, Donaldson S (2006) Hodgkin's disease. In: Pizzo P, Poplack D (eds) Principles and practise of pediatric oncology, 5th edn. Lippincott-Raven, Philadelphia, pp 695–721
9. Donaldson S, Link M, Weinstein H et al (2007) Final results of a prospective clinical trial with VAMP and low-dose involved-field radiation for children with low-risk Hodgkin's disease. J Clin Oncol 25:332–337
10. Oguz A, Karadeniz C, Okur F et al (2005) Prognostic factors and treatment outcome in childhood Hodgkin disease. Pediatr Blood Cancer 45:670–675
11. Hudson M, Krasin M, Link M et al (2004) Risk-adapted, combined-modality therapy with VAMP/COP and response based, involved-field radiation for unfavorable pediatric Hodgkin's disease. J Clin Oncol 22:4541–4550
12. Brusamolino E, Carella A (2007) Treatment of refractory and relapsed Hodgkin's lymphoma: facts and perspectives. Haematologica 92:6–10
13. Bartlett N (2008) Modern treatment of Hodgkin lymphoma. Curr Opin Hematol 15:408–414
14. Hudson M, Donaldson S (1997) Chapter 21. Hodgkin's disease. In: Pizzo P, Poplack D (eds) Principles and practice of pediatric oncology, 3rd edn. Lippincott-Raven Publishers, Philadelphia, pp 523–543

15. Kluge R, Körholz D (2011) Role of FDG-PET in staging and therapy of children with Hodgkin lymphoma. Klin Padiatr 223:315–319
16. Carbone PP, Kaplan HS, Musshoff K, Smithers DW, Tubiana M (1971) Report of the committee on Hodgkin's disease staging classification. Cancer Res 31(11):1860
17. Lister TA, Crowther D, Sutcliffe SB, Glatstein E, Canellos GP, Young RC, Rosenberg SA, Coltman CA, Tubiana M (1989) Report of a committee convened to discuss the evaluation and staging of patients with Hodgkin's disease: Cotswolds meeting. J Clin Oncol 7(11):1630
18. Seth R, Puri K, Singh P, Selvam P, Kumar R (2012) The role of fluorodeoxyglucose positron emission tomography-computerized tomography in resolving therapeutic dilemmas in pediatric Hodgkin lymphoma. Indian J Nucl Med 27:141–144
19. Cheson BD, Pfistner B, Juweid ME, Gascoyne RD, Specht L, Horning SJ et al (2007) Revised response criteria for malignant lymphoma. J Clin Oncol 25:579–586
20. Rathore N, Eissa HM, Margolin JF et al (2012) Pediatric Hodgkin lymphoma: are we over-scanning our patients? Pediatr Hematol Oncol 29:415–423
21. Biasotti S, Garaventa A, Padovani P et al (2005) Role of active follow-up for early diagnosis of relapse after elective end of therapies. Pediatr Blood Cancer 45: 781–786

19 Lymphoblastic Lymphoma in Children and Adolescents: Introduction

Apostolos G. Pourtsidis, Helen Dana, Alexandra V. Nikaki and Nikolaos V. Kritikos

Lymphoblastic lymphomas (LBL), like acute lymphoblastic leukemia (ALL), comprise of high-grade neoplasms arising from precursor lymphocytes of B- or T-cell lineage. In the great majority they are of T-cell lineage (more than 75 %) and localize to the mediastinum (more than 80 %), whilst the less frequent B-cell lineage lymphomas have various primary sites. Mediastinal, bone marrow, and CNS involvements are more common in T-LBL, whilst skin, lymph node, and bone involvements are observed most frequently in B-LBL [1]. The incidence of LBL remains relatively constant across ages for both males and females.

A.G. Pourtsidis, MD
Pediatric Oncology Department,
P. & A. Kyriakou Children's Hospital,
Levadias 8 Street, Athens 11527, Greece
e-mail: tolispou@gmail.com; tolisp@otenet.gr;
ap-pourts@ath.forthnet.gr

H. Dana
Pediatric Oncology Department,
"MITERA" Hospital, Kifissias Av. &
E. Stavrou 4, Maroussi 15123, Greece
e-mail: danaeleni@hotmail.gr

A.V. Nikaki
Department of Nuclear Medicine and PET-CT,
"HYGEIA" Hospital, Kifissias Av. & E. Stavrou 4,
Maroussi 15123, Greece
e-mail: anikaki@gmail.com

N.V. Kritikos
Department of Radiology, "MITERA" Hosptial,
Kifissias Av. & E. Stavrou 4, Maroussi 15123, Greece
e-mail: nikkr68@yahoo.gr

The simplest and least invasive procedure should be used to establish diagnosis, and staging evaluation should be done as quickly as possible, because lymphoblastic lymphomas have usually an aggressive behavior with rapidly growing tumor masses that could cause life-threatening complications (i.e., tracheal compression or renal failure), attributed either to the mass effect or to metabolic consequences (i.e., tumor lysis syndrome).

The initial staging of LBL is accomplished with a careful history, detailed physical examination, laboratory tests, imaging, and bone marrow biopsy. Standard imaging studies, including ultrasound, CT, and MR scan, are widely used to determine disease extent, whereas more recent technologies, such as PET scan, are rarely used in the routine management of LBL [2]. Nevertheless, in mediastinal T-cell LBL, PET/CT may have a role similar to that observed in Hodgkin disease, in that residual CT or MRI lesions after chemotherapy may indicate the need for radiation therapy. In this case, PET/CT may be used to distinguish inactive disease from viable tumor residue [3]. There is very limited data for the prognostic value of PET scan in assessing the rapidity of response to treatment. Numerous studies have demonstrated that PET scan has poor predictive value for detecting recurrence for LBL.

Treatment of pediatric lymphoblastic lymphomas is based on intensive, prolonged, multidrug chemotherapy protocols, that include CNS

J.A. Andreou et al. (eds.), *PET/CT in Lymphomas: A Case-Based Atlas*,
DOI 10.1007/978-3-319-27380-8_19

prophylaxis, already applied in ALL treatment. Long-term overall survival (OS) arises up to 80–90 %, with no need for radiation therapy, although with some late relapses [4]. In the adolescent and young adult group, OS varies from 40 to 60 %. In the adult population, improvements have also been achieved by using leukemia-like protocols, though results are generally worse compared to pediatric series [5]. Impressive results in advanced stage disease have also been noted recently within the BFM90 protocol, achieving EFS of 90 %, with no need for additional radiotherapy [6].

19.1 Cases Presentation

Apostolos G. Pourtsidis, Helen Dana, Alexandra V. Nikaki, and Nikolaos V. Kritikos

Case 1: Peripheral Lymph Nodes

We describe a rare case of B precursor LBL: A 12-year-old boy presented with a slowly growing submandibular mass, not responding to antibiotics, having emerged at least six months from diagnosis. He had no general symptoms as fever or weight loss. Physical examination revealed a painless, moving with swallowing, walnut in size mass without signs of inflammation. Lymphadenopathy and hepatosplenomegaly were not present and hematologic laboratory tests were non-contributory. Bone marrow aspiration and bone marrow biopsy showed good marrow cellularity, without malignant involvement. Cerebrospinal fluid cytology was negative as well. Magnetic resonance imaging (MRI) (Fig. 19.1) showed a large mass of 3.7×2.2×1.9 cm with homogenous enhancement.

Left submandibular lymph node excision was performed, and pathology revealed nodal architecture totally disrupted by an immature and malignant lymphoid neoplasm, characterized by diffuse growth pattern and numerous mitoses, constituted by lymphoid blasts. Immunostaining was positive for TdT, CD19, CD10, CD79a, HLADR, CD45, CD43, CD99, CD34, bcl2, and CD20 (~10 %) and negative for CD3, CD4, CD7, CD8, EMA, bcl6, CD15, CD30, and CD21. MIB-1 (Ki-67) index was 50–80 %. Pathology findings were conclusive for lymphoblastic lymphoma of B-cell precursor origin.

PET/CT imaging for initial staging revealed heterogeneous increased uptake of the radiopharmaceutical at the medium left cervical (SUVmax−2.6) and supraclavicular (SUVmax−3.5) lymph nodes, suggesting the presence of active disease at these sites (Fig. 19.2). Increased 18F-FDG uptake and hypermetabolic state (SUVmax−5.3) was also noted at the posterior wall of the nasopharynx on the left, finding which could be attributed to inflammation and required further clinical co-evaluation.

After complete staging, patient was treated as per Berlin-Frankfurt-Münster (BFM) NHL protocol for localized LBL (without the re-induction protocol II) [7]. After 9 weeks of induction, he was reevaluated for disease response with CT and PET/CT, and all the involved lymph nodes had disappeared (Fig. 19.3).

At present, 24 months after the initial diagnosis, patient is under oral maintenance therapy (daily mercaptopurine and weekly methotrexate) and remains in complete remission of his disease.

Discussion

Lymphoblastic lymphoma, as acute lymphoblastic leukemia (ALL), is a high-grade neoplasm arising from precursor lymphocytes of B- or T-cell lineage. According to the revised European-American Classification of Lymphoid Neoplasms, ALL and LBL account for 80 % and 20 % of lymphoblastic malignancies, respectively. Less than 10 % of LBL are of B-cell lineage, whilst 85 % of ALL express B-cell markers. B-cell precursor lymphoblastic lymphoma (B-LBL) is a rare subtype of lymphoblastic lymphoma (LBL), accounting for only 3 % of all NHL. Clinically, B-LBL usually involves skin, lymph nodes, testes, and bone [7, 8]. Systemic symptoms are not common [9]. B-LBL has a good prognosis and is curable with current multi-agent systemic chemotherapy, as in the ALL protocols. Correct diagnosis, including histopathology, immunophenotyping, and tumor genetics, is needed in order to differentiate B-LBL from other subtypes of LBL and therefore provide appropriate treatment and the chance for a better prognosis. Our patient was treated as per BFM-NHL protocol, which has been proven efficacious for localized B-LBL, with a 5-year event-free survival of approximately 85 %.

Most pediatric NHL are aggressive, therefore with a high FDG avidity, correlated with the histological subtype [10]. Lymphoblastic lymphoma is reported to be FDG-avid, although large studies have not been carried out particularly for B-cell lymphoblastic lymphomas [10]. For NHL pediatric population, FDG-PET/CT's sensitivity has been reported to be 88.3 % (vs. 69.1 % for CT), detecting 42.9 % of additional lesions and leading to upstaging in 7 out of 21 cases [11]. Moreover, FDG-PET/CT in initial staging of NHL may be useful for the exclusion of extranodal disease, since such an involvement (particularly splenic) is a common manifestation in children and young patients [12]. FDG-PET is emerging in pediatric oncology as both an integral part of the staging process and an essential tool in assessing therapy response [13], though more research is still required.

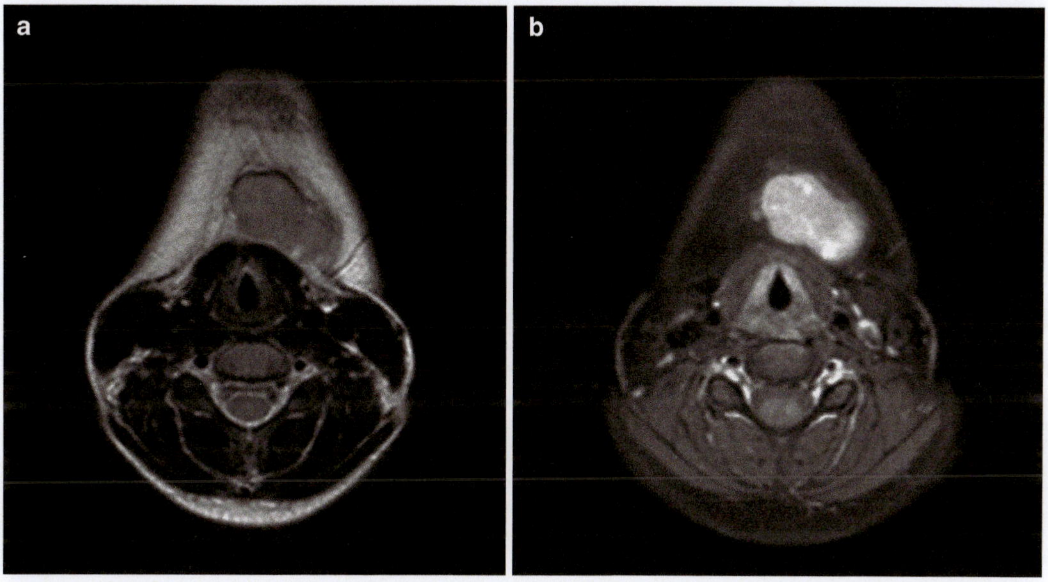

Fig. 19.1 T2W (**a**) and enhanced T1W fat saturated (**b**) images show an ovoid well-defined enhancing mass in the left subdental region

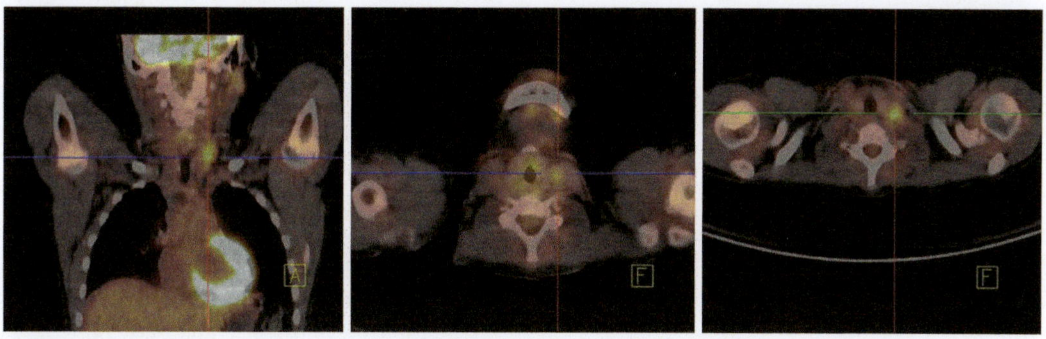

Fig. 19.2 Fused PET/CT images: Hypermetabolic lesions at the neck and the supraclavicular area consistent with active disease

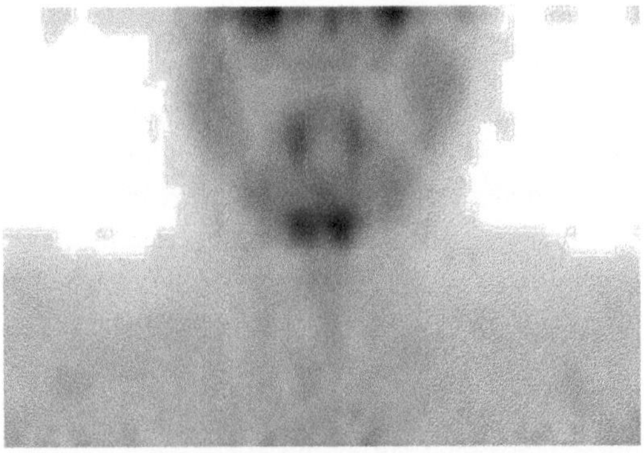

Fig. 19.3 MIP-PET of the neck: No lesions of increased uptake of the radiopharmaceutical are noted, evidence of complete response

Case 2: Mediastinum

A 13.5-year-old boy was referred to the pediatric oncology department in April 2014 with the diagnosis of a mediastinal mass. Symptoms started 3 months before diagnosis with chest pain, weight loss, and night sweating. Chest X-ray and cardiology survey at that time were normal. 15 days before diagnosis, patient presented with fever and cough and a new chest X-ray revealed a mediastinal enlargement. Chest CT confirmed the presence of an anterior mediastinum mass, with concomitant pleural and pericardial infusion. Bone marrow aspiration revealed infiltration with a 4 % of atypical lymphocytes, though bilateral bone marrow trephine biopsies were inconclusive. CT-guided biopsy of the mass was then performed and histology revealed mediastinal T-precursor lymphoblastic lymphoma/leukemia, as per WHO 2008 (immunochemistry positive for Tdt, CD3, CD5, CD8, CD1a, CD99, CD10, and CD79 and negative for CD34, PAX-5/BSAP, CD22, CD20/L-26, CD56/NCAM and myeloperoxidase, Ki-67/MIB-1 >80 %).

A PET/CT survey for disease staging before starting treatment was also performed (Fig. 19.4), which confirmed the presence of a mediastinal lymphatic mass with SUVmax of 10.2, together with the presence of several lymph nodes of the frontal mediastinum (SUVmax 5.6). Moreover, PET/CT revealed a hypermetabolic posterior cervical lymph node (SUVmax 2.6) and hypermetabolic retrocrural lymph nodes. There also was an increased uptake at the lateral nasopharynx (SUVmax 6.1), which was attributed to infection and a mild diffuse uptake of the bone marrow, indicative of metabolic hyperactivity.

Patient started chemotherapy as per EURO-LMB 02 protocol. He had a very good partial response after one month of induction chemotherapy, as proven by conventional imaging. At the end of the six-month induction therapy, there was a further imaging response, though with a residual mediastinal mass in conventional imaging. Since it could not be clarified if this mass represented residual active disease, inactive disease, or thymus rebound, a PET/CT scan was performed

(Fig. 19.5), which was indicative of residual active mediastinal disease (SUVmax 2.8).

An open biopsy was then performed and pathology revealed necrotic material, nuclear shadows, and moderate long-lasting inflammation, all conclusive for necrotic T-lymphoblastic lymphoma/leukemia.

Since then, patient is under consolidation oral chemotherapy as indicated by the treatment protocol, and remains in complete remission of his disease.

Discussion

T-cell pediatric lymphomas are a complex group of malignancies arising from precursor T-lymphoblasts or other mature T- and NK-cell subsets. In the current WHO classification, there are over 20 distinct entities of pediatric T-cell lymphomas, with T-cell lymphoblastic lymphoma being the most common and representing the one-third of all pediatric and adolescent non-Hodgkin lymphomas (NHL) [14–15]. Overall survival has improved over the past 30 years and arises up to 85–90 %, with no need of local surgery or irradiation, mainly due to the introduction of treatment protocols derived from regimens already proposed for children with acute lymphoblastic leukemia [6, 14]. The role of PET-CT in staging and estimating response to treatment for pediatric T-lymphomas remains controversial [12, 16, 17]. Though it has become a standard of care modality for tailoring treatment intensity in pediatric and adolescent Hodgkin lymphoma, its role in pediatric NHL is not yet well clarified [12]. As Bhojwani et al. have shown by analyzing a large series of 73 children and adolescents with NHL, in the case of residual disease suspected after conventional imaging, PET-CT has an 100 % sensitivity and negative predictive value in indicating residual tumor also detected by biopsy; however its specificity and positive predictive value are low (60 % and 25 %, respectively), and therefore a positive FDG-PET/CT examination is not reliable enough. Further investigation of hypermetabolic active disease with biopsy needs to be carried out when residual disease is detected both by conventional imaging and PET-CT, as it is the only warranted approach to accurately assess the nature of any residual mass [16].

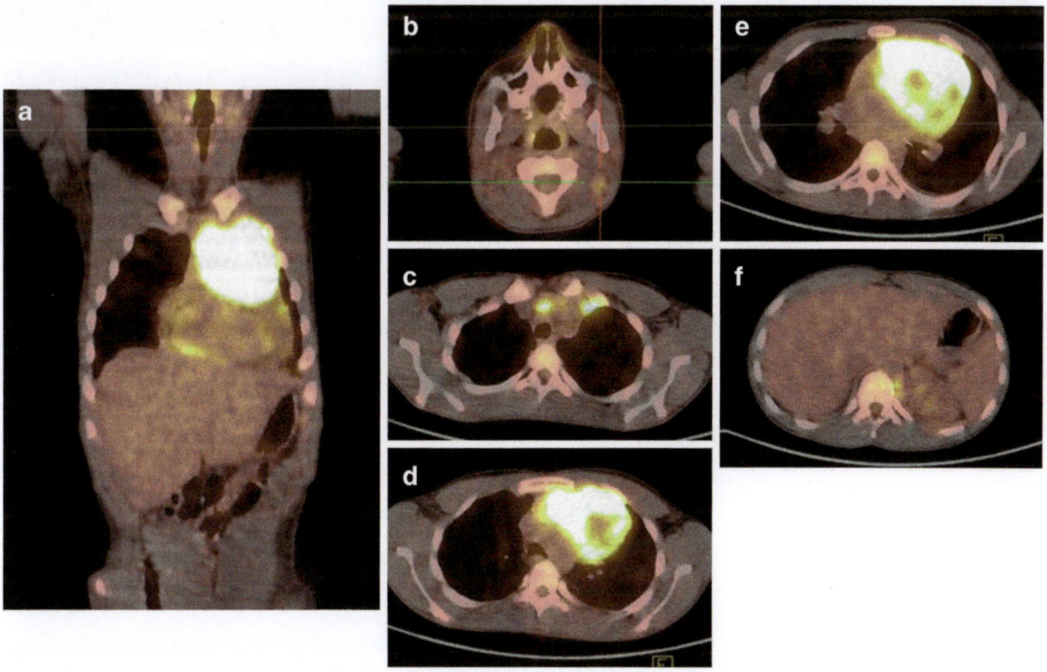

Fig. 19.4 Fused FDG-PET/CT: Hypermetabolic lymph node mediastinal mass (**a**, **c**–**e**). Small hypermetabolic lymph node at the left posterior cervical region (**b**); small hypermetabolic retrocrural node (**f**)

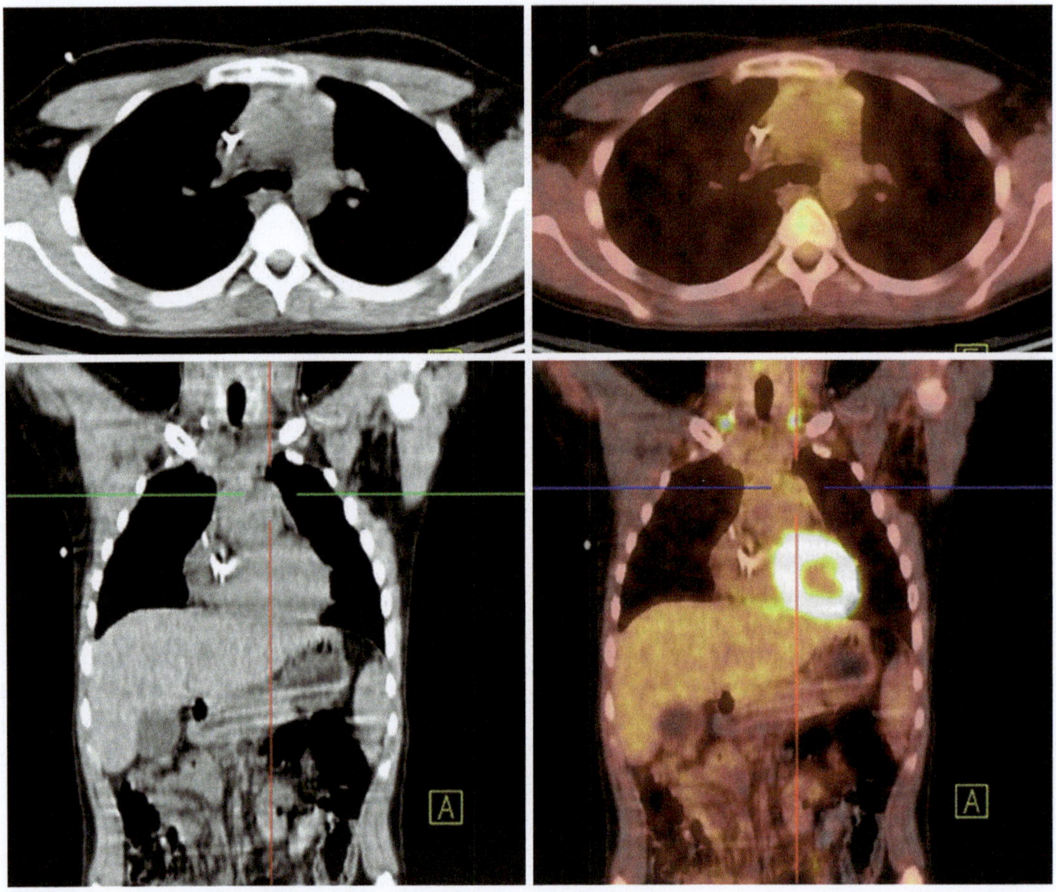

Fig. 19.5 CT and fused PET/CT: Residual, mildly hypermetabolic mass at the upper mediastinum (SUVmax of 2.8)

Acknowledgments The authors thank Sophia Polychronopoulou and Vassilios Papadakis, Department of Pediatric Hematology-Oncology of "Aghia Sofia" Children's Hospital, Athens, Greece, and Kalliopi Stefanaki, Department of Pathology of "Aghia Sofia" Children's Hospital, Athens, Greece, for their contribution by sharing the clinical and imaging data of their patient.

References

1. Jaffe ES, Harris NL, Stein H et al (2008) Introduction and overview of the classification of the lymphoid neoplasms. In: Swerdlow SH, Campo E, Harris NL et al (eds) WHO classification of tumours of haematopoietic and lymphoid tissues, 4th edn. Int Agency Res Cancer, Lyon, pp 157–166
2. Kostakoglu L, Cheson BD (2013) State-of-the-art research on "lymphomas: role of molecular imaging for staging, prognostic evaluation, and treatment response". Front Oncol 3:Article 212
3. Montravers F, McNamara D, Landman-Parker J et al (2002) [(18)F]-FDG in childhood lymphoma: clinical utility and impact on management. Eur J Nucl Med Mol Imaging 29:1155–1165
4. Rosolen A, Gross T (2012). Chapter 17. Malignant non-Hodgkin lymphomas in children. In: Stevens M, Caron H, Biondi A (eds). Cancer in Children. Clinical Management, 6th ed. New York: Oxford University Press, pp 203–219
5. Hoelzer D, Gokbuget N, Digel W et al (2002) Outcome of adult patients with T-lymphoblastic lymphoma treated according to protocol for acute lymphoblastic leukemia. Blood 99:4379–4385
6. Reiter A, Schrappe M, Ludwig WD et al (2000) Intensive ALL-type therapy without local radiotherapy provides a 90% event-free survival for children with T-cell lymphoblastic lymphoma: a BFM group report. Blood 95:416–421
7. Atlas M (2005) Non-Hodgkin lymphoma. In: Lanzkowsky P (ed) Manual of pediatric hematology and oncology. Elsevier Academic Press, London, pp 500–502
8. Maitra A, McKenna RW, Weinberg AG et al (2001) Precursor B-cell lymphoblastic lymphoma. A study of nine cases lacking blood and bone marrow involvement and review of the literature. Am J Clin Pathol 115:868
9. Neth O, Seidemann K, Jansen P et al (2000) Precursor B-cell lymphoblastic lymphoma in childhood and adolescence: clinical features, treatment, and results in trials NHL-BFM 86 and 90. Med Pediatr Oncol 35:20–27
10. Weiler-Sagie M, Bushelev O, Epelbaum R et al (2010) (18)F-FDG avidity in lymphoma readdressed: a study of 766 patients. J Nucl Med 51(1):25–30
11. Cheng G, Servaes S, Zhuang H (2013) Value of (18) F-fluoro-2-deoxy-D-glucose positron emission tomography/computed tomography scan versus diagnostic contrast computed tomography in initial staging of pediatric patients with lymphoma. Leuk Lymphoma 54(4):737–742
12. Kluge R, Kurch L, Montravers F, Mauz-Körholz C (2013) FDG PET/CT in children and adolescents with lymphoma. Pediatr Radiol 43(4):406–417
13. Cistaro A, Saglio F, Asaftei S et al (2011) The role of 18F-FDG PET/CT in pediatric lymph node acute lymphoblastic leukemia involvement. Radiol Case Rep 6(4):503
14. Cairo MS (2010) Non Hodgkin's lymphoma and lymphoproliferative disorders in children. In: Carrol WL, Finlay J (eds) Cancer in children and adolescents. Jones and Bartlett Publishers, Sudbury
15. El-Mallawany NK et al (2012) Pediatric T- and NK-cell lymphomas: new biologic insights and treatment strategies. Blood Cancer J 2(4):e65. doi:10.1038/bcj.2012.8, Epub 2012 Apr 13
16. Bhojwani D et al (2015) The role of FDG-PET/CT in the evaluation of residual disease in paediatric non-Hodgkin lymphoma. Br J Haematol 168(6):845–853
17. Sandlund JT et al (2015) International pediatric non-Hodgkin lymphoma response criteria. J Clin Oncol. doi:10.1200/JCO.2014.59.0745

20 Burkitt and Burkitt-Like Lymphomas in Children and Adolescents (Sporadic or Endemic B Mature): Introduction

Marina K. Servitzoglou, Helen Dana, Theodore A. Pipikos, and Georgia Ch. Papaioannou

Burkitt and Burkitt-like lymphomas (BL) account for 30–40 % of childhood NHL [1, 2]. It is the most common childhood cancer in equatorial Africa [3]. About 2.5 new cases per one million individuals occur every year worldwide. There is a definite predominance of boys over girls, with the ratios ranging from 1.3 to 8.8:1 [2, 4]. The peak age is between 4 and 7 years [4].

The BL cells have characteristically very high proliferation rate and a pathognomonic "starry sky" pattern, under low-power microscopy [5]. They show a mature B-cell phenotype and they typically bear surface immunoglobulins. They also express a variety of B-cell antigens and, practically all, CALLA and BCL6 antigens. The proliferation antigen Ki-67 is massively expressed. BCL2 may be occasionally weakly positive [5]. BL cells are usually characterized by chromosomal translocation t(8;14) and, more rarely, by t(8;22) or t(2;8), juxtaposing the c-myc oncogene, which is involved in cellular proliferation, with an immunoglobulin gene locus, resulting in inappropriate, constitutive expression of c-myc [6].

The clinical characteristic feature of BL is its aggressive behavior [2]. It is considered the most rapidly developing and growing malignant tumor in children, with a doubling time of approximately 24 hours. In the WHO Classification, three clinical variants of BL are described: endemic, sporadic, and immunodeficiency-associated types. Endemic BL occurs in African children, usually 4–7 years old, with estimated incidence 50 times higher than in the western world, and the site most often involved is the jaw. EBV is found in nearly all cases. Sporadic BL occurs worldwide, with no specific geographic or climatic association. The typical presentation is associated with an abdominal mass, mainly in the ileocecal region. Other sites of primary involvement are the lymph nodes of the head and neck region and Waldeyer's ring, the gonads, the kidneys, the omentum, the bones, or the skin [2]. Patients may also have

M.K. Servitzoglou
Department of Oncology, Children's Hospital "P. and A. Kyriakou", Thivon and Levadias, Athens 11527, Greece
e-mail: mservitzoglou@gmail.com

T.A. Pipikos (✉)
Department of Nuclear Medicine and PET/CT, "HYGEIA" Hospital, Erythrou Stavrou 4 and Kifissias, Maroussi 15123, Greece
e-mail: tpipikos@hygeia.gr

G.Ch. Papaioannou • H. Dana
Department of Pediatric Radiology, Hospital "MOTHER", Kifissias Av. and Q. Cross 4, Maroussi 15123, Greece
e-mail: gpapaio@hotmail.com; danaeleni@hotmail.gr

J.A. Andreou et al. (eds.), *PET/CT in Lymphomas: A Case-Based Atlas*,
DOI 10.1007/978-3-319-27380-8_20

malignant pleural effusion or ascites. Spread to the bone marrow and the central nervous system (CNS) at diagnosis is not uncommon [7]. Immunodeficiency-associated BL mainly occurs in HIV-infected patients, but might also occur in allograft recipients or individuals with congenital immunodeficiency deficits. The sites often involved are lymph nodes, bone marrow, and extranodal sites, mainly abdomen [8].

The evolution of treatment for childhood and adolescent BL has led to excellent survival rates, with chemotherapy alone, regardless of the disease stage. There are subtle differences in risk stratification across pediatric oncology cooperative groups and a near consensus in treatment agents. Basic principles of all groups have been the frequent, with short interval, intensive chemotherapy cycles to fight the extremely high proliferative activity of BL; the combination of chemotherapy agents with different mechanism of action and toxicity profile; and the efficient CNS-directed therapy in view of the strong tendency of BL for CNS infiltration [9]. Chemotherapy, among all pediatric oncology cooperative groups, is based on doxorubicin, cyclophosphamide, and methotrexate. The monoclonal antibody anti-CD20 (rituximab) has been relatively recently introduced in the treatment of childhood BL with so far promising results in advanced stage disease [10].

The cure rates for childhood BL with the modern treatments are higher than 80 %. One of the most important prognostic factors remains the response to the initial prophase treatment [11]. The combination of CNS and bone marrow involvement appears to have the worse impact on BL survival [12]. Additionally, cytogenetic abnormalities different than c-myc rearrangement, like gain of 7q or deletion of 13q, are associated with an inferior outcome [13].

20.1 Cases Presentation

Marina K. Servitzoglou, Helen Dana,
Theodore A. Pipikos,
and Georgia Ch. Papaioannou

Case 1: Abdomen

A 12.5-year-old girl was transferred to the Pediatric Oncology Department from a local hospital for investigation of an abdominal mass. Her history started weeks earlier with recurrent abdominal pain, abdominal distension, and episodes of vomiting.

The U/S and CT revealed a voluminous mass occupying the entire peritoneal cavity down to the pelvis, which pushed adjacent structures and encased ileus loops, sigmoid colon, and bladder in the right iliac fossa. Both kidneys and ureters were enlarged. Renal function was impaired. There were also bilateral pleural effusions, larger in the right side.

The biopsy of the mass, which was performed together with placement of bilateral ureteral stents, established the diagnosis of Burkitt lymphoma. The diagnosis was also confirmed by pleuritic fluid cytology. All malignant cells expressed c-myc translocation. Bone marrow aspirate and CSF cytology were negative.

The patient started prophase chemotherapy with COP, according to FAB LMB group B protocol, together with supportive care. Abdominal U/S performed a week later to assess response to treatment showed more than 20 % reduction in tumor burden. She continued chemotherapy, and she had a reassessment, following two courses of COPADM and one course of CYM.

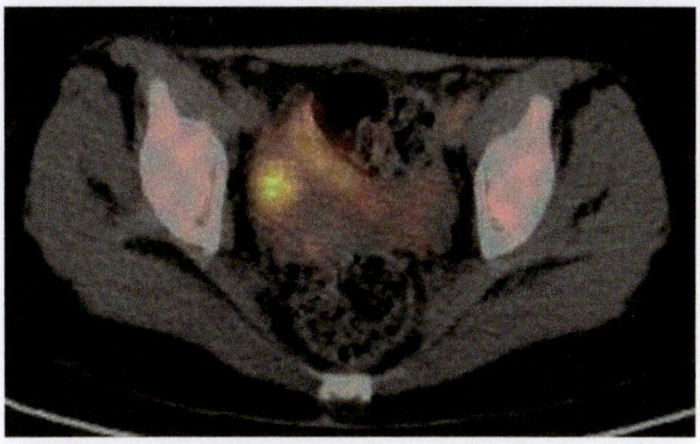

Fig. 20.1 Increased metabolic activity in the pelvis corresponding to the right ovary

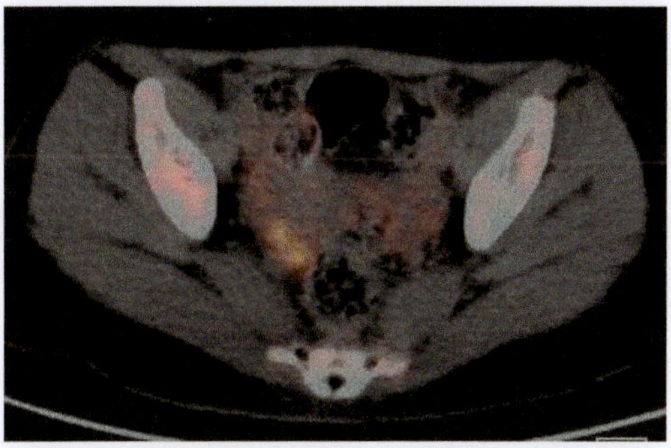

Fig. 20.2 Two pelvic lesions with mildly increased radiopharmaceutical uptake in the right side of the pelvis

CT revealed a residual pelvic mass. A PET/CT was then performed, which showed increased FDG uptake (SUVmax = 4,1) in the right ovary and two pelvic lesions (SUVmax = 2,8). Inguinal lymph nodes bilaterally (SUVmax = 1,0) were considered as inflammatory (Figs. 20.1 and 20.2).

Consequently, the treatment of the patient was upgraded, and she continued chemotherapy, according to the protocol, as group C. She

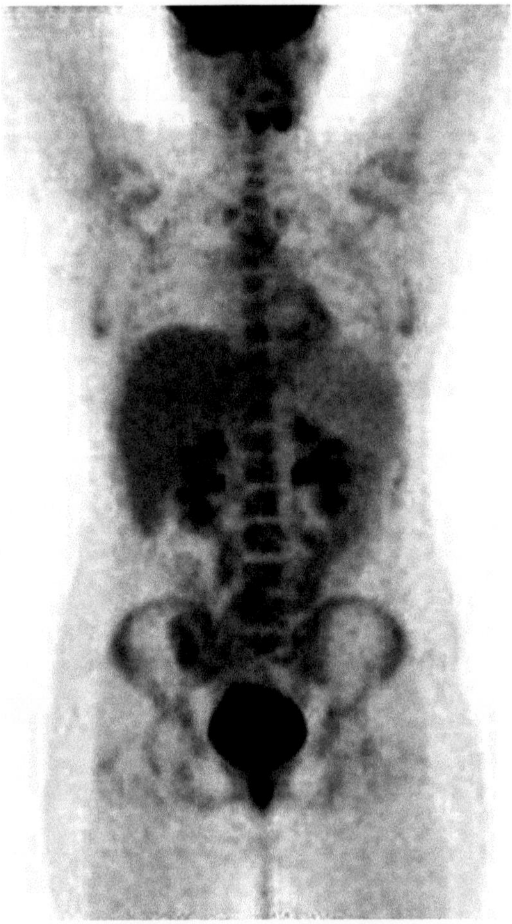

Fig. 20.3 End of therapy MIP image with no abnormal findings

received two cycles of CYVE, followed by four cycles of maintenance. PET/CT at the end of treatment was negative (Fig. 20.3), as so was the CT. The patient remains in complete remission, almost 2 years now, with no further therapy.

Discussion

The evaluation of treatment response, at specific time points during chemotherapy and at the completion of treatment, is critical for children with Burkitt lymphoma [9]. Children with unsatisfactory response to therapy, and specifically following prophase and first consolidation course, seem to have dismal prognosis, and protocol needs to be upgraded [9, 10, 14]. PET/CT is more likely to be accurate than CT/MRI, when the findings regarding residual lesions are discordant. PET scan, at reassessment and at completion of treatment, is a valuable imaging modality, which can predict disease status. Not only lymph node but also extranodal manifestations of Burkitt lymphoma can be detected with this molecular imaging modality, and ^{18}FDG uptake is getting reversed after successful treatment [15–17]. However, the evaluation of PET scan in childhood NHL, under the scope to replace histological documentation, is less advanced than in adult lymphoma.

Case 2: Abdomen

An 11-year-old boy was transferred to the Pediatric Oncology Department from another hospital for investigation of an abdominal mass. He had a 3-week history of recurrent abdominal pain, malaise, and weight loss. CT revealed a large right abdominal mass, with extensive hypodense central lesions, retro- and intraperitoneal, which pushed bowel loops at the left. The biopsy of the mass confirmed the diagnosis of Burkitt lymphoma. All malignant cells expressed c-myc translocation. Bone marrow aspirate and CSF cytology were negative.

The patient started prophase chemotherapy with COP, according to FAB LMB group B protocol. A week later, response to treatment was considered satisfactory and he continued his outlined chemotherapy.

At the second reassessment time point, following two courses of COPADM and one course of CYM, PET/CT was positive, showing an area of increased uptake (SUVmax = 6,0) below the liver, in contact with the right lateral abdominal wall, without increased metabolic activity in the residual abdominal mass (Figs. 20.4 and 20.5) respectively.

In view of the residual mass, the patient continued chemotherapy according to group C protocol and received two cycles of CYVE. At this stage, the CT did not reveal any change in the residual mass, and the PET showed minor reduction of the metabolic activity of the hypermetabolic lesion described above (SUVmax = 5,4), with new hypermetabolic areas noted in the interior cecal wall (Fig. 20.6).

Following these findings, he underwent, initially, an exploratory laparotomy for tumor biopsy and then a colonoscopy for cecal biopsy. The histology showed only necrotic tissue in both cases.

He continued with the first two maintenance cycles, but before the third, he presented with back pain. CT of the chest revealed an extensive condensation in the lower left lobe with a large pleural effusion. The cytology confirmed the recurrence of his disease. He continued salvage chemotherapy with three cycles of rituximab-ICE.

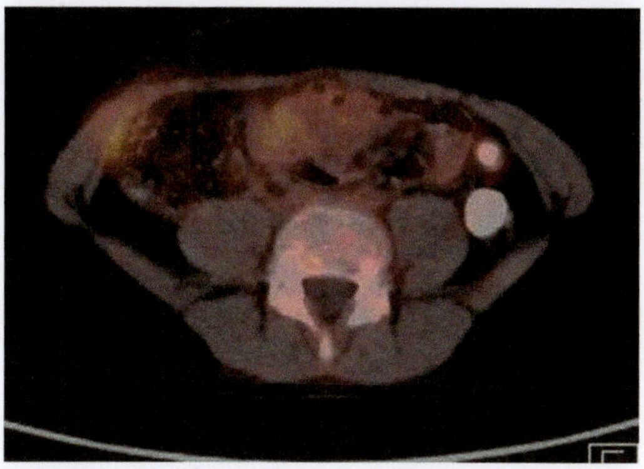

Fig. 20.4 Abdominal residual mass without increased metabolic activity

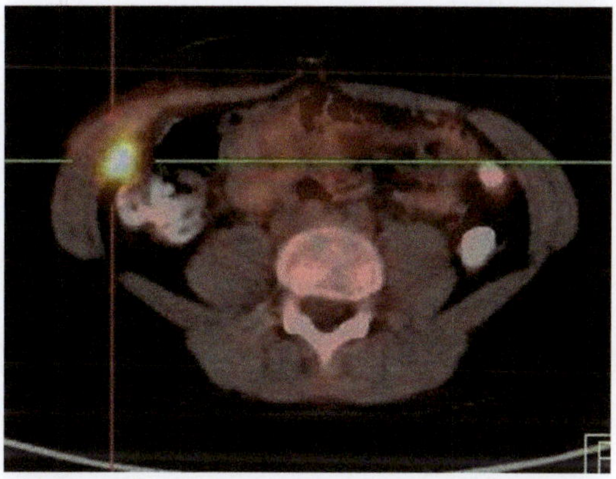

Fig. 20.5 Area of increased metabolic activity just below the right liver lobe, in contact with the abdominal wall

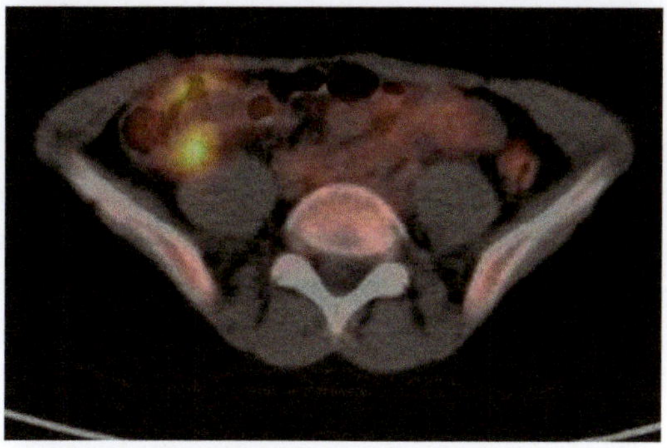

Fig. 20.6 New findings of increased metabolic activity in the posterior cecal wall

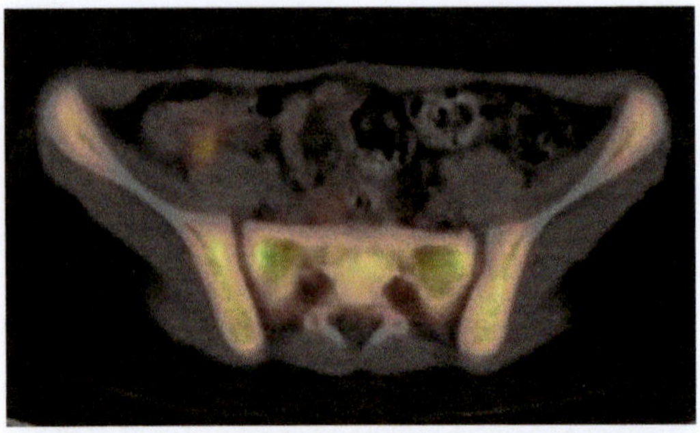

Fig. 20.7 Area of slightly increased residual metabolic activity in the posterior cecal wall

Following these courses, PET/CT showed a slight hypermetabolic area (SUVmax = 2,8) in the cecal wall (Fig. 20.7).

The patient was therefore referred for autologous stem cell transplantation (ASCT). At present, few months following ASCT, he remains in remission.

Discussion

PET/CT is more reliable than conventional imaging in detecting residual malignant lesions in childhood NHL and in establishing poor response to treatment [18]. However, it has not yet been formally introduced in pediatric B-cell NHL protocols, replacing histology in the assessment of residual mass viability. The sensitivity and negative predictive value of PET to indicate residual tumor detectable by biopsy are very high, but specificity and positive predictive value are significantly lower [19]. Thus, a negative PET can indicate complete remission, but since false-positive results are relatively common, biopsy and close monitoring are essential to determinate the presence of residual disease in children with NHL [19]. On the other hand, PET/CT has shown high sensitivity and specificity for the diagnosis of disease relapse in HL and NHL [20–22].

Case 3: Head and Neck and Bone Marrow

An 11-year-old girl presented in August 2013 with a 3-week painful swelling of the right mandible. Anorexia and loss of weight (4 kg in 3 weeks) were also present. Antibacterial and anti-inflammatory treatment had no result, so a regional MRI was performed, which revealed floating teeth and a large soft tissue mass, extending from the right mandible to the right maxilla, the right sinus, and the visceral skull (Fig. 20.8).

Mass was biopsied and histology revealed Burkitt lymphoma (immunochemistry positive for CD20, CD79a, Cd10, bcl-6, and κ light immunoglobulin chains, weakly and regionally positive for MUM1, and negative for bcl-2, Tdt, cyclin D1, and myeloperoxidase – MIB-1 index (Ki67): 100 %). Bone marrow aspiration was negative for metastatic disease; nevertheless bilateral trephine bone marrow biopsies revealed 15–20 % infiltration of the right iliac bone by Burkitt cells (immunochemistry positive for CD20, CD10, and bcl-6 and negative for CD3, CD34, bcl-2, CD68/PGM-1, myeloperoxidase, and light κ and λ immunoglobulin chains – MIB-1 index (Ki67) >80 %). CSF cytology was negative for CNS metastatic disease. Abdominal ultrasound and CT revealed multiple hypodense liver lesions (Fig. 20.9).

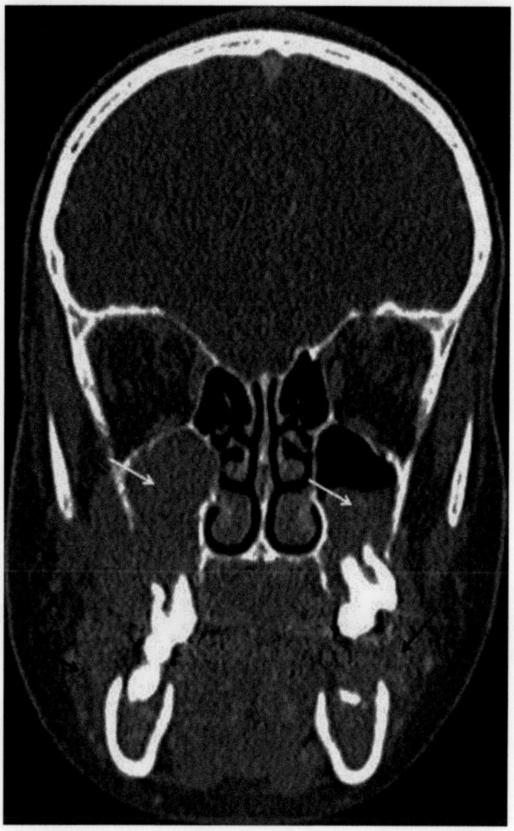

Fig. 20.8 Coronal MPR at the level of the mandible reveals extensive soft tissue mass occupying the bone marrow in the body and the mandibular arm and causing cortical lysis with extension to the adjacent soft tissues (*black arrows*) and the maxillary antra (*white arrows*) and appearances of floating teeth

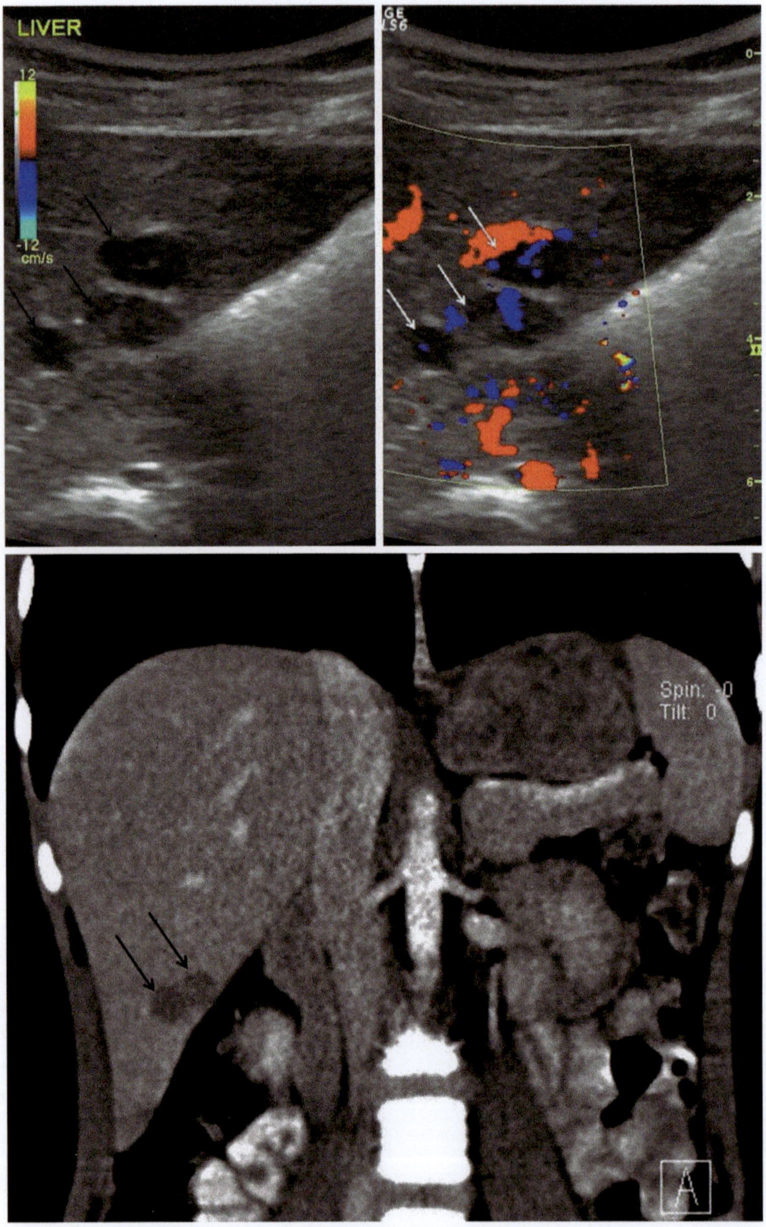

Fig. 20.9 Abdominal U/S (**a** B-mode and color Doppler) and CT (**b** coronal MPR post iv injection of contrast) reveal multiple focal lesions suggestive of hepatic infiltrates (*arrows*)

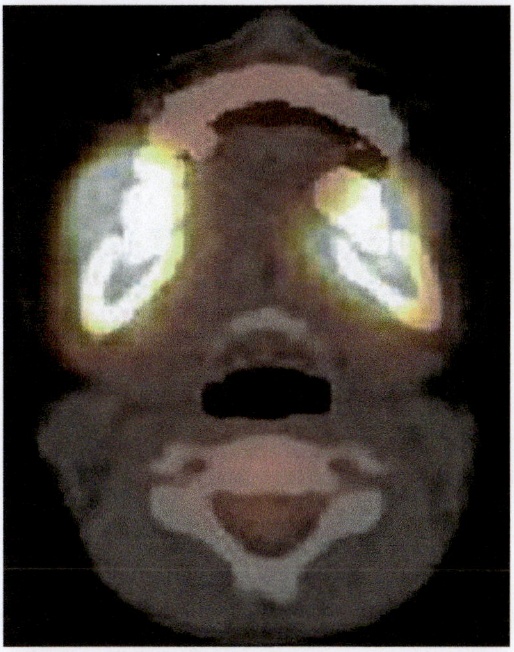

Fig. 20.10 Many intensely hypermetabolic lesions in the skull and the adjacent soft tissues

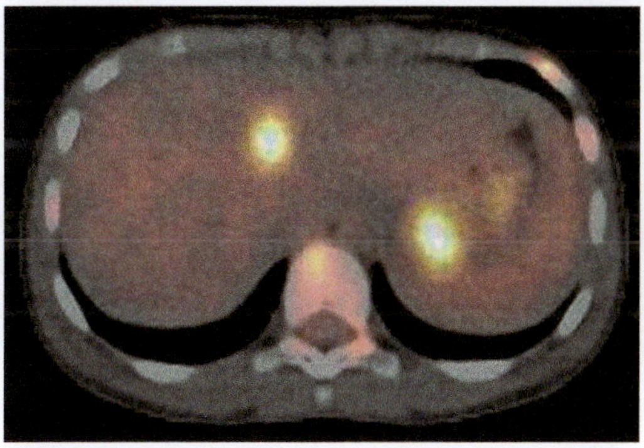

Fig. 20.11 Hypermetabolic liver lesions

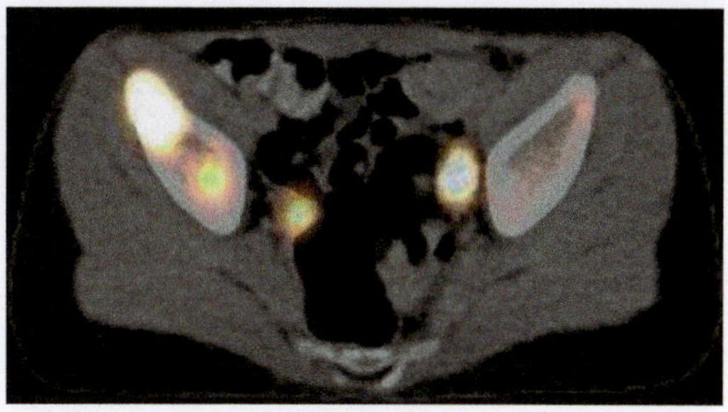

Fig. 20.12 Abnormal lymph nodes were found at the abdomen and pelvic area

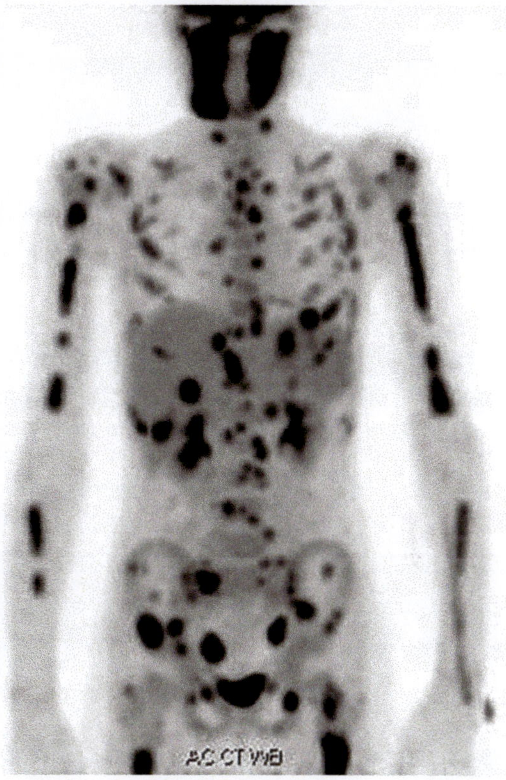

Fig. 20.13 Multiple hypermetabolic lesions were found through the whole skeleton including the extremities, as seen in MIP image

Conventional imaging (brain, cervical, and chest CTs) did not reveal any other metastatic lesions; nevertheless PET/CT imaging revealed extended metastatic disease (Figs. 20.10, 20.11, 20.12, and 20.13).

Patient started chemotherapy according to FAB LMB 96 (group B) protocol (stage IV, CNS negative, bone marrow infiltration <25 %). Conventional imaging showed good partial response after the pre-induction (COP) and the first induction schema (COPADM1). At the end of induction chemotherapy (COPADM2), conventional imaging was still indicative of residual disease, although bone marrow aspiration and trephine biopsies were normal. A PET/CT scan performed at that time confirmed the presence of residual disease at the right mandible, right sinus,

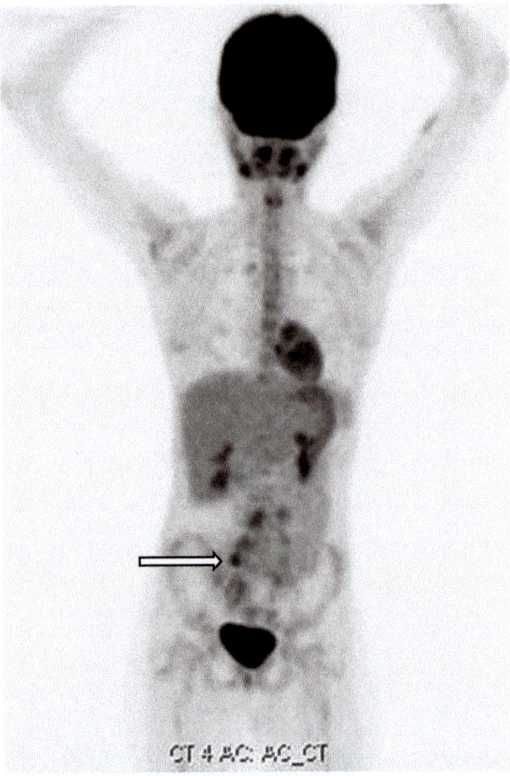

Fig. 20.14 MIP image showing small residual hypermetabolic lesions at the skull and peritoneal mass at the level of the pelvis after induction chemotherapy. The *arrow* points at the hypermetabolic pelvic lesion

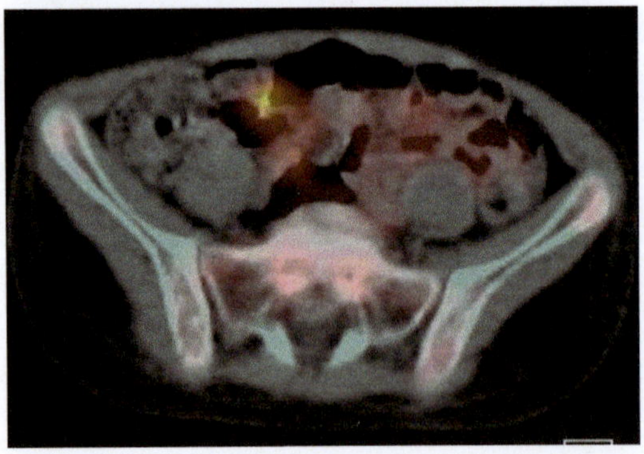

Fig. 20.15 Fused image showing a pelvic hypermetabolic lesion

and right pelvis (Figs. 20.14 and 20.15), so chemotherapy was intensified as per FAB LMB 96 (group C) protocol.

After intensified re-induction (CYVE1, CYVE2), a new PET/CT scan was performed (Fig. 20.16) which was negative for hypermetabolic lesions.

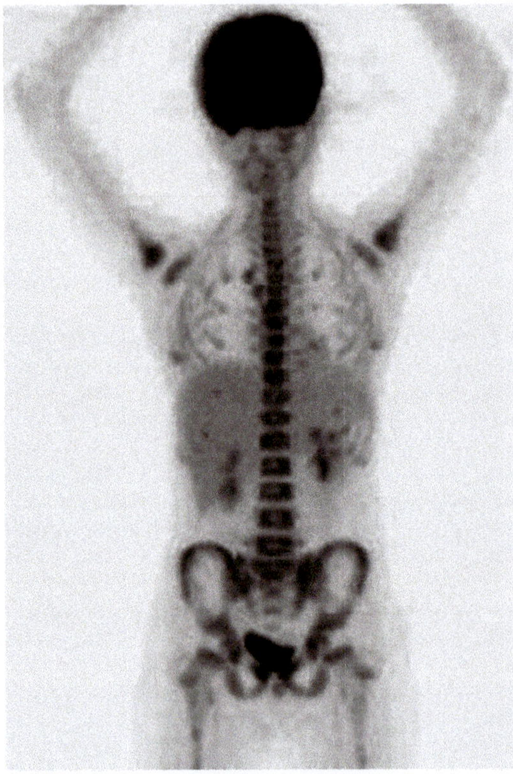

Fig. 20.16 MIP image after re-induction chemotherapy with no abnormal findings

PET/CT scan was also negative at the end of consolidation chemotherapy (M1-M4) (Fig. 20.17), 8 months after the initial diagnosis. Patient is in complete disease remission since (1 year off treatment).

Discussion

Burkitt lymphoma/leukemia (BL) accounts for about 40 % of all childhood and adolescence non-Hodgkin's lymphomas (NHL) and exhibits an aggressive clinical behavior. Cytogenetic evidence of c-myc rearrangement is the gold standard of molecular diagnosis. High proliferation rate (Ki-67/MIB-1) is also pathognomonic [9, 23]. Disseminated disease on diagnosis is not rare, with bone marrow involvement accounting for more than 20 % of all patients, even though this is not an adverse prognostic factor [24]. In contrast with adults, the prognosis of disseminated disease in childhood BL has raised up to a 5-year EFS of 85–90 % during the last decades, and this is due to the introduction of very intensive and of

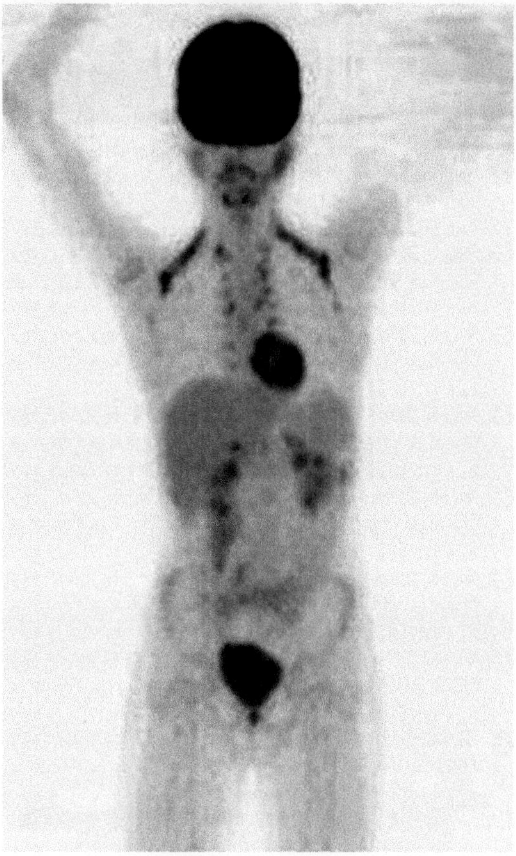

Fig. 20.17 MIP image after consolidation chemotherapy with no pathological findings. Adipose brown fat radiopharmaceutical accumulation

small duration (6–8 months) pediatric multiagent chemotherapy protocols, tailored to the tumor burden [9, 24, 25]. Response to initial treatment is one of the most important predictive factors [23, 25].

Primary sites are usually extranodal [23]. When floating teeth and teeth pain or numbness are present, visceral skull primary involvement should be suspected. Bone marrow involvement may confuse, as to whether lymphoma or leukemia is the appropriate diagnosis. Traditionally, patients with more than 25 % blasts in bone marrow aspiration are considered to have mature B leukemia, and those with less than 25 % blasts are considered to have lymphoma [23]. Even though it is not clear whether that numerical distinction represents a biological one, bone marrow involvement should justify choices of more intensive treatment. In the clinical case presented above, bone marrow infiltration was less than 20 % in the bone marrow biopsy, although bone and bone marrow disease seemed much more extended in the PET/CT imaging.

However, the role of PET/CT imaging in diagnosis and staging of the pediatric Burkitt lymphoma/leukemia is not yet well established. Imaging and dosing protocols and interpretive guidelines are nonstandardized for pediatric populations, and there is a tendency to follow the adult literature [26]. Regarding bone marrow involvement in adult lymphomas, recent studies have proved PET's sensitivity in identifying bone and bone marrow lesions, although further studies are needed to identify whether that makes bone marrow biopsy dispensable or both approaches are complementary [27].

What is better established in the case of pediatric NHL is the role of PET/CT in the evaluation of early response to treatment and the evaluation of residual disease during or after treatment, where its sensitivity and negative predictive value arises to 100 % [28, 29]. As in the case described above, early detection of hypermetabolic residual disease after two cycles of induction chemotherapy confirmed the aggressiveness of the disease and guided the therapeutic decision to intensifying chemotherapy and achieving better therapeutic results.

Acknowledgements

Case 2: Abdomen The authors thank N. Tourkantoni, A. Vlachou, A. Kattamis, First Department of Pediatrics, National and Kapodistrian University of Athens, Division of Hematology–Oncology for their contribution, by sharing clinical and imaging data of their patients.

Case 3: Head and Neck & Bone Marrow The authors thank Antonios Kattamis and Natalia Tourkantoni, 1st University Department of Pediatrics and Kalliopi Stefanaki, Pathology Laboratory of Athens "Aghia Sofia" Children's Hospital for their contribution by sharing the clinical, pathology, and imaging data of their patient.

References

1. Percy CL, Smith MA, Linet M et al (1999) Lymphomas and reticuloendothelial neoplasms. In: Ries LA, Smith MA, Gurney JG et al (eds) Cancer incidence and survival among children and adolescents: United States SEER Program 1975–1995. National Cancer Institute, SEER Program, Bethesda, pp 35–50, NIH Pub.No. 99–4649
2. Leoncini L, Raphael M, Stein H (2008) Burkitt lymphoma. In: Swerdlow SH, Campo E, Harris NL et al (eds) WHO classification of tumours of haematopoietic and lymphoid tissues, 4th edn. International Agency for Research on Cancer, Lyon, pp 262–264
3. Dong HY (2010) Aggressive B-cell lymphomas: diffuse large B-cell lymphoma and Burkitt lymphoma. In: Jones D (ed) Neoplastic hematopathology: contemporary hematology, vol Part 3. Humana Press, New York, pp 303–322.
4. Mbulaiteye SM, Biggar RJ, Bhatia K et al (2009) Sporadic childhood Burkitt lymphoma incidence in the United States during 1992–2005. Pediatr Blood Cancer 53(3):366–370
5. Diebold J, Jaffe ES, Raphael M et al (2001) Burkitt lymphoma. In: Jaffe ES, Harris NL, Stein H et al (eds) World health organization classification of tumours: pathology and genetics of tumours of haematopoietic and lymphoid tissues. IARC Press, Lyon, pp 181–184
6. Dave SS, Fu K, Wright GW et al (2006) Molecular diagnosis of Burkitt's lymphoma. N Engl J Med 354:2431–2442
7. Cairo MS, Sposto R, Perkins SL et al (2003) Burkitt's and Burkitt-like lymphoma in children and adolescents: a review of the Children's Cancer Group experience. Br J Haematol 120:660–670
8. Knowles DM (2003) Etiology and pathogenesis of AIDS-related non-Hodgkin's lymphoma. Hematol Oncol Clin North Am 17:785–820
9. Miles R, Arnold S, Cairo M (2012) Risk factors and treatment of childhood and adolescent Burkitt lymphoma/leukaemia. Br J Hematol 156:730–743
10. El-Mallawany N, Cairo M (2015) Advances in the diagnosis and treatment of childhood and adolescent B-cell non-Hodgkin lymphoma. Clin Adv Hematol Oncol 13(2):113–123
11. Mussolin L, Pillon M, d'Amore ES et al (2011) Minimal disseminated disease in high-risk Burkitt's lymphoma identifies patients with different prognosis. J Clin Oncol 29(13):1779–1784
12. Cairo MS, Sposto R, Gerrard M et al (2012) Advanced stage, increased lactate dehydrogenase, and primary site, but not adolescent age (≥15 years), are associated with an increased risk of treatment failure in children and adolescents with mature B-cell non-Hodgkin's lymphoma: results of the FAB LMB 96 study. J Clin Oncol 30(4):387–393
13. Poirel HA, Cairo MS, Heerema NA et al (2009) Specific cytogenetic abnormalities are associated with a significantly inferior outcome in children and adolescents with mature B-cell non-Hodgkin's lymphoma: results of the FAB/LMB 96 international study. Leukemia 23(2):323–331
14. Reiter A (2007) Diagnosis and treatment of childhood non-Hodgkin lymphoma. Am Soc Hematol Educ Program 1:285–296
15. Uslu L, Donig J, Link M et al (2015) Value of ^{18}F-FDG PET and PET/CT for evaluation of pediatric malignancies. J Nucl Med 56:274–286
16. Sioka C (2013) The utility of FDG PET in diagnosis and follow-up of lymphoma in childhood. Eur J Pediatr 172(6):733–738
17. Bailly C, Eugene T, Couec M-L et al (2014) Prognostic value and clinical impact of 18FDG-PET in the management of children with Burkitt lymphoma after induction chemotherapy. Front Med (Lausanne) 1:54
18. Mody R, Bui C, Hutchinson R et al (2007) Comparison of ^{18}F Flurodeoxyglucose PET with Ga-67 scintigraphy and conventional imaging modalities in pediatric lymphoma. Leuk Lymphoma 48(4):699–707
19. Bhowjani B, McCarville MB, Choi JK et al (2015) The role of FDG-PET/CT in the evaluation of residual disease in pediatric non-Hodgkin lymphoma. Br J Haematol 168(6):845–853
20. Qiu L, Chen Y, Wu J (2013) The role of ^{18}F-FDG PET and ^{18}F-FDG PET/CT in the evaluation of pediatric Hodgkin's lymphoma and non-Hodgkin's lymphoma. Hell J Nucl Med 16(3):230–236
21. Riad R, Omar W, Kotb M et al (2010) Role of PET/CT in malignant pediatric lymphoma. Eur J Nucl Med Mol Imaging 37:319–329
22. Kluge R, Kurch L, Montravers F, Mauz-Korholz C (2013) FDG PET/CT in children and adolescents with lymphoma. Pediatr Radiol 43(4):406–417
23. Childhood non-Hodgkin lymphoma treatment (PDQ). www.cancer.gov/types/lymphoma/hp/child-nhl-treatment-pdq
24. Patte C et al (1986) Improved survival rate in children with stage III and IV B cell non-Hodgkin's lymphoma and leukemia using multi-agent chemotherapy: results of a study of 114 children from the French Pediatric Oncology Society. J Clin Oncol 4(8):1219–1226

25. Patte C et al (2007) Results of the randomized international FAB/LMB96 trial for intermediate risk B-cell non-Hodgkin lymphoma in children and adolescents: it is possible to reduce treatment for the early responding patients. Blood 109(7):2773–2780
26. Binkovitz L PET/CT imaging of pediatric lymphoma: what's the evidence? www.snmmi.files.cms-plus.com/
27. Moulin-Romsee G et al (2010) (18)F-FDG PET/CT bone/bone marrow findings in Hodgkin's lymphoma may circumvent the use of bone marrow trephine biopsy at diagnosis staging. Eur J Nucl Med Mol Imaging 37(6):1095–1105
28. Bhojwani D et al (2015) The role of FDG-PET/CT in the evaluation of residual disease in paediatric non-Hodgkin lymphoma. Br J Haematol 168(6):845–853
29. Rhodes MM et al (2006) Utility of FDG-PET/CT in follow-up of children treated for Hodgkin and non-Hodgkin lymphoma. J Pediatr Hematol Oncol 28(5):300–306

21 Diffuse Large B-Cell Lymphoma in Children and Adolescents (B Mature): Introduction

Marina K. Servitzoglou, Helen Dana, Apostolos G. Pourtsidis, Fani J. Vlachou, and Demetrios N. Exarhos

Diffuse large B-cell lymphoma (DLBCL) is a mature B-cell neoplasm, which accounts for approximately 10–20 % of paediatric NHL [1]. In fact, this definition represents a morphologically, immunologically and clinically heterogeneous group of lymphoid neoplasms, rather than one entity [2]. In contrast to other childhood NHL, there is no specific genetic feature for DLBCL. The recent WHO classification delineated some newly defined entities on the basis of distinctive clinical, pathologic or biologic features.

M.K. Servitzoglou (✉)
Oncology Department, Children's Hospital "P. & A. Kyriakou", Levadias 8, Athens 11527, Greece
e-mail: mservitzoglou@gmail.com

H. Dana
Pediatric Oncology Department, "MITERA" Hospital, Kifissias Av. & E. Stavrou 4, Maroussi 15123, Greece
e-mail: danaeleni@hotmail.gr

A.G. Pourtsidis
Oncology Department, Children's Hospital P.& A. Kyriakou, Levadias 8 Street, Athens 11527, Greece
e-mail: tolispou@gmail.com; tolisp@otenet.gr; ap-pourts@ath.forthnet.gr

F.J. Vlachou
Department of Nuclear Medicine, "HYGEIA" Hospital, Kifissias Av. & E. Cross 4, Maroussi 15123, Greece
e-mail: fanivlachou@yahoo.com

D.N. Exarhos
Radiology Department, "EVANGELISMOS" General Hospital, Ipsilantou 45-47, Athens 10676, Greece
e-mail: jimexarhos@yahoo.com

DLBCL occurs more often in adolescents. About nine new cases per one million individuals until 19 years old occur every year. There is no variation in different world regions [3]. There is a slight predominance of boys over girls with male-to-female ratio of 1.4:1. DLBCL and BL are the most common NHL subtypes occurring in individuals with congenital or acquired immunodeficiency syndromes.

In DLBCL, the lymph node architecture or the extranodal tissue is replaced by a diffuse infiltrate of B-lineage blasts with variable morphology. Most of DLBCL are CD20 positive. The CD20-negative DLBCL can express other B-cell markers. The majority of paediatric DLBCL cases also express CD10 and BCL6 and about 40 % BCL2 [4, 5]. The expression of germinal centre-associated antigens, such as CD10 and BCL6, suggests the germinal centre cell as origin cell for DLBCL. Two principal subtypes have been identified by gene expression profiling, the germinal centre cell-like (GCB) and the activated B-cell-like (ABC) forms of DLBCL, which are associated with specific genetic alterations, different molecular signalling pathways and clinical outcomes. The GCB cases show a much better prognosis than ABC. It seems that the developmental stage of the primary B cell of the DLBCL influences the biologic and clinical behaviour of the lymphoma [5, 6].

In the new WHO classification, primary mediastinal large B-cell lymphoma (PMBL), DLBCL of the CNS and primary cutaneous DLBCL, leg type, are recognized as distinct entities [2, 7].

J.A. Andreou et al. (eds.), *PET/CT in Lymphomas: A Case-Based Atlas*,
DOI 10.1007/978-3-319-27380-8_21

PMBL has a distinctive gene expression profile and a closer relationship with Hodgkin lymphoma [8, 9]. The vast majority of paediatric DLBCL have a germinal centre B-cell phenotype and rarely demonstrate the t(14;18) translocation. Approximately 30 % of children younger than 14 years with DLBCL have a gene profile similar to Burkitt lymphoma.

The clinical presentation of paediatric DLBCL may be similar to BL, but it is more often localized and less often involves the bone marrow or CNS. About 20 % of DLBCLs present as PMBL, which is more common in adolescents. About 40 % of children present with extranodal mass, often stage I or II. The most frequent extrathoracic manifestations are tumours of the kidney and, more rarely, the liver, spleen and pancreas, whilst spread to other extranodal organs is rare. Bone marrow involvement occurs in about 15 % of DLBCL. There are two main types of bone marrow infiltration, either with large cells, generally associated with poorer prognosis, or with small cells, characteristic of low-grade lymphoma.

The treatment of DLBCL is the same as the treatment of BL, and the current strategies are based on risk stratification. The outcome of children with DLBCL is not different to that of patients with BL, and DLBCL histology has not been proved to be an adverse prognostic factor in international studies. However, PMBL carries a worse prognosis [9]. Additionally, adolescents have been reported to have inferior outcome compared with younger children [10]. The prognosis, also, for relapsed DLBCL is dismal, due to chemoresistance.

21.1 Case Presentation

Helen Dana, Apostolos G. Pourtsidis,
Marina K. Servitzoglou, Fani J. Vlachou,
and Demetrios N. Exarhos

Case 1: Mediastinum

A 13.5-year-old girl was referred to the paediatric oncology department in March 2013 with the diagnosis of a mediastinal mass. History had started 1 month ago with breathlessness at exercise and weight loss (3 kgs in 1 month). For the last 10 days, numbness and redness of the left arm and neck pain and torticollis were added to her symptoms. She also had cervical and supraclavicular oedema, without palpable lymph nodes. A cervical spine MRI was ordered, which revealed left internal jugular vein thrombosis. Then a chest and cervical CT were performed, which revealed a large mass of the anterior mediastinum, plus thrombosis of left internal jugular vein and superior and inferior vena cava. Abdomen imaging was normal. Blood count and serum biochemistry were also normal, including serum AFP and β-HCG. Patient was homozygous for the MTHFR mutation. Bone marrow aspiration and bilateral trephine biopsies were not indicative of any hematologic malignancy.

A CT-guided biopsy of the mediastinal mass was then performed, with histology being conclusive for non-Hodgkin diffuse large B-cell primary mediastinal lymphoma, as per WHO 2008. Immunochemistry was positive for CD20/L-26, PAX5/BSAP, CD79a, CD22, OCT-2, BOB-1, CD30/BerH2, MUM-1, bcl-6, bcl-2 and CD23 and negative for keratin AE1/AE3, CD15/Leu-M1, CD3, Tdt, ALK-1/p-80, CD10, CD138, κ light immunoglobulin chains and LMP-1(EBV). Ki-67 (MIB-1) index was greater than 70 %.

Before starting chemotherapy, a PET/CT scan was performed, which confirmed the diagnosis of primary mediastinal lymphoma (Fig. 21.1).

Patient underwent chemotherapy with 6 cycles of DA-EPOCH-R (dose adapted – etoposide, prednisone, vincristine, cyclophosphamide and rituximab), together with anticoagulant treatment. She tolerated therapy well. Disease was in remission after the first two chemotherapy cycles, with a normal chest CT and a normal PET/CT scan (Fig. 21.2).

10 months after the end of treatment (14 months since diagnosis), the patient remains in complete remission.

Discussion

Primary mediastinal diffuse large B-cell lymphoma (PMDLBCL) accounts for 1–2 % of all paediatric non-Hodgkin lymphomas (NHL) and is more often seen in female adolescents [11, 12]. Although it is used to be considered as a subtype of diffuse large B-cell lymphoma, the most recent WHO's classification recognizes it now as a distinct entity. Tumour cells arise from the putative thymic medulla B-cell and evolve to a bulky, invasive mediastinal tumour that may cause pressure and obstructive effects (i.e. superior vena cava syndrome). Morphologically, tumour shows a diffuse large cell proliferation with sclerosis and compartmentalization of tumour cells that may confound differential diagnosis with nodular sclerosis Hodgkin lymphoma. Immunochemistry markers are similar to the ones found in DLBCL, but certain distinct chromosomal changes (i.e. 9p and 2p gains) may lead to diagnosis. Eventually, it is suggested that PMDLBCL has a distinct molecular profile that may reflect a distinct clinical entity with distinct response to treatment [8, 11, 13, 12].

Furthermore, it has been shown that, when treated with the standard paediatric NHL protocols, children and adolescents with PMDLBCL do worse than those with other B-cell lymphomas (5-year EFS of 66 % vs. 5-year EFS of 85 %) [9, 13, 12]. Dose-adjusted multi-agent regimen (etoposide, doxorubicin, cyclophosphamide, vincristine, prednisone) with gradually escalating chemotherapy doses, plus immunotherapy with anti-CD20 (rituximab), seems to be the most promising therapeutic option [12], with the probable cost of more toxic late effects in the future.

The role or PET/CT in diagnosis, staging and following up of paediatric PMDLBCL is not well clarified, and paediatric protocols do not include it in their routine imaging techniques. Nevertheless, upcoming data from adult studies suggest that it may have a promising contribution as a prognostic factor in PMDLBCL and that its interim use may guide risk-adapted dose immunochemotherapy and/or radiotherapy in the future [14–16].

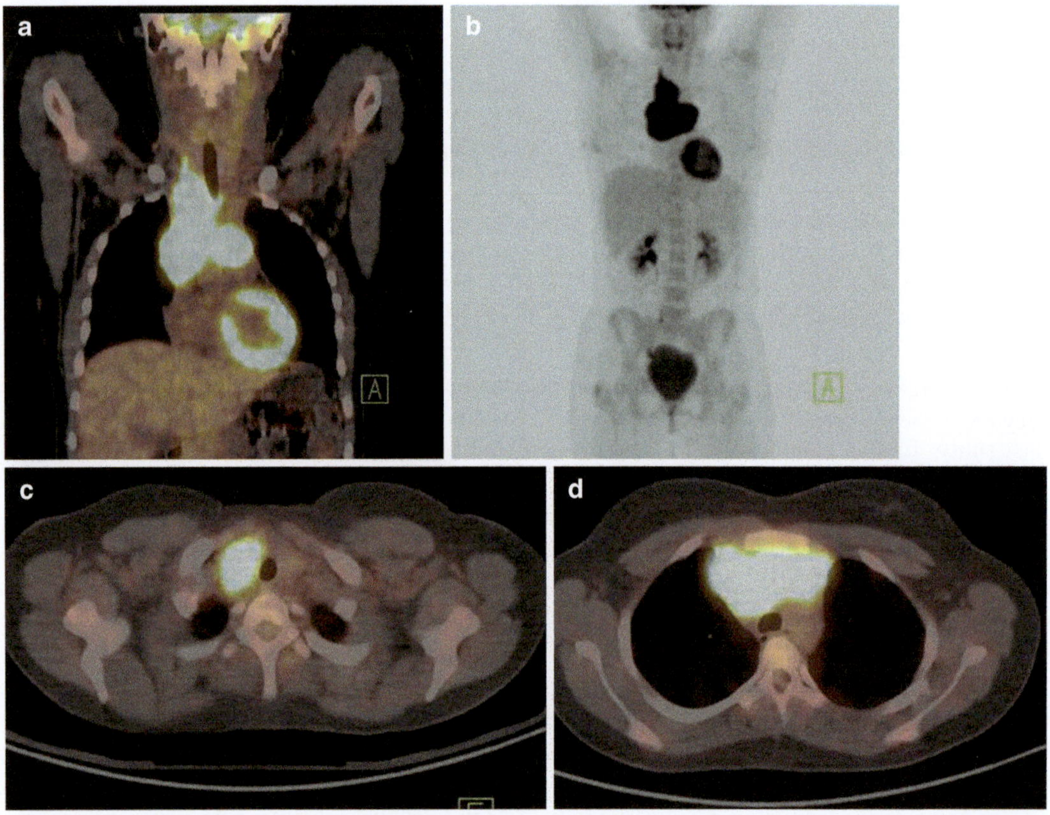

Fig. 21.1 Coronal PET/CT image (**a**), MIP image (**b**) and axial PET/CT images (**c**, **d**) show a large hypermetabolic lymphatic mass extending from the right supraclavicular area to the anterior mediastinum (SUV_{max} 16.4)

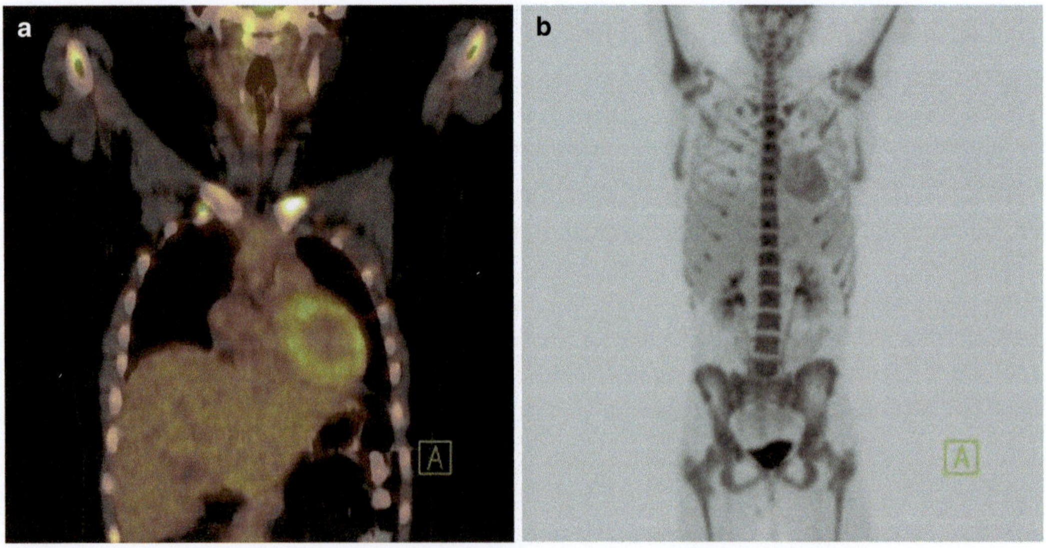

Fig. 21.2 Interim PET/CT (**a**, **b**), after two chemotherapy cycles, shows complete remission of the disease. The hypermetabolic visualization of the bone marrow is attributed to G-CSF administration

Case 2: Abdomen

An 8-year-old girl presented with a 2-month history of low-grade fever, malaise, reduced appetite and weight loss. Full blood cell count showed severe anaemia, with haemoglobin 7.1 g/dl and hematocrit 22.5 %. Abdominal US and the subsequent CT showed a large mass located in the area of the uterus, left ovary and upper part of the vagina. Both kidneys were enlarged with multiple parenchymal lesions. Biopsy of the pelvic mass revealed the diagnosis of diffuse large B-cell lymphoma (DLBCL). Bone marrow aspirate and CSF cytology were negative for lymphoma.

PET/CT showed increased FDG uptake (SUV_{max}=5,6) in the pelvis, the renal lesions (SUV_{max}=5,6) and the periportal area (SUV_{max}=2,4). The increased uptake in the left pelvis (SUV_{max}=4,2) was attributed to bowel uptake (Fig. 21.3).

Patient commenced chemotherapy with COP, according to FAB LMB 96, group B protocol. The response to treatment, a week later, was considered satisfactory and continued with 2 COPADM and 1 CYM. CT, at the 2nd re-evaluation timepoint, showed a sizable residual mass in the area of the left pelvis. Patient underwent a surgical removal of the left ovary and the residual mass. Histology revealed no viable tumour.

She continued chemotherapy with another course of CYM. PET/CT at the end of treatment was negative (Fig. 21.4). One year off therapy, patient continues to be in complete remission.

Discussion

Paediatric DLBCL is typically mediastinal. However, extranodal presentation is more frequent in children comparing to adults. Extrathoracic tumours more often occur in the kidneys and the liver, spleen and pancreas, whereas spread to other extranodal organs is rare [4]. Primary NHL of the genital tract is a rare entity. Specifically, the primary lymphomas of female genitalia represent less than 1 %, whilst the most common histological subtype is DLBCL [17]. The adnexa is more often involved, followed by the uterine body and cervix and, less commonly, the vulva and vagina. The prognosis seems to be favourable, and, with early diagnosis and appropriate therapy, radical surgery can be avoided [18].

The advantages of PET/CT for the staging and re-evaluation of lymphoma are mainly due to the detection of FDG-avid lymph nodes and of extranodal sites, previously missed at conventional CT (usually the liver, spleen, cortical bone, bone marrow and skin). In NHL, DLBCL and high-grade follicular lymphoma demonstrate the highest FDG metabolism [19]. PET/CT is an accurate method for end-of-treatment evaluation, because of its ability in differentiating between residual viable tumour and fibrosis. This ability is especially important in DLBCL, which often responds with fibrosis and necrosis, rather than tumour shrinkage. However, the correlation of PET/CT response at the end of first-line therapy with progression-free survival and overall survival in DLBCL has not yet been established [20].

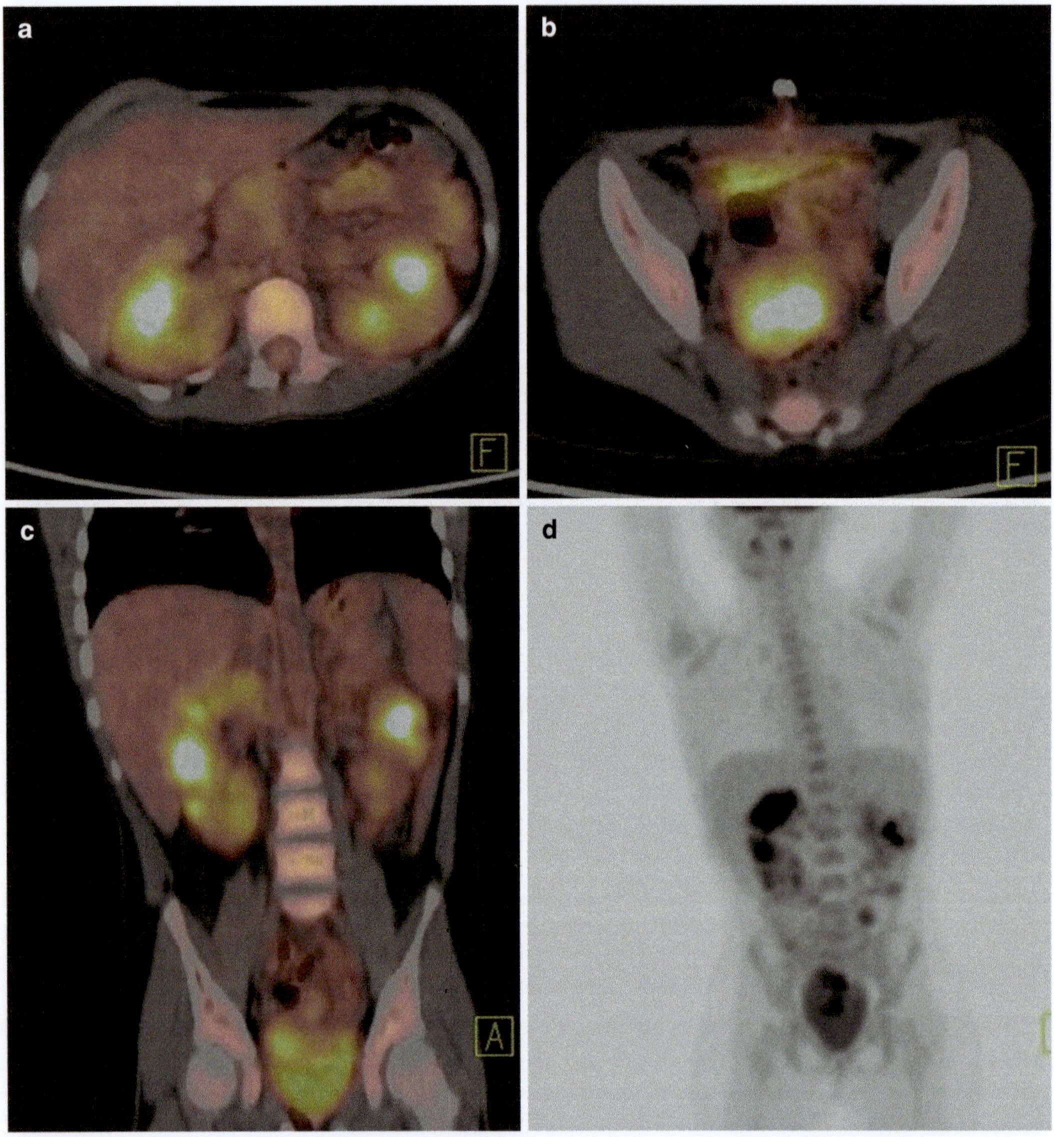

Fig. 21.3 Axial (**a**, **b**) and coronal (**c**) PET/CT images show multiple parenchyma hypermetabolic renal lesions (SUV_{max} 5,6) as well as a hypermetabolic pelvic mass in the area of the uterus (SUV_{max} 5,6). MIP image (**d**) shows the extent of the disease in the abdomen and pelvis

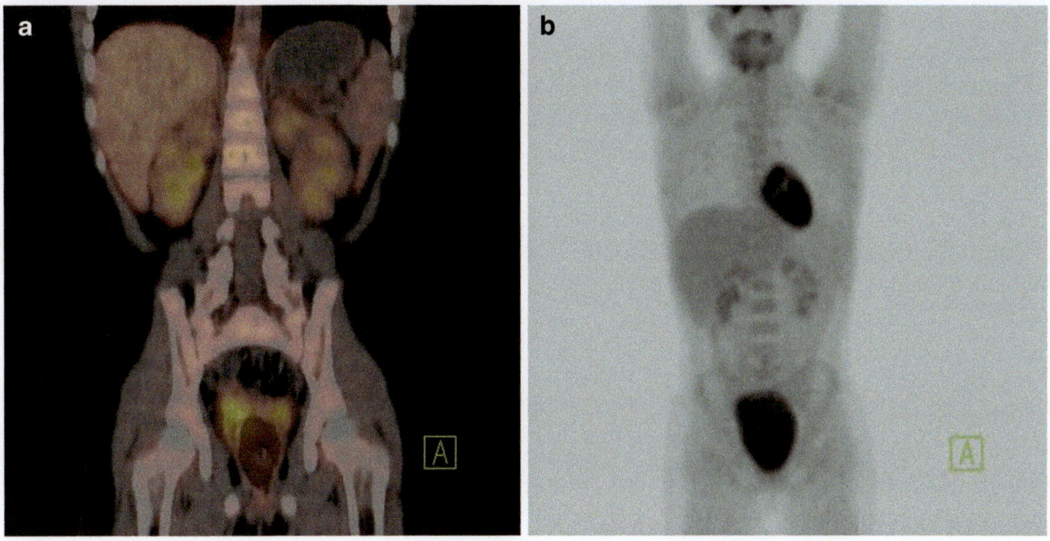

Fig. 21.4 PET/CT images (**a**, **b**) at the end of treatment show complete remission of the disease

Case 3: Bones

A male adolescent, 15 years old, presented at our department in July 2014 with the diagnosis of a B-cell lymphoma of the right femur. Tumour was incidentally diagnosed in a plain femur X-ray (Fig. 21.5), which was performed in the context of following up a fracture of the right femoral head, which had occurred after a fall during school gymnastics 3 months ago. Right femur MRI and CT confirmed the presence of a large intertrochanteric mass, occupying the whole upper third of the right femur (Fig. 21.6a, b).

Open (true cut) biopsy was then performed, and histology revealed high-grade non-Hodgkin lymphoma of B-cell origin (DLBCL as per WHO). Immunophenotype was positive for CD20, PAX5, BCL6 and MUM1, regionally and weekly positive for BCL2 and CD10 and negative for CD5, CD30, TdT, CD34, CD99, CD38, CD138, CD56, CD3, CD21, CD23, EBR and LMP. There was also a mixture of T-origin lymphocytes (CD3, CD5 positive and CD20 negative) and of fewer histiocytic cells (CD68 positive). MIB1 index (Ki67) was higher than 90 %. Immune stain against c-myc was positive in less than 40 % of neoplastic cells. FISH tumour cytogenetics for IGH, BCL2, BCL6 and MYC were negative.

Metastatic survey with chest CT, abdominal MRI, bone marrow aspiration, trephine biopsy and CSF cytology was negative. Initial staging was completed with a whole-body PET/CT, which confirmed the diagnosis of right femur lymphoma with no distant metastases (Fig. 21.7).

Patient started chemotherapy according to FAB LMB 96 (group B) protocol. He tolerated therapy excellently, with a very good tumour response, confirmed by conventional imaging (plain X-rays and MRI of the right femur) (Fig. 21.8a, b) performed at the required by the protocol timepoints, during induction chemotherapy (COP, COPADM1 and COPADM2).

He had an interim PET/CT performed during consolidation chemotherapy (CYM1, CYM2) with improved, but not negative, findings (Fig. 21.9).

At the end of chemotherapy (4 months since diagnosis), he had a very good partial response confirmed by conventional imaging (right femur CT and MRI), (Fig. 21.10), though with a serious suspicion of residual disease. The results of a new PET/CT performed at that timepoint did not exclude this possibility, on the contrary reinforced the suspicion (Fig. 21.11).

An open biopsy of the residual mass was then decided, which revealed foci of necrosis fulfilled with necrotic 'ghost cells' consistent with necrotic lymphoma, marrow areas consistent with cavity fibrosis and chronic inflammation and no morphologic or immunophenotypic evidence of viable tumour.

Five months after the end of therapy, patient is under close imaging and clinical follow-up, in excellent general condition, with good mobilization of the right femur and with no evidence of disease progression or relapse. The latest PET/CT shows further improvement, though still not negative (Fig. 21.12).

Discussion

Primary non-Hodgkin lymphoma of the bones (PLB) is a rare subgroup (4 % of all paediatric NHLs), usually occurring at the second decade of life (median age at diagnosis 11.5 years), with male predominance. The femur and pelvis are the most frequently involved bones [21, 22, 23]. Paediatric PLBs are more heterogeneous and consist of lymphoblastic lymphoma, Burkitt lymphoma, and DLBCL. DLBCL is the most common histological subtype and, in contrast with adults, the one with the most favourable outcome, arising at a 5-year overall survival greater than 95 % [23].

DLBCL is one of the most consistently PET-avid lymphomas. The standard uptake value (SUV) is typically high, with most lymphomas having an SUV_{max} greater than 10. In adults, its contribution in the accuracy of initial staging, the estimation of early response to treatment and the evaluation of complete response after treatment are well documented [21, 24].

In contrast with adults, PET results are challenging to interpret in paediatric patients with NHLs, especially in the case of identifying viable residual disease [24, 25, 26]. Interpretation may become more ambiguous in the case of paediatric DLBCLs, particularly those of the bones, which respond to treatment with intra-tumoral necrosis and/or fibrosis rather than with complete imaging regression. In that case, a biopsy is often warranted to confirm the presence or absence of viable tumour [21, 24].

PET's sensitivity and negative predictive value in paediatric NHLs arises to 100 %; nevertheless, its specificity is low (60 %) and so is its positive predictive value (25 %). False-positive PET/CT studies are relatively common in paediatric clinical practice, with reported rates between 50 and 75 % in paediatric NHLs. Reasons commonly include infection/inflammation and thymic rebound, whilst fibrosis and necrosis are the most common causes during or after chemotherapy. Therefore, changing the therapeutic plan on the basis of a positive PET alone is not recommended and a biopsy confirmation should be required. On the other hand, because false-negative rate of PET is extremely low, avoiding biopsy may be an option for children with residual disease in conventional imaging and a negative PET/CT [27, 24, 25, 26].

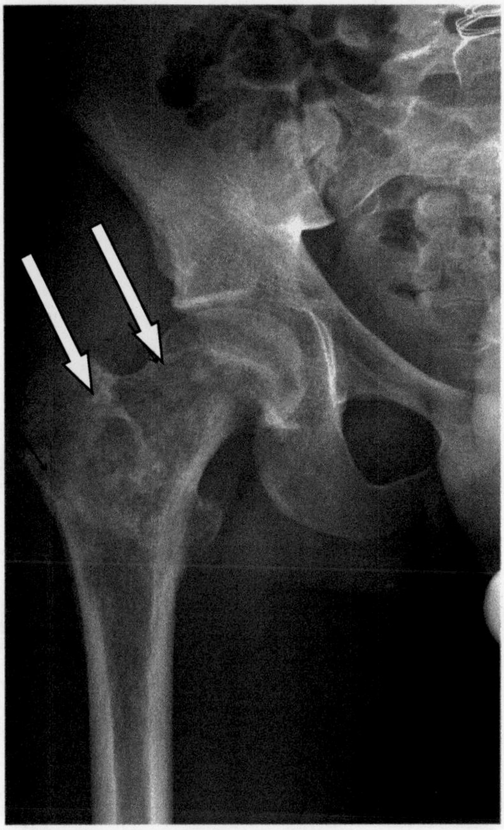

Fig. 21.5 Radiograph of the right hip shows loss of normal architecture and moth-eaten pattern in the proximal metadiaphysis of the right femur (*arrows*) and coexistent unilayer periosteal reaction

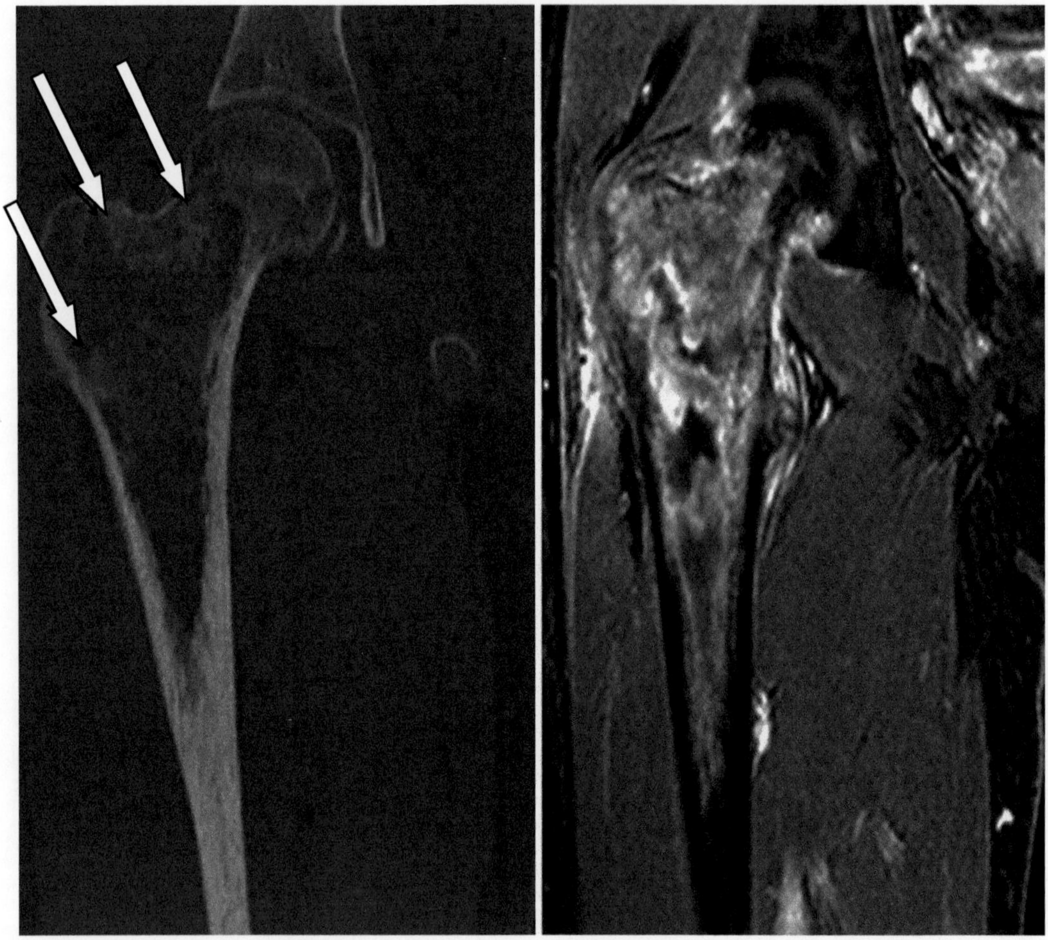

Fig. 21.6 Similar findings with Fig. 21.5 are evident on CT (**a** coronal MPR) and MRI (**b** T1-weighted fat-saturated imaged post iv injection of contrast)

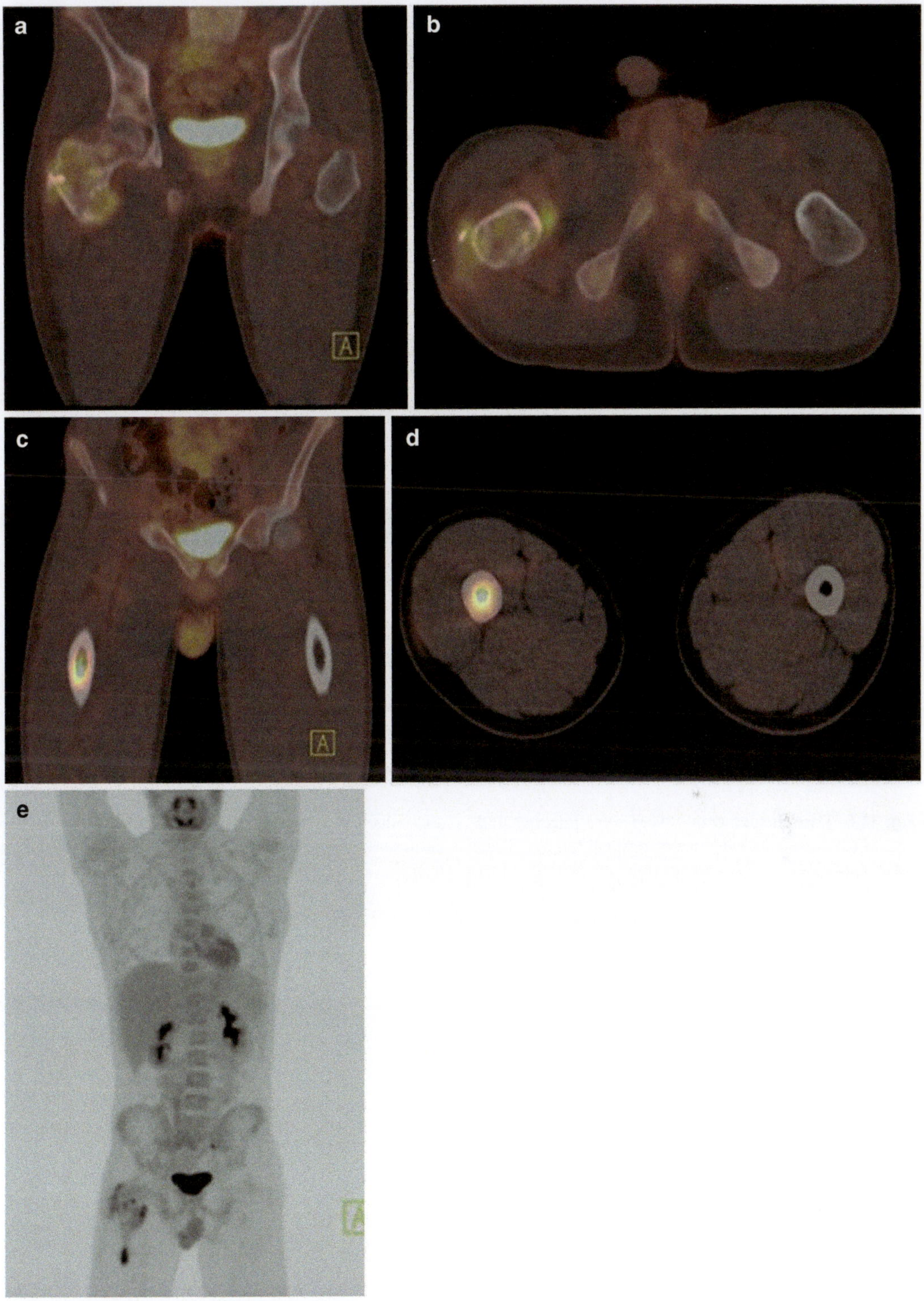

Fig. 21.7 Coronal and axial PET/CT images (**a**, **b**) show disorder of the normal structure of the neck of the right femur, with increased metabolic activity (SUV_{max} 3,7) and disruption of the cortical continuity at the minor trochanter. An area of increased metabolic activity (SUV_{max} 7) in the bone marrow of the upper third of the right femur is seen in coronal and axial PET/CT images (**c**, **d**). No other foci of increased metabolic activity are seen. MIP image (**e**) shows the extent of the disease at the right femur

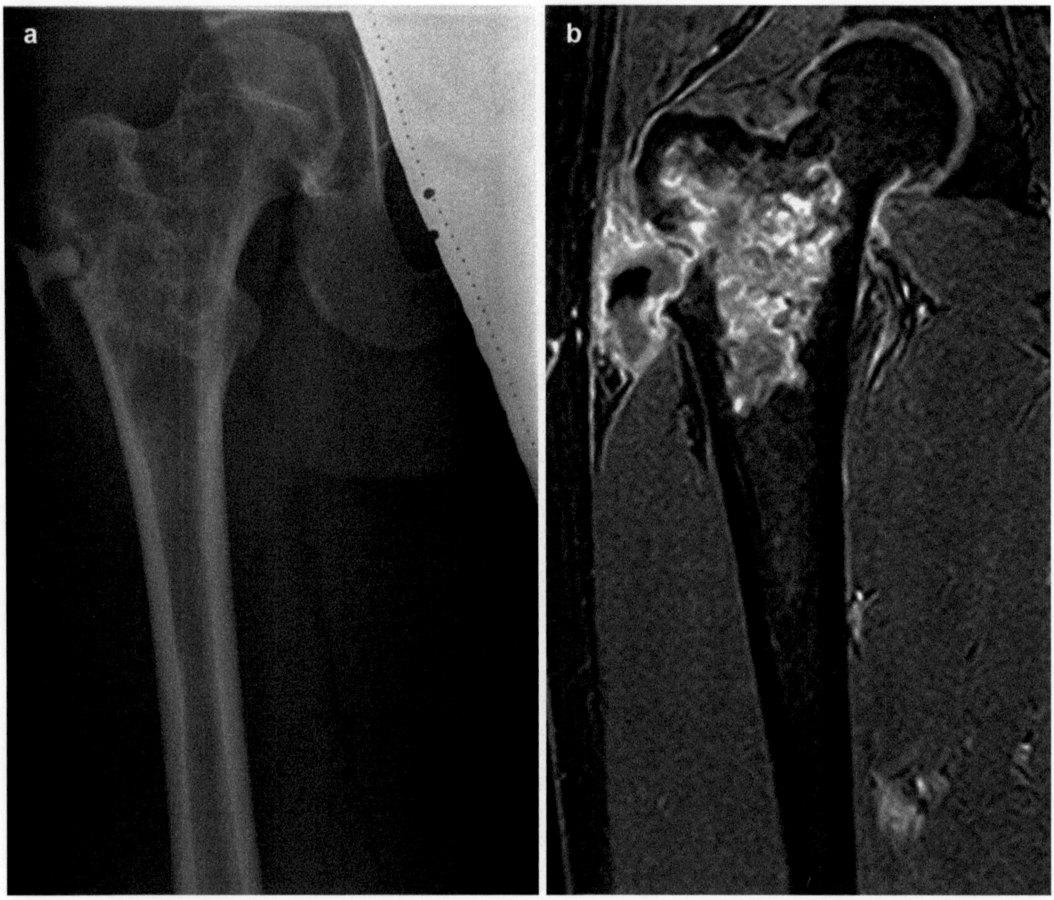

Fig. 21.8 Post-chemotherapy, there were imaging findings of response with evidence of residual tumour. There was improvement of the architecture on radiograph (**a**) and reduction of the extent of the lesion of abnormal signal intensity on T1-weighted fat-saturated image post iv injection of contrast (**b**)

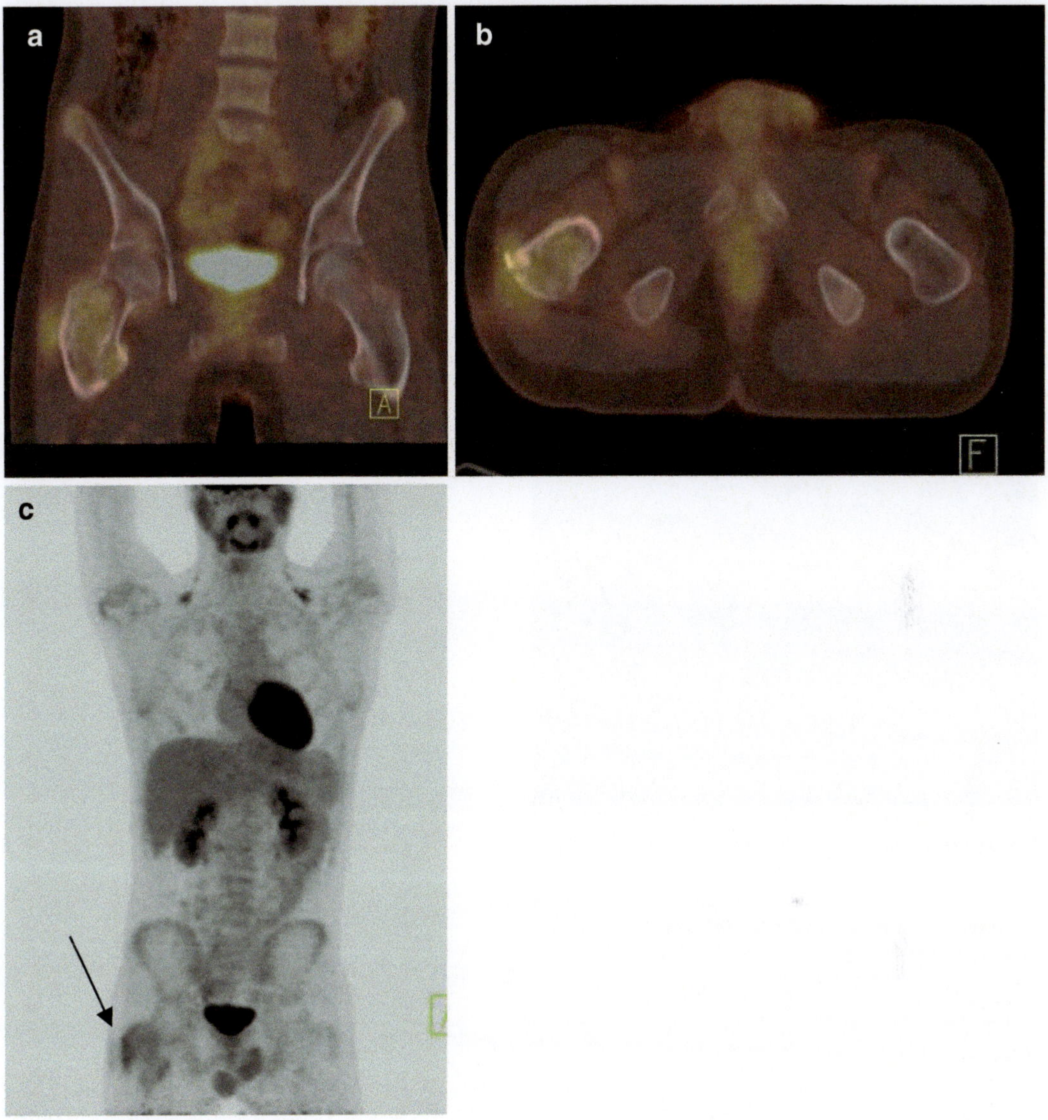

Fig. 21.9 In coronal and axial PET/CT images (**a**, **b**), there is still disorder of the normal structure of the neck of the right femur, but the metabolic activity is reduced compared to the previous examination (SUV_{max} 2,4), and the region of minor trochanter is more sclerotic. Increased FDG uptake at the adjacent soft tissue (SUV_{max} 5) is also observed. MIP image (**c**) shows the improvement (*arrow*) of the disease after therapy

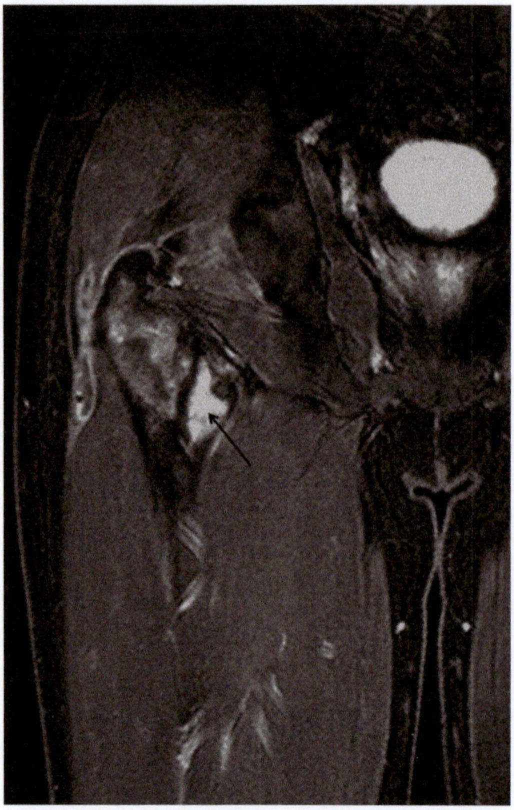

Fig. 21.10 At the completion of chemotherapy, MRI of the hip revealed residual area of enhancement in the proximal right femur with a region of intense enhancement at the level of the lesser trochanter (*arrow*), highly suspicious of residual infiltrate

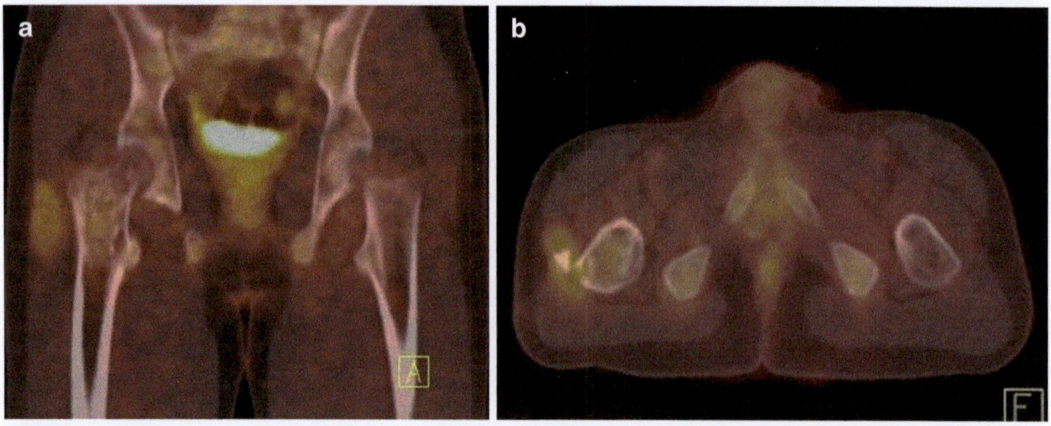

Fig. 21.11 Coronal and axial PET/CT images (**a**, **b**) show a combination of lytic and sclerotic areas in the region of the neck of the right femur with slightly increased FDG uptake as well as increased uptake of the radiopharmaceutical at the adjacent soft tissue

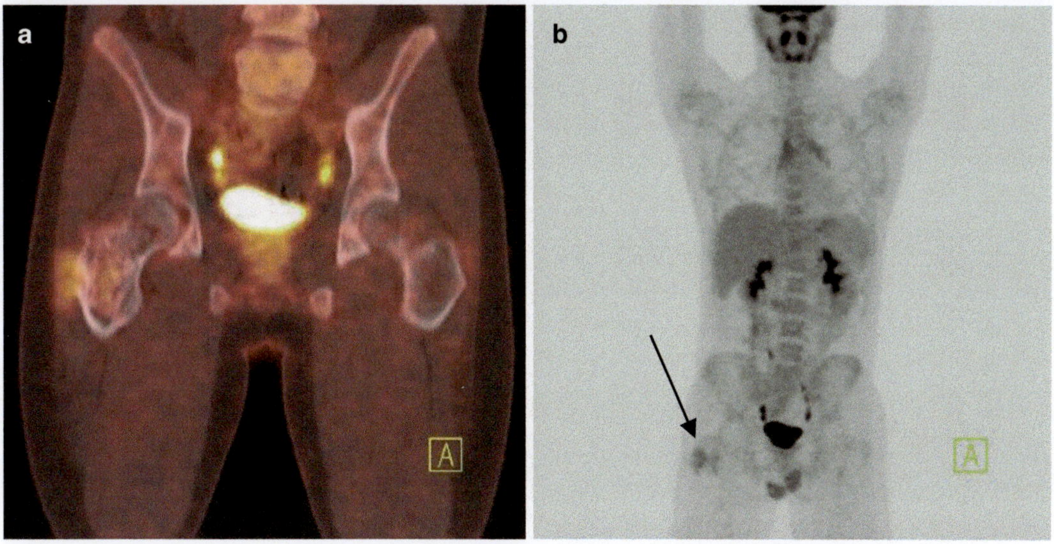

Fig. 21.12 Coronal PET/CT image (**a**) and MIP image (**b**) 5 months after the end of therapy show further improvement in the region of the neck of the right femur and slightly increased FDG uptake at the adjacent soft tissue (SUV_{max} 2, 5)

Case 4: Bones and Bone Marrow

A 10-year-old boy presented in January 2013 with pain along the lateral aspect of his right heel without any history of injury. In March 2013 he suffered from persisting limping due to pain in his right leg and swelling of soft tissue in heel region. At this time, plain X-ray (Fig. 21.13) and magnetic resonance imaging of the foot showed lytic and sclerotic areas, and 3-phase bone scan was positive for increased uptake and increased osteoblastic activity in the right heel.

Open biopsy of the lesion was done with surgical excision and curettage. Pathology revealed chronic inflammation and tissue culture grew Staph. epidermidis. After review of history, clinical, radiological and histopathology data, a diagnosis of acute osteomyelitis was made and antibiotics IV and orally were prescribed for 10 weeks, plus physiotherapy and muscle strengthening. For the next 3 months, the patient continued to have pain and limitation in his daily activities. In July 2013 he presented with neck pain and low-grade fever and deterioration of his general clinical condition. He was then hospitalized and was treated with combinations of antibiotics for 2 months. At this time MRI of the spine revealed multiple inflammatory-like lesions involving cervical and thoracic vertebras. Further workup, including bone marrow aspiration and biopsy; US of the neck, abdomen and pelvis; and bone scan, was normal. Despite treatment, he periodically had recurrent episodes of symptoms, and finally, in September 2013 he clinically deteriorated and was readmitted with fever, fatigue, decreased appetite, restricted neck movements and pain in the lumbar region. Lymphadenopathy and hepatosplenomegaly were not present.

Whole-body MRI and CT revealed increased number of lesions involving cervical, thoracic and lumbar vertebras typical of secondary localizations (Fig. 21.14), worse appearance in the right foot (Fig. 21.15), a new lytic lesion in the sternum (Fig. 21.16) and kidney swelling with multiple solid hypoechoic oval lesions (Fig. 21.17).

Bone marrow aspiration revealed decreased cellularity without any malignant involvement, but bone marrow biopsy showed infiltration with small- and medium-sized abnormal lymphoid cells. Immunohistochemical studies revealed positivity of these cells for CD20, PAX-5, CD79a, Bcl-6 and MIB-1 and negativity for CD3 and CD10.

An ^{18}F-fluorodeoxyglucose positron emission tomography scan revealed the presence of heterogeneous uptake of the sternum body ($SUV_{max}=3.3$), thoracic and lumbar vertebras, iliac bones ($SUV_{max}=3.4$) and right heel, suggesting the presence of disease with high metabolic activity in these sites (Figs. 21.18, 21.19, and 21.20). There were multiple focal lesions in both iliac bones, which could be suggestive of bone marrow infiltration, interpretation consistent with the result of the bone marrow biopsy. No abnormal uptake was observed in other sites.

At this time a fine needle biopsy from the sternum lesion was also performed. Pathology showed the marrow cavity completely infiltrated from malignant cells with excessive focal fibrosis. Bone architecture was almost totally replaced by large lymphoid in origin cells with abnormalities in the nuclear surroundings and increased number of multilobulated nuclei. Immunochemistry demonstrated positive staining for CD79a, CD20, PAX-5, bcl2pr, bcl6 and LCA and negative staining for CD3, CD10, CD30 and CD23. Mib-1 (Ki-67) index was sufficiently increased. These findings confirmed the diagnosis of a high-grade B-cell lymphoma of large cells or else a primary bone diffuse large B-cell lymphoma (DLBCL) with bone marrow involvement.

Patient commenced chemotherapy as per FAB LMB 96 group C (due to bone marrow involvement) protocol. Bone marrow examination showed remission at the due per protocol time period. Further imaging studies during and after chemotherapy indicated complete imaging remission; nevertheless, 18 F-fluorodeoxyglucose positron emission tomography scan revealed only mild improvement (Figs. 21.21 and 21.22).

It was therefore decided to proceed to autologous stem cell transplantation (ASCT) after receiving BEAM as conditioning regimen. Four months after the autologous stem cell transplantation, a new PET/CT study showed complete remission (Fig. 21.23).

At present, 15 months after transplantation, patient remains in complete remission of his lymphoma.

Discussion

Diffuse large B-cell lymphoma (DLBCL) accounts for approximately 10 % of non-Hodgkin lymphomas (NHL) of childhood. Whereas lymphoblastic lymphoma (LBL), Burkitt lymphoma (BL) and anaplastic large cell lymphoma (ALCL) are rather homogeneous clinicopathologic subentities of childhood NHL, DLBCL represents a heterogeneous group of lymphoid neoplasms. In DLBCL, a diffuse neoplastic infiltrate composed of B-lineage blasts with variable morphology replaces the normal lymph node architecture or the normal extranodal tissue. In the majority of paediatric DLBCL cases, it is the morphology, resembling centroblasts, together with the expression of germinal centre-associated antigens, such as CD10 and BCL6, which suggest a germinal centre cell origin [4]. DLBCL is rarely diagnosed in children less than 4 years of age, after which its incidence increases throughout childhood. Compared to BL patients, children with DLBCL more frequently present with localized disease and focal lesions in the liver, spleen, lung and mediastinum, whereas increased lactate dehydrogenase (LDH), pleural effusions and ascites are less frequently observed. Bone marrow (BM) and central nervous system (CNS) are rarely affected. Primary DLBCL bone lymphoma involving numerous bones and bone marrow involvement is not common. Moreover, paediatric PLB-DLBCL with or without bone marrow involvement has a favourable prognosis, though remaining poorly characterized [23]. From recent multicentre trials on paediatric B-NHL including DLBCL, event-free survival (EFS) of over 90 % was reported for the subgroup of patients diagnosed with DLBCL. Thus, outcome of children with DLBCL was similar to outcome of patients with BL, and DLBCL histology was not an adverse prognostic factor [28]. Therapeutic approaches are identical to the ones used for B mature NHL (i.e. FAB LMB 96 or B-NHL of the BFM group). Although high-dose chemotherapy followed by autologous bone marrow rescue is known to improve the outcome of relapsed lymphoma, the role of upfront ASCT for patients with DLBCL is controversial [29]. In patients with primary bone marrow DLBCL, the high risk of autograft contamination with lymphoma cells is of major concern; therefore, the role of ASCT has to be further explored.

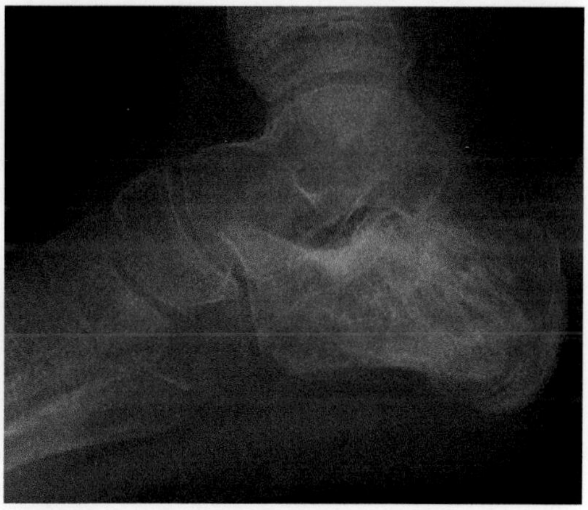

Fig. 21.13 Plain X-ray of the right heel

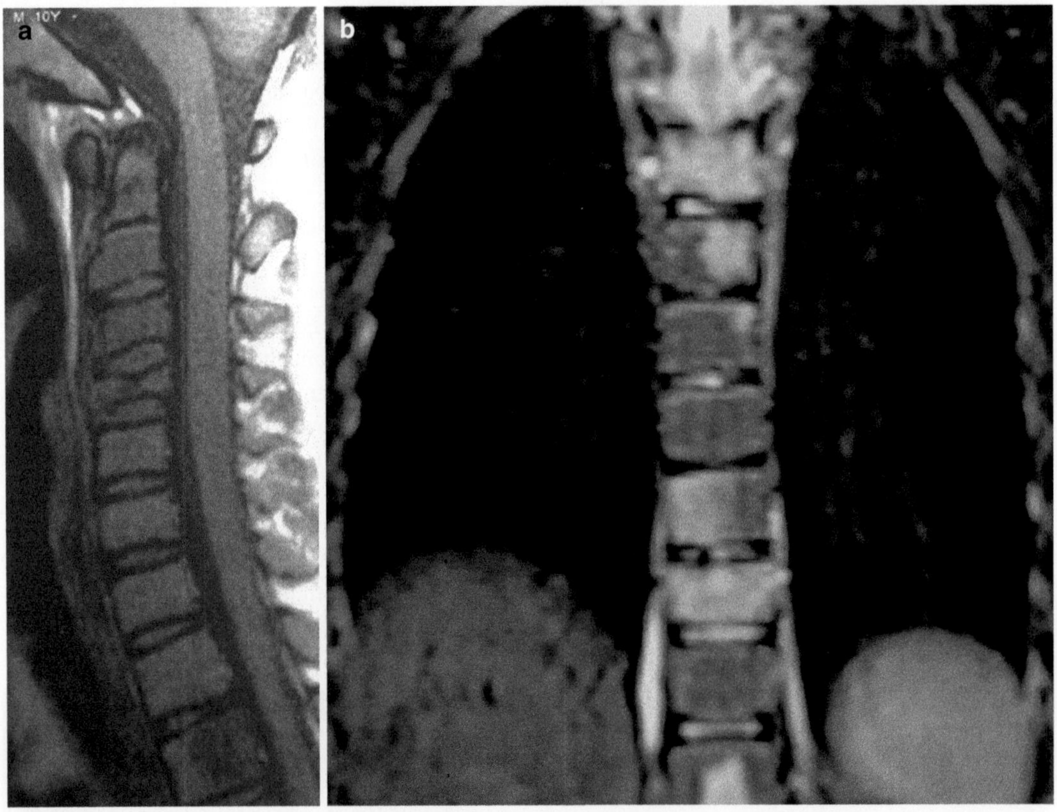

Fig. 21.14 (**a**, **b**) Vertebral lesions, T1 sagittal image of the cervical spine and T2 coronal image of thoracic spine

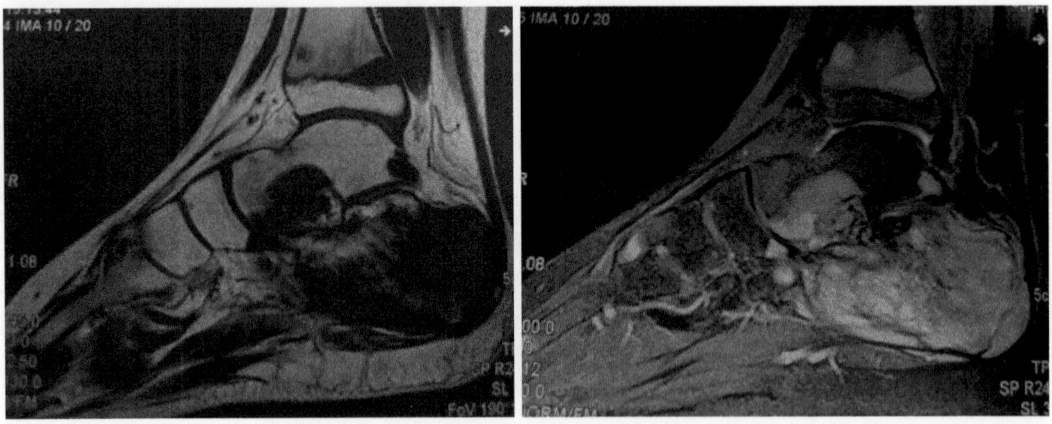

Fig. 21.15 T1 sagittal and T2 sagittal images of the right foot

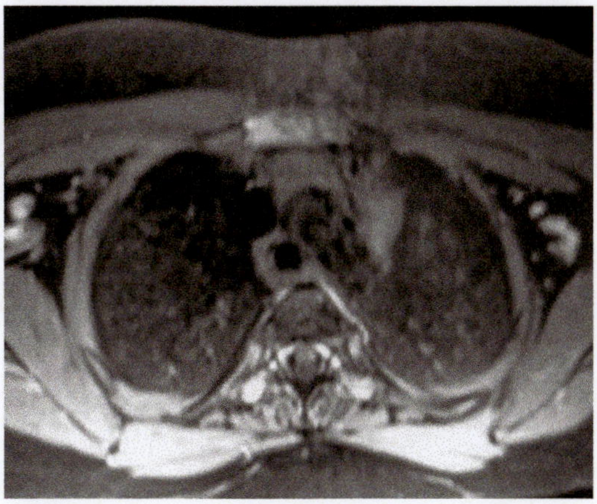

Fig. 21.16 Axial postcontrast MRI of the sternum

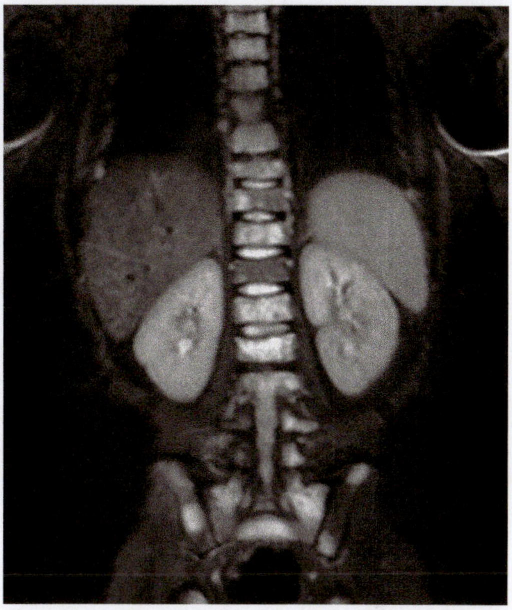

Fig. 21.17 Kidney swelling, coronal MRI of the kidneys

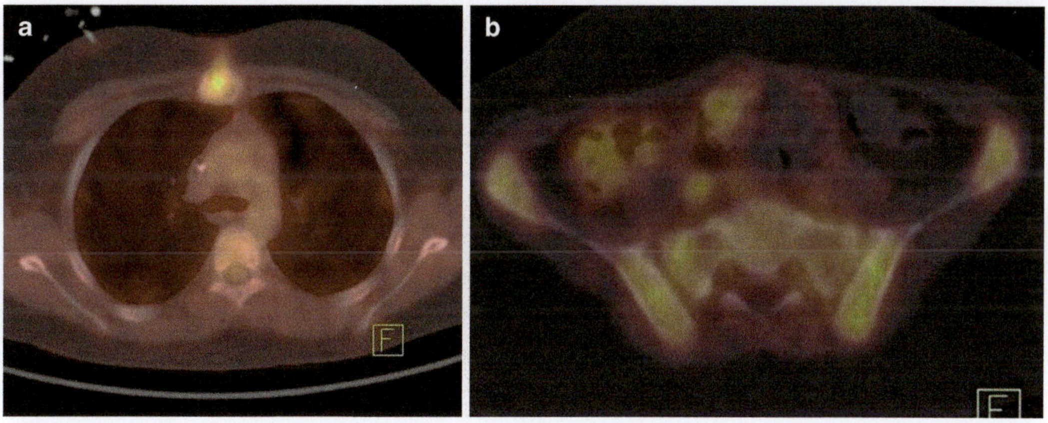

Fig. 21.18 Axial PET/CT images (**a**, **b**) show a lytic lesion at the sternum with increased metabolic activity (SUV_{max}3,3) and diffusely increased FDG uptake in the iliac bones (SUV_{max}3,2)

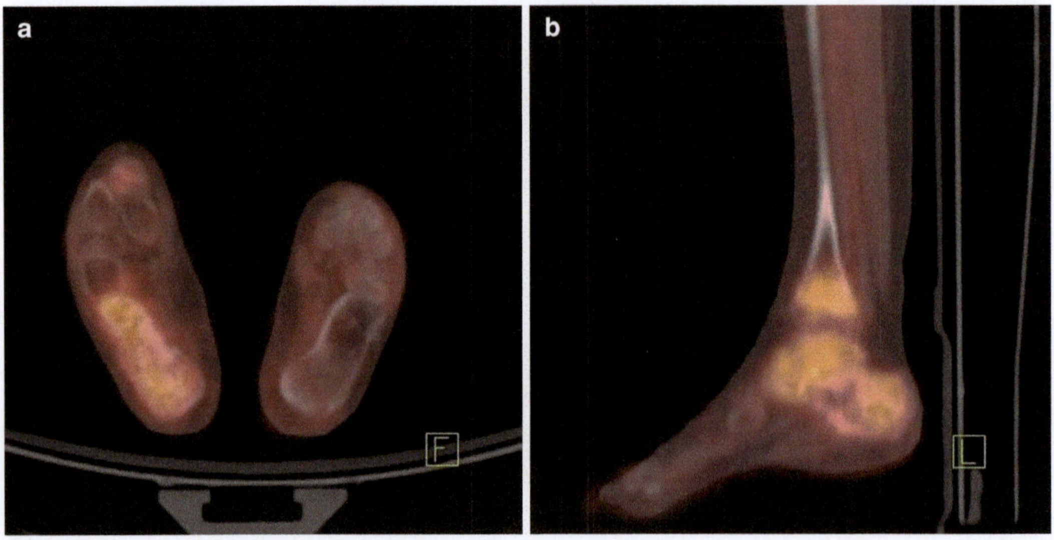

Fig. 21.19 Axial and sagittal PET/CT images (**a**, **b**) show lytic and sclerotic areas in the right heel with increased radiopharmaceutical uptake (SUV_{max} 3,3)

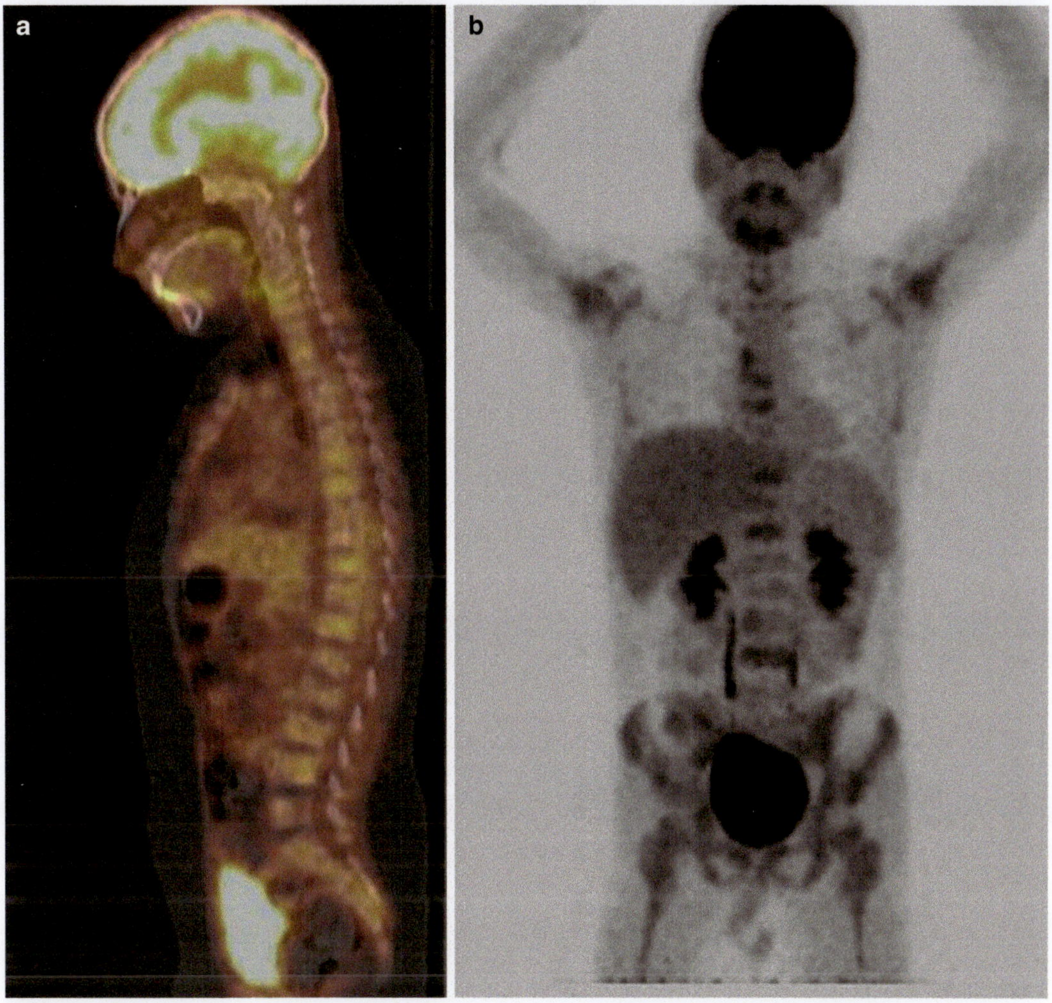

Fig. 21.20 Sagittal PET/CT image (**a**) shows sclerotic lesions with increased FDG uptake in cervical, thoracic and lumbar vertebras (SUV_{max} 3,5). MIP images of the body (**b**) and of the legs (**c**) show the extent of the disease

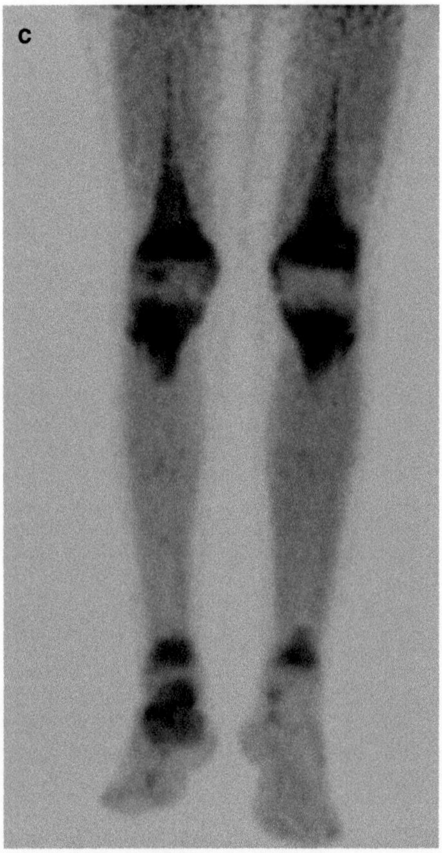

Fig. 21.20 (continued)

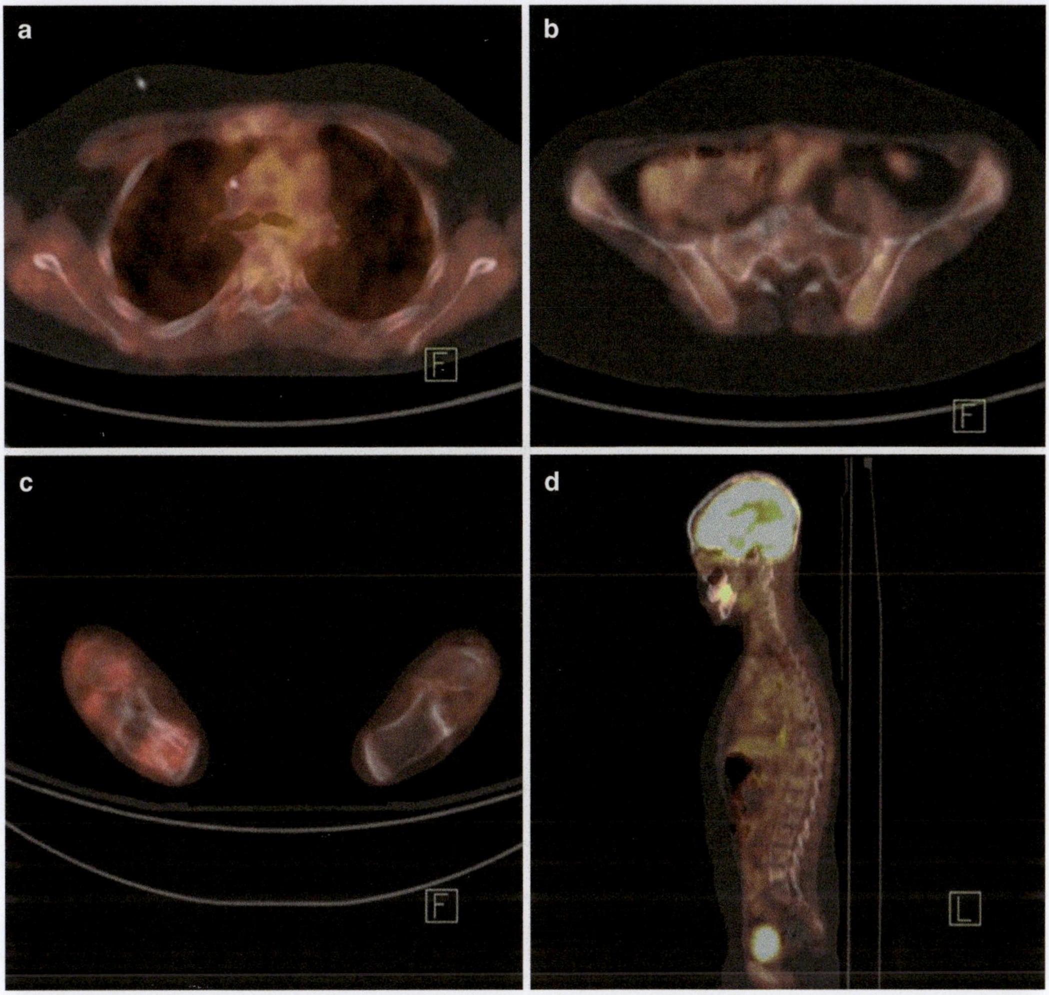

Fig. 21.21 PET/CT study shows improvement at the end of therapy. Axial PET/CT images (**a–c**) and sagittal PET/CT image (**d**) show sclerotic lesions at the sternum, at the right heel, at vertebras and iliac bones with slightly increased metabolic activity (SUV_{max} 2,4)

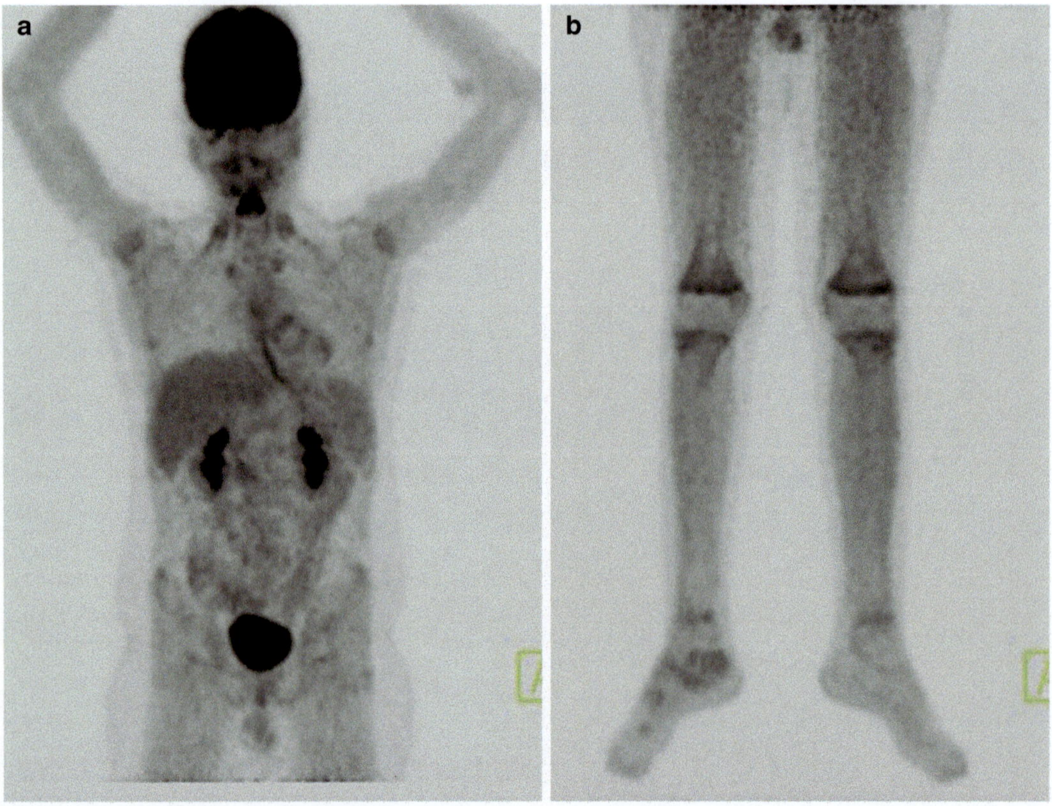

Fig. 21.22 Whole-body MIP images (**a**, **b**) show improvement

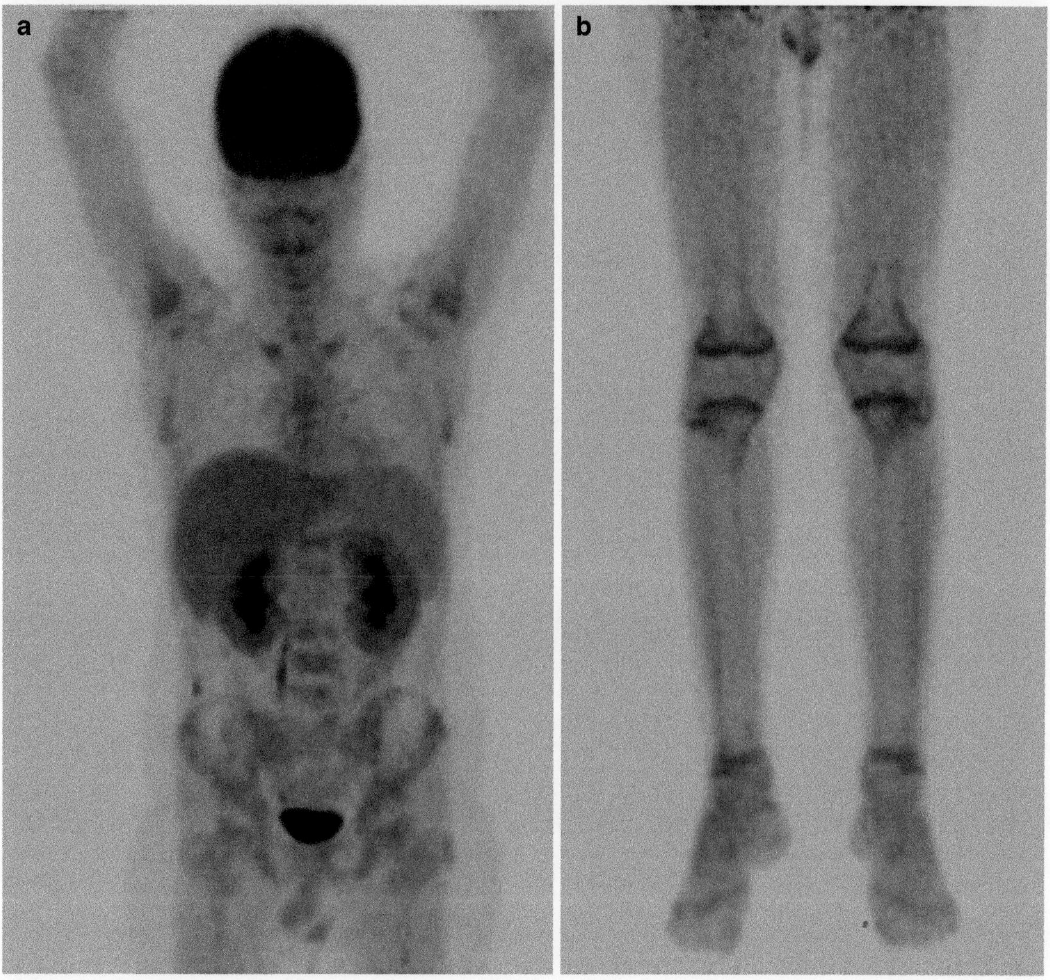

Fig. 21.23 Four months after ASCT PET/CT study shows complete remission. In whole-body MIP images (**a**, **b**), no foci of increased metabolic activity are seen

Case 5: Peripheral Lymph Nodes

A rare case of paediatric follicular lymphoma is here described: a 13-year-old child was admitted to the hospital with a history of a slowly growing mass on his preauricular region for the previous 6 months. His medical history was otherwise unremarkable, and he was not on any medication. He had no fever, weight loss or other symptoms. Physical examination revealed a non-tender mass in the parotid area without pain or redness. Cervical lymphadenopathy was not recognized. There were no other palpable lymph nodes or hepatosplenomegaly. There were no abnormalities in laboratory findings, including ESR 15 mmHg, lactate dehydrogenase (LDH) 545 IU/l and uric acid 3.6 mg/dl.

Ultrasonography (US) and magnetic resonance imaging (MRI) showed a sizeable lymphatic mass in the left parotid region. Bone marrow biopsy and aspiration and cerebrospinal fluid cytology were negative. PET/CT imaging revealed increased uptake of the radiopharmaceutical on the left parotid region ($SUV_{max}=5.6$) and in two left jugular lymph nodes ($SUV_{max}=3.9$), suggesting the presence of disease with high metabolic activity in these sites (Fig. 21.24). There were no other regions with increased FDG uptake and high metabolic activity.

After complete staging lymph node excision was done. On histological examination, features were compatible with non-Hodgkin B-cell nodular follicular lymphoma, paediatric type, according to WHO Classification 2008, that is, a lymph node with abnormal, severe follicular hyperplasia, effacement of the architecture and focal invasion of the adjacent part of the major salivary gland. Immunochemistry demonstrated that neoplastic cells strongly expressed B-cell markers [CD20/L-26], with germline-centred detection of CD10 and bcl-6 and no detection of bcl-2, CD43 or monotypic κ and λ immunoglobulin light chains. There was no expression of LMP-1 protein for Epstein-Barr virus. The detection of clonal rearrangement of the heavy immunoglobulin chains contributed to the confirmation of the diagnosis.

Patient underwent chemotherapy with 2 induction cycles of R-CHOP (rituximab, prednisone, vincristine, cyclophosphamide), according to the NHL protocol for FL [30]. All involved lymph nodes had regressed as assessed by MRI at the end of induction; therefore, PET/CT was not repeated. At present, 12 months after the initial diagnosis, patient remains in complete remission.

Discussion

Follicular lymphomas (FL) are among the most common non-Hodgkin lymphomas (NHLs) in adults (22 %). However, they are very rare in children, making up less than 3 % of paediatric NHL cases. Major reports show a male predominance of close to 4:1 and an age range of occurrence of 7.5–11.7 years. They are most commonly located in the head and neck region, in the lymph nodes or the tonsils, whereas rare are documentations of extranodal occurrences, such as gastrointestinal tract, parotid gland, kidney, epididymis and testis [31].

Paediatric FL(pFL) is a rare disease. In adults FL is considered an incurable disease, and thus, its clinical course differs from that of DLBCL, if treated with comparable therapy. However, the outcome of both diseases, FL and DLBCL in children, is equivalent when treated with NHL, mature B-cell lymphomas' protocols. Relapses, which are frequent in adult FL, are rare in children. Data suggest that paediatric FL is a disease that differs from its adult counterpart, both genetically and clinically [30]. The genetic hallmark of adult FL, the translocation t(14;18)(q32;q21), is typically not detectable in paediatric FL. Nodular follicular lymphomas of paediatric type do not express bcl-2 protein, and they are not characterized by bcl-2 rearrangements. Clonality detection of the rearrangement of the heavy chain immunoglobulin gene contributes to the confirmation of the diagnosis [32].

The molecular mechanisms involved in the pathogenesis of paediatric FL still remain to be elucidated. In one study, pFL was found to be associated with male gender (3:1), older age (72 % ≥10 years old), low serum LDH levels (<500 U/l in 75 %), grade 3 histology (in 88 %) and limited disease (87 % stage I/II disease), mostly involving the peripheral lymph nodes. Forty-four out of sixty-three patients received polychemotherapy and one out of sixty-three rituximab only, whilst seventeen out of sixty-three underwent a 'watch-and-wait' strategy. Of 36 stage I patients, 30 had complete resections. Only one patient relapsed, and 2-year event-free survival and overall survival were 94 ± 5 and 100 %, respectively, after a median follow-up of 2.2 years.

Conclusively, treatment outcome in pFL seems to be excellent with risk-adapted chemotherapy or with complete surgical resection and observational strategy only [33]. In contrast to adult FL, clinical course is not characterized by relapses. Furthermore, a simultaneous presence of DLBCL can frequently be detected at initial diagnosis in paediatric FL, but this does not indicate a more aggressive clinical course.

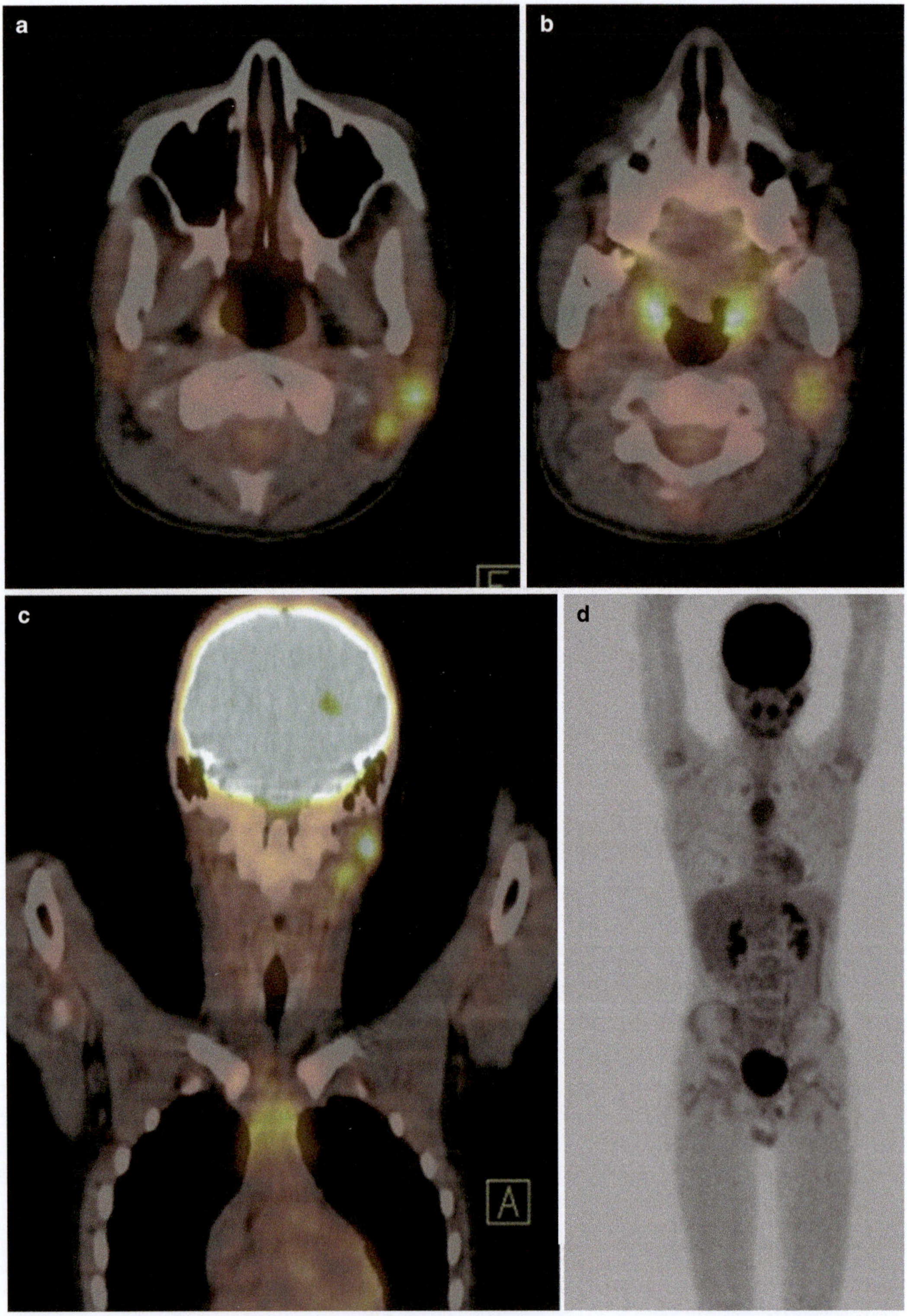

Fig. 21.24 Axial and coronal PET/CT images (**a–c**) show hypermetabolic lymph nodes in the left parotid region (SUV_{max} 5,6) and on the left side of the neck (SUV_{max} 3,9). PET MIP image (**d**) shows the extent of the disease in the neck and the absence of other foci of increased metabolic activity. The hypermetabolic depiction of the thymus is compatible with patient's age

Acknowledgments
Case 1: Mediastinum The authors thank Antonios Kattamis and Natalia Tourkantoni, 1st University Department of Pediatrics, and Kalliopi Stefanaki, Pathology Laboratory, of Athens 'Aghia Sofia' Children's Hospital, for their contribution by sharing the clinical, pathology and imaging data of their patient.

Case 2: Abdomen The authors are indebted to N. Tourkantoni, K. Katsibardi and A. Kattamis, First Department of Pediatrics, National and Kapodistrian University of Athens, Division of Hematology – Oncology, for sharing clinical and imaging information of their patient.

Case 5: Peripheral Lymph Nodes The authors thank Antonios Kattamis, Natalia Tourkantoni, Tania Vlachou, First Department of Pediatrics, University of Athens 'Aghia Sofia' Children's Hospital, and Kalliopi Stefanaki, Pathology Laboratory of Athens 'Aghia Sofia' Children's Hospital, for their contribution by sharing the clinical, pathologic and imaging data of their patient.

References

1. Percy CL, Smith MA, Linet M et al (1999) Lymphomas and reticuloendothelial neoplasms. In: Ries LA, Smith MA, Gurney JG et al (eds) Cancer incidence and survival among children and adolescents: United States SEER Program 1975–1995. National Cancer Institute, SEER Program, Bethesda, pp 35–50, NIH Pub.No. 99–4649
2. Jaffe ES, Harris NL, Stein H et al (2008) Introduction and overview of the classification of the lymphoid neoplasms. In: Swerdlow SH, Campo E, Harris NL et al (eds) WHO classification of tumours of haematopoietic and lymphoid tissues, 4th edn. International Agency for Research on Cancer, Lyon, pp 157–166
3. Stein H, Warnke RA, Chan WC (2008) Diffuse large B-cell lymphoma (DLBCL), NOS. In: Swerdlow SH, Campo E, Harris NL et al (eds) WHO classification of tumours of haematopoietic and lymphoid tissues, 4th edn. International Agency for Research on Cancer, Lyon, pp 233–237
4. Reiter A, Klapper W (2008) Recent advances in the understanding and management of diffuse large B-cell lymphoma in children. Br J Haematol 142(3):329–347
5. Miles RR, Raphael M, McCarthy K et al (2008) Pediatric diffuse large B-cell lymphoma demonstrates a high proliferation index, frequent c-Myc protein expression, and a high incidence of germinal centre subtype: Report of the French-American-British (FAB) international study group. Pediatr Blood Cancer 51(3):369–374
6. Oschlies I, Klapper W, Zimmermann M et al (2006) Diffuse large B-cell lymphoma in pediatric patients belongs predominantly to the germinal-centre type B-cell lymphomas: a clinicopathologic analysis of cases included in the German BFM (Berlin-Frankfurt-Munster) Multicenter Trial. Blood 107(10):4047–4052
7. Campo E, Swerdlow S, Harris N et al (2011) The 2008 WHO classification of lymphoid neoplasms and beyond: evolving concepts and practical applications. Blood 117(19):5019–5032
8. Oschlies I, Burkhardt B, Salaverria I et al (2011) Clinical, pathological and genetic features of primary mediastinal large B-cell lymphomas and mediastinal gray zone lymphomas in children. Haematologica 96(2):262–268
9. Gerrard M, Waxman I, Sposto R et al (2013) Outcome and pathologic classification of children and adolescents with mediastinal large B-cell lymphoma treated with FAB/LMB96 mature B-NHL therapy. Blood 121(2):278–285
10. Burkhardt B, Oschlies I, Klapper W et al (2011) Non-Hodgkin's lymphoma in adolescents: experiences in 378 adolescent NHL patients treated according to pediatric NHL-BFM protocols. Leukemia 25(1):153–160
11. Klapper W et al (2012) Patient age at diagnosis is associated with the molecular characteristics of diffuse large B-cell lymphoma. Blood 119(8):1882–1887
12. Childhood Non-Hodgkin Lymphoma Treatment (PDQ). www.cancer.gov/types/lymphoma/hp/child-nhl-treatment-pdq
13. Poirel HA et al (2009) Specific cytogenetic abnormalities are associated with a significantly inferior outcome in children and adolescents with mature B-cell non-Hodgkin's lymphoma: results of the FAB/LMB 96 international study. Leukemia 23(2):323–331
14. Martelli M et al (2014) [^{18}F]fluorodeoxyglucose positron emission tomography predicts survival after chemoimmunotherapy for primary mediastinal large B-cell lymphoma: results of the international extranodal lymphoma study group IELSG-26 study. J Clin Oncol 32(17):1769–1775
15. Moskowitz GH et al (2010) Risk-adapted dose-dense immunochemotherapy determined by interim FDG-PET in advanced-stage diffuse large B-cell lymphoma. J Clin Oncol 28(11):1896–1903
16. Nagle SJ et al (2015) The role of FDG-PET imaging as a prognostic marker of outcome in primary mediastinal B-cell lymphoma. Cancer Med 4(1):7–15
17. Heeren JHM, Croonen AM, Pijnenborg JMA (2008) Primary extranodal marginal zone B-cell lymphoma of the female genital tract: a case report and literature review. Int J Gynecol Path 27:243–246
18. Ahmad AK, Hui P, Litkouhi B et al (2014) Institutional review of primary non-Hodgkin lymphoma of the female genital tract: a 33-year experience. Int J Gynecol Cancer 24(7):1250–1255
19. Schoder H, Noy A, Gonen M et al (2005) Intensity of 18fluorodeoxyglucose uptake in positron emission tomography distinguishes between indolent and aggressive non-Hodgkin's lymphoma. J Clin Oncol 23:4643–4651
20. Coughlan M, Elstrom R (2014) The use of FDG-PET in diffuse large B cell lymphoma (DLBCL): predicting outcome following first line therapy. Cancer Imaging 14:34

21. Armitage JO (2012) My treatment approach to patients with diffuse large B-cell lymphoma. Mayo Clin Proc 87(2):161–171
22. Glotzbecker MP et al (2006) Primary non-Hodgkin's lymphoma of bone in children. J Bone Joint Surg Am 88(3):583–594
23. Zhao XF et al (2007) Pediatric primary bone lymphoma – diffuse large B-cell lymphoma. Morphologic and immunohistochemical characteristics of 10 cases. Am J Clin Pathol 127:47–54
24. Bhojwani D et al (2015) The role of FDG-PET/CT in the evaluation of residual disease in paediatric non-Hodgkin lymphoma. Br J Haematol 168(6):845–853
25. Qiu L et al (2013) The role of 18F-FDG PET and 18F-FDG PET/CT in the evaluation of pediatric Hodgkin's lymphoma and non-Hodgkin's lymphoma. Hell J Nucl Med 16(3):230–236
26. Rhodes MM et al (2006) Utility of FDG-PET/CT in follow-up of children treated for Hodgkin and non-Hodgkin lymphoma. J Pediatr Hematol Oncol 28(5):300–306
27. Bakhshi S et al (2012) Pediatric nonlymphoblastic non-Hodgkin lymphoma: baseline, interim, and post-treatment PET/CT versus contrast-enhanced CT for evaluation – a prospective study. Radiology 263(3): 956–968
28. Patte C, Auperin A, Gerrard M, Michon J, Pinkerton R, Sposto R, Weston C, Raphael M, Perkins SL, McCarthy K, Cairo MS (2007) Results of the randomized international FAB/LMB96 trial for intermediate risk B-cell non-Hodgkin lymphoma in children and adolescents: it is possible to reduce treatment for the early responding patients. Blood 109:2773–2780
29. Kazama H, Teramura M, Yoshinaga K, Masuda A (2012) B-cell lymphoma treated with high-dose chemotherapy rescued by in vivo rituximab-purged autologous stem cells. Case Rep Med 2012:Article ID 957063
30. Oschlies I, Salaverria I, Mahn F, Meinhardt A, Zimmermann M, Woessmann W, Burkhardt B, Gesk S, Krams M, Reiter A, Siebert R, Klapper W (2010) Pediatric follicular lymphoma – a clinico-pathological study of a population-based series of patients treated within the non-Hodgkin's Lymphoma – Berlin-Frankfurt-Münster (NHL-BFM) multicenter trials. Haematologica 95:253–259
31. Swerdlow SH (2004) Pediatric follicular lymphomas, marginal zone lymphomas, and marginal zone hyperplasia. Am J Clin Pathol 122(Suppl 1):S98–S109
32. Louissaint A Jr, Ackerman AM, Dias-Santagata D, Ferry JA, Hochberg EP, Huang MS et al (2012) Pediatric-type nodal follicular lymphoma: an indolent clonal proliferation in children and adults with high proliferation index and no *BCL2* rearrangement. Blood 120(12):2395–2404
33. Attarbaschi A, Beishuizen A, Mann G, Rosolen A, Mori T, Uyttebroeck A, Niggli F, Csoka M, Krenova Z, Mellgren K et al (2013) Children and adolescents with follicular lymphoma have an excellent prognosis with either limited chemotherapy or with a "watch and wait" strategy after complete resection. Ann Hematol 92(11):1537–1541

Anaplastic Large Cell Lymphoma in Children and Adolescents

22

Margarita S. Baka-Kagia, Vassilios K. Prassopoulos, and Georgia Ch. Papaioannou

22.1 Introduction

Margarita S. Baka-Kagia, MD

Anaplastic large cell lymphoma (ALCL) is a distinct form of non-Hodgkin lymphoma (NHL), which accounts for 10–15 % of all childhood lymphomas [1, 2]. First described in 1985 by Stein et al., ALCL is characterized by the malignant cell expression of CD30 [3]. Clinically, ALK-positive ALCL occurs most frequently in the first three decades of life with a slight male predominance [4]. The median age at diagnosis for children and adolescents with ALCL is approximately 12 years with only very rare cases below 1 year of age. Pediatric ALCL is characterized by advanced disease at presentation (75 % of cases), a high incidence of nodal involvement (>90 %), frequent association with B symptoms (75 %), and frequent extranodal involvement, including skin (25 %), lung (10 %), bone (17 %), and liver (8 %) [1, 5, 6, 7]. Coexisting skin involvement is common with systemic ALCL, so careful evaluation for systemic disease must be undertaken before the diagnosis of primary cutaneous ALCL is made. Central nervous system involvement is rare. Bone marrow involvement varies, depending on the mode of detection utilized. Basic morphology has a low level of detection (<10 %), which increases to 15–30 % when immunohistochemical staining with CD30 and ALK is utilized. Molecular studies have demonstrated even higher bone marrow involvement, with >50 % having detectable disease by polymerase chain reaction (PCR) [8–10]. Rarely, ALCL can present in a leukemic phase with leukocytosis and circulating lymphoma cells [11–13]. No correlation between ALCL and immune deficiencies has been reported.

All ALCL are CD30 positive and most (>90 %) pediatric ALCLs have a chromosomal rearrangement involving the ALK gene. Their prognosis tends to be superior to adults, who generally have an ALK-negative disease [14].

Radiographic imaging is essential in the staging of patients with NHL. CT scan and, more recently, MRI have been used for staging. Data support that PET identifies more abnormalities than CT scanning, but it is unclear whether this should be used to change therapy [15]. The use of

M.S. Baka-Kagia, MD
Department of Pediatric Oncology, P. and A. Kyriakou Children's Hospital, Thivon and Livadias Str., Athens 11527, Greece
e-mail: margbaka@hotmail.com

V.K. Prassopoulos, MD
Department of Nuclear Medicine and PET/CT, "HYGEIA" Hospital, 4, E. Stavrou and Kifissias Av., Maroussi 15123, Greece
e-mail: vprasso@otenet.gr

G.Ch. Papaioannou, MD, PhD (✉)
Department of Pediatric Oncology, "MITERA" Hospital, 4, E. Stavrou and Kifissias Av., Maroussi 15123, Greece
e-mail: gpapaio@hotmail.com

J.A. Andreou et al. (eds.), *PET/CT in Lymphomas: A Case-Based Atlas*,
DOI 10.1007/978-3-319-27380-8_22

PET to assess rapidity of response to therapy appears to have prognostic value in HL and some types of NHL observed in adult patients but requires further investigation in pediatric NHL. Caution is also required for surveillance scanning, because false-positive results are common. At these cases, a biopsy to prove residual or recurrent disease should be required [16].

22.2 Case Presentation

Margarita S. Baka-Kagia, MD,
Vasilios K. Prassopoulos, MD,
and Georgia Ch. Papaioannou, MD, PhD

Case 1

History and figures are taken after permission of Dr *Luciana Barbosa*, first author of the paper entitled *Anaplastic Cutaneous Lymphoma Mimicking Infection,* published in *J Radiol Case Rep 2014;8(3):39–47* [17].

A 17-year-old adolescent presented with a 2-week history of pain, swelling, and vesicular skin lesions of the anterior aspect of the left thigh. Imaging studies then revealed the presence of a solid well-circumscribed space-occupying lesion below the subcutaneous fat and between the medial and intermedius vastus muscles. It presented peripheral vascularization and contrast enhancement with surrounding edema. Its features were nonspecific, however suggestive of rather an infectious lesion (i.e., abscess). With the diagnosis of a possible abscess, he was admitted for IV antibiotics. During hospitalization he developed fever as well. He then underwent biopsy, and the histology of the partially excised lesion showed large cell anaplastic lymphoma of the soft tissue, strongly positive for CD30 and CD5, indicating T-immunophenotyping, although EMA and ALK were negative. Following surgery and partial excision, an FDG-PET/CT scan was obtained. It revealed increased uptake of the radiopharmaceutical within the residual lesion, which presented growth in size to the preoperative dimensions (Fig. 22.1). Patient was treated as per the BFM NHL protocol.

Discussion

Anaplastic large cell lymphoma (ALCL) is a distinct form of non-Hodgkin lymphoma (NHL) which accounts for 10–15 % of all childhood lymphomas [18]. Pediatric ALCLs are characterized by advanced disease at presentation, high incidence of nodal involvement, frequent presence of B-symptoms and frequent extranodal involvement, such as the skin (25 %), lung (10 %), bone (17 %), and liver (8 %). Coexisting skin involvement is common in systemic ALCL, so that careful evaluation for systemic disease must be undertaken before the diagnosis of primary cutaneous ALCL is made [4, 18]. Children, in the contrary to the presented patient, are usually ALK positive, and this has a positive impact in the prognosis [18]. Conventional imaging studies are crucial in order to determine areas initially involved as well as for estimation of response to therapy. FDG-PET/CT is a useful modality for the estimation of visceral involvement in cutaneous ALCL [19].

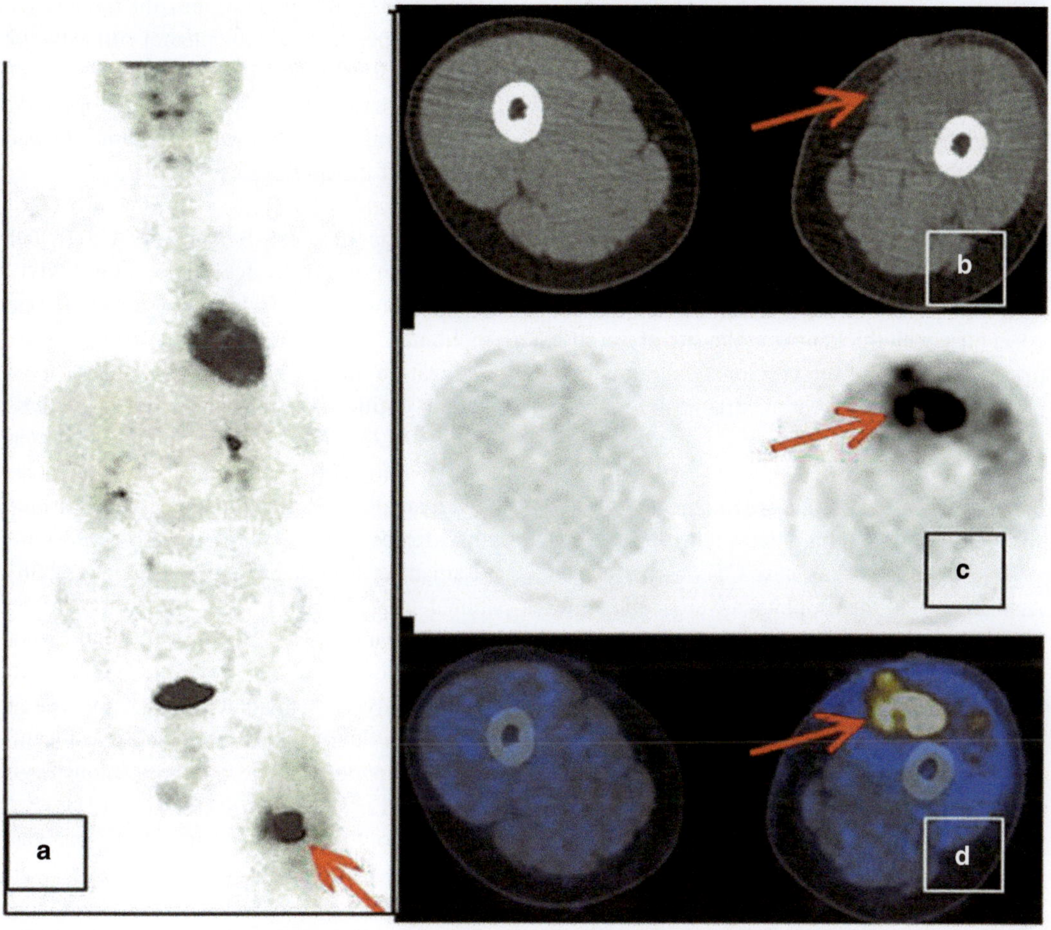

Fig. 22.1 (**a**) FDG-MIP imaging, (**b**) CT imaging, (**c**) FDG-PET imaging, (**d**) fused FDG-PET/CT imaging. Increased FDG uptake at the left thigh is observed

Case 2

History and figures are taken after permission of Dr *Edward Y. Lee*, one of the authors of the paper entitled *Anaplastic Large Cell Lymphoma of the Esophagus in a Pediatric Patient: Case Report,* published in *Pediatr Radiol* (2012) 42:627–631 [20].

A 3-year-old boy presented to the hospital with abdominal pain and vomiting. He was discharged with the diagnosis of gastroenteritis. Due to the persistence of symptoms, he came back to the hospital. An esophagram and CT of the thorax were obtained and revealed a long, rather smooth stricture in the mid-esophagus and extraluminal collection of barium contrast. Axial images and MPRs demonstrated a significant concentric wall thickening at the site of the stricture and pooling of the previously administrated oral contrast. Differential diagnosis included recent caustic ingestion causing esophageal perforation, or an ingested foreign body with secondary inflammation. He was managed with IV antibiotics and total parenteral nutrition.

Twelve days later, a new CT was performed. Appearances of the esophagus were stable; however, right axial and mediastinal adenopathy were new findings of uncertain etiology. A second esophagram demonstrated the unchanged stricture; however, there were no findings of leak. In conclusion, caustic ingestion seemed more likely the diagnosis at this point.

He continued with the same conservative therapy, but 1 month later he presented with progressive difficulty in swallowing and increased drooling. An esophageal endoscopy was undertaken, which revealed a complete obstruction of the esophagus from intraluminal granulated tissue, without suspicion of malignancy. However, a biopsy was obtained from the right axillary lymph node found on CT. Histology showed anaplastic lymphoma, small cell variant, and ALK positive.

FDG-PET/CT scan that was then performed for staging revealed increased uptake of the radiopharmaceutical at the esophagus and the right supraclavicular space, as well as hypermetabolic lesions at the mediastinum, the right axilla, the right upper arm, and the pleural surfaces, not visible to prior CT examinations (Fig. 22.2). Patient was treated with chemotherapy for ALCL stage 3. Evaluation following therapy showed resolution of the findings.

Discussion

Anaplastic large cell lymphoma (ALCL) is a distinct form of non-Hodgkin lymphoma (NHL) which accounts for 10–15 % of all childhood lymphomas [1, 21]. The World Health Organization now classifies ALCL into three separate entities: ALK-positive ALCL, ALK-negative ALCL, and primary cutaneous ALCL [22]. Histological examination of our patient showed anaplastic lymphoma, small cell variant, and ALK positive.

Lamant et al. has published a review of 361 patients treated on ALCL99 protocol. Among them, 114 patients (32 %) have had small cell or lymphohistiocytic variant, as in this case. In multivariate analysis, patients with either subtype or a composite subtype with some features of small cell or lymphohistiocytic pattern demonstrated an increased risk for relapse ($P = .002$) [21].

The role of PET/CT in pediatric ALCL remains unclarified. As its avidity correlates to the lymphoma aggressiveness, it may be a useful modality for accurate staging on diagnosis and evaluation during or after treatment [19]. In the case described above, PET/CT imaging revealed more extensive disease than conventional imaging; nevertheless disease disappeared in conventional and functional imaging after successive therapy.

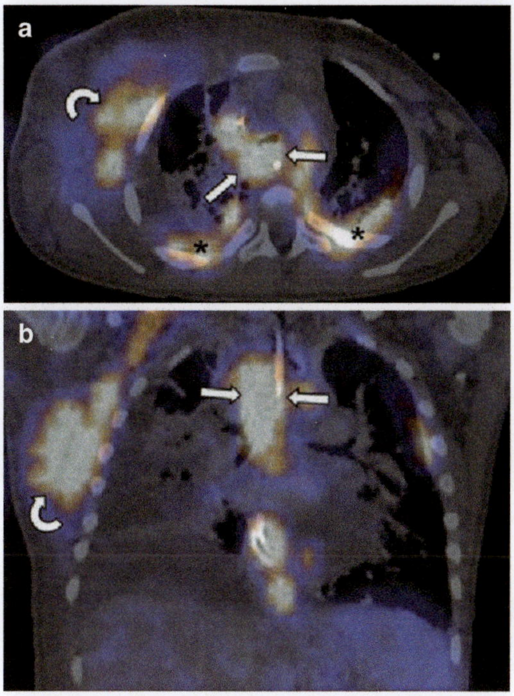

Fig. 22.2 (**a**) sagittal, (**b**) coronal fused PET/CT imaging. Hypermetabolic activity is observed in soft tissue around the esophagus (*white arrows*), at multiple sites of the mediastinum, at the right axilla (*curved arrow*), as well as at pleural surfaces (*asterisks*)

Acknowledgments

Case 1 The authors are indebted to Dr L. Barbosa and collaborators, Radiology Department Centro Hospitalar e Universitario de Coimbra, Quinta dos Vales, S. Martinho do Bispo, Coimbra, Portugal, for sharing clinical and imaging information of their patient.

Case 2 The authors are indebted to Dr *Edward Y. Lee* and collaborators, Department of Radiology, Children's Boston, and Harvard Medical School, for sharing clinical and imaging information of their patient.

References

1. Sandlund JT, Downing JR, Crist WM (1996) Non-Hodgkin's lymphoma in childhood. N Engl J Med 334(19):1238–1248
2. Seidemann K, Tiemann M, Schrappe M et al (2001) Short-pulse B-non-Hodgkin lymphoma-type chemotherapy is efficacious treatment for pediatric anaplastic large cell lymphoma: a report of the Berlin-Frankfurt-Munster Group Trial NHL-BFM 90. Blood 97(12): 3699–3706
3. Stein H, Mason DY, Gerdes J et al (1985) The expression of the Hodgkin's disease associated antigen Ki-1 in reactive and neoplastic lymphoid tissue: evidence that Reed-Sternberg cells and histiocytic malignancies are derived from activated lymphoid cells. Blood 66(4):848–858, 36
4. Ferreri AJ, Govi S, Pileri SA, Savage KJ et al (2012) Anaplastic large cell lymphoma. ALK-positive. Crit Rev Oncol Hematol 83(2):293–302
5. Seidemann K, Tiemann M, Schrappe M et al (2001) Short-pulse B-non-Hodgkin lymphoma-type chemotherapy is efficacious treatment for pediatric anaplastic large cell lymphoma: a report of the Berlin-Frankfurt-Munster Group Trial NHL-BFM 90. Blood 97(12): 3699–37
6. Lowe EJ, Sposto R, Perkins SL et al (2009) Intensive chemotherapy for systemic anaplastic large cell lymphoma in children and adolescents: final results of Children's Cancer Group Study 5941. Pediatr Blood Cancer 52(3):335–339
7. Le Deley MC, Reiter A, Williams D et al (2008) Prognostic factors in childhood anaplastic large cell lymphoma: results of a large European intergroup study. Blood 111(3):1560–1566
8. Damm-Welk C, Busch K, Burkhardt B et al (2007) Prognostic significance of circulating tumor cells in bone marrow or peripheral blood as detected by qualitative and quantitative PCR in pediatric NPM-ALK

positive anaplastic large-cell lymphoma. Blood 110(2):670–677
9. Damm-Welk C, Schieferstein J, Schwalm S et al (2007) Flow cytometric detection of circulating tumour cells in nucleophosmin/anaplastic lymphoma kinase-positive anaplastic large cell lymphoma: comparison with quantitative polymerase chain reaction. Br J Haematol 138(4):459–466
10. Mussolin L, Pillon M, d'Amore ES et al (2005) Prevalence and clinical implications of bone marrow involvement in pediatric anaplastic large cell lymphoma. Leukemia 19(9):1643–1647
11. Bayle C, Charpentier A, Duchayne E et al (1999) Leukaemic presentation of small cell variant anaplastic large cell lymphoma: report of four cases. Br J Haematol 104(4):680–688
12. Onciu M, Behm FG, Raimondi SC et al (2003) ALK-positive anaplastic large cell lymphoma with leukemic peripheral blood involvement is a clinicopathologic entity with an unfavorable prognosis. Report of three cases and review of the literature. Am J Clin Pathol 120(4):617–625
13. Villamor N, Rozman M, Esteve J et al (1999) Anaplastic large-cell lymphoma with rapid evolution to leukemic phase. Ann Hematol 78(10):478–482
14. Savage KJ, Harris NL, Vose JM et al (2008) ALK-anaplastic large-cell lymphoma is clinically and immunophenotypically different from both ALK1 ALCL and peripheral T-cell lymphoma, not otherwise specified: report from the International Peripheral T-Cell Lymphoma Project. Blood 111(12):5496–5504
15. Cheng G, Servaes S, Zhuang H (2013) Value of (18) F-fluoro-2-deoxy-D-glucose positron emission tomography/computed tomography scan versus diagnostic contrast computed tomography in initial staging of pediatric patients with lymphoma. Leuk Lymphoma 54(4):737–742
16. Eissa HM, Allen CE, Kamdar K et al (2014) Pediatric Burkitt's lymphoma and diffuse B-cell lymphoma: are surveillance scans required? Pediatr Hematol Oncol 31(3):253–257
17. Barbosa L, Brito MJ, Balaco I et al (2014) Anaplastic cutaneous lymphoma mimicking infection. J Radiol Case Rep 8(3):39–47
18. Jaffe ES, Harris NL, Stein H et al (2008) Classification of lymphoid neoplasms: the microscope as a tool for disease discovery. Blood 112(12):4384–4399
19. Bhojwani D, McCarville MB, Choi JK et al (2015) The role of FDG-PET/CT in the evaluation of residual disease in paediatric non –Hodgkin lymphoma. Br J Haematol 168(6):845–853
20. Hryhorczuk AL, Harris MH, Vargas SO, Lee EY (2012) Anaplastic large cell lymphoma of the esophagus in a pediatric patient. Pediatr Radiol 42(5):627–631
21. Lamant L, McCarthy K, d'Amore E et al (2011) Prognostic impact of morphologic and phenotypic features of childhood ALK-positive anaplastic large-cell lymphoma: results of the ALCL99 Study. J Clin Oncol 29(35):4669–4676
22. Swerdlow SH, Campo E, Harris NL et al (2008) WHO classification of tumours of haematopoietic and lymphoid tissues, 4th edn. IARC, Lyon

Appendix

Table A.1 2014 Revised criteria for response assessment in malignant lymphomas

	Complete response (CR)	Partial response (PR)	No response/stable disease (SD)	Progressive disease (PD)
PET-based criteria[a]				
Lymph nodes	D5-PS score 1, 2, or 3 (±residual masses)	D5-PS score 4 or 5 – but reduced compared to baseline- and residual mass(es) of any size At interim evaluation: responding disease At final evaluation: residual disease (treatment failure)	D5-PS score 4 or 5 – but no significant change in FDG uptake compared to baseline (applicable at both interim and final evaluation)	D5-PS score 4 or 5 and increase in FDG uptake compared to baseline (applicable at both interim and final evaluation) *and/or* New FDG-avid lesions consistent with lymphoma (applicable at both interim and final evaluation) Biopsy or follow-up PET encouraged if lymphomatous nature of the lesion(s) is uncertain
Extralymphatic sites	D5-PS score 1, 2, or 3 (±residual masses)*			
Non-measured lesions	Not applicable	Not applicable	Not applicable	
Organ enlargement	Not applicable*	Not applicable	Not applicable	
Bone marrow	No FDG-avid disease*	Residual uptake higher than normal marrow but less than baseline (diffuse uptake permitted)**	No change from baseline	New or recurrent FDG-avid foci

(continued)

J.A. Andreou et al. (eds.), *PET/CT in Lymphomas: A Case-Based Atlas*,
DOI 10.1007/978-3-319-27380-8

Table A.1 (continued)

	Complete response (CR)	Partial response (PR)	No response/stable disease (SD)	Progressive disease (PD)
Conventional (CT) criteria[a]				
Target lymph nodes/masses and/or extralymphatic sites	Nodal regression to LDx ≤1.5 cm No extralymphatic sites	Up to 6 sites in total: ≥50 % decrease in SPD***	Up to 6 sites in total): <50 % decrease in SPD and no progressive disease criteria met	PPD progression of ≥1 individual node/lesion, which should be abnormal (all the following): LDx >1.5 cm Increase by ≥50 % from PPD nadir Increase of LDx or SDx (compared to nadir) by 0.5 or 1.0 cm for lesions ≤2 and >2 cm, respectively And/or new sites, defined as: Regrowth of previously resolved lesions New node >1.5 cm in any axis New extranodal site >1.0 cm in any axis; if <1.0 cm, it should be unequivocal and attributable to lymphoma
Non-measured lesions	Absent	No increase (regressed or absent/ normal)	No increase falling into the definition of progression (see below)	Clear progression or new lesions
Organ enlargement	Regression to normal	Spleen regression by >50 % (in its length beyond normal)	No increase falling into the definition of progression (see below)	Prior splenomegaly: increase of splenic length by >50 % of the extent of its prior increase beyond baseline No prior splenomegaly: increase ≥2 cm from baseline
Bone marrow	Morphologically normal; negative IHC, if indeterminate	Not applicable	Not applicable	New or recurrent involvement

Adapted and modified from Cheson BD, Fisher RI, Barrington SF, et al. Recommendations for initial evaluation, staging and response assessment of Hodgkin and non-Hodgkin lymphoma: the Lugano classification. *J Clin Oncol* 2014; 32:3059–3067; (Table 3)

Terms used throughout this table:

1. Target lesions (target lymph nodes/masses and/or extralymphatic sites) or measured dominant lesions: They include the dominant lesions, i.e., those, which are the major determinants of response. They should include up to 6 of the largest nodes/nodal masses or extranodal lesions, being representative of the total tumor burden. Further selection criteria include: (a) to be clearly measurable bidimensionally; (b) to be located at as much as disparate anatomic regions is possible, including both mediastinal and retroperitoneal areas, if involved. Measurable nodes and extranodal lesions should have an LDx of >1.5 cm and >1.0 cm, respectively

2. Non-measured lesions: They include: (a) any nodal or extranodal disease, which has not been selected as "Measured Dominant Disease" according to the above definition; (b) lesions considered abnormal, but failing to fulfill the requirements for measurability; (c) any site of suspected disease, which is assessable but is difficult to be followed by quantitative measurements (serous effusions, bone lesions, leptomeningeal disease, etc)

*An uptake higher than mediastinum or liver can be compatible with complete metabolic response, if observed at sites that might have high physiologic uptake or high uptake due to "activation" (i.e., chemotherapy or growth factor-induced), such as the Waldeyer's ring, GI tract, spleen, or marrow. In such cases, FDG uptake at sites of initial involvement should not exceed the surrounding normal tissue, even if this is "physiologically" high

** Caution: Persistent focal lesions might be further evaluated by MRI, biopsy, or a new PET

***Further instructions to assess partial response, when small residuals are present, are provided in the corresponding article (see below)

Abbreviations: *PET* positron emission tomography, *D5-PS* Deauville 5-point scale, *CT* computed tomography, *FDG* fluorodeoxyglucose, *IHC* immunohistochemistry, *LDx* longest transverse diameter of a lesion, *MRI* magnetic resonance imaging, *PET* positron emission tomography, *PPD* cross product of the LDx and perpendicular diameter, *SDx* shortest axis perpendicular to the LDx, *SPD* sum of the product of the perpendicular diameters for multiple lesions
[a]PET-based criteria are recommended for FDG-avid lymphoma subtypes (defined in Chap. 4). Conventional (CT) criteria are recommended for non-FDG-avid lymphoma subtypes (defined in Chap. 4)

Table A.2 Deauville 5-point scale (D5-PS) for the evaluation of interim and final PET/CT scan in patients with malignant lymphomas (Deauville criteria)

1: No abnormal FDG uptake (above background)
2: FDG uptake ≤ mediastinum
3: Mediastinum < FDG uptake ≤ liver
4: FDG uptake moderately increased above the liver
5: FDG uptake markedly increased at any site including new sites of disease
X: New areas of uptake unlikely to be related to lymphoma

Table A.3 The recently revised "Modified Ann Arbor Staging System" (Lugano) for primary nodal lymphomas

Stage	Definition	Extranodal (E) status
Limited		
I	One nodal group of adjacent nodes (including a single node only)	Single extranodal lesion without nodal involvement
II	≥2 nodal groups on the same side of the diaphragm	Nodal stage I/II with limited contiguous extranodal involvement
II bulky*	II with "bulky" disease	As above
Advanced		
III	Nodal involvement on both sides of the diaphragm or only above the diaphragm plus spleen involvement	Not applicable
IV	Noncontiguous extralymphatic involvement	Not applicable

Adapted and modified from Cheson BD, Fisher RI, Barrington SF, et al. Recommendations for initial evaluation, staging and response assessment of Hodgkin and non-Hodgkin lymphoma: the Lugano classification. *J Clin Oncol* 2014; 32:3059–3067; (Tables 1 and 2)
Notes:
1. Regarding imaging methods, the extent of the disease is evaluated and determined by positron emission tomography/computed tomography (PET/CT) for FDG-avid histologies (see Chap. 4) and only by CT for non-FDG-avid histologies (see Chap. 4)
2. Tonsils, Waldeyer's ring, and spleen are considered nodal tissue
3. B-symptoms have been retained in the current staging classification only for Hodgkin lymphoma, because they may guide treatment only in this specific setting. The designation "B", as proposed in the Ann Arbor classification, is used to declare the presence of fever >38.3 °C, drenching night sweats and unexplained weight loss (>10 % over 6 moths)
4. * Whether bulky stage II should be treated as limited or advanced disease may be determined by histology and prognostic factors. The designation X is not recommended to declare bulk as it used to be the case in Ann Arbor staging. Instead, the longest disease measurement by CT scan is encouraged. The definition of bulk may vary according to histology
5. Criteria for involvement of various anatomic structures by clinical and imaging methods:
   a. Lymph nodes: Palpable by clinical examination; increased FDG uptake by PET/CT for FDG-avid histologies; unexplained node enlargement by CT for non-FDG-avid histologies
   b. Spleen: Palpable by clinical examination; increased diffuse FDG uptake, solitary mass, nodules or miliary lesions by PET/CT for FDG-avid histologies; vertical length >13 cm, mass or nodules by CT for non-FDG-avid histologies
   c. Liver: Increased diffuse FDG uptake or mass lesions by PET/CT for FDG-avid histologies; nodules by CT for non-FDG-avid histologies. Liver size by physical examination or CT is not considered as reliable to assess lymphomatous involvement
   d. Central nervous system (CNS): Relevant signs or symptoms clinically; not defined by PET/CT; mass lesion(s) by CT; mass lesion(s) and/or leptomeningeal infiltration by MRI; cerebrospinal fluid positive by cell morphology and/or flow cytometry
   e. Other extranodal sites, including skin, lung, gastrointestinal tract, bone, bone marrow: Site-dependent symptoms/signs clinically; positivity on PET/CT (adequate for bone marrow and highly suggestive for other sites) – biopsy can be considered if necessary

Index

J.A. Andreou et al. (eds.), *PET/CT in Lymphomas: A Case-Based Atlas*,
DOI 10.1007/978-3-319-27380-8

CPI Antony Rowe
Chippenham, UK
2017-01-24 10:15